Shame 4.0

Claude-Hélène Mayer • Elisabeth Vanderheiden •
Paul T. P. Wong
Editors

Shame 4.0

Investigating an Emotion in Digital Worlds and the Fourth Industrial Revolution

Springer

Editors
Claude-Hélène Mayer
Department of Industrial Psychology and People Management
University of Johannesburg
Auckland Park, Johannesburg, South Africa

Kulturwissenschaftliche Fakultät
Europa Universität Viadrina
Frankfurt (Oder), Germany

Paul T. P. Wong (*emeritus*)
Trent University
Toronto, ON, Canada

Elisabeth Vanderheiden
Global Institute for Transcultural Research
Römerberg, Germany

ISBN 978-3-030-59526-5 ISBN 978-3-030-59527-2 (eBook)
https://doi.org/10.1007/978-3-030-59527-2

This Springer imprint is published by the registered company Springer Nature Switzerland AG.
The registered company address is: Gewerbestrasse 11, 6330 Cham, Switzerland

Revolutionaries do not make revolutions!
The revolutionaries are those who know when
power is lying in the street and when they can pick it up.

—Hannah Arendt (1972). Crises of the Republic, *p. 206. Houghton Mifflin Harcourt*

Foreword

In the Mesopotamian city-state of Eshnunna (ca. 1770 BC), men who were paid one shekel of silver to harvest but failed to harvest were fined ten shekels of silver. Meanwhile, in the Soviet Union, managers understated their productivity and overstated their resource requirements to secure safe production targets. Closer to home, getting on the wrong side of a social media audience can cost workers their jobs. The relationship between shame and the economy is ancient, because shame and economic activities are ancient.

Shame is the common thread running through these chapters—shame in the workplace, shame and policing, cyber bullying and mobbing, honor killings, shame in human-machine interactions, and more. Shame is sometimes viewed as an ugly, maladaptive emotion. However, a close look at this emotion reveals a lot of engineering sophistication. To appreciate the functional logic of shame it helps to consider the social-evaluative psychology of audiences—the environment that would have selected for shame over evolutionary time and that shame targets in its moment-to-moment operation.

Human social life is intensely evaluative. We are consumed by what's hot and what's not, what's cool and what's uncool. We can evaluate other people because the human brain is equipped with neurocognitive mechanisms that evolved to evaluate others and, more broadly, to regulate one's interactions with others. The way we evaluate others shapes the extent to which we attend to, associate with, defer to, and help others. Social evaluations in aggregate shape the way people form, cultivate, negotiate, and dissolve various types of partnerships: economic partnerships, romantic partnerships, political alliances, and others.

To generate social evaluations, the brain uses as input information about a target individual that probabilistically indicates (1) the degree to which the target will make positive contributions to the fitness of the self, and (2) the degree to which the target will aggressively inflict costs on the self if not propitiated. Inputs to social-evaluative computations include, for example: cues of the target's skills and productivity, cues of the target's inclination to help the self when in need, and cues of the target's physical formidability. Based on these and other inputs, the relevant mechanisms deliver evaluations of the target as social partner, as well as internal representations of the degree to which the individual will value the target's welfare when making decisions.

In sum, people value or disvalue, respect or disrespect, specific other individuals as a function of the probable extent to which the actions and characteristics of others will improve (or damage) the valuer's own welfare and fitness.

When others (an audience) detect new information about an individual that is at odds with how much they value the individual, they recalibrate their valuation of the individual either upward or downward, with correspondingly positive or negative effects on their disposition to aid or defer to that individual. This recalibrational dynamic would have selected, on the receiver's end, for neurocognitive mechanisms to minimize the transmission of negative information about the self and the cost of being devalued when negative information spreads. The emotion of shame seems to be a primary defense against the threat of information-triggered devaluation. (This regime would also have selected for motivational mechanisms to incentivize others to place more weight on the welfare of the focal individual—the pride system).

If the adaptive function of shame is to limit the threat of devaluation, the computational structure of shame might reflect this function the way a key fits its lock. Indeed, the evidence suggests that shame is packed with design features to minimize the threat of devaluation. For example, when facing the prospect or actuality of being devalued, people feel pain, avoid taking acts that could cause or exacerbate devaluation, and conceal damaging information. When others discover reputation-damaging information, the individual withdraws, appeases, and produces a stereotyped nonverbal display that mollifies audiences by signaling subordination. When the discrediting actions or traits become known by others, people behave more cooperatively, a predicted response for a system designed to restore one's reputation as a good cooperative partner. If cooperative overtures are not successful or cost-effective, the system can switch to countering devaluation by deceit or force—shame sometimes leads to lies, blaming, and verbal and physical aggression.

The operation of shame varies over development and across situations, individuals, and cultures. At the same time, however, there are regularities in shame across cultures and throughout history. For example, the intensity of anticipatory shame that study participants from the United States and India report regarding each of various offenses closely tracks the actual punishments (fines, in copper chin) that the Tang Code (China, AD 653) established for those who committed those offenses.

The present volume is a fascinating exploration of shame in the era of the internet, genome editing, and self-driving cars. The actors, technologies, and forms of organization are modern. But beneath the new garbs lies an old and recognizably human drama.

Montreal, Canada Daniel Sznycer

Acknowledgement

In the light of the Fourth Industrial Revolution, far-reaching changes are to be expected in all areas of life and fields of action globally. After having intensively examined the topic of shame as a resource from various cultural and multiple scientific perspectives in our previous publications, our aim in this book is to trace Shame 4.0. We aim at investigating how digitalization and the transition from the Third towards the Fourth Industrial Revolution affect development and forms of appearance and perception. We are also interested to explore future ways of dealing with shame in various contexts and new media.

Such a publication is always the work of many people. We are grateful for the intense cooperation: We thank our co-authors for contributing their manifold theoretical and empirical works. We would also like to thank the University of Johannesburg, in particular the Department of Industrial Psychology and People Management with Professor Freddie Crous as Head of Department, for supporting research on the Fourth Industrial Revolution and making it a core topic of the University to explore the future trends for the new, global generations.

We are particularly pleased that this publication project is realized within the scope of the recently founded Global Institute for Transcultural Research (GITR) in Germany.

We would also like to thank Springer International for the extraordinary cooperation: special thanks go to Shinjini Chatterjee, Ameena Jafaar and Shanthi Ramamoorthy and her team for their professional and dedicated support.

Additional thanks go to Ruth Coetzee for the careful and thoughtful language editing of the editors' chapters.

We would also like to thank our families and friends for their patience and their many inspiring conversational impulses.

During the completion phase of this book, the COVID-19 pandemic is keeping the world in suspense in a way never seen before. We can only guess at the moment what this pandemic will mean in the medium and long term for the development of Shame 4.0 and the Fourth Industrial Revolution, as addressed in our concluding chapter. We hope that this publication will also provide you, the reader, with inspiring impulses to perceive the diversity of Shame 4.0 in a fresh and more differentiated way, to transform it and to develop it further in your contexts.

We dedicate this book to all those people and organisations who are now taking advantage of the Fourth Industrial Revolution as an opportunity to achieve social, political and economic justice, while respecting the creation and human rights.

Johannesburg, South Africa — Claude-Hélène Mayer
Römerberg, Germany — Elisabeth Vanderheiden

Contents

Editors and Contributors

About the Editors

Claude-Hélène Mayer, (Dr. habil., PhD, PhD) is a Professor in Industrial and Organisational Psychology at the Department of Industrial Psychology and People Management at the University of Johannesburg, an Adjunct Professor at the European University Viadrina in Frankfurt (Oder), Germany and a Senior Research Associate at Rhodes University, Grahamstown, South Africa. She holds a Ph.D. in Psychology (University of Pretoria, South Africa), a Ph.D. in Management (Rhodes University, South Africa), a Doctorate (Georg-August University, Germany) in Political Sciences (socio-cultural anthropology and intercultural didactics), and a Habilitation (European University Viadrina, Germany) in Psychology with focus on work, organizational, and cultural psychology. She has published several monographs, text collections, accredited journal articles, and special issues on transcultural mental health and well-being, sense of coherence, shame, transcultural conflict management and mediation, women in leadership in culturally diverse work contexts, constellation work, coaching, and psychobiography.

Elisabeth Vanderheiden is a pedagogue, theologian, intercultural mediator. She is the CEO of the Global Institute for Transcultural Research and the President of Catholic Adult Education in Germany. Her publishing activities focus on pedagogy, in particular on the further education of teachers and trainers in adult education, vocational and civic education, but also on the challenges of digitalisation. She has also edited books on intercultural and transnational issues. Her most recent publications deal with shame as a resource as well as with mistakes, errors and failures and their hidden potentials in the context of Culture and Positive Psychology 1.0 and 2.0. Current research projects deal with love in transcultural contexts, with life crises as well as humour in the context of Positive Psychology 2.0. Another focus of her work is Design Thinking in transcultural contexts.

Paul T. P. Wong, Ph.D., C.Psych. is Professor Emeritus of Trent University and Adjunct Professor at Saybrook University. He is a Fellow of APA and CPA and President of the International Network on Personal Meaning (www.meaning.ca) and the Meaning-Centered Counselling Institute. Editor of the International Journal of Existential Psychology and Psychotherapy, he has also edited two influential volumes on The Human Quest for Meaning. A prolific writer, he is one of the most cited existential and positive psychologists. The originator of Meaning Therapy and International Meaning Conferences, he has been invited to give keynotes and meaning therapy workshops worldwide. He is the recent recipient of the Carl Rogers Award from the Society for Humanistic Psychology (Div. 32 of the APA).

Contributors

Hendriati Agustiani Faculty of Psychology, Universitas Padjadjaran, Bandung, West Java, Indonesia

Athira Alex Department of Psychology, Don Bosco Arts and Science College, Kannur, India

Kenichi Asano Department of Psychological Counseling, Mejiro University, Tokyo, Japan

Trina Banerjee Department of Psychology, Mount Carmel College, Bangalore, India

Dharm P. S. Bhawuk University of Hawai'i at Manoa, Honolulu, HI, USA

Simon Cozens Worldview Center for Intercultural Studies, St. Leonards, TAS, Australia

Hijriyati Cucuani Psychology Faculty of Padjadjaran University of Bandung, Bandung, West Java, Indonesia

Tony Brian D'souza Department of Psychology, St. Joseph's College (Autonomous), Bangalore, Karnataka, India

A. T. P. Farisha Ramana Vidyalaya, Chennai, India

Paul J. P. Fouché Department of Psychology, University of the Free State, Bloemfontein, Republic of South Africa

Pauline Green Enterprise Centre, Derby, UK

Diana Harding Faculty of Psychology, Universitas Padjadjaran, Bandung, West Java, Indonesia

Kwang-Kuo Hwang Department of Psychology, National Taiwan University, Taipei, Taiwan

Grace Maria Jochan Department of Psychology, Mount Carmel College, Bangalore, India

Anita Kasabova Department of History & Theory of Culture, Sofia University 'St. Kliment of Okhrid', Sofia, Bulgaria

Thula U. Koops Institut für Sexualforschung, Sexualmedizin und Forensische Psychiatrie, Universitätsklinikum Hamburg-Eppendorf, Hamburg, Germany

Yasuhiro Kotera Enterprise Centre, Derby, UK

Barbara Lewandowska-Tomaszczyk State University of Applied Sciences in Konin, Konin, Poland

Xiaochen Luo School of Psychology, Fuller Theological Seminary, Pasadena, CA, USA
Department of Psychology, Michigan State University at East Lansing, East Lansing, MI, USA

Claude-Hélène Mayer Department of Industrial Psychology and People Management, University of Johannesburg, Auckland Park, Johannesburg, South Africa
Kulturwissenschaftliche Fakultät, Europa Universität Viadrina, Frankfurt (Oder), Germany

Gillian McKay Department of Politics and International Studies, University of Leeds, Leeds, UK

Rudolf M. Oosthuizen Department of Industrial and Organisational Psychology, University of South Africa, Pretoria, South Africa

Grace Perry Division of Epidemiology, University of Utah, Salt Lake City, UT, USA

Justine Pistorius Department of Industrial and Organisational Psychology, University of Johannesburg, Johannesburg, South Africa

Sowmya Puttaraju Jain University, Bangalore, Karnataka, India
Department of Psychology, Mount Carmel College, Bangalore, Karnataka, India

Wei Gabriel Qi School of Psychology, Fuller Theological Seminary, Pasadena, CA, USA
Department of Psychiatry, Stony Brook University, Stony Brook, NY, USA

Shereen H. Shaw Department of Secondary and Further Education, Edge Hill University, Ormskirk, UK

David Sheffield Enterprise Centre, Derby, UK

Sergio A. Silverio Department of Women & Children's Health, King's College London, St. Thomas' Hospital, London, UK

Marina Sulastiana Faculty of Psychology, Universitas Padjadjaran, Bandung, West Java, Indonesia

Yoshiyuki Takano University of Prince Edward Island, Charlottetown, Canada

Michael Uebel University of Texas, Austin, TX, USA

Leona M. Ungerer Department of Industrial and Organisational Psychology, University of South Africa (Unisa), Pretoria, South Africa

Elisabeth Vanderheiden Global Institute for Transcultural Research, Römerberg, Germany

Zixuan Wang Kennedy Krieger Institute, Department of Behavioral Psychology, Baltimore, MD, USA
Quince Orchard Psychotherapy, Gaithersburg, MD, USA

Catherine Wilkinson School of Education, Liverpool John Moores University, Liverpool, UK

Samantha Wilkinson Department of Natural Sciences, Manchester Metropolitan University, Manchester, UK

Paul A. Wilson Institute of English Studies, University of Lodz, Lodz, Poland

Paul T. P. Wong Trent University, Toronto, ON, Canada

Piers Worth Buckinghamshire New University, Bucks, UK

Leila Z. Wu Department of Psychology, The Pennsylvania State University, Pennsylvania, PA, USA

Chapter 1
Shame in the Fourth Industrial Revolution, Industry 4.0, and the Age of Digitalisation

Claude-Hélène Mayer and Elisabeth Vanderheiden

1 Asking the Relevant Questions of Our Times

What is the meaning of shame in a new and rapidly changing world? How does the concept of shame change in digital worlds, the Fourth Industrial Revolution (4IR) and Industry 4.0? What are its new dimensions? How does this emotion change when realities are becoming virtual and when communication is technologised and digitalised? How does shame manifest in human–machine interactions? Is shame still an important emotion when new technological systems are being created, automated systems are going viral, and the Internet of Things (IoT) becomes important? How does shame fit into the value chain and the process of the hybridisation of products? Where does shame and shaming come into the context of security, police, and other protective services? How does shame relate to ethics and the new field of machine and information ethics?

In the context of Industry 4.0 and 4IR, endless new questions are being asked. Certainly, the 4IR and Industry 4.0 are concepts primarily related to business and technology and might be experienced as far from the context of emotions, dealing with emotional impact or with emotional intelligence or competence. Shame, as an emotion that is often experienced as negative and which can unfold manifold destructive effects on individual, organisational, and collective levels, needs to be

C.-H. Mayer (✉)
Department of Industrial Psychology and People Management, University of Johannesburg, Auckland Park, Johannesburg, South Africa

Kulturwissenschaftliche Fakultät, Europa Universität Viadrina, Frankfurt (Oder), Germany

E. Vanderheiden
Global Institute for Transcultural Research, Römerberg, Germany
e-mail: ev@keb-rheinland-pfalz.de

C.-H. Mayer et al. (eds.), *Shame 4.0*, https://doi.org/10.1007/978-3-030-59527-2_1

transformed into a positive resource which can contribute to self-development and growth in an individual, a group, or society.

As in their previous books (*The Value of Shame: Exploring a Health Resource in Cultural Contexts* (Vanderheiden & Mayer, 2017) and *The Bright Side of Shame: Transforming and Growing Through Practical Applications in Cultural Contexts* (Mayer & Vanderheiden, 2019)), the authors and editors of this book use a resource-orientated perspective. This is a point of view which focuses on the positive and potential growth and development aspects of individuals, organisations, societies, and finally also global contexts, to overcome and transform negative, painful, and shadow qualities into light, towards positive and growth-orientated emotions.

In *Psychology Today*, Moore (2020) asks whether, in the US context, it is time to reskill employees, while the World Economic Forum (WEF, 2020) announces that by 2025, machines "will complete more jobs than humans". According to Schwab (2016) (WEF, 2016), it is particularly important that individuals and organisations take on a proactive role in redesigning their skills, their perspectives, and ideas about the world and how it is changing, while governments and political and governing bodies need to support the change to enable the transformation of the workforce to facilitate successful change. Being proactive means that people are driven to engage with the topic and deal with it, if possible, in a positive, constructive, and strength- and growth-orientated way. This requires dealing actively with negative experiences and emotions, such as fear of the new and insecure times, shame about a lack of knowledge in terms of technology, or sadness with regard to the loss of what has gone before.

At times when the focus of attention shifts from human–human interaction, towards questions of how best to programme robots for successful human–machine interaction, we need to ask new questions and develop reflexive and participative responses. These questions and responses must arise not only at the level of how to deal with the changes technologically but also with regard to how best to address the changes on intra-psychological, inter-psychological, social, and cultural levels.

First, however, we will discuss what 4IR and Industry 4.0 actually mean and where state-of-the-art discourses lead.

2 What Meanings Do the Concepts of the "Fourth Industrial Revolution" and "Industry 4.0" Hold?

During the past years, 4IR discourse has greatly increased, and many scientists, researchers, and practitioners question what the 4IR and Industry 4.0 refer to Mayer and Oosthuizen (2020).

There are different ways to define the 4IR and Industry 4.0. Speringer and Schnelzer (2019), for example, describe the 4IR as a digitally enabled and technologically driven pragmatic change. These authors see Industry 4.0 as the 4IR's representation. The term "Industry 4.0" was first described in 2011 by Henning

Kagermann, the head of the German National Academy of Science and Engineering (Kagermann, Anderl, Gausemeier, Schuh, & Wahlster, 2018; Kagermann, Lukas, & Wahlster, 2011).

Often researchers use the terms 4IR and Industry 4.0 interchangeably, and even in scientific contexts, the terms suffer from a lack of distinctiveness and a vast number of non-uniform definitions. However, Speringer and Schnelzer (2019) point out that although the concepts are defined ambiguously, 4IR and Industry 4.0 need to be differentiated. These authors suggest that "Industry 4.0 basically represents the economic point of view, which primarily takes manufacturing/production into consideration" (Speringer & Schnelzer, 2019, p. 6).

They further describe five features which play a considerable role in Industry 4.0, namely:

- Digitalisation of manufacturing
- Decentralisation of manufacturing
- Vertical and horizontal integration of the value chain
- Increased productivity
- Flexibility

The authors explain that in terms of components of Industry 4.0, cyber-physical systems and the Internet of Things as well as technical innovations are major drivers of Industry 4.0. Technical innovation accordingly refers to various inventions, such as cloud computing, big data, virtual realities, augmented reality, and artificial intelligence (AI). Speringer and Schnelzer (2019) provide a well-researched state of the art of technological terms and concepts. They point out that 4IR emerging technologies are described by some authors in a similar way to Industry 4.0 concepts; however, in their opinion, the 4IR refers rather to the "systemic change with a holistic view that also takes effects on society, governance, environment, etc. into consideration" (Speringer & Schnelzer, 2019, p. 7). Industry 4.0 is therefore a specific aspect of the 4IR and needs to be differentiated.

Klaus Schwab, the pioneer and inventor of the concept of the 4IR and chairperson of the WEF, highlights that humankind stands at the brink of a technological revolution that will fundamentally alter the way people live, work, and relate to one another (Schwab, 2016). This new way of living and working is at the core of the new era. It is both an extension of the Third Industrial Revolution and completely new. It builds on the previous revolutions: The First Industrial Revolution used water and steam power to mechanise production. In the Second, it was electricity that made mass production possible. The Third made use of electronics and information technology to automate production. Now the 4IR builds on the Third with the digital revolution that began in the middle of the last century. It is characterised by the merging of technologies, in that the boundaries between physical, digital, and biological spheres are blurring (Schwab, 2016).

Schwab is convinced that the 4IR is also a revolution of its own kind and not simply an extension of the previous revolution. He argues that the 4IR is drastically influenced by its speed, its breadths, and its systemic effect and is therefore a revolution in itself (Schwab, 2016). Schwab (2017) points out that the 4IR needs to be developed in a way that it is:

> empowering and human-centered, rather than divisive and dehumanizing, is not a task for any single stakeholder or sector or for any one region, industry or culture. The fundamental and global nature of this revolution means it will affect and be influenced by all countries, economies, sectors and people. It is, therefore, critical that we invest attention and energy in multistakeholder cooperation across academic, social, political, national and industry boundaries. These interactions and collaborations are needed to create positive, common and hope-filled narratives, enabling individuals and groups from all parts of the world to participate in, and benefit from, the ongoing transformations.

Schwab's (2016, 2017, 2019) understanding of the new era has become a milestone in discourses around the new digital worlds and developments, based on an understanding of development which is primarily coined in the Western developed world. Schwab (2019) views the changes as a societal transformation at a global scale, bringing not only economic change but also new and strong developments on political, community, and identity construction levels and which need to be monitored, driven, and guided well to be globally successful.

Researchers from all over the world have begun to explore the changes of the 4IR and their impact on various levels and in different sub-contexts. Nankervis, Connell, Cameron, Montague, and Prikshat (2019), for example, present their understanding of the 4IR as being an era of rapid change, immense challenges, and incredible opportunities for the current and future workforce. Several researchers (see Hirschi 2018) point out that the 4IR is drastically influenced by new emerging or rapidly expanding technologies, such as automation, cybernation, and high technologies, but also by nanotechnology, biotechnology, artificial intelligence, new information technology systems and 3D printing, as well as cloud computing. Other scholars such as Baheti and Gill (2011) mention that integrating computational and physical capabilities in the interaction of machines and humans is a core of the 4IR. Still others already speak of the Fifth Industrial Revolution when taking into account nanotechnologies, expanded global boundary-spanning communication, and advanced human–machine interactions (Pathak, Pal, Shrivastava, & Ora, 2019; Rai & Rai, 2015). Therefore, one can say that a varied and extensive number of definitions and concepts exist which relate to the 4IR concepts, taking different areas of development into account. The large spread of definitions and concepts is reflected in this book (see Sect. 7 in this chapter).

Bendel (2019) contends that the 4IR—and in particular Industry 4.0—is first and foremost a "marketing term" which is primarily being used in economic communication. For Bendel (2019), the term represents a "future project" (German: *Zukunftsprojekt*) which primarily deals with the hybridisation of products (combination of products and services) and the individualisation and integration of clients, customers, and business partners into the value chain systems. Further, the 3D printer development and advancements of (semi-)automated machines, as well as cyber-physical systems and the Internet of Things, advance industry and human–machine interaction. Bendel (2019), based on his experience as a professor in economic information systems, information ethics, and machine ethics, focuses primarily on the economic and information sector.

However, the 4IR is not bound to any specific areas of society, but rather penetrates the ideas and approaches of thinking and behaving on individual, organisational, social, and global levels. Most obviously, the 4IR seems to manifest in the changes in industry with particular focus on digitalisation, logistics, production, and manufacturing areas (Bogner, Voelklein, Schroedel, & Franke, 2016). An important aspect of the 4IR in industry is the transformation into new value sets and workforce behaviour, such as the flexibility of working times, but also flexibility in terms of products and processes which are now more than ever driven by automation, extensive networking, and decentralised control mechanisms, as well as a data acquisition and integration through information and communication technologies (Weisbecker, Burmester, & Schmidt, 2015). Other studies point out that in the 4IR, the entire value chain changes and needs to be adjusted to contribute to an organisation's success (Bogner et al., 2016). Within the entire context of 4IR organisational changes, new technologies are tested, new machines are developed, and new ways of production, communication, and networking replace conventional ways at a high speed (Pardi, 2019; Pardi, Krzywdzinski & Lüthje, 2019).

Speringer and Schnelzer (2019), in their report for the United Nations Industrial Development Organization, present different models of Industry 4.0 and show that there are different regional perspectives in the Global North and Global South[1] on how to define and differentiate the 4IR and Industry 4.0. Often, only the positions of the developed countries on Industry 4.0 and the 4IR are taken into account. Several international key players, such as the European Commission (2017) and the United Nations (2016), emphasise that the 4IR and Industry 4.0 can help to address the challenges of these times, such as poverty, growing inequalities, and increasing unemployment, but also climate change, escalating conflict, violence and extremism, and environmental destruction, and bring positive new approaches to tackle all of these challenges. Norton (2017) and Schwab (2017) also point out that the new technologies might bring equalising effects on wages or enhance smallholder production on global levels. The 4IR can therefore become a positive force in reaching the 2030 sustainability goals. Speringer and Schnelzer (2019), however, state that there is a high risk that developing countries and low-income countries are being left behind in the 4IR process. The transformational process might even bring more inequality into the world, based on a growing global economic split (United Nationals Development Program, 2018).

Organisations and institutions which are influencing the way individuals think and act, such as early childhood education institutions, schools, and higher education organisations, need to play a crucial role in the 4IR and prepare the future workforces to meet the demands of the world of work (Gleason, 2018). Bendel (2019) notes that

[1]Global North and Global South are here defined as primarily geographical and socio-economic concepts (Trefzer, Jackson, McKee, & Dellinger, 2014) which influence the management of 4IR processes in the future.

the challenge to really prepare well for the 4IR lies in the hands of the educational system and particularly the school system. However, the 4IR also impacts strongly on the mobility of people, on health, on the energy sector, and on the climate. According to Bendel (2019), these are and will become the most important contexts of application of the 4IR. Further fields of application are data collection and big data, automated cars, service robots and robotics, e-health and e-medical records, as well as smart systems and energy management (Bendel, 2019). These fields of application need to be supported by corporate politics, global leadership which takes various cultural and socio-economic viewpoints into consideration, policy change and awareness, as well as inclusion and mobilisation (Norton, 2017). Further, recent research suggests to develop universal standards and targets on a global level (Singh, 2016).

Based on the rapidly changing world, global connections, and the new fields of application, the quality and the quantity of employees' workloads are expected to change drastically, as well as the skills that are needed (Webber-Youngman, 2017). Several authors predict that technological skills will be particularly important to success in the 4IR and Industry 4.0 contexts and that a radical change in skill requirements can already be seen (Morgan, 2019; World Economic Forum, 2018a, b). In addition to these hard skills, soft skills such as creativity (DiLiello & Houghton, 2008), systemic thinking, and the transformation of negative towards positive emotions (Mayer & Viviers, 2016) need to be developed. Stichter (2020) even argues that virtues, like skills, need to be developed and trained. Virtues, in this sense, are developed by learning from one's failures, and according to Stichter (2020), it is a challenge to develop skills based on moral failures. Therefore, emotion regulation as a moral skill needs to be taken into account, particularly when individuals deal with moral challenges. Other studies have further indicated that employees will need creativity, expertise (ability to find solutions, to learn), and well-being (positive emotions, engagement) to adapt to the fast development characterised by the 4IR (Ghislieri, Molino, & Cortese, 2018; Kour, El-Den & Sriratanaviriyakul, 2019; Mayer, 2019; Palti, 2017). The findings of Mayer (2020, 2021) show that in particular creativity, positive emotions, and focus on solutions are skills and mindsets that are needed to drive Industry 4.0 and to be innovative and successful in the 4IR.

The change in work lives, talent management, recruitment, and skill management will profoundly affect industries which transform into the 4IR (Wilke, 2020 in press). Obviously, 4IR and Industry 4.0 carry consequences with regard to political and legislative approaches within different countries, such as in South Africa (see Oosthuizen and Mayer 2019). Therefore, it is argued here that it is necessary to allow for different approaches to define and respond to the transformational processes of the 4IR and Industry 4.0. This needs to be done in order to finally construct a concept of the 4IR that is driven by a global movement and inclusive definitions, rather than a concept that is restrictive, led only by a few selected countries with a high economic impact. This book accordingly supports previous research (e.g. Speringer and Schnelzer 2019) who propose that approaches to shape 4IR and Industry 4.0 need to be driven not only by the Global North—where most of the research and political strategies regarding the concept originate—but also by the Global South and the developing countries. By including the Global South in new discourses, the focus from Global North discourses can shift towards more equalised global communication and participation and thereby should change towards a more social and economically just world.

3 Why a Positive View of the Fourth Industrial Revolution and Industry 4.0?

Shamim, Cang, Yu, and Li (2016) emphasise that 4IR changes are viewed as contributing to the improvement of the human species and the human functioning and condition, anchoring the processes in developing a new set of values. Other authors (Mayer & Oosthuizen, 2020) point out that the 4IR focuses on the optimal functioning of the individual, the organisation, and even the world. The positive psychology perspective might be useful on the path of developing further by using the lens of optimal human functioning and strengths. Other authors such as Alkatheeri et al. (2020) also point out that flow, happiness, meaningfulness, and health and hope are important concepts in the development of the new world of the 4IR.

A great deal of literature focuses on positive organisational behaviour within organisations and from cross-cultural and cultural perspectives (Ramlall, Al-Kahtani & Damanhouri, 2014). But scarcely any research has been carried out with regard to positive organisational behaviour and management in the context of the 4IR. Barmeyer and Mayer (2020) argue that in the 4IR, particularly management skills need to change, and a focus is needed on positive intercultural competence in global and cross-cultural collaboration. This means that employees need to have intercultural competence while engaging with what is positive and constructive in rapidly changing environments. Other research supports this perspective and highlights that the increasing ambiguities arising in the 4IR need to be managed by individuals as well as workforces. The ability of these individuals and groups to cope with ambiguities and adversaries is vital for success (Berger, 2018; WEF, 2018c).

Mayer and Oosthuizen (2020) argue in their recent publication that employees and organisations heading towards the 4IR should explore positive psychology 1 (PP1.0) and positive psychology 2 (PP2.0) approaches to create an awareness of the dialectical interplay of negative and positive mindsets and their impacts on the individual, but also on the organisation as such. A positive outlook on the change could support the creation of positive rather than negative emotions which accompany the development of and transitions into the 4IR. Lomas and Ivtzan (2016), for example, point out that fear and anxieties in organisations with regard to negative impacts of the 4IR could interfere with the aim of organisations to transform. In this book, it is argued that a positive approach to the transformations of the 4IR can support individuals and organisations to create meaning (Ivtzan, Lomas, Hefferon, &

Worth, 2016) and a new, transformed, integrated, and interconnected approach to meaning in life and at work. This could create a higher degree of resilience and happiness, as promoted by Mayer and Oosthuizen (2020), and could also contribute to structural changes on social and political levels (see f. e. McKay, Shaw and Silverio, Wilson and Lewandowska-Tomaszczyk, and Vanderheiden on The Terror of Being Judged, and Vanderheiden and Mayer Outlook in this book).

4 Emotions and Shame Within a Changing World

The present book explores new views and perspectives from various disciplines and boundary-crossing transcultural fields and presents the 4IR not only as a process of technological advantages but also as a possible process of transition with regard to the development of awareness, mindfulness, and growth and development as a human species. Thereby, emotions play a particular role.

It has been previously highlighted that both positive and negative emotions are crucial in human interactions. It is argued here that specifically when times are changing and transitions are in progress, emotions need to be taken into consideration, since they are an important part of human life, influencing thoughts and behaviour (Honegger, 2015; Nunez & Jäger, 2015; see Mayer Shame 4.0: Empirical Evidence of the Importance of Emotions in a Technologising World of Work), as well as of organisational and individual life (Pratt & Doucet, 2000). Emotions further impact on mental health and well-being, and it has been pointed out that negative emotions can lead to ill-health or psychological problems, while positive emotions usually contribute to increased mental health and well-being (see Mayer Shame 4.0: Empirical Evidence of the Importance of Emotions in a Technologising World of Work). Often emotions in organisational contexts are influenced by unconscious systems psychodynamics (Oosthuizen & Mayer, 2019), and several authors concur that in rapid transformations, such as in Industry 4.0, emotional intelligence and positive emotions can support coping (Barber, 2019).

Shame has been described as an emotion which, along with guilt, manifests unconsciously (Werden, 2015) and which is often experienced as negative (Nunez & Jäger, 2015). It has been characterised as an often negatively experienced emotion, needing to be transformed into a resource-orientated emotion which can support the individual in individual growth and self-development (Mayer & Vanderheiden, 2019; Vanderheiden & Mayer, 2017). Emotion regulation is therefore, as proposed by Stichter (2020), an important skill in managing emotions. If applied, emotion regulation can support and encourage the individual to self-develop and self-motivate. Besides emotional regulation, individuals also need to be skilled in emotion differentiation in order to explore their emotions in depth and know what kind of emotions are felt and experienced and how to react to these emotions (Cameron, Payne & Doris, 2013). Bigman, Sheppes, and Tamir (2017) emphasise that emotion regulation is possible and increases mental health and well-being. At the same time, emotions are always interrelated with the cultural context and play an important role in relationships, identity formation, and the construction of meaning (Küpers & Weibler, 2008).

Several researchers have recently started to study emotions within the context of the 4IR and Industry 4.0 (Glikson & Erez, 2013; Jonker, 2019; Temekova, 2018). Mayer (in this book chapter—Shame 4.0: Empirical Evidence of the Importance of Emotions in a Technologising World of Work) argues that shame is an important emotion to focus on when moving into Industry 4.0, particularly with regard to new human–technological interaction, skill and failure in skill management, performance-related evaluations, and failure to deal with technological innovation in organisations. Wong (2019) argues that shame and shaming need to be taken into consideration to shape Industry 4.0 and the 4IR and the changes it is bringing about.

Schwab, among others, draws attention to the fundamental and global character of the 4IR. Even if it is not possible at this point to describe conclusively how far-reaching and profound these changes will be, it must be assumed that the way in which shame manifests itself in this context will be affected. The editors of this book have created the term Shame 4.0 for this purpose. It describes all the facets of shame that result from the contexts and phenomena associated with the 4IR. In this respect, Shame 4.0 describes various phenomena, some of which are identified below;

1. One recent form of shame is that which results from automation, in other words, shame about being a human who is replaceable by a machine or robot. For example, a manager may experience shame that employees prefer to trust the decision of an artificial intelligence rather than that of a manager (Schreier, 2020).
2. Shame is resulting from being a victim of discriminatory algorithms (see Mayer on Bias in this book; see Vanderheiden on The Terror of Being Judged).
3. Shame often arises from the fact that very private and possibly sensitive information about lifestyles, purchasing behaviour, and preferences is frequently collected and stored in large quantities without the knowledge of the users. Security-relevant systems such as smart home systems are also secured via this information. The Internet of Things, in particular, is extremely vulnerable to botnets and other malware. This can quickly lead to invasion of privacy and publication of very private information and shameful situations and experiences.
4. Cloud solutions will continue to grow in the wake of the 4IR. This will also increase the vulnerability of such systems, for instance, through external hacker attacks or other criminal activities, which can lead to the publication of sensitive personal data and therefore to a potential exposure of shame.
5. We still know very little about how the friendly and even intimate relations between humans and machines will change. But there are already first marriages between humans and holograms or robots, as well as relationships of humans with dolls equipped with artificial intelligence (Die Welt, 2020; ZEIT, 2018). Apps already exist that suggest friendships, in which, for example, a deceased friend is "replicated" (Bovermann and Bastiaens, 2020). It remains to be seen, and is an exciting subject of research, to what extent a Shame 4.0 phenomenon will develop here.

6. Numerous applications are currently developing using artificial intelligence, in the context of which, interactions between algorithms and people in very sensitive contexts take place. Examples of these are medicine, therapy, and counselling contexts, but also diets or help in overcoming addiction (Loerzer, 2020). There are potentially enormous opportunities associated with this, but there are also potential Shame 4.0 risks, because an imbalance can arise between the all-encompassing knowledge algorithms and people in vulnerable situations who may not be aware of what data about them is collected, by whom, or how it is processed and sold.
7. Another facet of Shame 4.0 could show itself as the shame of algorithms and robots themselves (Spektrum, 2020). This is still a long way off, but numerous projects around the world are working on enabling algorithms and robots to simulate emotions, which could include shame (Azeem, Iqbal, Toivanen & Samad, 2012; Wolfangel, 2019).

This is only a first incomplete approximation of possible facets of a possible Shame 4.0 concept, but already it indicates essential implications and trends.

5 Critical Voices on the Fourth Industrial Revolution and Industry 4.0 Transitions

Some authors (e.g. Ghislieri et al. 2018) call on the need for advanced debate and discourse concerning the changes of the 4IR. Xu, David, and Kim (2018) comprehensively highlight the opportunities and challenges of the 4IR, while Butollo and Lüthje (2017) recommend that open discourses are needed and that the aims and ways of the 4IR need to be critically discussed.

It has been pointed out that the terms and concepts of Industry 4.0 and 4IR have scarcely yet been defined or discussed scientifically (Bendel, 2019). The science of 4IR is in its infancy, and the concept and term lack scientific and rigorous discourses on a transdisciplinary science level. Although many articles and chapters start addressing conceptual and theoretical issues of the 4IR, empirical evidence is still rare (Mayer & Oosthuizen, 2020, in this book chapter—Shame 4.0: Empirical Evidence of the Importance of Emotions in a Technologising World of Work). Further, the questions are: What is part of a common industrialisation process, and what in truth are 4IR and Industry 4.0?

Bendel (2019) points out that the 4IR comes with different disadvantages which need to be explored and addressed. On one hand, Industry 4.0 is highly complex in terms of structures and systems, and its complexity is extremely delicate and susceptible to faults. Automated systems need to be carefully controlled in case they make mistakes, make the wrong decisions, are fed with unsuitable algorithms, or follow the wrong information or regulations. Ethics, according to Bendel (2019), must be developed further to deal with problems such as hacking, job loss due to the increase in semiautomated machines, or automated decision-making. Another critical point is that through smart systems, individuals become transparent citizen.

With regard to global, regional, and cultural influences, the 4IR mainly fosters an understanding of the world which is contextually influenced, with culture-specific perceptions of the times and spaces. By advancing the global understanding of the new era and by aiming to create a global 4IR, marginalised regions—particularly those lacking technological advancements, with slow digitalisation processes and minimal digitalised infrastructure—are disadvantaged in the 4IR processes which rapidly change in the developed countries in the world. Speringer and Schnelzer (2019, p. 42) have found in their research an outstanding difference between countries in the Global North and Global South regarding 4IR developments. For Global North countries, the motivation to transform into a 4IR society is seen as a new technological development and innovation, while it seems for Global South countries to offer a possibility to advance and "catch up with the global competition".

Countries and regions—which are already challenged by minimal technological infrastructure, poor educational and skill levels, poverty, hunger, low income, and other typical challenges which developing countries often experience—might suffer from a growing gap between the developed and the developing countries and might not become equal partners or counterparts of the 4IR. Authors such as Norton (2017), Schwab (2017), and Singh (2016) comment that there is a chance that developing countries might be excluded from the transformation and led into mode inequality. The implementation and development of the 4IR requires clear midterm and long-term strategies and planning to avoid becoming a threat to societies which have to cope with all the potential downhills of the 4IR, such as increasing unemployment, growing gaps in equality, and making educational curricula obsolete (Speringer & Schnelzer, 2019).

At the same time, research has already shown that the use of modern technology (computers, smart phones) has a negative impact on mental and physical health and well-being, particularly when used in leisure time (see Derks, van Mierlo, and Schmitz (2014) and Ghislieri, Emanuel, Molino, Cortese, and Colombo (2017)). The health and well-being implications of increased human–machine interaction and the full impact of technology on humans are not yet clear, but need to be considered (Ghislieri et al., 2018). Increasing use of the internet, remote working, and technology-based learning already have detectable health implications based on the overlap of life–work contexts and an imbalance of increasing workloads (Ghislieri et al., 2017). This means that individuals and employees working in the new home office need to learn new coping mechanisms and strategies to keep boundaries between leisure time and work and also to restructure their life and work.

Another critical issue in the 4IR is the fact that countries and regions undergoing transition into a 4IR workforce will need far fewer low-skilled workers, instead requiring a particular set of highly specialised and skilled employees in certain segments of specific industries. The 4IR might include the risk of high rates of unemployment and also the risk of the loss of quality of life (Botlik, 2020). Also, Frey and Osborne (2017) emphasise that many jobs will be susceptible to computerisation and will be at risk. This means that employees need to upskill or change jobs within the coming years (Ghislieri et al., 2018). The health implications of this situation are not yet clear; it can be assumed that with a higher speed of change in organisations and societies and in more competitive and technologically advanced workplaces, employees might be challenged or even over-challenged.

This subsection does not present a complete or comprehensive overview of the critical voices which are raised with regard to the 4IR and Industry 4.0 developments. However, it provides a first glimpse into the critical aspects of these transformational times.

6 Cultural Voices in the Fourth Industrial Revolution and in Industry 4.0

By taking into account many perspectives from different cultural contexts, countries, and disciplines, this book aims to contribute to the global discourse on 4IR and Industry 4.0 processes.

The editors of this book have therefore chosen to present various cultural perspectives by defining culture broadly as "the coordination of meaning and action within a bounded group" (Bennett, 2017). By using such an open definition, the editors ensure the inclusion of specific subgroups (e.g. teams in organisations, mental health cultures, or youth cultures), regional and country cultures (see Cucuani in this book), and specific disciplinary cultures (e.g. Industrial Psychology Oosthuizen in this book), as well as new professional cultures which are bound to new technological developments (e.g. predictive policing cultures Mayer in this book, etc.) or new developments in social media (e.g. Anita Kasabova).

Further, the book provides spaces for the exploration of intercultural, transcultural, and cross-cultural approaches, referring to the space in which "members of the culturally bounded groups meet to create new meaning and action in the in-between of their cultural groups" (Mayer & Mayer, 2020, p. 165).

Schwab (2017) postulates that the 4IR could and should be orientated as a new "empowering and people-centred" era (see Sect. 2 of this chapter). It is not yet known how this chance for reorientation and transformation of global contexts can actually be used as a culture-building opportunity. This will depend decisively on how national parliaments, leaders, global and national corporations, NGOs, and citizens will shape these interrelationships in their respective areas of responsibility. According to Mayer (2016), culture is a construct that can change at any time, is constructed, and is therefore always new and different. To this extent, cultures construct themselves anew in this understanding through perspectives, communication, and encounters (Mayer, 2016). With this in mind, the editors associate the 4IR with the hope that individuals and collectives will use the opportunity to create humane, empowering, peaceful, and just transcultural connections.

In the following paragraphs, the different chapters will be briefly presented to provide an insight into the content of the book.

7 Exploring New Perspectives on Shame in Cultures of the Fourth Industrial Revolution and Industry 4.0

The book focuses at shame and shaming in a number of contexts which are affected by the 4IR. The authors in this book variously explore shame in different contexts, by taking on the question of how shame and shaming come into play in cultures affected by the 4IR.

The book consists of five parts:

Part I: Shame 4.0 in the 4IR Workplace
Part II: Shame 4.0 in Therapy, Counselling, and Health
Part III: Shame 4.0 in Philosophy, Religion, and Belief Systems
Part IV: Shame 4.0 in the Media
Part V: Outlook (This final part offers an outlook on Shame 4.0 in the face of COVID-19.)

To begin, *Claude-Hélène Mayer* and *Elisabeth Vanderheiden* provide an overview chapter titled "Meaning of Shame in Cultures of the Fourth Industrial Revolution" and present a first insight into the topic. This chapter is followed by the five different parts of the book which are now introduced.

Part I: Shame 4.0 in the 4IR Workplace

In Part I, chapters refer mainly to workplaces, workplace experiences, and related topics such as leadership within the context of the 4IR and with regard to shame. Shame can be an impactful emotion in workplaces, organisations, and leadership in the 4IR, as discussed in Part I of this book.

Claude-Hélène Mayer and *Rudolf M. Oosthuizen* explore the transformation of shame through (compassionate) love in leadership in the workplace. This chapter presents empirical findings from a qualitative study conducted in the hermeneutical research paradigm. Methodologically, the study used structured interviews of 22 leaders from different countries and cultural backgrounds to inquire about shame and love in leadership, workplace, and organisations. The authors discuss the findings that leaders' (compassionate) love transforms shame in the workplace in four ways: through a change towards a positive attitude, by helping to understand others, by seeing love as a transcultural experience, and by seeing love as a positive transformational force. Findings also relate to love and shame interlinkages and show which strategies of loving leadership leaders chose to transform toxic shame in the workplace.

Authors *Yasuhiro Kotera*, *David Sheffield*, *Pauline Green*, and *Kenichi Asano* present a "Cross-Cultural Comparison of Mental Health Shame: Negative Attitudes and External, Internal, and Reflected Shame About Mental Health in Japanese and

UK Workers". They present insights on Japan and the UK and the commodities of the "shame culture" of these economically developed countries, within the rapid advancement of technologies in the 4IR.

The authors examine mental health shame in UK and Japanese workers. The results show interesting links between mental health and shame. Family-reflected shame was a significant predictor of mental health in Japanese workers, while self-reflected shame was a significant predictor in UK workers. In this chapter, the authors discuss the implications of these findings with particular reference to how to reduce mental health shame in Japanese and UK workplaces and the provision of solutions for mental well-being, relating to the advantages of technologies.

Shame has a special place for Malay people, so is learned from the earliest childhood. This is what the authors *Hijriyati Cucuani*, *Marina Sulastiana*, *Diana Harding*, and *Hendriati Agustiani* state in their chapter on Malay people and the role played by shame for tackling counterproductive work behaviour. The concept of *malu* is described as shame and is viewed by the participants of their study as an emotion and trait in which a person feels uncomfortable, discouraged, and guilty for mistakes or violations of regulations, religious values, and social norms. Their empirical study shows that shame-proneness in Malay workers in Pekanbaru is considered quite important in working and that workers should be ashamed to do things that are not in accordance with the rules, religious values, and social norms. The study shows that technology affects one's shame-proneness. The negative impacts of the shift into shame-proneness in Malay people in 4IR include openness beyond borders, less sensitive to the environment, difficult to filter out foreign cultures that are inappropriate. The authors discuss their findings in the light of the literature on 4IR and cultures of the Malay people.

Claude-Hélène Mayer presents in her chapter "Shame 4.0: Empirical Evidence of the Importance of Emotions in a Technologising World of Work" findings from a qualitative study within a single case study of an engineering organisation. The study shows that managers experience shame in the context of Industry 4.0. It further highlights shame, as a rather negatively experienced emotion can be transformed into a positive and constructive transformation into Industry 4.0. Conclusions and recommendations are given with regard to future research and practice from an industrial and organisational psychology perspective.

The following chapter by *Claude-Hélène Mayer* reflects on prejudice, bias, and shame in the context of predictive policing. Predictive policing is one emerging field in crime science, investigation, and intelligence. It uses specific computer programmes, algorithms, and big data to categorise individuals and groups as potential offenders or victims. This can evoke shame in the person concerned. The aim of this chapter is to reflect on the interlinkages of predictive policing and shame, present a state-of-the-art intervention, and reflect on a possible way forward.

Part II: Shame 4.0 in Therapy, Counselling, and Health

Paul Wong and *Kwang-Kuo Hwang* open Part II of this book with their article on cross-cultural perspectives on shame and their impact on mental health and social control. They emphasise that the new technologies have given individuals enormous power to shame others and authoritarian governments the ability to socially control citizens on an unthinkable scale. This chapter focuses on cultural differences between the East and the West in two major types of shame: relational shame and moral shame. For both cultures, the violation of personal identity leads to shame. The authors review shame with regard to concepts of shyness and humiliation in China and the ambivalences of the terms and concepts connected to shame and place it into a positive psychology framework and the 4IR contexts.

Yoshiyuki Takano discusses shame in the context of the 4IR and technological advancements in Japanese culture. The 4IR bring new experiences of shame through, for example, cyberbullying on Facebook. The author explains that traditional concepts of shame in Japanese culture have shifted over the years, but simply attributing such differences to "historical circumstance" and "technological advancement" can be misleading. The chapter examines two key concepts that explore the meaning of shame in Japanese culture through the 4IR: firstly, through the Deleuzian concept of deterritorialisation, and secondly, through the meaning of shame in relation to culture, history, subjectivity, and human connection with technology to allow for the possibility of constructing new meaning and understanding in regard to shame. The author finally defines shame as a critical component of therapy and transformational processes within the Japanese society.

Piers Worth explores Erik Erikson's theory who is the creator of the life cycle. The author outlines Erikson's theory of the life cycle and places "shame" in a dynamic relationship with many other aspects of life, such as the 4IR, and more broadly our growth and development. The author then provides a reconceptualisation of the theory and proposes aspects of positive psychology practice to transform shame.

Athira Alex and *A.T.P. Farisha* reflect on shame in the context of ethical standards and existential theory. The authors discuss shame in the light of Wong's as well as Gilbert's theory. The chapter contributes a new explanation of shame and what it means in the context of positive psychology and existential theory and in times of the 4IR while following existential principles.

The team of authors *Thula U. Koops*, *Catherine Wilkinson*, *Grace Perry*, *Samantha Wilkinson*, and *Sergio A. Silverio* focus on public exposure through naming and shaming in cyberspace. Digital discourses have become an important side effect of the advancement of the digitalisation during the 4IR. The authors present contemporary debates, referring to forms of shaming used to re-enforce social norms with regard to mass media and the growing desire for genital cosmetic surgery by young women and girls.

Elisabeth Vanderheiden presents in her chapter on shame, life-crises, and digitalisation findings from an international study which examined the role of shame in life crises. The aim of this chapter is to describe the concept of life crisis, its connection to and what significance digital media have in coping with this life crisis. The author explores the concepts of shame in life crisis and coping with these crises with regard to the cultural background of the participants. She further studies the impact of the 4IR on life crises and shame and the transformation of shame by using technologies of the 4IR.

Part III: Shame 4.0 in Philosophy, Religion, and Belief Systems

In Part III of this book, authors focus on shame in the context of philosophy, religion, and belief systems in the 4IR.

The next chapter approaches shame in the context of the 4IR through the lens of Baruch Spinoza (1632–1677), a Dutch, Portuguese-born Jewish philosopher, who focused developed concepts of enlightenment and innovative concepts of self and the universe. The authors, *Claude-Hélène Mayer* and *Paul J.P. Fouché*, explore Spinoza's life through the notions of shame and faith development from a psychobiographical perspective, contributing to the theory of shame and faith development and its potential positive effect when transformed into a source of growth, self-development, and understanding. The chapter finally draws a conclusion how the theories and experiences of Spinoza can be used as lessons and potential learnings for individuals living through the challenges of the 4IR.

Dharm P.S. Bhawuk explains the Indian worldview, *lajjA*, which is a virtue that has both internal and external manifestations, and it is different from embarrassment, social anxiety, poor self-concept, or guilt. As a virtue to be cultivated, lajjA is the guide and guard for monitoring personal responsibility and is closer to conscience, rather than shame or guilt. In this chapter, the author examines lajjA and conscience from positive psychological perspectives for managing shame and guilt in the globalised world that is progressing towards the 4IR. The chapter ends with providing implications for global psychology frameworks.

Sowmya Puttaraju and *Tony Brian D'Souza* start of this part of the book by focusing on shame, the interconnectivity through the internet, and the internet being the medium of digital surveillance and privacy, a questionable possession. The authors present internet-based shaming behaviour, such as internet shaming, digital lynch mobs, and digital vigilantism. The chapter identifies how digital tools increase disciplinary surveillance in a wider social space, using the theories of surveillance and theories of shame.

Simon Cozens also deals with shame on the internet and its connection to the permanent nature of digital identities and their longevity. Shame can no longer be hidden or evaded, and so innovative approaches are now required which the author finds in Christian theology and pastoral practice. The author suggests to firstly deconstruct social identity as derived from the gaze of the other, before reconfiguring it as derived from the gaze of the other, and discusses this procedure with regard to the permanent digital record created online.

Part IV: Shame 4.0 in the Media

The next part of this book, Part IV, focuses on shame in the context of the media in the 4IR.

The first author in this part, *Anita Kasabova*, writes in her chapter about Aristotle's idea on shame in the *Rhetoric* and the *Nicomachean Ethics* and his emphasis on the eyes. Analysing his use of the words *aiskhyne* and *aidos*, the author portrays how these two concepts relate to shame in social media. Aristotle's *aiskhyne* oscillates between painful self-focused feelings accompanied by public humiliation and allowing us to reflect on our actions. *Aidos* denotes a fear of disgrace while adapting our behaviour to social norms. The author argues that the Greek words provide a paradigm which can be used for analysing shame situations in social media culture. She further discusses social media culture and how it impacts people's well-being in 4IR.

The public exposure through naming and shaming in cyberspace has become an important side effect of the advancement of the digitalisation and technologisation during the 4IR. The authors, *Claude-Hélène Mayer* and *Elisabeth Vanderheiden*, provide the reader with insights on forms of shaming, effects of shaming, and counter-strategies to shaming and naming in online contexts. They explore how online and offline realities interact and present contemporary debates on shaming in the 4IR. They provide two selected examples, namely, slut-shaming (the exposure and shaming of individuals for their perceived or actual sexual behaviour) and body shaming—by referring to "pro-ana" (anorexia nervosa) and "pro-mia" (bulimia nervosa) movements, glorifying shame-based eating disorders which are interlinked with shame and shaming online. The authors reflect how shame and shaming impact on global, social, and individual levels.

In this chapter, shame in the context of Chinese students is explored. The authors, *Zixuan Wang*, *Wei Gabriel Qi*, *Leila Z. Wu*, and Xiaochen Luo, provide an overview of the scarce literature on the issues of shame pertaining to the perception of body shape in social media, from a culturally specific framework that is comprised of Chinese urban young adults. They further present findings from a qualitative study of Chinese undergraduate participants attending colleges in the USA, to examine the interplay between one's cultural identity and the experience of shame with body image within the context of social media use. The findings shed light on the concept of shame from a cultural perspective in association with social media and the benefits of continued research on this subject.

Grace Maria Jochan and *Trina Banerjee* explore shaming behaviour in the context of expression and have subsequently led to neologisms like internet shaming, digital lynch mobs, and digital vigilantism. The historical and contemporary notions of individualism-collectivism and the dynamic cosmopolitan culture and its influence on social media behaviour, according to the authors, require scrutiny when concerned with shaming behaviour. The chapter identifies how digital tools increase disciplinary surveillance in a wider social space, using the theories of surveillance and theories of shame. The authors use a qualitative axiological assumption in understanding the concept of shaming.

Paul A. Wilson and *Barbara Lewandowska-Tomaszczyk* explore social media which offer online spaces within which individuals can launch protests that can be less restricted by offline cultural influences. However, the blurred boundary between these two spaces, the permeability of which is dependent on contextual factors, means that the total separation between the two is illusory. The authors analyse the honour killing of the Pakistani social media star; Qandeel Baloch, who campaigned against the oppression of women in Pakistan, was killed by her brother, Waseem. The authors investigate the role of shame in online vis-à-vis offline spaces for both siblings and discuss this in the light of *fight*, *flight*, and *fright* responses to the social threat of shame that correspond to anger, fear, and depression.

Paul A. Wilson and *Barbara Lewandowska-Tomaszczyk* reflect on the role of shame as a resource in the honour killing of Qandeel Baloch, the Pakistani social media star who campaigned against the oppression of women in Pakistan. She was killed by her brother, Waseem. The authors investigate the role of shame in online vis-à-vis offline spaces for both siblings and argue that her enforced devirtualised presence in the offline Pakistani honour culture was particularly instrumental in her demise. The authors further assess the possible effects of *fight*, *flight*, and *fright* responses to the social threat of shame that correspond to anger, fear, and depression, Finally, they examine the interplay between these factors and the utilisation of shame as a resource.

Shame has been often been argued as a culturally bound emotion which can affect a country's citizens to varying degrees. *Shereen H. Shaw* and *Sergio A. Silverio* explore shame in Arab societies which are often regarded as being heteronormative, masculinist, and patriarchal. These cultures are themselves in turn often synonymous with particular shame narratives associated with the suppression of women and sexuality. This chapter explores the reclamation of sexuality by Arab women and how their rebellion against centuries of suppression is tackling the culture of shame in which they continue to exist during the 4IR.

Gillian McKay discusses shame within the context of returning migrants and 4IR processes, highlighting positive as well as possible negative effects of the 4IR and migrants. The authors emphasise in particular the emotional and psychosocial effects of returning to one's country of origin, as well as the potential push and pull factors. By exploring these topics and interrelationships, the author investigates the power of digital media in overcoming the negative emotions experienced by returnees, including feelings of shame. This chapter explores the experiences of shame in returning migrants and discusses how the 4IR may be useful in overcoming these negative emotions, ultimately transforming them into something that is beneficial not only for their psychosocial well-being but also for potential migrants to make informed decisions about their intent to migrate.

Elisabeth Vanderheiden is exploring public shaming as a resource and strategic tool in this chapter. She refers to the growing awareness of public shaming as a resource for empowerment and self-efficiency, as well as a strategic tool against discrimination in (political) conflicts. Shame as a political instrument is particularly relevant when no formal punishment. The author presents the state of the art and discusses when shame can become a tool of legitimisation of political participation, e.g. in grassroots campaigning. Finally, a case study is being analysed and interpreted, leading to general and specific conclusions and recommendations.

Author *Rudolf M. Oosthuizen* writes in his chapter about the changing aspects in human life and human–machine interaction in the 4IR. He presents a critical review of shame for artificial cognitive systems, which must or may not be able to interact with human beings in the context of the 4IR. He further criticises that shame has been neglected in most of research cases by researchers of robotics, computer sciences, or artificial intelligence, and the author investigates in his chapter the literature on shame in artificial devices, as well as the culture of future human–machine interactions.

Leona Ungerer focuses on cyber-shaming and its consequences in virtual spaces. She sees cyber-shaming as shaming via electronic means and focuses on enforcing established or perceived social norms. Progress in electronic communication channels, however, has radically changed the role of social norm enforcement in constraining behaviour, with norm enforcement potentially being indiscriminate, reflecting inaccuracies, and involving behaviour that deserves punishment in itself. This chapter provides a description of digital culture and elaborates on the shallowing hypothesis as part of this culture in the 4IR. It further distinguishes cyber-shaming from related and provides suggestions how to deal with cyber-shaming in a resourceful way.

This speculative essay of author *Michael Uebel* proposes an account of shame phenomena in the Fourth Industrial Revolution that traces the origin and meaning of shame to technology. The author refers to Norbert Elias (1939/2000) and reflects upon the imbrication of human agency, identities, and visibility as it relates to the historically shifting threshold of shame from pre-industrial to post-industrial societies. The essay has four main concerns: outlining the history of shame and its moralities from a sociological perspective, identifying the technological origins of shame, considering some transformations of shame by technology, and speculating upon the future of shame as a moral construct embedded in technology, with some consideration of the binary divisions such as technology/society and subject/object that have traditionally structured the cultural significance of shame.

Part V: Outlook

In Part V of this book, the editors provide a future-orientated outlook with regard to shame in the context of COVID-19 and the way forward. In their outlook, *Elisabeth Vanderheiden* and *Claude-Helene Mayer ask*: "Who could breathe without hope?" They then present "Some Theses on Shame and Shaming 4.0 in the Age of the Corona Pandemic". The authors aim at stimulating reflection and asking of further questions with regard to shame and shaming in the face of COVID-19. The chapter refers to global and diverse cultural contexts and, from the particular perspective of Positive Psychology 2.0, pays special attention to the efforts that individuals and collectives are making to constructively manage and transform the global crisis.

Finally, *Justine Pistorius*, a Johannesburg artist, presents in this book her artwork "The Shame Warrior". She describes her artistic approach and reflection on the different facets of shame in the context of the 4IR, thereby paying particular attention to the spiritual aspects and positive psychology. Through her art, she calls for a more holistic approach to shame, not only through words but also through artistic approaches and expressions.

8 The Contribution of This Book

The aim of the book is to explore the concept of shame and its potential meaning in the context and cultures of the 4IR and Industry 4.0. Thereby, the editors further aim at bringing scientists and research from different disciplines, cultures, and scientific traditions together, given them a voice, thereby contributing to the discourses on shame, 4IR, Industry 4.0, and culture.

The introduction shows that a large number of concepts and definitions exist in relation to the 4IR and Industry 4.0. This book is an attempt to bring researchers and scientists from different disciplines, cultures, societies, and science and knowledge traditions together. Therefore, the reader will find chapters in this book which use different approaches and definitions across all chapters with regard to the book's main concepts, namely, the 4IR, Industry 4.0, shame, and culture. Thereby, the foci of the different chapters vary, and the main perspectives might focus either on the 4IR, some on Industry 4.0, some on shame, and some on culture. The main focus of each chapter is defined by the authors themselves. From a holistic viewpoint, this book on the one hand presents overlapping ideas across sciences, cultures, and applications while on the other hand might create awareness on the crossroads of the diverse viewpoints. The book thereby reflects to breadths of research under the umbrella of the 4IR movement. This kind of "patchwork" approach is seen as an important aspect of creating a "global" approach to the 4IR since we deal with various ways of understanding what the 4IR and Industry 4.0 are. This book can therefore only, on the one hand, be an approach to contributing to listening to the different voices and narrations within the context of the 4IR and, on the other hand, become a contribution to a formation of a new, holistic, and global understanding of these transformational concepts which is anchored in the (cultural) realities of the researchers. To a large extent, it might reflect the breadths of the concepts, maybe even their "fuzziness", as described by Speringer and Schnelzer (2019).

While some of the chapters explore aspects which have hardly been discussed in the concepts of the 4IR before, others stay in more known and previously studied areas of research.

Some chapters focus on specific research topics, such as the role of humanitarian data brokering in migrant shame and shaming, technology as a historical and culturally situated mediator of shame, and also shame induced by AI-driven profiling algorithms on marginalised and/or vulnerable communities. Other chapters explore the relationship between emerging technologies and shame which has rarely been discussed in the business world outside of a future of work, education, and/or training context. Further on, the aspect of emotions and management in the context of the 4IR and especially Industry 4.0 is often overlooked when dealing with the technological and business aspects.

A majority of the chapters focuses on shame and shaming in specific cultural contexts, such as in Pakistan, or they explore shame in the context of cyberbullying, digital manufacturing, digital tools, and digital technology, such as in social media. It might be argued that shame in the context of digitalisation is not necessarily

4IR- or Industry 4.0-related, as partly described in literature and theory on the 4IR and Industry 4.0. This focus might be rather seen as part of the 3IR movement. Digitalisation is generally often viewed as a 3IR concept and practice. However, it plays a major part in the transition towards the 4IR. However, digitalisation is a pillar in the 4IR and in Industry 4.0 might change and expand its meaning in the 4IR context. It is therefore included in this book.

The chapters presented focus on the concepts of shame and cultures and are anchored in different theoretical and cultural traditions, scientific perspectives, and disciplines. The authors present their preferred viewpoints and definitions for the perspective taken in their chapters. Common, however, for all chapters is that the authors focus on a positive, constructive, and resource-orientated perspective.

Finally, the work presented in this book is "work in progress". It reflects the viewpoints of the authors and editors in momentum and will surely be developed and advanced in future research and practice.

References

Alkatheeri, Y., Ameen, A., Isaac, O., Nusari, M., Duraisamy, B., & Khalifa, G. S. (2020). The effect of big data on the quality of decision-making in Abu Dhabi government organisations. In *Data management, analytics and innovation* (pp. 231–248). Singapore: Springer.

Azeem, M. M., Iqbal, J., Toivanen, P., & Samad, A. (2012). Emotions in robots. *Communications in Computer and Information Science, 281*, 144–153.

Baheti, R., & Gill, H. (2011). The impact of control technology: Cyber-physical systems. *IEEE Control Systems Society, 12*(1), 161–166.

Barber, S. (2019). *A truly 'transformative' MBA: Executive education for the fourth industrial revolution*. University of Bedfordshire, UK. Retrieved from http://hdl.handle.net/10547/622822

Barmeyer, C., & Mayer, C.-H. (2020). Positive intercultural management in the fourth industrial revolution: managing cultural otherness through a paradigm shift. *International Review of Psychiatry, 32*(7–8), 638–650.

Bendel, O. (2019). *Definition: Industrie 4.0.* Retrieved February 22, 2020, from https://wirtschaftslexikon.gabler.de/definition/industrie-40-54032

Bennett, M. (2017). *Culture*. Defined in an email communication on 30 April 2017.

Berger, R. (2018). *The Fourth Industrial Revolution – Industrie 4.0*. Munich: Roland Berger. Retrieved from https://www.rolandberger.com/en/Insights/Global-Topics/Industry-4.0/.writing of the paper.

Bigman, Y. E., Sheppes, G., & Tamir, M. (2017). When less is more: Effects of the availability of strategic options on regulating negative emotions. *Emotion, 17*(6), 993–1006.

Bogner, E., Voelklein, T., Schroedel, O., & Franke, J. (2016). Study based analysis on the current digitalization degree in the manufacturing industry in Germany. *Procedia CIRP, 57*, 14–19.

Botlik, J. (2020). Movement of autonomous systems after selected infrastructure as a globalization effect induced by initiate Industry 4.0. *SHS Web of Conferences, 74*. https://doi.org/10.1051/shsconf/20207402001.

Bovermann, K., & Bastiaens, T. (2020). Towards a motivational design? Connecting gamification user types and online learning activities. *RPTEL, 15*, 1. https://doi.org/10.1186/s41039-019-0121-4.

Butollo, F., & Lüthje, B. (2017). Made in China 2025: Intelligent manufacturing and work. In *The new digital workplace. How new technologies revolutionise work* (pp. 42–61). London: Palgrave.

Cameron, C. D., Payne, B. K., & Doris, J. M. (2013). Morality in high definition: Emotion differentiation calibrates the influence of incidental disgust on moral judgments. *Journal of Experimental Social Psychology, 49*, 719–725.
Derks, D., van Mierlo, H., & Schmitz, E. (2014). A diary study on work-related smartphone use, psychological detachment and exhaustion: Examining the role of the perceived segmentation norm. *Journal of Occupational Health Psychology, 19*, 74–84. https://doi.org/10.1037/a0035076.
Die Welt. (2020). *Ro(bo)mantik: Ingenieur "heiratet" seine selbstgebaute Robo-Freundin - WELT.* Retrieved May 10, 2020, from https://www.welt.de/kmpkt/article163506203/Ingenieur-heiratet-seine-selbstgebaute-Robo-Freundin.html
DiLiello, T. C., & Houghton, J. (2008). Creative potential and practiced creativity: Identifying untapped creativity in organizations. *Creativity and Innovation Management, 17*, 37–46.
European Commission. (2017). *Key lessons from national industry 4.0 policy initiatives in Europe, Digital Transformation Monitor.* European Commission, Brussels, Belgium.
Frey, C. B., & Osborne, M. A. (2017). The future of employment: How susceptible are jobs to computerisation? *Technological Forecasting Social Change, 114*, 254–280. https://doi.org/10.1016/j.techfore.2016.08.019.
Ghislieri, C., Emanuel, F., Molino, M., Cortese, C. G., & Colombo, L. (2017). New technologies smart, or harm work-family boundaries management? Gender differences in conflict and enrichment using the JD-R theory. *Frontiers in Psychology, 8*, 1070. https://doi.org/10.3389/fpsyg.2017.01070.
Ghislieri, C., Molino, M., & Cortese, C. (2018). Work and organizational psychology looks at the fourth industrial revolution: How to support workers and organizations? *Frontiers in Psychology, 9*. https://doi.org/10.3389/fpsyg.2018.02365.
Gleason, N. W. (2018). Singapore's higher education systems in the era of the fourth industrial revolution: Preparing lifelong learners. In *Higher education in the era of the fourth industrial revolution* (pp. 145–169). Singapore: Palgrave Macmillan.
Glikson, E., & Erez, M. (2013). Emotion display norms in virtual teams. *Journal of Personnel Psychology, 12*(1), 22–32.
Hirschi, A. (2018). The fourth industrial revolution: Issues and implications for career research and practice. *Career Development Quarterly, 66*, 192–204.
Honegger, M. (Ed.). (2015). *Schreiben und Scham: Wenn ein Affekt zur Sprache kommt.* Gießen: Psychosozial-Verlag.
Ivtzan, I., Lomas, T., Hefferon, K., & Worth, P. (2016). *Second wave positive psychology.* London: Routledge. https://doi.org/10.4324/9781315740010.
Jonker, C. (2019). Emotion experiences and management within digital work contexts. In M. Coetzee (Ed.), *Thriving in digital workspaces* (pp. 131–144). Cham: Springer.
Kagermann, H., Anderl, R., Gausemeier, J., Schuh, G., & Wahlster, W. (2018). *Industrie 4.0 in a global context strategies for cooperating with international partners (Acatech Study).* München, Germany: National Academy of Science and Engineering.
Kagermann, H., Lukas, W.-D., & Wahlster, W. (2011). Industrie 4.0: Mit dem Internet der Dinge auf dem Weg zur 4. Industriellen Revolution. *VDI Nachrichten, 13*, 2.
Kour, J., El-Den, J., & Sriratanaviriyakul, N. (2019). The role of positive psychology in improving employees' productivity: An experimental study. *Procedia Computer Science, 161*, 226–232.
Küpers, W., & Weibler, J. (2008). Emotions in organization: An integral perspective. *International Journal of Work Organizations and Emotions, 2*(3), 256–287.
Loerzer, S. (2020). *Caritas in München: Diese App soll Suchtkranken helfen.* Retrieved 10 May 2020, from https://www.sueddeutsche.de/muenchen/muenchen-sucht-caritas-app-1.4567140
Lomas, T., & Ivtzan, I. (2016). Second wave positive psychology: Exploring the positive-negative dialectics of well-being. *Journal of Happiness Studies, 17*(4), 1753–1768.
Mayer, C.-H. (2016). *Von Brillen, Rücksäcken und Eisbergen…Was ist eigentlich Kultur?* Retrieved 10 May 2020, from https://www.trainerscut.com/home/von-brillen-rucksäcken-und-eisbergen/

Mayer, C.-H. (2019). Reflections on key factors of creativity and the art of collaboration in the 21st century workspaces. In M. Coetzee (Ed.), *Thriving in digital workspaces: Innovations in theory, research and practice* (pp. 147–166). Cham: Springer.

Mayer, C.-H. (2020). Key concepts for managing organizations and employees turning towards the fourth industrial revolution. *International Review of Psychiatry, 32*(7–8), 673–684.

Mayer, C.-H. (2021). Shame 4.0 – empirical evidence of the importance of emotions in a technologising world of work. In C.-H. Mayer, E. Vanderheiden, & P. T. P. Wong (Eds.), *Shame 4.0: Investigating an emotion in digital worlds and the fourth industrial revolution* (pp. 91–108). Cham: Springer.

Mayer, C.-H., & Mayer, L. J. (2020). On being "outside the box" or being "inside": Intercultural communication, relationship-building and identity ascription failures. In E. Vanderheiden & C.-H. Mayer (Eds.), *Mistakes, errors and failures across cultures: Navigating potentials* (pp. 163–181). Cham: Springer.

Mayer, C.-H., & Oosthuizen, R. (2020). Positive transformation towards the fourth industrial revolution: Empirical evidence from a technology company. *International Review of Psychiatry, 32*(7-8), 659–672. https://doi.org/10.1080/09540261.2020.1763927.

Mayer, C.-H., & Vanderheiden, E. (2019). *The bright side of shame. Transforming and growing through practical applications in cultural contexts*. Cham: Springer.

Mayer, C.-H., & Viviers, R. (2016). Systemic thinking and transcultural approaches in coaching psychology: Introducing a new coaching framework. In L. E. Zyl, M. W. Stander, & A. Odendaal (Eds.), *Coaching psychology: meta-theoretical perspectives and applications in multi-cultural contexts* (pp. 205–230). Cham: Springer.

Moore, J. (2020, January 5). The Fourth Industrial Revolution. Is it time to re-skill our employees? *Psychology Today*. Retrieved from https://www.psychologytoday.com/us/blog/putting-america-work/202001/the-fourth-industrial-revolution

Morgan, J. (2019). Will we work in twenty-first century capitalism? A critique of the fourth industrial revolution literature. *Economy and Society, 48*(3), 371–398.

Nankervis, A., Connell, J., Cameron, R., Montague, A., & Prikshat, V. (2019). Are we there yet? Australian HR professionals and the Fourth Industrial Revolution. *Asia Pacific Journal of Human Resources*.

Norton, A. (2017). *Automation and inequality. The changing world of work in the global South, IIED Issue Paper*. London, UK: International Institute for Environment and Development (IIED).

Nunez, D. G., & Jäger, M. (2015). Scham, Schuld, Schreiben. Fehlerkulturen im Schreibprozess. In M. Honegger (Ed.), *Schreiben und Scham: Wenn ein Affekt zur Sprache kommt* (pp. 20–47). Gießen: Psychosozial-Verlag.

Oosthuizen, R. M., & Mayer, C.-H. (2019). At the edge of the fourth industrial revolution: Employees' perceptions of employment equity from a CIBART perspective. *SA Journal of Industrial Psychology/SA Tydskrif vir Bedryfsielkunde, 45*(0), a1695. https://doi.org/10.4102/sajip.v45i0.1695.

Palti, I. (2017). Creativity will be the source of our next industrial revolution, not machines. *Quartz, 11*. Retrieved from https://qz.com/954338/creativity-will-be-the-source-of-our-next-industrial-revolution-not-machines/

Pardi, T. (2019). Fourth industrial revolution concepts in the automotive sector: Performativity, work and employment. *Journal of Industrial and Business Economics, 46*(3), 379–389.

Pardi, T., Krzywdzinski, M., & Lüthje, B. (2019). *Digital manufacturing revolutions as political projects and hypes: Evidences from the auto sector*. In ILO Research Department Working Paper.

Pathak, P., Pal, P. R., Shrivastava, M., & Ora, P. (2019). Fifth revolution: Applied AI & human intelligence with cyber physical systems. *International Journal of Engineering and Advanced Technology, 8*(3), 23–27.

Pratt, M. G., & Doucet, L. (2000). Ambivalent feelings in organizational relationships. In *Emotion in organizations* (2nd ed., pp. 204–226). London: Sage.

Rai, S., & Rai, A. (2015). Nanotechnology – The secret of fifth industrial revolution and the future of next generation. *Nusantara Bioscience, 7*(2), 61–66.

Ramlall, S., Al-Kahtani, A., & Damanhouri, H. (2014). Positive organizational behavior in the workplace: A cross-cultural perspective. *International Journal Of Management & Information Systems (IJMIS), 18*(3), 149. https://doi.org/10.19030/ijmis.v18i3.8700.

Schreier, J. (2020). *Künstliche Intelligenz oder emotionale Intelligenz ist hier die Frage*. Retrieved May 10, 2020, from https://www.industry-of-things.de/kuenstliche-intelligenz-oder-emotionale-intelligenz-ist-hier-die-frage-a-876261/

Schwab, K. (2016). Davos 2016: Die Vierte Industrielle Revolution. In *Handelsblatt*. Retrieved February 22, 2020, from https://www.handelsblatt.com/politik/international/davos-2016/davos-2016-die-vierte-industrielle-revolution/12836622.html?ticket=ST-46596007-ZgWruoD7u5eChRgd6Yfo-ap2

Schwab, K. (2017). *The Fourth Industrial Revolution: What it means, how to respond. 2016*. In World Economic Forum.

Schwab, K. (2019). *The Fourth Industrial Revolution | Special Feature*. Retrieved February 22, 2020, from https://www.britannica.com/topic/The-Fourth-Industrial-Revolution-2119734

Shamim, S., Cang, S., Yu, H. and Li, Y. (2016). *Management approaches for Industry 4.0: A human resource management perspective*. IEEE Congress on Evolutionary Computation, CEC 2016. Retrieved from https://pureportal.strath.ac.uk/en/publications/management-approaches-for-industry-40-a-human-resource-management

Singh, Z. (2016). Sustainable development goals: Challenges and opportunities. *Indian Journal of Public Health, 60*, 247–250. https://doi.org/10.4103/0019-557X.195862.

Spektrum. (2020). *Künstliche emotionale Intelligenz: Das richtige Gefühl*. Retrieved May 10, 2020, from https://www.spektrum.de/news/emotionen-perfektionieren-kuenstliche-intelligenz/1566366

Speringer, M., & Schnelzer, J. (2019). Differentiation of Industry 4.0 Models. The 4th Industrial Revolution from different Regional Perspectives in the Global North and Global South. In Regional Academy on the United Nations (RAUN) (Eds.) *Innovations for development: Towards sustainable, inclusive, and peaceful societies*, Vienna. Retrieved from http://www.ra-un.org/publications

Stichter, M. (2020). Learning from failure: Shame and emotion regulation in virtue as skill. *Ethical Theory and Moral Practice*. https://doi.org/10.1007/s10677-020-10079-y.

Temekova, M. (2018). Studying the leadership style of business organizations' management under the conditions of the fourth industrial revolution. *Asia Pacific Journal of Research and Business Management, 9*(2), 1–15.

Trefzer, A., Jackson, J. T., McKee, K., & Dellinger, K. (2014). *Introduction: The global south and/in the global north: Interdisciplinary investigations* (pp. 1–15). Bloomington, IL: Indiana University Press.

UNDP. (2018). *Development 4.0: Opportunities and challenges for accelerating progress towards the sustainable development goals in Asia and the Pacific, Sustainable Development Series*. New York: UN Development Programme.

United Nations. (2016). *Sustainable development goals (SDGs)*. United Nations Sustainable Development.

Vanderheiden, E., & Mayer, C.-H. (2017). *The value of shame - Exploring a health resource in cultural contexts*. Cham: Springer.

Webber-Youngman, R. C. W. (2017). Life skills needed for the 4th industrial revolution. *Journal of the Southern African Institute of Mining and Metallurgy, 117*(4), iv–v.

Weisbecker, A., Burmester, M., & Schmidt, A. (2015). *Mensch und computer. Workshopband*. Berlin: De Gruyter Oldenbourg.

Werden, R. (2015). *Schamkultur und Schuldkultur. Revision einer Theorie*. Münster: Aschendorff Verlag.

Wilke, K. (2020). *Managing talent in the automotive industry: Gaining competitive advantage in times of change*. Doctoral Thesis, Europa Universität Viadrina, Frankfurt (Oder), Germany.

Wolfangel, E. (2019). ZEIT ONLINE | *Die Angst der Maschine*. Retrieved May 10, 2020, from https://www.zeit.de/2019/33/robotik-kuenstliche-intelligenz-emotionen-angst

Wong, P. T. P. (2019). Foreword: From shame to wholeness: An existential positive psychology perspective. In C.-H. Mayer & E. Vanderheiden (Eds.), *The bright side of shame. Transforming and growing through practical applications in cultural contexts* (pp. v–xi). Cham: Springer.

World Economic Forum (WEF). (2016). *The Fourth Industrial Revolution.* Retrieved February 22, 2020, from https://www.youtube.com/watch?v=o0ipIV7ZJ74

World Economic Forum (WEF). (2018a). *The future of jobs report 2018.* Retrieved October 7, 2019, from http://www3.weforum.org/docs/WEF_Future_of_Jobs_2018.pdf

World Economic Forum (WEF). (2018b, September 17). *Machines will be more tasked than humans by 2025, but Robot Revolution will still create 58 million net new jobs in the next five years.* Retrieved from https://www.weforum.org/press/2018/09/machines-will-do-more-tasks-than-humans-by-2025-but-robot-revolution-will-still-create-58-million-net-new-jobs-in-next-five-years/

World Economic Forum (WEF). (2018c). *Agile governance. Reimagining Policy-making in the Fourth Industrial Revolution.* Working Paper. World Economic Forum.

World Economic Forum (WEF). (2020). Machines will do more tasks than humans by 2025 but robot revolution will still create 58 million net new jobs in next five years. [online] World economic forum. Retrieved February 11, 2021.

Xu, M., David, J., & Kim, S. (2018). The fourth industrial revolution: Opportunities and challenges. *International Journal of Financial Research, 9*(2), 90. https://doi.org/10.5430/ijfr.v9n2p90.

ZEIT. (2018). *ZEIT ONLINE. Sie haben die Wahl.* Retrieved May 10, 2020, from https://www.zeit.de/digital/2018-09/manga-fs

Claude-Hélène Mayer (Dr. habil., Ph.D., Ph.D.) is a Professor in Industrial and Organisational Psychology in the Department of Industrial Psychology and People Management at the University of Johannesburg; an Adjunct Professor at the European University Viadrina in Frankfurt (Oder), Germany; and a Senior Research Associate at Rhodes University, Grahamstown, South Africa. She holds a Ph.D. in Psychology (University of Pretoria, South Africa), a Ph.D. in Management (Rhodes University, South Africa), a Doctorate (Georg-August University, Germany) in Political Sciences (socio-cultural anthropology and intercultural didactics), and a Habilitation (European University Viadrina, Germany) in Psychology with focus on work, organisational, and cultural psychology. She has published several monographs, text collections, accredited journal articles, and special issues on transcultural mental health and well-being, sense of coherence, shame, transcultural conflict management and mediation, women in leadership in culturally diverse work contexts, constellation work, coaching, and psychobiography.

Elisabeth Vanderheiden is a Pedagogue, Theologian, and Intercultural Mediator. She is the CEO of the Global Institute for Transcultural Research and the President of Catholic Adult Education in Germany. Her publishing activities focus on pedagogy, in particular on the further education of teachers and trainers in adult, vocational, and civic education but also on the challenges of digitalisation. She has also edited books on intercultural and transnational issues. Her most recent publications deal with shame as a resource as well as with mistakes, errors, and failures and their hidden potentials in the context of Culture and Positive Psychology 1.0 and 2.0. Her current research projects deal with love in transcultural contexts, with life crises, as well as with humour in the context of Positive Psychology 2.0. Another focus of her work is design thinking in transcultural contexts.

Part I
Shame 4.0 at the Workplace

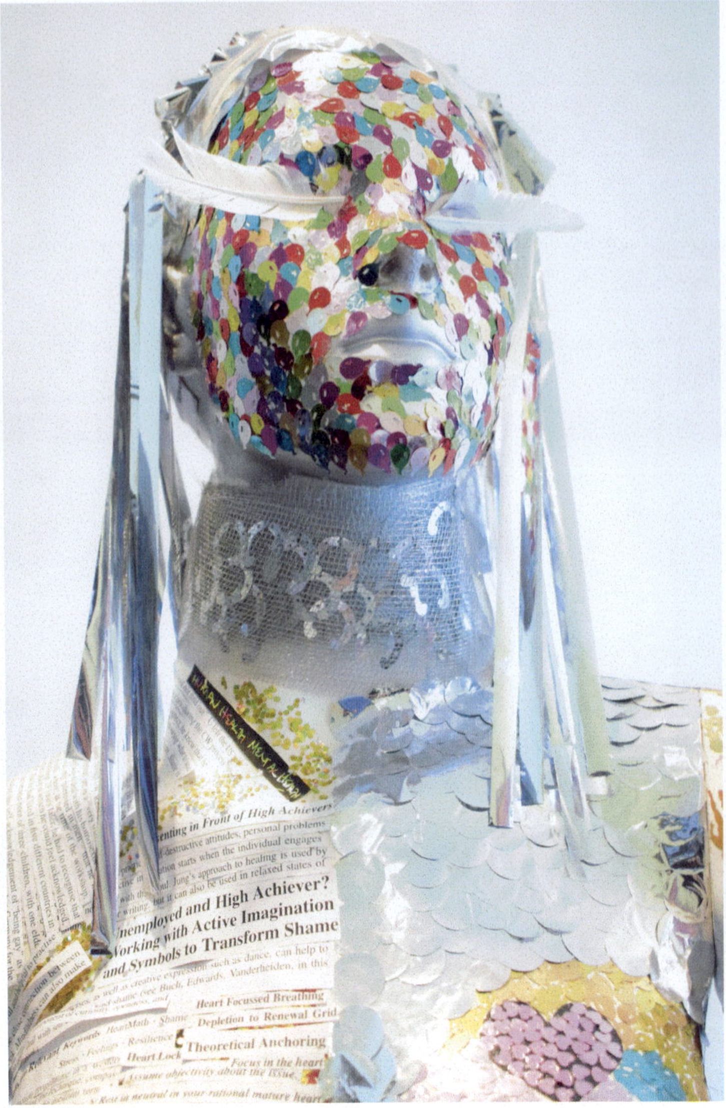

Chapter 2
Transforming Shame Through Love: Envisioning Positive Transcultural Leadership in Contemporary and Future Workplaces

Claude-Hélène Mayer and Rudolf M. Oosthuizen

1 Introduction

Shame has advanced to become an important issue within the leadership contexts of contemporary workplaces (Mayer & Tonelli, 2017; Oosthuizen, 2017). It was previously assumed that the positive transformation of negative emotions such as shame in workplaces might become even more important when contemporary workplaces transform into future-orientated workplaces, integrating rapid technological changes, digitalisation, and smart systems (see Mayer and Vanderheiden on Investigating an Emotion in Digital Worlds and the Fourth Industrial Revolution in this book).

Industry 4.0 workplaces are defined by rapid changes in the move to a higher degree of technology usage. The Fourth Industrial Revolution (4IR) is coalescing, thanks to an expansive array of disruptive technologies such as artificial intelligence (AI), Internet of Things (IoT), and autonomous vehicles (AVs) (Kruger, 2020; Tan, 2016; Tan & Wu, 2017). Today's digital era challenges organisations not only to follow the technological trajectories, by developing new technological solutions and/or adopting the latest disruptive technology, but most importantly to become resilient organic systems that are open to changes and keen to experiment and

C.-H. Mayer (✉)
Department of Industrial Psychology and People Management, University of Johannesburg, Auckland Park, Johannesburg, South Africa

Kulturwissenschaftliche Fakultät, Europa Universität Viadrina, Frankfurt (Oder), Germany

R. M. Oosthuizen
Department of Industrial and Organisational Psychology, University of South Africa, Pretoria, South Africa
e-mail: oosthrm@unisa.ac.za

C.-H. Mayer et al. (eds.), *Shame 4.0*, https://doi.org/10.1007/978-3-030-59527-2_2

innovate continuously. The view of the organisation as a techno-human system points out that organisations need to integrate the traditional rational-based principles and technology assets with the emotive features of human life, such as shame and love, and understand that emotions play a fundamental role in the organisational life and in the pursuit of business excellence (Schiuma, 2017).

Recently, it has been suggested that transcultural management during the 4IR may profit from a paradigm shift to concepts of "positive intercultural management (PIM)", particularly within changing, new 4IR workplaces (Barmeyer & Mayer, 2020). The authors here argue that PIM particularly needs to include the ability of leaders in contemporary organisations to focus on the positive aspects in general. However, specifically with regard to the increase in transcultural employment relations and transcultural teamwork and the growing diversity in organisations, as well as the transformation to 4IR workspaces which are based on increased digitalisation, AI, machine learning, robotics, and remote workplaces (Guoping, Yun, & Aizhi, 2017), leaders should be prepared to detect negative behaviour, attitudes, and emotions and support employees to transform these negative emotions for both personal and organisational growth (Pol & Reveley, 2017) (see also Oosthuizen in this book).

Further, it is argued here that leadership in this realm should focus not only on being transcultural but also on being transculturally orientated, thus taking systemic, dynamic perspectives into account which use the potential and synergies of cultural complex workspaces. According to Treichel und Mayer (2011), transcultural concepts and workspaces are primarily concerned with a systemic rather than a unit-orientated perspective, strengths and interests rather than structures and efficiency, transformation rather than transaction, potentials rather than knowledge, competencies rather than skills, diversity rather than self and other dualisms, and synergy rather than exchange. Transcultural contexts are therefore viewed as more complex and demanding than monocultural contexts and workspaces (Treichel & Mayer, 2011). It is thus assumed here that these more complex transcultural workplaces are a well-received reflection of and response to the increasing systemic complexities constructed and demanded by the 4IR changes, which also foster growth in transcultural interactions and systemic interwoven aspects.

In recent studies and research on shame, it has been pointed out that negative emotions and particularly shame can be transformed to become a force for self-development and personal growth (Mayer & Vanderheiden, 2019; Velotti, Garofalo, Bottazzi, & Caretti, 2017; Wong, 2019). It is argued in this chapter that this development and growth can become particularly important for leaders across cultures. It is further assumed that not just any emotion can support the transformation of shame to a constructive force but that love in particular may be supportive in transforming shame and other negative emotions into an experience of personal growth and development (Mayer & Vanderheiden, 2020).

Based on the empirical findings of a qualitative study, this chapter aims at exploring the relationship between love and shame within the leadership context of contemporary workplaces from the perspective of international leaders. It further proposes love as a relevant emotion for transforming shame in Industry 4.0

workplaces. In this chapter, the findings attempt to respond to the following research questions:

- How can love support overcoming shame?
- How are love and shame interlinked?
- When did you overcome shame through love (narrations)?
- What loving strategies do you use as a leader to transform toxic shame in the workplace?

In the following section, the authors will present the relevant literature on love and leadership in transcultural 4IR contexts, as well as shame. The research methodology will then be presented, and the findings will be indicated and discussed. Finally, the chapter presents a conclusion and makes a number of recommendations.

2 Transforming Shame Through Compassionate Love in Leadership

2.1 Conceptualisation of Shame

Shame is an influential, self-conscious, multifaceted feeling. It tends to be experienced by leaders who are inclined to disguise it. It is often related to feelings of being immobilised and mediocre and is linked to an awareness of social unpleasantness (Tangney, Miller, Flicker, & Barlow, 1996). It often merges with other primary feelings (e.g. anxiety or anger; Gilbert, 1998) and has been discovered to be highly correlated with symptoms of psychopathology (Irons & Lad, 2017; Kim, Thibodeau, & Jorgensen, 2011). Furthermore, shame is a penetrating negative feeling personified by the discernment of an inclusive deflation of the self by the leader (Tangney & Dearing, 2002). Feelings of shame are often sparked by social and organisational occasions in which a decline in personal and professional status or feelings of rejection are perceived by leaders.

Shame may essentially refer to diverse features of the self, such as behaviours or physical characteristics, as well as to the broader identity (Andrews, Qian, & Valentine, 2002; Hejdenberg & Andrews, 2011). Explicitly, a multidimensional conceptualisation of shame has been proposed (Andrews et al., 2002) in order to ascertain (1) experiences of characterological shame (e.g. regarding personal habits, manner with others, and personal skills), (2) experiences of behavioural shame (e.g. referring to doing something wrong, saying something stupid, and failing in competitive contexts), and (3) physical shame (e.g. referring to being ashamed of one's physical appearance) (Velotti, Elison, & Garofalo, 2014; Velotti et al., 2017) (see Mayer and Vanderheiden on Naming and Shaming in this book).

2.2 Conceptualisation of Transformational and Transcultural Leadership

Transformational leadership is tracked in the research of Bass and Riggio (2006) and Riggio (2009), who expand their ideas on the innovative concepts of Burns (1978). Dimitrov (2015) provides the following four Is of transformational leaders: (1) idealised inspiration (being the role model for followers), (2) inspirational enthusiasm (inspiring and motivating followers), (3) individualised kindness (showing genuine concern about the needs and feelings of followers), and (4) intellectual encouragement (challenging followers to be creative and innovative).

Transcultural leadership is a blend of transformational leadership and multiculturalism, as proposed by Derungs (2011), and is further described as a viable leadership approach in a globalised environment. Transcultural leadership abilities and practices that have been proven to be generally effective are the ability to encourage organisational employees and ethical decision-making and create tactical visualisations that extend across cultural peripheries (Northouse, 2016). Other critical transcultural leadership abilities and practices include the skill to develop oneself and others and strong collective and interpersonal skills and the skill to elucidate multifaceted, equivocal difficulties. However, the crucial leadership abilities and practices for efficient transcultural leadership include the skill to incorporate other cultures and develop a universal mindset (Perez, 2017) that is able to deal with ambiguities, resolve conflicts constructively, and create transcultural identities and which has strong competencies in relationship-building, communication across cultures, and self-management (Mayer, 2011).

2.3 Conceptualisation of Compassionate Love

Compassion refers to concern for the sufferings of the self and others, with an obligation to attempt to relieve or counteract them. There are two significant psychological theories that reinforce this description. The first encompasses cultivating the skill to observe and turn towards and connect with misery (as opposed to avoiding or dissociating from it). Connecting with sorrow and pain is often problematic; the first psychological theory of compassion comprises a form of strength and courage to do this (Gilbert, 2014). The second psychological theory of compassion comprises developing insight and dedication to find modes to lighten and avoid suffering. This necessitates training in developing abilities and methods that support leaders' ability to manage suffering and advance well-being (Irons & Lad, 2017).

Compassionate love is "an attitude toward other(s), either familiar others or outsiders or all of humanity; including emotions, perceptions, and actions that are concentrated on loving concern, sensitivity, and an alignment toward supporting, assisting, and appreciating the other(s), particularly when the other(s) is (are) perceived to be hurting or in hardship" (Monin, Schulz, & Feeney, 2015). It has been asserted that compassionate love may be the kind of love that advocates the most prominent social gain (Fehr & Sprecher, 2009). This kind of love has been categorised in distinctive ways. In any case, most definitions accentuate caring, valuing, and concern for the recipient. Sprecher and Fehr (2005) characterise compassionate love as feelings, cognitions, and behaviours that are centred on caring, concern, and tenderness and an inclination to comforting, making a difference and understanding other individuals.

This kind of love is usually stimulated by the realisation that another individual is in distress. Consequently, Berscheid (2010) affirms that it is this antecedent that separates compassionate love from other kinds of love (e.g. passionate/romantic love). Compassionate love is furthermore characterised by an emotion centred on advancing the well-being of another (Berscheid, 2006). In spite of the fact that it is similar to empathy (Batson, 2009), it is considered to be a longer-lasting, prosocial feeling/orientation that can be experienced in both a social setting and with outsiders (Collins et al., 2014; Oosthuizen, 2020).

2.4 *Love and Shame in 4IR Workplaces*

Researchers have long sought ways to operationally describe love and to determine different kinds of love. When people articulate communal care for and interest in one another (in either a romantic or non-romantic context), these daily social connections may develop into the experience of ephemeral increases in emotions of love (Fredrickson, 2016). Corresponding to this context, employees experience positive meaning in their daily work lives via bio-behavioural synchrony—shared fleeting experiences of positive feelings—and mutual sensitivity. Positivity resonance has been previously indicated to have an important effect on well-being in organisations (Major, Le Nguyen, Lundberg, & Fredrickson, 2018). At its core, the construct of love is recognised as a feeling or as a combination of feelings with a sense of collective connectedness. Izard (1977) states that love is a mixture of a feeling of joy and the interest that individuals feel in relation to others, which underpins the impression that love is multilayered and not restricted to just romantic love. This broader perspective on organisational love, as stemming generally from positive emotion and social connectedness amongst employees in organisations, and not only from romantic relationships, may be viewed as a blend of organisational research in the working relationship between employees and emotion science (Oravecz, Dirsmith, Heshmati, Vandekerckhove, & Brick, 2020).

By means of culture-general approaches, transcultural leaders can transform shame through compassionate love by changing attitudes and using identity-based and self-development-related approaches in the following ways:

1. Transcultural leaders develop their *attentional and mindfulness skills* as a way to notice "loops in the mind" and unhelpful (although understandable) ways of

managing their shame and distress. Developing skills in mindfulness facilitates groundedness in the here and now and helps to facilitate emotion regulation.
2. Transcultural leaders are encouraged to *develop a compassionate part of themselves*, linked to the qualities of wisdom, strength, and commitment. This involves various skills training, including the training of those skills linked to memory, imagery, and acting (Gilbert, 2014). Once developed, transcultural leaders are encouraged to use this part of themselves to relate to their trauma memories, sense of shame, and self-criticism. Although self-compassion is a key focus, it is important that transcultural leaders are also able to relate to others in caring and compassionate ways and are also open to the care, kindness, and compassion of others. Collectively, these are referred to as the three flows of compassion.
3. Transcultural leaders should also cope with common fears and blocks. These *resistances need to be transformed to compassion in leaders* (Gilbert, 2014). In a qualitative study, Lawrence and Lee (2014) found that leaders with trauma experiences initially had aversive and fearful responses to attempts to become more compassionate with themselves. However, over time and with support, they were able to experience more positive feelings associated with self-compassion and have a more positive outlook generally on their future (Irons & Lad, 2017).

Focusing on the transformation of the 4IR workplace and the emotions involved, it may be said that people have a love–hate relationship with new technologies like AI, IoT, 3D printing, and AVs (Van Rensburg, 2019). In some cases, people welcome change with open arms; in others, people resist or try to escape it. People love change when the immediate benefits are obvious but hate it when the situation is demanding of them—when they feel it threatens their comfort, security, or way of life (Kruger, 2020). According to Van Rensburg (2019), the 4IR is all happening too fast, is too unpredictable, and is complex so that individuals are anxious and insecure about it.

Researchers have recognised the theoretical possibility for shame and anxiety to be transformed through loving encounters, but whether the affective force of love emerges is seemingly determined by kindness. Loving encounters do not arise at will (Pullen, Rhodes, & Thanem, 2017; Thanem & Wallenberg, 2015). Pouthier and Sondak's (2019) indicate the critical role played by the mutual recognition and the acceptance of fundamental vulnerability in the emergence of new smart technologies, algorithms, AI, robotics, and machine learning. This dynamic differs from the underlying shared awareness of a common and specific vulnerability. This vulnerability may emerge from the 4IR resonances of frustration and anger. It may follow specific shaming episodes and may lead to collective outrage and mobilisation: employees who feel ashamed that they do not cope with new technological advancements might, for example, feel ashamed. The struggle (Vachhani & Pullen, 2019) is against employees' own desire to maintain the myth of self-mastery (Kenny & Fotaki, 2015). The emergence of loving encounters occurs through a process of self-fragilisation (Ettinger, 2006), where individuals expose the hurt they experienced in the pursuit of recognition and open themselves to be respected and admired by others. When organisational members become mutually aware of their fundamental vulnerability and mutual interdependence, they may become more disposed to act lovingly or generously (Rushing, 2010).

Emotions denote all those factors of human expression that cannot be reduced to rules/procedures or technological components; rather they need to be disclosed and channelled for contributing to the organisational value mechanisms. On the other hand, technology guarantees efficiency and control. Both rationality and emotions, technology and humanity, matter for the success of an organisation, and in the new Digital Age, they need to be integrated. For this reason, organisations need to shape a loving environment in which technology and love are fused and intertwined. The successful organisations of the Digital Age will be those recognising that as much as they will become more technologically advanced, the people will still be at the heart of organisational life and actually the most human distinguishing factors will become even more fundamental for the creation and delivery of value. A loving environment is capable of engaging employees in their daily work activities, of inspiring executives to build igniting visions and energise people, and of making organisations more aware of the value propositions delivered to stakeholders (Schiuma, 2017).

Pouthier and Sondak (2019) elucidate that organisational cultural conditions may facilitate the emergence of loving encounters (Pullen & Rhodes, 2015). In loving encounters, employees resist the impulse to make value judgements—involving aggression and exclusion. Such a culture supports the resistance to 4IR, as well as the experience and display of compassion. Dominant forms of organising divert attention from such dynamics (Acker & Webber, 2016), numbing people to the lives of others, for whose lack of well-being they refuse to take responsibility. Additionally, a climate of psychological safety facilitates the admission of sad affects, without which the recognition of human vulnerability in the context of 4IR and the effort to alleviate each other's suffering may not happen. In the absence of a safe climate, employees may dismiss exposure of their own weaknesses as too interpersonally risky, thus precluding the emergence of loving encounters. The identification of contextual features that make loving encounters more likely deserves additional scholarly exploration.

Pouthier and Sondak (2019) clarify the emancipatory potential of loving encounters. Researchers have proposed that ethico-political acts of love matter (Lund & Tienari, 2019), even if they do not "change the world in one fell swoop" (Pullen et al., 2017). Employees could, through reiterated acts of love, disrupt the tight grip of 4IR anxiety. It is not surprising that employees express their marvel at the possibilities of what the near future may bring, mixed in with anxiety about disruptive change and potential work loss. This supports the notion that the affirmative politics of love may constitute a real challenge to dominant discriminatory norms (Kenny & Fotaki, 2015; Pullen & Rhodes, 2014), in part perhaps because unlike individual acts of resistance they do not rely on an illusion of autonomy (Mumby, Thomas, Martí, & Seidl, 2017).

The key to the efficacy of communal laughter and reciprocal generosity may be the deep nurturing sense of connection and positive regard that people experience in such loving encounters and the resulting increase in felt vitality. Such experiences create the possibility of thinking and doing otherwise (Mumby, 2009) through certain practical ideas shared to start love-based leadership in a 3D printing company, mobile supercomputers, intelligent robots, and virtual assistants, such as Siri, and relating to each other in more joyful and authentic ways (Vlieghe, 2014). Employees experience an increase in joy through love, which may induce them to seek out and repeat those encounters (Thanem & Wallenberg, 2015). Given how critical the repetition of loving encounters seems to be to employees and the overall potency of emancipating organisational members, scholars are encouraged to elaborate on the potentially self-reinforcing nature of the affirmative politics of love in the 4IR context (Ojansivu, 2019).

3 Research Methodology

The research design of this study is hermeneutical and interpretative, and its foundation is qualitative in nature, exploring relationships between people, situations, and objects and their allocated meanings (Ashworth, 2015; Denzin, 2017).

3.1 Research Instrument

Data collection was conducted by means of 22 online survey interviews involving an online survey conducted with male and female leaders working in global, transcultural organisational work settings. Clearly, cross-cultural and transcultural differences are part of this research and need to be taken into account with regard to bias in interpretation (Runyan, 1994). Questions included, for example, the following: "What is love?" "How are love and leadership connected" "How does love impact in your work context?" "How are love and shame in the workplace interlinked?" "Which strategies do you use to transform negative emotions, e.g. shame or shaming in the workplaces?" Data were analysed using content analysis, specifically the five-step process of Terre Blanche, Durrheim, and Painter (2006, pp. 322–326). This process includes the following: Step 1, familiarisation and immersion; Step 2, inducing themes; Step 3, coding; Step 4, elaboration; and Step 5, interpretation and checking. Data quality was ensured through a rigorous, trustworthy research approach (Yin, 2013), taking the context, research process, and bias into account (Lincoln & Guba, 2000) and applying the quality criteria of credibility, dependability, transferability, and conformability (Yin, 2013).

3.2 Sample and Sampling

The study used purposeful and snowball sampling (Naderifar, Goli, & Ghaljaie, 2017). The sample consisted of 22 individuals, ranging in age from 33 to 80 years. The 9 females and 13 males indicated their religious affiliation as follows: 7 were Christian, 4 Roman Catholic, 2 Protestant, and 1 each atheist, agnostic, atheist/agnostic, Buddhist, Muslim, Jew, and Jesuit, while 1 indicated no religious affiliation. In terms of first language, interviewees spoke German (10 participants), English (5), Afrikaans (2), Japanese (1), Tswana (1), Hebrew (1), and Romanian (1). National affiliation was indicated subjectively as the following: eight Germans, five US citizens, two Japanese, two South Africans, and one participant each with White, German-Iranian, Israeli, Romanian, and Bavarian (region in Germany) origin. Highest level of education was mentioned as follows: nine doctoral degrees, six master's degrees, three "Diplom" degrees (equivalent to master's degree in Germany), two habilitations (postdoctoral degree), one national diploma, and one high school certificate. The sample further included seven professors, three academics, three directors, two consultants, one professor/entrepreneur, one entrepreneur, one executive manager, one project manager, one teacher, one psychologist, and one educational officer.

3.3 Ethics and Limitations

Ethical guidelines were followed, promoting voluntary participation, transparency; application of informed consent and explanations about the study, as well as the right to withdraw at any point in time; respectful communication; and anonymity (Roth & Von Unger, 2018). Ethical approval for this research study was given by the German university to which one of the authors of this chapter is affiliated. The study was limited to a qualitative research design, and the research and sampling methods are described here. There is the potential for bias in the data and in its interpretation with regard to the sample, owing to the participation of a majority of German first-language speakers and the relatively strong educational background of most of the participants. The study could therefore be criticised as being elitist. As a result, it is not possible to generalise from these findings; however, the data provide valuable insights into aspects of love and shame which should be followed up in future studies.

4 Research Findings

The research findings respond to the following questions: How can love support overcoming shame? How are love and shame interlinked? When did you overcome shame through love (narrations)? What loving strategies do you use as a leader to transform toxic shame in the workplace? The findings will be reported in the following sections.

4.1 How Does Love Support Transforming Shame in the Workplace?

Leaders in 4IR workplaces believe to a strong degree that love has a positive impact on transforming shame in four different ways, as shown in Fig. 2.1.

When leaders talked about the transformational force of love, 29 of their statements referred to the idea that love leads to a positive attitude, including respectful and trusting behaviour, acceptance, a positive attitude in general, and compassion. By leading to a positive attitude, shame is transformed either within the self or with regard to others. For example, P2, a US male entrepreneur, highlighted:

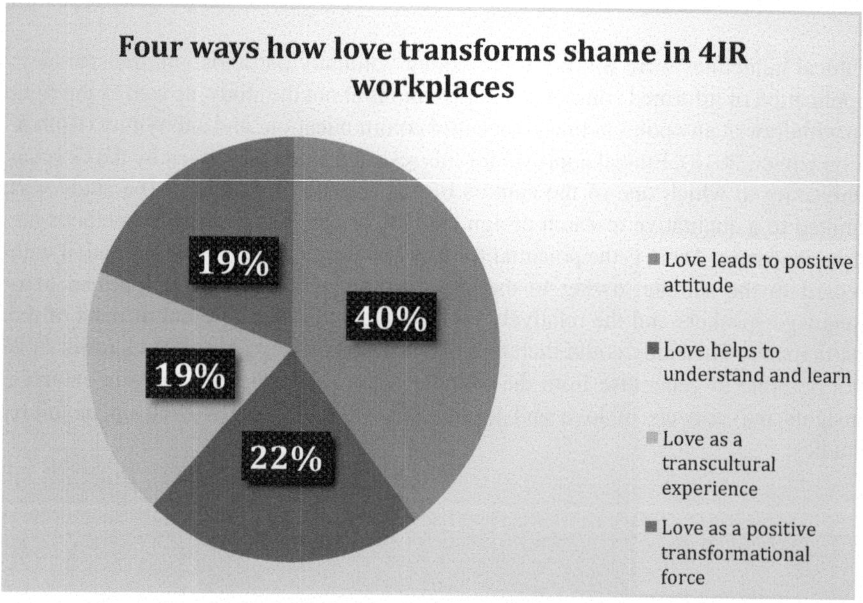

Fig. 2.1 Four ways in which love transforms shame in 4IR workplaces

Table 2.1 Love transforms shame in 4IR workplaces I

Frequency	Category	Participants
Love leads to a positive attitude—29 statements		
8	Respectful and trusting behaviour	P2, P3, P6, P9, P10, P14, P18, P22
8	Acceptance	P2, P3, P14, P8, P16, P18, P20, P22
7	Positive attitude	P2, P5, P9, P10, P14, P16, P19
6	Compassion	P2, P9, P15, P16, P21, P22

Table 2.2 Love transforms shame in 4IR workplaces II

Love helps to understand and learn—16 statements		
9	Helps to understand, accept, respect, and value the contexts of the other	P4, P5, P6, P8, P10, P11, P13, P18, P22
7	Learn about others	P4, P5, P8, P11, P14, P18, P19

> By facilitating love, trust and respect among teams and organisational members a leader can engage, empower, and enable a caring and loving workplace in multiple small places. It's about the attitude.

Love can support leaders to develop relationships with employees and thereby foster positive interactions and a loving workplace which contributes to productivity and the creation of positive work relationships (Table 2.1).

Sixteen of the leaders' statements mention that love helps to understand and learn and, through the new ways of understanding and learning, contributes to the transformation of shame and shameful experiences. P6, an American male professor, emphasised:

> In general, my approach has always been to communicate to people I am leading that they are okay, good, loveable people, worthy of respect, and we are all humans, with our human imperfections, mistakes, insufficient learning. And even if they feel shamed or ashamed, I am committed to them. Love helps to learn about and to accept the others—the way they are.

Furthermore, love is viewed as being a transcultural experience, referring to the perspective that love is transcendental and universal and can thus have an impact on individuals in intercultural or cross-cultural interactions. Since leaders seem to see love in the sense of compassionate love as a universal emotion, love is seen as having a positive impact across cultures (Table 2.2).

Additionally, five individuals highlighted that love, as an experienced, compassionate emotion, helps individuals to see with the heart rather than to stereotype individuals of different cultural origins. Finally, 14 statements were identified as referring to love as a positive transformational force. Here, leaders emphasised that just through loving and having a loving attitude, problems can be transformed to transcultural solutions. Love has a further impact on experiences of shame by creating positive relationships and thereby transforming shameful experiences. Last but not least, love fosters open communication and thereby transforms the shameful experiences.

Table 2.3 Love transforms shame in 4IR workplaces III

Love connects through being a transcultural experience—14 statements		
9	Love is a transcultural experience	P1, P7, P9, P10, P13, P18, P19, P20, P21
5	Love helps not to stereotype "the other"	P3, P5, P6, P11, P20
Love is a positive transformational force—14 statements		
8	Transform problems in transcultural solutions	P1, P7, P8, P9, P14, P18, P19, P20
3	Love creates positive relationships	P3, P10, P19
3	Open communication	P7, P9, P14

In his interview, P5, an American male professor, related to both aspects, seeing love as a compassionate transcultural and transformational experience:

> I think love can support positive transcultural interaction in at least two ways. Firstly, love between two specific individuals of different cultures can be a powerful way to challenge prejudice and racism when they make an effort to understand each other's cultural worldview and accept that worldview as valid, though I suspect there are many intercultural relationships in which the pair love one another in some ways but don't make the effort to fully understand each other or challenge their stereotypes and biases, but if love can't get someone to challenge their prejudices I'm not sure what would.
>
> Secondly, I think promoting a love for humanity itself, promoting in our cultures the idea that we should respect and value other human lives no matter how different they are from our own, that developing such an ideology would improve transcultural relations. I am thinking of those feelings that encourage one to sacrifice for strangers who are persecuted, such as Europeans who protected Jews during the Holocaust, or Americans running the underground railroad to free slaves in the south.

Love is seen as an overall positive force which supports the leaders to manage and overcome challenging interactions and situations and create accommodating and transformational and transcultural workplaces (Table 2.3).

4.2 *How Are Love and Shame Interlinked?*

During the interviews, the leaders referred to the concepts of love and shame and their interlinkages. Of all the statements, 18 relate to the idea that negative love experiences cause shame. Four individuals highlighted that they felt shame either as a result of rejected love or when love became toxic and violent or that a deprivation of love could become an instrument of power and would be shameful. Two statements each refer to the idea that it is shameful when love is unreciprocated and it can become very shameful when love makes you vulnerable. Furthermore, love creates shame when it is connected to a demand from the other and it is shameful when a loved one is being hurt. P8, a male Iranian-German professor, pointed out:

> Love is no isolated feeling—the affection must somehow be shown to the loved person. Otherwise love is unlikely to survive and might only be an admiration of an imaginary person. Showing love to someone always bears the risk that the love is not returned. This can

lead to shame, because I do not receive the affection that I wanted from a person whom I value. The more I open myself to that person, the more I might feel shame when this love is rejected or unreflected.

This statement shows that compassionate love also comes with potential vulnerabilities and challenges and that it requires courage. Moreover, the effects of loving may be complex and difficult to deal with. Altogether 11 statements reflect the interconnection of love and shame as positive and powerful. Furthermore, six statements refer to the fact that love, as an attitude, can help to overcome public shame. Five people highlighted that love is expressed to counteract shame. A female Japanese leader in an educational context had this to say (P10):

In order to wipe off shame and restore pride, love for oneself as well as love for one's surroundings is necessary. Love can wipe off self-shame and public shame.

Finally, ten statements see love and shame as further interconnected with concepts of the self. Six individuals highlighted that one way to overcome shame is to love oneself, as already mentioned in P10. In addition, two statements each highlight that one does not feel love when one feels ashamed and that it is a shame if one cannot contain love. One of these statements is shown in the following:

Loving oneself first can provide a pathway out of shame and such can be facilitated by the expression of love by another. Self-esteem is often a reflection of some source beyond yourself who expressed confidence and love in you first. Hence, the role of leadership includes such expressions to others or simply by delegating, supporting, and trusting in other's work.

Besides love, different concepts such as pride, confidence, and self-esteem are important for strengthening loving and compassionate leadership and responding to shame or preventing shame. The discourses on love and shame show the complex concepts and emotions involved in these powerful interactions of emotions (Table 2.4).

4.3 Narrations of Love-Transformed Shame

Three leaders told stories relating to the fact that shame happens in (love) relationships and that in this kind of relationship in particular, shame can emerge very strongly. Another three narrations refer to the idea that shame is caused by publicly inadequate shameful behaviour. Some leaders highlighted that shame is caused by the experience of inadequate behaviour; however, not every leader referred to love as a possibility to transform toxic shame. P20, a Japanese male leader, stated (P20):

I think that shame is possible without love. Soldiers can feel a shame if they fail in a task for example. Samurais made hara-kiri when they were ashamed even though they did not value the emotion of love so much.

A black African male leader pointed out:

Table 2.4 Interlinking love and shame

Frequency	Category	Participants
Negative love experiences cause shame—18 statements		
4	Feel shame as a result of rejected love	P7, P8, P9, P14
4	Shame happens when love becomes toxic and violent	P1, P14, P16, P18
4	Deprivation of love and application of shame = instrument of power	P1, P18, P19, P20
2	Shame when you love without reciprocity	P18, P19
2	Love makes vulnerable = shame	P7, P9, P12
1	If love requires something from the other = shame	P4
1	Shame when I hurt someone	P8
Love as a resource to overcome shame—12 statements		
6	Loving attitude helps to overcome (public) shame	P1, P6, P7, P9, P10, P11, P14
5	Love is expressed to counteract shame	P2, P14, P15, P16, P19, P21
Shame, love, and the self—10 statements		
6	Self-love is a way out of shame	P2, P7, P11, P14, P15, P16
2	If you feel shame, you do not feel love	P13, P19
2	It is shameful if one cannot contain love	P4, P7

Table 2.5 Transforming shame in love narrations

Frequency	Overall category	Participants
Shame caused in relationships		
1	Shame of being left and divorced	P1
1	When I love someone, I can feel the love of a person	P22
1	Partner feels less loved than daughter from previous relationship	P4
Shame caused by public inadequate shameful behaviour		
1	Hara-kiri is based on shame	P20
1	Kiss of stranger in childhood	P7
1	Failed examination	P10

> Professionalism is one of the key facts, I proclaim so that as a leader I may not find myself been manipulated by pity, and shame and professionalism are neutral selected emotions that will be compulsory at workplace and emotion that expose weakness as shameful have potential to deceive.

The participants' narrations indicate that as soon as leaders were asked to narrate their own shame and love experiences, they referred to personally experienced emotions, mainly within a private context, and removed their organisational or leadership perspective, preferring to relate to love within their own private spheres (Table 2.5). This may indicate that love and shame are deeply anchored emotions and are often experienced in a personal and private setting when relationships are close and when a person seems to be at their most vulnerable.

4.4 *Leadership Strategies to Transform Toxic Shame in the Workplace*

According to the leaders, there are three possibilities for transforming toxic shame through love in leadership, as presented in Fig. 2.2.

Altogether, the leaders emphasised in 39 statements that a loving strategy in terms of a loving attitude can transform shame. They particularly highlighted love as being a foundational attitude, thereby supporting the transformation of toxic shame into healthy shame. Furthermore, shame is transformed through a generalised kind and loving attitude. As an emotion, love supports individuals in respecting and accepting negative emotions and thereby builds a basis for transforming them. Others stated that love also displays dignity and thereby transforms shame into a resource. Thus, when in a loving state, one can love everyone; love helps to value everyone, even oneself, and thereby transforms shame. Finally, a loving attitude connects the individual to the greater good and thereby helps to transform toxic shame. Moreover, according to four of the leaders, even if one decides to love consciously, this is the first step to transforming negative emotions such as shame. A Japanese female leader had this to say (P10):

> In our leadership culture, jintokku (benevolence) is valued. Leaders should be competent, but competence only does not necessarily serve as a requirement for a great leader. Of course, leaders should be competent. But at the same time, they have to be kind and considerate towards others, transform the negative into dignity. And this needs a loving attitude.

The leader refers to a loving attitude as a basis for transcultural leadership which is linked in her Japanese culture to benevolence. On the other hand, a black male leader from South Africa (P12) emphasised:

> In my culture, a loved leader is the one who has love or living love and who cannot be feared for love lived within . . . and love is the great thing that human beings are gifted with and it is valued.

Within the African context, love as a concept is viewed as a human gift which goes beyond the cultural context to be seen as universal and thereby reaching out across cultures. Love counters fear and other negative emotions and therefore brings to the fore positive, interpersonal relationships (Table 2.6).

Fig. 2.2 Strategies of love in leadership

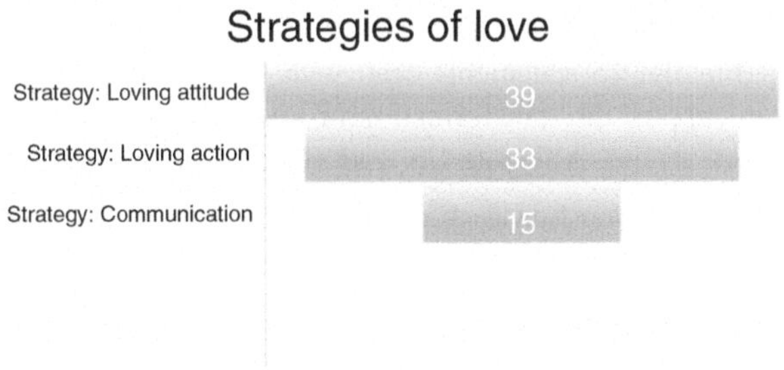

Table 2.6 A loving attitude

Frequency	Category	Participants
Strategies of love to transform shame: attitude—39 statements		
9	Takes love as the foundational attitude	P1, P6, P7, P9, P10, P14, P15, P16, P21
7	Transforms shame through a general positive attitude (warmth, forgiving, love)	P1, P4. P5, P7, P14, P16, P22
6	Helps to respect or accept negative emotions	P1, P3, P6, P14, P16, P18
5	Displays dignity	P3, P10, P11, P14, P16
4	Value every person	P10, P13, P16, P22
4	Connects to the greater good	P7, P8, P16, P18
4	Decides consciously to love	P1, P7, P14, P16

Table 2.7 Loving actions

Frequency	Category	Participants
Strategies of love to transform shame: actions—33 statements		
8	Show respect	P1, P6, P8, P10, P14, P15, P16, P21
5	Provide opportunities	P4, P13, P16, P18, P21
5	Love unconditionally	P5, P10, P13, P19, P21
4	Show commitment	P6, P11, P16, P19
4	Self-reflect and internalise	P7, P16, P18, P22
3	Keep away from negative feelings and thoughts	P9, P12, P13
2	Invite the other out (coffee, ice cream)	P11, P21
2	Act professionally	P12, P14

Furthermore, 33 statements refer to loving actions in order to transform toxic shame successfully. One German male leader explained:

> When we have got conflict at work and it turns out to be toxic, negative or even shameful, I try to relax the situation with my employees and invite them for tea, coffee or ice cream. I change the context and we do something together to have a new perspective on the situation.

Actions of leaders to counteract toxic shame vary but include outings and an active change of context and perspective, showing respect by different acknowledging actions, and professional actions which relate to the task on hand rather than to the emotions (Table 2.7).

Finally, 15 statements dealt with the idea that loving communication strategies can support the transformation of toxic shame to healthy and resourcefully experienced shame. A female US leader commented (P18):

> Love requires individuals to seek understanding of the object of their love—it allows for miscommunication because the assumption is that the other person is an individual whose own feelings matter—it crosses the boundaries of culture insofar as love exists for us all, although the way in which that love is expressed differs across cultures. Therefore, we need strategies to communicate our love in a comprehensive way across cultures.

Table 2.8 Loving communication

Frequency	Category	Participants
Strategies of love to transform shame: communication—15 statements		
6	Communicate that we are all human beings and accept that we all are	P6, P8, P10, P16, P18, P21
5	Communicate irritations openly	P11, P13, P14, P21, P22
4	Communicate positively (listen, show care, ask etc.)	P13, P14, P18, P21

Leaders use different communication techniques which they either assume to be universal or aim at helping them to understand the other person better. They aim at being open, listening carefully, showing care and concern, and asking questions to minimise conflict and maximise strengths and well-being in difficult situations (Table 2.8).

5 Discussion

This study follows the call by Ojansivu (2019) for a focus on loving encounters which may then provide deeper insight and an overall potency in emancipating organisational employees and leaders. Such positive and loving leadership in organisations contributes to self-reinforcing affirmative politics of love in the 4IR context (as in Ojansivu, 2019), supports mental health and well-being in transcultural management and leadership (as in Mayer, 2011), and could provide a stable base for human interactions which are nowadays filled with insecurities, vulnerabilities, and anxieties (Lund & Tienari, 2019). This research is therefore viewed as being part of developing leadership in the 4IR context, not only by advancing technologies but also by advancing competencies in transcultural leadership (Treichel & Mayer, 2011). Such competencies include problem-solving, emotional regulation, systemic viewpoints, and the management of ambiguities.

The findings show that from the international leaders' perspective, compassionate love is a positive force for overcoming shame and promoting constructive transcultural leadership which has a positive impact on transcultural encounters and might even reaffirm further loving relationships (as described by Pouthier and Sondak, 2019). Love is viewed as leading to a general positive attitude, helping to understand others better and to learn new things. It is viewed as a transcultural experience that reinforces the building of bridges across cultures and is described as being a general, positive transformational force which has an impact on happiness and authenticity (Vlieghe, 2014).

These views on compassionate love in leadership are in the main supported by the literature, which highlights that compassion and compassionate love counteract sorrow (Gilbert, 2014). As described in the main body of literature, love can support the transformation of shame by connecting with the pain, working through it, and overcoming it. The second theory suggests the use of compassionate love to find modes to support and lighten the pain. This is the approach generally referred to in the findings. In terms of theories of positive psychology, this approach relates to methods which work with the positive to relieve the pain. As highlighted by Monin et al. (2015), compassionate love in transcultural leaders connects leaders and employees in a sensitive, supportive, assistive, and appreciative way to the self and to others, thereby overcoming the difficulties in relationships with others, as well as the hardships caused by the changes brought about by the 4IR (Pullen et al., 2017).

The findings also support Fehr and Sprecher's (2009) idea that compassionate love—through powerful kind-heartedness and the aspect of connectivity—brings social gain. It may be assumed that, particularly with regard to transforming shame, this social gain supports the reintegration of the individual after an act or experience of shame, thereby transforming the relationship with others and contributing to the overall well-being of others (as in Berscheid, 2006).

Data on the interlinkages between love and shame further strengthen the idea that love, as a compassionate and general feeling, is a resource for overcoming negative experiences and is a transformational force for dealing with negativity, sorrow, and pain (as in Gilbert, 2014). As highlighted by Oosthuizen (2020), love can support the transformation of shame in a social setting, as well as with outsiders outside a specific social setting. Compassionate love has, furthermore, various forms of expression, as described in the leaders' narrations presented in this chapter, which refer to two main categories, namely, shame caused by interpersonal relationships and shame caused by inadequate shameful behaviour in public. Here, love transforms shameful experiences in the personal and public spheres. The narrations—all positive in nature—provide the narrator with the idea that love, as a positive emotion and a positive force, helps to transform negativity and thereby provides the reader with the idea of trust, hope, and a positive outlook, as well as the advancement of well-being (as in Irons & Lad, 2017).

Finally, leaders describe different ways in which transcultural leaders transform shame through compassionate love. In this study, leaders referred to three main strategies: having a loving attitude, displaying loving actions, and engaging in loving communication. These strategies for transforming shame in transcultural leadership are bound to cultural concepts and may be presented and experienced in culture-specific ways (e.g. the Japanese concept of benevolence). The strategic ways mentioned by the leaders correspond with ways of showing compassionate love described in the literature, for example, through attention and mindfulness, compassionate self-development (Gilbert, 2014), and coping with resistance to develop compassion with the self and others. Like the leaders in this study, the literature on compassionate love focuses mainly on an inner attitude and a loving attitude, followed by loving action and loving communication, thereby showing that compassionate love transforms actions and situations as well as communication when it becomes an authentic part of the self and part of the individual's values and norms.

If a loving attitude is present, it appears that loving action and communication develop by themselves. In other words, the strengths of compassionate love are anchored within the individual and their self-development rather than within the leadership actions. The location of passionate love within the self and particularly the attitude of individuals relate further to Major et al.'s (2018) idea that this inner attitude of compassionate love resonates with the social connections and the environment and thereby is seen as a sense of connection to others. Love, although often considered in the context of romantic love, has been accepted in the literature as an important aspect of organisational life and culture as well as leader–employee interactions (as in Oravecz, Dirsmith, Heshmati, Vandekerckhove, & Brick, 2020).

The study at hand supports the view that love is not just an emotion found in romantic relationships and contexts but one which underpins social connectedness in general while contributing to other underlying feelings. The leaders in this study also referred to connected feelings regarding compassionate love and thereby showed that compassionate love can be seen as a positive anchor for the individual and for leaders specifically in building a comprehensive and multilayered web of positive emotions and social connections in organisations through compassionate leadership (supporting Fredrickson, 2016).

Within the rapidly changing contexts of the 4IR and the experiences of disruptive, unpredictable, and complex processes (Van Rensburg, 2019), compassionate love for self and others can become an even more important resource in leadership than in the previous three industrial revolutions, since it may help not only to overcome shame in workplaces and in leadership but also to transform other negative feelings, such as fears, anxieties, and vulnerabilities—as supported by the leaders of this study. This general positive influence of compassionate love on leadership underlies the data set and the findings pertaining to the transcultural leaders, thereby supporting the idea that love emphasises the interdependence of individuals in the 4IR world and their fundamental vulnerability, which can be addressed by compassionate love and positive mindsets (as in Rushing, 2010).

Lund and Tienari (2019) highlight that love narrations can support employees in organisations to overcome anxieties. This study actually expands on this idea of Lund and Tienari (2019) by presenting love narrations to overcome shame. At the same time, although the study was conducted on love in transcultural leadership, the love narrations in this study refer to interpersonal relationships (family and friends) and to overcoming public shaming incidents or other pressurised situations. Accordingly, these compassionate love narrations appear to anchor and stabilise the individual by connecting to positive (self) feelings and trustful relationships. Compassionate love, on this different level, therefore appears to provide the individual with a positive general mindset, trust, and a steadying effect, allowing them to tackle the challenges in the 4IR workplace. This may indicate once more that compassionate love not only supports an individual with a specific focus but also is a general emotion that supports others on a broad, underlying level in the form of a positive mindset.

By providing such a positive, stable mindset through personal narrations, the references to positive incidents seem to create possibilities of thinking in new, different, and positive creative ways, as highlighted by Mumby (2009), thereby supporting the overcoming of shame. The study supports the perspectives of

Thanem and Wallenberg (2015), as well as of Vlieghe (2014) and Ojansivu (2019), who all in their own right highlight that loved-based leadership in 4IR settings has a positive impact on leadership and organisations and might particularly support employees in dealing with the upcoming challenges of the 4IR in general and human–machine interaction in particular.

6 Conclusions

This chapter aimed to explore the concepts of love and shame in leadership from the perspective of leaders from different cultural background working in 4IR leadership contexts. Four main questions were asked and responded to. In conclusion, it may be highlighted that the leaders interviewed focused mainly on the topic of love and shame with regard to their work contexts and their ideas on how love can contribute to managing the 4IR successfully in the context of transcultural diverse work settings and 4IR settings.

Leaders highlight that love can support transforming shame through a positive attitude, understanding others and learning about others, seeing love as a transcultural experience that can bridge differences across cultures, and seeing it as a positive transcultural force. For the 4IR, love appears to be very important as a stabilising and connecting influence, since diverse workforces will grow and communication and interaction across distances, with flexible work arrangements, technologised and digitalised workplaces, and working from remote areas, will increase while bringing instabilities, anxieties, and vulnerabilities which need to be managed sympathetically. Love, as a compassionate emotion, can contribute in such cases to improved self-management and cooperation with others based on mutual respect, dignity, and benevolence.

Since shame is viewed as a negative emotion which is interlinked with love, it seems to be extremely important in 4IR workplaces to be aware of negative emotions such as shame since these emotions may not be directly displayed to the other but rather technologically mediated and may create conflict (across cultures) over time. In digitalised and technologised workplaces, these emotions may remain unrecognised and unattended to for longer than in, for example, regular de-technologised, face-to-face interactions. Love—and particularly a loving attitude—would seem to be a strong resource for overcoming shame in these new settings in particular; moreover, self-love may play a major role in overcoming shame in technologised social interactions and incidents of public shaming, such as in cyber-shaming and cyberbullying (see the chapter by Mayer and Vanderheiden in this book).

In this study, shame is viewed as happening particularly in (negative) relationships and resulting from publicly inadequate and shameful behaviour; it may be caused by failing examinations or unrequited love. When narrating experiences of shame and love, the leaders preferred to talk about personal and private experiences than about workplace experiences, which might be because stability, security, and love are primarily related to close, stabilising, and intimate relationships which are often regarded as a stabilising resource in challenging situations, in general, as well as in shameful situations, in particular.

It may be concluded that shame and love are such in-depth experiences that they are particularly powerful in the context of personal experiences. In terms of leadership experiences and the transformation of toxic shame in transcultural situations, leaders point out that attitudes, actions, and communication need to be adjusted to become loving and compassionate when shame is at play. Again, this appears to be particularly important when leaders are dealing with highly complex situations and workplaces where change is rapid and which are often remote and technologised. Therefore, leaders count a general loving attitude and mindset as very important for transforming shame in the self and others across cultures.

7 Recommendations for Theory and Practice

Many open questions still need to be addressed in future research, such as how love and shame and emotions in general can be dealt with most efficiently and healthily when it comes to working with human–machine interaction and AI in highly complex, diverse, and rapidly changing (remote) workplaces and transcultural situations. Research should address the role of emotions in 4IR and how to deal with them in a healthy, digitalised, or technologised manner. It may be assumed that in micro-level interactions, the key to transforming negative emotions and strengthening positive emotions lies in the attitude of the self and the self-management practices and transcultural competencies of the employees and the leaders themselves. On the meso-level—that is, the organisational level—in 4IR transforming organisations, interactions should address the need for self-development and the strengthening of the individual employee and leader within the workplaces to manage insecurities, anxieties, and vulnerabilities. This can happen through research and research-based training, as well as programmes on how to deal with negative emotions and how to lead in a transformational and transculturally positive way.

Employees need to be trained specifically in how to work in 4IR workplaces that are increasingly digitalised and influenced by machine learning, robotics, and remote workplaces. They need to be encouraged to stay healthy, loving, and compassionate while dealing with challenges. Furthermore, the researchers and practitioners of the future will need to address issues related to the programming of machines and the human–machine interfaces to communicate in a compassionate and loving way with one another: Is that even possible? It may be that compassionate love is key not only to competent 4IR leadership in organisations but also to a global approach to bigger issues and challenges that need to be addressed within engineering and computer engineering contexts for expanding compassionate love in leadership not only in human–human interactions but also in human–machine interactions.

Acknowledgements We thank all the participants of the study for their voluntary participation and for sharing their views on compassionate leadership, shame, and future-orientated workplaces.

References

Acker, S., & Webber, M. (2016). Discipline and publish: The tenure review process in Ontario universities. In L. Schultz & M. Viczko (Eds.), *Assembling and governing the higher education institution* (pp. 233–255). London: Palgrave Macmillan.

Andrews, B., Qian, M., & Valentine, J. D. (2002). Predicting depressive symptoms with a new measure of shame: The experience of shame scale. *British Journal of Clinical Psychology, 41*, 29–42.

Ashworth, P. (2015). Conceptual foundations of qualitative psychology. In J. A. Smith (Ed.), *Qualitative psychology: A practical guide to research methods* (3rd ed., pp. 4–25). London, UK: Sage.

Barmeyer, C., & Mayer, C.-H. (2020). Positive intercultural management in the fourth industrial revolution: Managing cultural otherness through a paradigm shift. *International Review of Psychiatry, 32*(7-8), 638–650.

Bass, B., & Riggio, R. (2006). *Transformational leadership* (2nd ed.). Mahwah, NJ: Lawrence Erlbaum Associates.

Batson, C. D. (2009). *These things called empathy: Eight related but distinct phenomena.*

Berscheid, E. (2006). Searching for the meaning of "love". In R. J. Sternberg & K. Weis (Eds.), *The new psychology of love* (pp. 171–183). New Haven, CT: Yale University Press.

Berscheid, E. (2010). Love in the fourth dimension. *Annual Review of Psychology, 61*, 1–25.

Burns, J. (1978). *Leadership*. New York, NY: Harper & Row.

Collins, N. L., Kane, H. S., Metz, M. A., Cleveland, C., Khan, C., Winczewski, L., et al. (2014). Psychological, physiological, and behavioural responses to a partner in need: The role of compassionate love. *Journal of Social and Personal Relationships*, 1–29. https://doi.org/10.1177/0265407514529069.

Denzin, N. K. (2017). Critical qualitative inquiry. *Qualitative Inquiry, 23*(1), 8–16.

Derungs, I. M. (2011). *Trans-cultural leadership for transformation*. Basingstoke, UK: Palgrave Macmillan.

Dimitrov, D. (2015). Leadership in a humane organization. *European Journal of Training and Development, 39*(2), 122–142. https://doi.org/10.1108/EJTD-07-2014-0051.

Ettinger, B. (2006). From proto-ethical compassion to responsibility: Besideness and the three primal motherphantasies of not-enoughness, devouring and abandonment. *Athena: Philosophical Studies, 2*, 100–135.

Fehr, B., & Sprecher, S. (2009). Compassionate love: Conceptual, measurement, and relational issues. In B. Fehr, S. Sprecher, & L. G. Underwoods (Eds.), *The science of compassionate love: Theory, research, and applications* (pp. 27–52). Malden, MA: Wiley/Blackwell.

Fredrickson, B. L. (2016). Love: Positivity resonance as a fresh, evidence-based perspective on an age-old topic. In L. F. Barrett, M. Lewis, & J. M. Haviland-Jones (Eds.), *Handbook of emotions* (pp. 847–858). New York, NY: Guilford Press.

Gilbert, P. (1998). What is shame? Some core issues and controversies. In P. Gilbert & B. Andrews (Eds.), *Shame: Interpersonal behavior, psychopathology and culture* (pp. 3–38). New York, NY: Oxford University Press.

Gilbert, P. (2014). The origins and nature of compassion focused therapy. *British Journal of Clinical Psychology, 53*(1), 6–41.

Guoping, L. I., Yun, H. O. U., & Aizhi, W. U. (2017). Fourth industrial revolution: Technological drivers, impacts and coping methods. *Chinese Geographical Science, 27*(4), 626–637. https://doi.org/10.1007/s11769-017-0890-x.

Hejdenberg, J., & Andrews, B. (2011). The relationship between shame and different types of anger: A theory-based investigation. *Personality and Individual Differences, 50*, 1278–1282.

Irons, C., & Lad, S. (2017). Using compassion focused therapy to work with shame and self-criticism in complex trauma. *Australian Clinical Psychologist, 3*(1), 1743.

Izard, C. E. (1977). *Human emotions*. New York, NY: Plenum Press.

Kenny, K., & Fotaki, M. (2015). From gendered organizations to compassionate border spaces: Reading corporeal ethics with Bracha Ettinger. *Organization, 22*, 183–199.

Kim, S., Thibodeau, R., & Jorgensen, R. S. (2011). Shame, guilt, and depressive symptoms: A meta-analytic review. *Psychological Bulletin, 137*, 68–96.

Kruger, A. (2020, January 3). The rise of the robot workers – banking: Machines and artificial intelligence have been 'stealing' jobs for decades. *The Citizen* (Gauteng).

Lawrence, V. A., & Lee, D. (2014). An exploration of people's experiences of compassion focused therapy for trauma, using interpretative phenomenological analysis. *Clinical Psychology and Psychotherapy, 21*, 495–507.

Lincoln, Y. S., & Guba, E. G. (2000). Paradigmatic controversies, contradictions, and emerging confluences. In N. K. Denzin & Y. S. Lincoln (Eds.), *Handbook of qualitative research* (2nd ed., pp. 163–188). Thousand Oaks, CA: Sage.

Lund, R., & Tienari, J. (2019). Passion, care, and eros in the gendered neoliberal university. *Organization, 26*, 98–121.

Major, B. C., Le Nguyen, K. D., Lundberg, K. B., & Fredrickson, B. L. (2018). Well-being correlates of perceived positivity resonance: Evidence from trait and episode-level assessments. *Personality and Social Psychology Bulletin*. https://doi.org/10.1177/0146167218771324.

Mayer, C.-H. (2011). *The meaning of sense of coherence in transcultural management*. Münster: Waxmann.

Mayer, C.-H., & Tonelli, L. (2017). "Dream on – There is no salvation!" Transforming shame in the workplace through personal and organisational strategies. In E. Vanderheiden & C.-H. Mayer (Eds.), *The value of shame: Exploring a health resource in cultural contexts* (pp. 135–156). Cham, Switzerland: Springer.

Mayer, C.-H., & Vanderheiden, E. (2019). *The bright side of shame: Transforming and growing through practical applications in cultural contexts*. Cham, Switzerland: Springer.

Mayer, C.-H., & Vanderheiden, E. (2020). *Handbook of love in cultural and transcultural contexts*. Cham, Switzerland: Springer.

Monin, J. K., Schulz, R., & Feeney, B. C. (2015). Compassionate love in individuals with Alzheimer's disease and their spousal caregivers: Associations with caregivers' psychological health. *Gerontologist, 55*(6), 981–989. https://doi.org/10.1093/geront/gnu001.

Mumby, D. (2009). The strange case of the farting professor: Humor and the deconstruction of destructive communication. In P. Lutgen-Sandvik & B. Sypher (Eds.), *Destructive organizational communication: Processes, consequences, and constructive ways of organizing* (pp. 316–338). New York, NY: Routledge.

Mumby, D. K., Thomas, R., Martí, I., & Seidl, D. (2017). Resistance redux. *Organization Studies, 38*, 1157–1183.

Naderifar, M., Goli, H., & Ghaljaie, F. (2017). Snowball sampling: A purposeful method of sampling in qualitative research. *Strides in Development of Medical Education, 14*(3), e67670.

Northouse, P. (2016). *Leadership theory and practice* (3rd ed.). Thousand Oaks, CA: Sage.

Ojansivu, J. (2019). *Lead through love: Fourth Industrial Revolution with rising generations creating demands on better workplaces*.

Oosthuizen, R. M. (2017). Managing shame in organizations: Don't let shame become a self-destructive spiral. In E. Vanderheiden & C.-H. Mayer (Eds.), *The value of shame: Exploring a health resource in cultural contexts* (pp. 217–234). Cham, Switzerland: Springer.

Oosthuizen, R. M. (2020). The expression of compassionate love in cultural diversity contexts. In C. H. Mayer & E. Vanderheiden (Eds.), *Handbook of love in cultural and transcultural contexts*. Cham, Switzerland: Springer.

Oravecz, Z., Dirsmith, J., Heshmati, S., Vandekerckhove, J., & Brick, T. R. (2020). Psychological well-being and personality traits are associated with experiencing love in everyday life. *Personality and Individual Differences, 153*, 109620.

Perez, J. R. (2017). Global leadership and the impact of globalization. *Journal of Leadership, Accountability and Ethics, 14*(3).

Pol, E., & Reveley, J. (2017). Robot induced technological unemployment: Towards a youth-focused coping strategy. *Psycho-sociological Issues in Human Resource Management, 5*(2), 169–186.

Pouthier, V., & Sondak, H. (2019). When shame meets love: Affective pathways to freedom from injurious bodily norms in the workplace. *Organization Studies*. https://doi.org/10.1177/0170840619847722.

Pullen, A., & Rhodes, C. (2014). Corporeal ethics and the politics of resistance in organizations. *Organization, 21*, 782–796.

Pullen, A., & Rhodes, C. (2015). Is becoming-woman possible in organizations? In A. Pullen & C. Rhodes (Eds.), *The Routledge companion to ethics, politics and organizations* (pp. 355–367). London: Routledge.

Pullen, A., Rhodes, C., & Thanem, T. (2017). Affective politics in gendered organizations: Affirmative notes on becoming-woman. *Organization, 24*, 105–123.

Riggio, R. (2009). Are you a transformational leader? *Psychology Today*. Retrieved from www.psychologytoday.com/blog/cutting-edge-leadership/200903/are-you-transformational-leader

Roth, W. M., & Von Unger, H. (2018, September). Current perspectives on research ethics in qualitative research. *Forum Qualitative Sozialforschung/Forum: Qualitative Social Research, 19*(3).

Runyan, W. M. (1994). Coming to terms with the life, loves, and work of Henry A. Murray (review of F. Robinson, Love's story told: A life of Henry A. Murray). *Contemporary Psychology, 39*, 701–704.

Rushing, S. (2010). Preparing for politics: Judith Butler's ethical dispositions. *Contemporary Political Theory, 9*, 284–303.

Schiuma, G. (2017). Arts catalyst of creative organisations for the fourth industrial revolution. *Journal of Open Innovation: Technology, Market, and Complexity, 3*(4), 20.

Sprecher, S., & Fehr, B. (2005). Compassionate love for close others and humanity. *Journal of Social and Personal Relationships, 22*(5), 629–651. https://doi.org/10.1177/0265407505056439.

Tan, T. B. (2016). *The Fourth Industrial Revolution: Coping with disruptive change (RSIS Commentaries No. 264)*. Singapore: Nanyang Technological University.

Tan, T. B., & Wu, S. S. (2017, October). *Public policy implications of the fourth industrial revolution for Singapore. RSIS Policy Report*. Singapore: RSIS.

Tangney, J. P., & Dearing, R. L. (2002). *Shame and guilt*. New York, NY: Guilford Press.

Tangney, J. P., Miller, R. S., Flicker, L., & Barlow, D. H. (1996). Are shame, guilt and embarrassment distinct emotions? *Journal of Personality and Social Psychology, 70*, 1256–1269.

Terre Blanche, M., Durrheim, K., & Painter, D. (2006). First steps in qualitative data analysis. In *Research in practice: Applied methods for the social sciences* (pp. 321–344). Cape Town: UCT Press.

Thanem, T., & Wallenberg, L. (2015). What can bodies do? Reading Spinoza for an affective ethics of organizational life. *Organization, 21*, 235–250.

Treichel, D., & Mayer, C.-H. (2011). *Lehrbuch Kultur. Lehr- und Lernmaterialen zur Vermittlung kultureller Kompetenzen. Waxmann Studium*. Münster: Waxmann.

Vachhani, S. J., & Pullen, A. (2019). Ethics, politics and feminist organizing: Writing feminist infrapolitics and affective solidarity into everyday sexism. *Human Relations, 72*, 23–47.

Van Rensburg, G. (2019, November). Industry 4.0 and our love-hate relationship with change: 4th Industrial Revolution. *HR Future*, 28–31.

Velotti, P., Elison, J., & Garofalo, C. (2014). Shame and aggression: Different trajectories and implications. *Aggression and Violent Behavior, 19*, 454–461.

Velotti, P., Garofalo, C., Bottazzi, F., & Caretti, V. (2017). Faces of shame: Implications for self-esteem, emotion regulation, aggression, and well-being. *The Journal of Psychology, 151*(2), 171–184. https://doi.org/10.1080/00223980.2016.1248809.

Vlieghe, J. (2014). Laughter as immanent life-affirmation: Reconsidering the educational value of laughter through a Bakhtinian lens. *Educational Philosophy and Theory, 46*, 148–161.

Wong, P. T. P. (2019). Foreword: From shame to wholeness: An existential positive psychology perspective. In C.-H. Mayer & E. Vanderheiden (Eds.), *The bright side of shame: Transforming shame in cultural contexts* (pp. v–ix). Cham, Switzerland: Springer.

Yin, R. K. (2013). *Case study research: Design and methods* (5th ed.). Thousand Oaks, CA: Sage.

Claude-Hélène Mayer (Dr. habil., Ph.D.) is a Professor in Industrial and Organisational Psychology in the Department of Industrial Psychology and People Management at the University of Johannesburg; an Adjunct Professor at the European University Viadrina in Frankfurt (Oder), Germany; and a Senior Research Associate at Rhodes University, Grahamstown, South Africa. She holds a Ph.D. in Psychology (University of Pretoria, South Africa), a Ph.D. in Management (Rhodes University, South Africa), a Doctorate (Georg-August University, Germany) in Political Sciences (socio-cultural anthropology and intercultural didactics), and a Habilitation (European University Viadrina, Germany) in Psychology with focus on work, organisational, and cultural psychology. She has published several monographs, text collections, accredited journal articles, and special issues on transcultural mental health and well-being, sense of coherence, shame, transcultural conflict management and mediation, women in leadership in culturally diverse work contexts, constellation work, coaching, and psychobiography.

Rudolf M. Oosthuizen (DLitt et. Phil.) received a BA degree (Cum Laude) from the University of Pretoria in 1992 and obtained a BA (Honours) in Psychology at the same university in 1993. In 1999, he received an MA degree in Industrial and Personnel Psychology from the Potchefstroom University for Christian Higher Education. In 1999, he registered as Industrial Psychologist with the Health Professions Council of South Africa. In 2005, he completed a DLitt et. Phil. in Industrial and Organisational Psychology at the University of South Africa (UniSA). Currently, he is an Associate Professor in the Department of Industrial and Organisational Psychology at the University of South Africa. He is the Manager for the MComIOP programme and is responsible for the lecturing of honour subjects and the supervision of master's and doctoral students. He has presented conference papers at national and international conferences and published articles in accredited scientific journals. His fields of interests are (1) career psychology and career development and management from an individual and organisational perspective in the twenty-first-century world of work; (2) positive psychology, with the focus on salutogenesis, sense of coherence, locus of control, self-efficacy, the hardy personality, and learned resourcefulness; and (3) employment relations and the improvement of the quality of employment relations in organisations and in society in general.

Chapter 3
Cross-Cultural Comparison of Mental Health Shame: Negative Attitudes and External, Internal, and Reflected Shame About Mental Health in Japanese and UK Workers

Yasuhiro Kotera, David Sheffield, Pauline Green, and Kenichi Asano

1 Introduction

1.1 Challenging Work Mental Health

Poor mental health of workforce is a cause for concern in many countries (Kestel, 2019). In the UK, the government report identified that 15% of the UK workforce had some type of mental health problems and more than 300,000 workers lost their jobs due to mental illness every year, which was more than those who lost their jobs due to physical health problems (Stevenson & Farmer, 2017). The costs of workplace mental health on employers were estimated to be about £40 billion, half of which was incurred from presenteeism—reduced work productivity caused by poor mental health. Additionally, the costs on the government were estimated to be about £25 billion, including welfare, tax reduction, and national health service. Counting other expenses, the total costs of poor work mental health to the UK economy were approximately £80 billion per year (Stevenson & Farmer, 2017). Considering the UK's GDP is £2 trillion, £80 billion is not negligible.

Likewise, Japanese workers also suffer from poor mental health: 60% of the employees experience intense anxiety and stress (Ministry of Health, Labour and Welfare [MHLW], 2013), and the number of Japanese workers' compensation claims for mental health problems has been steeply increasing (200 in 2000 to

Y. Kotera (✉) · D. Sheffield · P. Green
Kedleston Road, Derby, UK
e-mail: y.kotera@derby.ac.uk; d.sheffield@derby.ac.uk; p.green1@derby.ac.uk

K. Asano
Department of Psychological Counseling, Mejiro University, Tokyo, Japan
e-mail: k.asano@mejiro.ac.jp

C.-H. Mayer et al. (eds.), *Shame 4.0*, https://doi.org/10.1007/978-3-030-59527-2_3

1500 in 2015; MHLW, 2016). The Japanese government passed a new policy that aims to prevent *karoshi* ('過労死' = death from overwork) and other (over)work-related health disorders in 2014 (MHLW, 2014). To facilitate its implementation, the government budget for preventive strategies against overwork-related disorders increased by 35% (5.5 billion JPY in 2015 to 7.4 billion JPY in 2016) (MHLW, 2016). The new policy defined (over)work-related disorders as (i) death by cerebrovascular/cardiovascular diseases (CCVD), (ii) suicide following the onset of mental illness caused by work, and (iii) CCVD and mental disorders due to work. This policy also emphasises the transparency of workers' physical and mental health, including work-life balance. More recently (2016), the government has initiated the work-style reform to help reduce overtime working, which in turn is aimed to help maintain the Japanese workforce (The Prime Minister of Japan and His Cabinet, 2016). Despite these radical attempts, the results remain ambiguous (Ito & Aruga, 2018).

1.2 Work Mental Health in the 4IR

Advancement in technologies is beneficial to work productivity, enhancing perceived autonomy over and flexibility in work (Kossek, Lautsch, & Eaton, 2006; Mazmanian, Orlikowski, & Yates, 2013). Today many organisations utilise technologies to allow employees to decide the time and location of work, to some degree, using virtual teams and telecommuting (Cascio, 2000; Townsend, DeMarie, & Hendrickson, 1998). However, disadvantages of using advanced technologies have also been reported, including negative impacts on workers' mental health. The long-term use of computers was associated with depression and insomnia in 25,000 Japanese workers in a 3-year longitudinal study (Nakazawa et al., 2002). Similar results were found in Korea too (Kim, Kang, Yoo, Lee & Hong, 2016). The 'always-on' culture in the 4IR yields more stress on workers by blurring the boundary between work and life: 59% of UK workers answer phone calls, and 55% check emails outside their working hours (AXA, 2017). Modern workers suffer from pressure that they must respond to queries right away even when not working (i.e. workplace telepressure; Barber & Santuzzi, 2015). This *autonomy paradox* (technologies that are intended to help work autonomy have resulted in reducing the autonomy; Mazmanian et al., 2013) adds more stress on workers by disrupting workers' recovery from work (Day, Scott, & Kelloway, 2010; Olson-Buchanan and Boswell, 2006). In America, 44% of workers check emails on vacation, and 54% do so during sick leave (American Psychological Association, 2013). Telepressure was associated with workaholism, work-life conflict, and burnout (Barber & Santuzzi, 2015). These findings suggest that maintaining good work mental health can be difficult in the 4IR, requiring organisations to adopt new approaches (e.g. turning off emails).

1.3 Mental Health Shame

Shame can deter people from asking for help and is directly related to poor mental health (Corrigan, 2004). Shame is a potent affect that can damage people's mental health (Kim, Thibodeau, & Jorgensen, 2011) and is related to depression (Matos & Pinto-Gouveia, 2010), anxiety (Tangney, Wagner, & Gramzow, 1992), paranoia (Matos, Pinto-Gouveia, & Gilbert, 2013), post-traumatic stress disorder (Harman & Lee, 2010), and eating disorders (Skårderud, 2007). Moreover, a recent meta-analysis reported that shame was strongly related to self-harm, while guilt was not (Sheehy et al., 2019). High shame about mental health problems (i.e. mental health shame) has been seen in both UK and Japanese working populations, associated with poor workplace mental health (Kotera, Adhikari, & Van Gordon, 2018; Kotera, Gilbert, Asano, Ishimura & Sheffield, 2018; Kotera, Green & Sheffield, 2019d).

Shame about mental health problems can be categorised into three types: internal, external, and reflected shame (Gilbert, 1998). External shame is pertinent to the feeling of being disdained by others, fearing rejection and isolation, regarding mental health problems. When one believes they are perceived negatively by others, because of their mental health problems, external shame is present. Internal shame refers to one's own negative self-judgements, associated with undesired self. When one believes that they are inadequate, because of their mental health problems, internal shame is present. Lastly, reflected shame is related to worries that their mental health problems may cause shame in their family (family-reflected shame) or that their family member's mental health problems may cause them a feeling of shame (self-reflected shame).

1.4 Shame Culture of Japan and the UK

People in both Japanese and British cultures are sensitive to shame. Japanese culture has been described as a shame culture (Benedict, 1946), emphasising shame based on social reputation, which leads to a strong focus on social appearances (Inoue, 2007). Japanese people tend to behave (or not to behave) based on how others will see them, rather than their internal judgements (Benedict, 1946). For instance, during WWII, to die in combat was seen as a virtue (rather than to come home alive) in Japanese society. A Japanese sergeant, Shoichi Yokota was found in Guam and sent back to Japan in 1972, 27 years after Japan's surrender. He did not know the war was over, and on his return to Japan, he said he felt shameful about returning home alive (Hikita, 2004) as he did not fulfil the virtue of dying on the field of combat. Shame is also emphasised in the chapter of 'Honor' in the book *Bushido: The Soul of Japan* (Nitobe, 1900), which describes the way of a samurai. Any infringement upon the integrity of one's reputation, also described as 'the immortal part of one's self', is felt as shame ('廉恥心 [Renchishin]') (Nitobe, 1900). Shame is seen strongly in today's Japanese workplaces: Japanese workers on average take half of the allowed annual leave days, as many of them (63%) feel ashamed to take many days off, making them the least rested workers in the developed countries (Saiidi, 2018).

Shame in modern Japan has also been captured in the science world. Japanese people feel strong shame about asking for help about their mental health problems, exacerbating their challenging mental health status even more (Ando, Yamaguchi, Aoki, & Thornicroft, 2013; Kotera, Gilbert, et al., 2018; Maekawa, Ramos-Cejudo, & Kanai, 2016; Tanaka, Ogawa, Inadomi, Kikuchi & Ohta, 2003) (see also Takano in this book).

Likewise, shame is also emphasised in the British culture. For example, in the eighteenth century, a notorious courtesan, Harriette Wilson used her memoir as a blackmailing tool to ask for more money from her clients for the fear of being shamed (Peakman, 2009). In the nineteenth century, as noted in the civilising process (Elias, 1979), educational institutions in Europe disciplined pupils through shaming rather than physical punishment. For example, in sexual education, girls were told to be careful not to listen to anything said about sex, conveying a sense of shame in them (von Raumer, 1857). Today, many UK doctors (72%) believe that education and training would help reduce the sense of shame in their workplace, by fostering openness in the culture (Moberly, 2015). Moreover, high levels of shame towards mental health problems were reported in UK students, who are afraid that seeking help would mean that they would violate some standard (Kotera, Conway & Van Gordon, 2019a; Kotera, Green & Sheffield, 2019c).

These findings and reports demonstrate that shame is an important construct in both Japanese and British cultures, suggesting a need for further investigation.

1.5 Aims

This study aimed to compare mental health and mental health shame in Japanese and UK workers. Firstly, we compared the levels of mental health problems, namely, depression, anxiety, and stress as these were most common in both populations, and mental health shame, namely, negative attitudes, external shame, internal shame, and reflected shame. Secondly, we compared relationships between mental health problems and mental health shame in each workforce. Lastly, we examined how much mental health shame could predict variance in mental health problems in each population group.

2 Methods

2.1 Participants

Opportunity sampling was employed to recruit Japanese workers, through online advertisement in researchers' networks. One hundred and thirty-one workers (73 males, 58 females; age mean = 40.31; standard deviation = 11.17;

range = 22–73 years) completed two self-report questionnaires about mental health problems and mental health shame. 21% were hospitality workers, 16% worked in manufacturing, and 15% worked in education; 12% were team leaders in a section, 11% were presidents of an organisation, and 10% were section chiefs. No incentives were given for participation.

UK workers consisted of two sectors: hospitality and construction. Online questionnaires on researchers' networks were used to recruit UK hospitality workers through opportunity sampling. One hundred and fourteen (52 males, 62 females; age mean = 28.24; standard deviation = 8.37; range = 18–55 years) hospitality workers completed the two self-report measures. Construction workers were recruited by the health and safety leaders in UK construction companies. These leaders distributed the study information to their organisations, which indicated the URL to the online questionnaires. One hundred and fifty-five (138 males and 17 females; age mean = 40.28; standard deviation = 11.05; range = 21–67 years) workers completed the scales. Half of them worked in transitory sites (i.e. site-based), 39% worked at office, and the remaining 11% worked at other places such as highways. Thirty-five per cent of them were managers, 23% were foremen/supervisors, and 20% were operatives/workers. No incentives were given for participation.

In both Japanese and UK participant groups, workers who (i) had a diagnosed mental health disorder, (ii) were under 18 years old, and (iii) had not worked for at least a year (in the industry for the UK workers) were excluded. Ethics approval was obtained from the University Research Ethics Committee.

2.2 Instruments

Mental health shame was evaluated using the Attitudes Towards Mental Health Problems (ATMHP) (Gilbert et al., 2007). This 35-item comprises 4 subsections: (i) Community and Family Attitudes apprise their perception of how their community and family view mental health problems (e.g. 'My community sees mental health problems as something to keep secret'), (ii) External Shame relates to their perception of how their community and family would see them if they had a mental health problem, respectively (e.g. 'I think my community would see me as inadequate'), (iii) Internal Shame considers how they perceive themselves if they had a mental health problem (e.g. 'I would see myself as a weak person'), and (iv) Reflected Shame evaluates how their family would be viewed if they had a mental health problem (family-reflected shame) and fears of reflected shame on themselves, associated with a close family member having a mental health problem (self-reflected shame). Each item was responded on a four-point Likert scale (from 0 = do not agree at all to 3 = completely agree; a higher score indicates stronger shame). All of the subscales had good internal consistency ($\alpha = 0.85$–0.97; Gilbert et al., 2007).

Mental health was evaluated by identifying the level of their mental health problems using the Depression Anxiety and Stress Scale (DASS21), a shortened form of the original DASS42 (Lovibond & Lovibond, 1995). DASS21 consists of three subscales (seven items each), measuring the levels of depression (e.g. 'I found it difficult to work up the initiative to do things'), anxiety (e.g. 'I was worried about situations in which I might panic and make a fool of myself'), and stress (e.g. 'I found myself getting agitated'). These three symptoms were most common mental health problems in the general public (European Community, 2005) and workforce (Office of Applied Studies, 2007) and thus were appropriate to be used in this study. Each item was responded on a four-point Likert scale (from 0 = did not apply to me at all to 3 = applied to me very much or most of the time). DASS21 had good reliability ($\alpha = 0.87$–0.94; Antony, Bieling, Cox, Enns, & Swinson, 1998).

2.3 Analysis Procedure

Firstly, all data collected was screened for outliers and the assumptions for parametric tests. Secondly, in order to compare mental health and mental health shame between Japanese and UK workers, t-tests were conducted. Finally, correlations between mental health and mental health shame were measured and compared between these two populations. IBM SPSS version 25 was used for these analyses.

3 Results

In the Japanese dataset, there was no outlier identified, using the outlier labelling rule (Hoaglin & Iglewicz, 1987). In the UK dataset, one score in family attitudes, six scores in family external shame, two scores in depression, and five scores in anxiety were identified as outliers using the outlier labelling rule (Hoaglin & Iglewicz, 1987), and so were winsorised (Tukey, 1962). All the subscales demonstrated good reliability ($\alpha \geqq 0.78$). Table 3.1 summarises the descriptive statistics of each sample.

3.1 Comparing the Levels of Mental Health and Shame

Because not all of the subscales were normally distributed (Shapiro-Wilk's test; $p < 0.05$), data were square-root transformed to satisfy the assumption of normality. Levene's test for equality of variances indicated that homogeneity of variances for all scores was not maintained ($p < 0.05$); therefore, Welch t-tests were conducted (Welch, 1947). Japanese workers had higher levels of mental health problems and mental health shame in all subscales than UK workers; anxiety had the greatest difference in the three mental health problems ($t = 17.84$), and family-relevant shame (family attitudes $t = 12.32$, family external shame $t = 12.55$, and

Table 3.1 Descriptive statistics and Welch t-tests of mental health and mental health shame between Japanese workers and UK workers

	Japanese workers		UK workers			
	M	SD	M	SD	*t*	*df*
Number (males, females)	131 (73, 58)		269 (190, 79)			
Age	40.31	11.17	35.18	9.91		
Depression (0–42)	**20.66**	6.60	11.81	9.52	12.69	393.65
Anxiety (0–42)	**18.34**	5.64	8.24	6.55	17.84	395.65
Stress (0–42)	**23.68**	7.38	12.64	7.02	15.71	352.58
Community attitudes (0–12)	**7.45**	2.59	4.70	3.10	10.52	397.78
Family attitudes (0–12)	**5.84**	2.26	3.28	3.40	12.32	379.03
Community external shame (0–15)	**10.62**	4.30	6.46	4.19	10.24	389.98
Family external shame (0–15)	**6.85**	2.96	3.86	4.60	12.55	369.15
Internal shame (0–15)	**11.14**	4.29	7.27	4.02	9.27	354.34
Family-reflected shame (0–21)	**12.6**	4.25	7.67	5.69	11.16	397.73
Self-reflected shame (0–15)	**6.96**	2.82	4.54	4.56	10.29	371.04

p **< 0.001**

family-reflected shame $t = 11.16$) had the greatest difference in all the mental health shame subscales (Table 3.1).

3.2 *Comparing Correlations Between Mental Health and Shame*

Pearson's correlation was performed to explore correlations between mental health and mental health shame in Japanese workers and UK workers, respectively.

In both populations, mental health and mental health shame were overall associated with each other (Table 3.2). Gender was related to depression, stress, family attitudes, community external shame, family external shame, family-reflected shame, and self-reflected shame in UK workers, while gender was not related to any variable in Japanese workers. Age was related to mental health problems in both populations, while significant correlations between age and mental health shame were only seen in UK workers. Other differences were that while (i) anxiety and family attitudes, (ii) self-reflected shame and family attitudes, and (iii) self-reflected shame and internal shame were significantly correlated in the UK workers, they were not in the Japanese workers.

Table 3.2 Correlations between mental health and shame

		Japanese workers (top triangle)											
		1	2	3	4	5	6	7	8	9	10	11	12
1	Gender (1 = M, 2 = F)	–	−0.06	−0.01	−0.04	−0.14	−0.07	0.02	0.00	0.00	0.01	0.08	0.02
2	Age	−0.35**	–	−0.25**	−0.25**	−0.24**	−0.02	−0.04	0.06	−0.14	−0.04	0.01	−0.01
3	Depression	0.13*	−0.18**	–	0.64**	0.67**	0.35**	0.27**	0.37**	0.29**	0.38**	0.36**	0.26**
4	Anxiety	0.10	−0.24**	0.75**	–	0.75**	0.30**	0.15	0.35**	0.25**	0.33**	0.43**	0.35**
5	Stress	−0.12*	−0.02	0.70**	0.71**	–	0.37**	0.19*	0.34**	0.26**	0.29**	0.38**	0.32**
6	Community attitudes	0.12	−0.19**	0.39**	0.41**	0.34**	–	0.23**	0.73**	0.17	0.43**	0.30**	0.24**
7	Family attitudes	0.22**	−0.30**	0.46**	0.45**	0.30**	0.67**	–	0.24**	0.62**	0.28**	0.43**	0.07
8	Community external shame	0.16**	−0.19**	0.35**	0.35**	0.30**	0.76**	0.64**	–	0.32**	0.49**	0.43**	0.33**
9	Family external shame	0.30**	−0.35**	0.48**	0.50**	0.28**	0.61**	0.85**	0.63**	–	0.27**	0.48**	0.32**
10	Internal shame	0.07	−0.07	0.35**	0.38**	0.26**	0.50**	0.48**	0.54**	0.48**	–	0.63**	0.23
11	Family-reflected shame	0.23**	−0.22**	0.48**	0.46**	0.29**	0.60**	0.64**	0.64**	0.69**	0.60**	–	0.38**
12	Self-reflected shame	0.25**	−0.32**	0.49**	0.52**	0.34**	0.55**	0.63**	0.55**	0.70**	0.42**	0.69**	–
$*p < 0.05$, $**p < 0.01$		UK workers (bottom triangle)											

3.3 *Comparing Shame's Predictions of Mental Health*

In order to compare how each type of mental health shame predicted the variance in mental health problems, multiple regression analyses were conducted. Firstly, the three subscales of mental health problems were combined to calculate the level of mental health (Lovibond & Lovibond, 1995). At step one, gender and age were entered to statistically adjust for their effects, and at step two, the mental health shame subscales were entered. Adjusted coefficient of determination (Adj. R^2) was reported. Multicollinearity was not a concern (VIF < 10). In the Japanese workers, ATMHP subscales accounted for 26% of the variance for mental health problems, indicating a medium effect size (Cohen, 1988), with age and family-reflected shame as significant predictors. By contrast, in the UK workers, ATMHP subscales predicted only 5% of the variance for mental health problems, indicating a small effect size (Cohen, 1988), with gender and self-reflected shame as significant predictors (Table 3.3).

4 Discussion

This chapter compared mental health shame and mental health problems between Japanese and UK workers. Japanese workers had higher levels of mental health problems and mental health shame than UK workers. In both populations, mental

Table 3.3 Multiple regression: mental health shame for mental health problems

	Japanese workers			UK workers		
	B	SE_B	*β*	*B*	SE_B	*β*
Step 1	5.34	0.26		5.33	0.49	
Gender (1 = M, 2 = F)	−0.13	0.11	−0.10	**−1.17****	0.21	−0.33
Age	**−0.02****	0.01	−0.28	**0.01***	0.01	0.07
Adj. R^2		0.07			0.13	
Step 2	2.75	0.46		4.02	0.57	
Gender	−0.14	0.09	−0.11	**−1.19****	0.21	−0.34
Age	**−0.02****	0.00	−0.28	0.02	0.01	0.10
Community attitudes	0.21	0.15	0.16	0.33	0.18	0.17
Family attitudes	0.06	0.14	0.04	−0.08	0.18	−0.05
Community external shame	0.09	0.12	0.09	−0.08	0.15	−0.05
Family external shame	0.00	0.13	0.00	−0.20	0.15	−0.16
Internal shame	0.05	0.10	0.06	0.24	0.14	0.12
Family-reflected shame	**0.27***	0.12	0.25	−0.01	0.14	−0.01
Self-reflected shame	0.20	0.11	0.15	**0.31****	0.11	0.23
Δ Adj. R^2		0.26			0.05	

A dependent variable: mental health problems
$^*p < 0.05$, $^{**}p < 0.01$

health problems and mental health shame were related to each other, except anxiety and family attitudes, self-reflected shame and family attitudes, and self-reflected shame and internal shame were not associated with one another in Japanese workers. Lastly, self-reflected shame was a significant predictor for mental health problems in UK workers, whereas family-reflected shame was a significant predictor for mental health problems in Japanese workers.

Higher levels of mental health problems in Japanese workers may imply severe working conditions in Japan. Despite the new initiatives forcing them to work shorter hours, e.g. leaving the building by 8 pm, many Japanese workers work outside of the office for many hours or do not take a lunch break (Muroi, 2019; Obic Business Consultants, 2019). Indeed, many workers still continued to work at a cafe or restaurant that opens late, enabled by the remote working technologies: these working hours are not on the company record, making their government report clean (Muroi, 2019; Obic Business Consultants, 2019). This suggests that policy changes alone do not change practice: cultural and societal changes are needed (Kawashima, 2018). Moreover, remote working technologies facilitate these increased work hours. This negative use of technologies can be explained by the collectivism in Japanese culture (e.g. in Japanese offices, no one wants to be the first one to leave; CNBC International, 2018). Advanced technologies offer us the *potential* to reduce working hours; however, when not used properly, they can extend working hours, damaging workers' mental health. Employers and policy-makers need to be aware of the impact of culture, as policies and/or technologies alone cannot implement meaningful changes. Global companies in Japan may be in a better position to make effective changes as their organisational culture is not entirely Japanese: more non-traditional organisational practice is possible. For example, recently, Microsoft Japan conducted the 'Work Life Choice Challenge 2019 Summer', where workers were paid for four Fridays in August without working (Jackman, 2019). The results were promising: their sales increased by 40%, pages printed dropped 59%, and electricity consumption dropped 23% compared with the same month last year. Microsoft workers used technologies effectively, limiting the length and frequency of face-to-face meetings by using collaborative tools such as Microsoft Teams: almost all employees (94%) were satisfied with this attempt (McGregor, 2019). Employee mental health was not reported, but given their high satisfaction, this type of attempt should be implemented broadly in Japanese organisations, and the mental health effects should be evaluated.

Strong associations between mental health and mental health shame were in line with previous findings (e.g. Kotera, Gilbert, Asano, Ishimura, and Sheffield, 2019b; Kotera et al., 2019c, 2019d). In both workforces, workers who felt strong shame tended to have mental health problems. This suggests that organisations need to consider how to reduce their employees' mental health shame. For example, self-compassion training was reported effective in reducing shame (Braehler et al., 2013; Kelly, Zuroff, Foa & Gilbert, 2010). Given the workers' high mental health shame, online self-compassion training, which is undertaken individually, may be more effective as they do not have to worry about colleagues knowing. Three-hour online self-compassion training attended by healthcare workers increased their self-compassion and mental wellbeing (Rao & Kemper, 2017). Such training should be implemented to Japanese and UK workers to reduce their mental health problems and mental health shame.

In Japanese workers, (i) anxiety and family attitudes, (ii) self-reflected shame and family attitudes, and (iii) self-reflected shame and internal shame were not associated with one another, whereas these variables were associated with one another in the UK workers. This may be related with rather Japan-unique phenomena, *hikikomori* (a severe form of social seclusion, where an individual does not leave the house for at least 6 months) among Japanese workers (Voiskounsky & Soldatova, 2019). *Hikikomori* is a serious problem in Japanese society (Cabinet Office, 2019). *Hikikomori* is associated with shame, where one feels ashamed of who they are, stopping them from going outside their home (Cole, 2013). Recent findings report that advanced technologies enable one to be a *hikikomori*, virtually communicating with others online (Voiskounsky & Soldatova, 2019). Parallel with the 'uchi-soto' notion in Japanese culture (Burt, Bachnik, & Quinn, 1995), Japanese workers are more conscious of how outsiders (e.g. colleagues) will see them than how insiders (e.g. family members) will see them. This may help explain why these family-related shame (i.e. family attitudes and self-reflected shame) variables were not related to other variables in Japanese workers.

In our regression analyses, self-reflected shame was a significant predictor for mental health problems in UK workers, whereas family-reflected shame was a significant predictor for mental health problems in Japanese workers. This suggests the difference of their cultural emphases: Japanese collectivism and UK's individualism. For many UK workers, their distress caused by worries that their family member's mental health problems would cause their image negatively (i.e. self-reflected shame) predicted high mental health problems. In an individualistic culture, it is important to have a strong identity that separates them from their belonging groups, and expressing such differences is welcomed (Markus & Kitayama, 1991). Therefore, negative influences on their image from family members can be a concern. On the other hand, in a collectivistic culture, where one's identity is often determined by the group they belong to, meeting social expectations is valued (Markus & Kitayama, 1991). Japanese workers may feel that they have failed a social expectation by having a mental health problem and may be afraid that such a disgrace may cause a negative perception towards their family. These differences can inform how organisations or in-house mental health practitioners need to approach their shame differently. For the UK workers, self-awareness training would be useful, as it helps them to have a strong sense of identity (O'Connor & Seymour, 2003). Having a clear identity can help them cope with self-reflected shame by reducing worries for being tarred by the same brush as other family members. For Japanese workers, providing clear and accurate information about mental health would be useful, noting that anyone could suffer from a mental health problem. For example, educating people that the heritability of depression is about one-third would be helpful (Matsumoto, Kunimoto, & Ozaki, 2013), and there are diverse causes for mental health problems (not only family but also other developmental, social, and environmental factors). These findings are especially useful for managers and HR staff in today's internationalised workplaces.

Lastly, it is noteworthy that recent studies and literature, employing the functionalist perspective of emotions, noted the positive aspects of shame (Mayer & Vanderheiden, 2019), which encourage positive changes in oneself (Lickel, Kushlev, Savalei, Matta & Schmader, 2014). Compared with regret and guilt, shame was an independent predictor for the desire for positive changes in oneself. Moreover, shame predicted creativity as a way to restore self-image in the workplace, and exposure to a creative team environment positively impacted on this shame-creativity relationship (González-Gómez & Richter, 2015). These findings suggest that the interventions discussed above (e.g. compassion training, mental health education) may benefit from discussing the positive aspects of shame. Shame in a globalised workplace can be transformed into positive resources through respect, empathy, and trust (Clarke & Takashiro, 2019). For example, Japanese senior managers noted that reframing (i.e. identifying positive aspects of what appears to be negative) was effective in their managerial practice (Kotera & Van Gordon, 2019). The authors' experience in developing workers' self-care attitudes using reframing accords this: this type of exercise could be used to promote positive perspectives and attitudes towards shame.

While this chapter offers useful insights into mental health shame in modern workplaces in Japan and the UK, several limitations should be noted. Firstly, the participants were collected through opportunity sampling, limiting the generalisability of the findings. Secondly, the industries they worked in were not controlled and differed in the two samples; there were some differences between the two UK samples ($p \geqq 0.03$), but these were much smaller than the country differences: however, future research should examine the contribution of industry and organisational culture. Thirdly, measuring shame using self-report scales might limit their accuracy (Fan et al., 2006), for example, the social desirability biases (Latkin, Edwards, Davey-Rothwell, & Tobin, 2017). Lastly, the causal direction of these relationships has not been analysed. Longitudinal data and intervention studies would help elucidate the temporal patterning of the observed relationships.

5 Conclusion

Work mental health is a primary concern in Japan and the UK, and their shame culture was thought to be related to their high shame about mental health problems. We cross-culturally compared their mental health and mental health shame between Japan and the UK and found that Japanese workers had higher levels of mental health problems and mental health shame. Mental health problems and shame were overall related to each other in both workforces. Mental health shame predicted medium effect size in the Japanese workers, while they predicted small effect size in the UK workers. Findings in this chapter can offer helpful insights into the importance of culture in terms of shame in the 4IR and how a sense of shame can impact on workers' mental health cross-culturally. Reducing shame in workers using modalities such as online self-compassion training may be essential to the global workforce today, especially for people who are suffering from poor mental health that is partly caused by the technology.

References

American Psychological Association. (2013). *Americans stay connected to work on weekends, vacation, and even when out sick*. American Psychological Association Press Room. Retrieved from http://www.apa.org/news/press/releases/2013/09/connected-work.aspx.

Ando, S., Yamaguchi, S., Aoki, Y., & Thornicroft, G. (2013). Review of mental-health-related stigma in Japan. *Psychiatry and Clinical Neurosciences, 67*, 471–482. https://doi.org/10.1111/pcn.12086.

Antony, M. M., Bieling, P. J., Cox, B. J., Enns, M. W., & Swinson, R. P. (1998). Psychometric properties of the 42-item and 21-item versions of the depression anxiety stress scales in clinical groups and a community sample. *Psychological Assessment, 10*(2), 176–181. https://doi.org/10.1037/1040-3590.10.2.176.

AXA. (2017). *Generation stress: 4 in 5 Brits could be suffering burnout as a result of stress, AXA research reveals*. Retrieved from https://www.axa.co.uk/newsroom/media-releases/2017/generation-stress-research/.

Barber, L. K., & Santuzzi, A. M. (2015). Please respond ASAP: Workplace telepressure and employee recovery. *Journal of Occupational Health Psychology, 20*(2), 172–189.

Benedict, R. (1946). *The chrysanthemum and the sword: Patterns of Japanese culture*. Boston, MA: Houghton Mifflin.

Braehler, C., Gumley, A., Harper, J., Wallace, S., Norrie, J., & Gilbert, P. (2013). Exploring change processes in compassion focused therapy in psychosis: Results of a feasibility randomized controlled trial. *British Journal of Clinical Psychology, 52*(2), 199–214. https://doi.org/10.1111/bjc.12009.

Burt, S. M., Bachnik, J. M., & Quinn, C. J. (1995). Situated meaning: Inside and outside in Japanese self, society and language. *Language, 71*(2), 402. https://doi.org/10.2307/416181.

Cabinet Office. (2019). *Survey in life conditions [Seikatsujoukyou ni kansuru chousa]*. Tokyo: Author.

Cascio, W. F. (2000). Managing a virtual workplace. *The Academy of Management Executive (1993-2005)*. Academy of Management. https://doi.org/10.2307/4165661.

Clarke, C. H., & Takashiro, N. (2019). Transforming shame to collective pride and social equity in bicultural organizations in Japan. In C. H. Mayer & E. Vanderheiden (Eds.), *The bright side of shame: Transforming and growing through practical applications in cultural contexts*. Basel: Springer.

CNBC International. (2018). *Why does Japan work so hard?* | CNBC explains [Video file]. Retrieved from https://www.youtube.com/watch?v=9Y-YJEtxHeo&t=182s.

Cohen, J. (1988). *Statistical power analysis for the behavioral sciences*. Mahwah, NJ: Lawrence Erlbaum Associates.

Cole, L.W. (2013). *Japanese culture-bound disorders: The relationship between "Taijin Kyofusho, Hikikomori," and shame*. Doctoral Thesis, Biola University.

Corrigan, P. (2004, October). How stigma interferes with mental health care. *American Psychologist*. https://doi.org/10.1037/0003-066X.59.7.614.

Day, A., Scott, N., & Kelloway, E. K. (2010). Information and communication technology: Implications for job stress and employee well-being. *Research in Occupational Stress and Well Being, 8*, 317–350. https://doi.org/10.1108/S1479-3555(2010)0000008011.

Elias, N. (1979). *The civilizing process: Sociogenetic and psychogenetic investigations*. Hoboken, NJ: Blackwell.

European Community. (2005). *Improving the mental health of the population: Towards a strategy on mental health for the European Union*. Brussels: Author.

Fan, X., Miller, B., Park, K.-E., Winward, B., Christensen, M., Grotevant, H., & Tai, R. (2006). An exploratory study about inaccuracy and invalidity in adolescent self-report surveys. *Field Methods, 18*, 223–244. https://doi.org/10.1177/152822X06289161.

Gilbert, P. (1998). What is shame? Some core issues and controversies. In P. Gilbert & B. Andrews (Eds.), *Shame: Interpersonal behaviour, psychopathology and culture* (pp. 3–36). New York, NY: Oxford University Press.

Gilbert, P., Bhundia, R., Mitra, R., McEwan, K., Irons, C., & Sanghera, J. (2007). Cultural differences in shame-focused attitudes towards mental health problems in Asian and non-Asian student women. *Mental Health, Religion & Culture, 10*(2), 127–141. https://doi.org/10.1080/13694670500415124.

González-Gómez, H., & Richter, A. (2015). Turning shame into creativity: The importance of exposure to creative team environments. *Organizational Behavior and Human Decision Processes, 126*, 142–161. https://doi.org/10.1016/j.obhdp.2014.09.004.

Harman, R., & Lee, D. (2010). The role of shame and self-critical thinking in the development and maintenance of current threat in post-traumatic stress disorder. *Clinical Psychology & Psychotherapy, 17*(1), 13–24. https://doi.org/10.1002/cpp.636.

Hikita, S. (2004). *Zenkiroku terebi sichouritsu 50 nen sensou [All the record for the 50-year- war of TV programme rating]*. Tokyo: Kodansha.

Hoaglin, D. C., & Iglewicz, B. (1987). Fine-tuning some resistant rules for outlier labeling. *Journal of the American Statistical Association, 82*(400), 1147. https://doi.org/10.2307/2289392.

Inoue, T. (2007). *Sekentei no kouzou-syakaishinrigakushi heno kokoromi [The structure of decency—Challenge for the history of social psychology]*. Tokyo: Kodansha.

Ito, H., & Aruga, T. (2018, August 1). Japan imposes a legal overtime cap, but mental health issues are complex. *The Lancet Psychiatry*. https://doi.org/10.1016/S2215-0366(18)30266-9.

Jackman, S. (2019). *Microsoft Japan says four-day work week boosted productivity 40%*. Retrieved from https://www.bloomberg.com/news/articles/2019-11-04/microsoft-japan-says-four-day-work-week-boosted-productivity-40.

Kawashima, Y. (2018). *Karoshi and Japan's work style reform*. Retrieved from https://ksr.hkspublications.org/2018/08/02/karoshi-and-japans-work-style-reform/.

Kelly, A., Zuroff, D., Foa, C., & Gilbert, P. (2010). Who benefits from training in self-compassionate self-regulation? A study of smoking reduction. *Journal of Social and Clinical Psychology, 29*(7), 727–755. https://doi.org/10.1521/jscp.2010.29.7.727.

Kestel, D. (2019). *Mental health in the workplace*. Retrieved August 19, 2019, from https://www.who.int/news-room/commentaries/detail/mental-health-in-the-workplace.

Kim, T., Kang, M. Y., Yoo, M. s., Lee, D., & Hong, Y. C. (2016). Computer use at work is associated with self-reported depressive and anxiety disorder. *Annals of Occupational and Environmental Medicine, 28*(1). https://doi.org/10.1186/s40557-016-0146-8.

Kim, S., Thibodeau, R., & Jorgensen, R. S. (2011). Shame, guilt, and depressive symptoms: A meta-analytic review. *Psychological Bulletin, 137*(1), 68–96. https://doi.org/10.1037/a0021466.

Kossek, E. E., Lautsch, B. A., & Eaton, S. C. (2006). Telecommuting, control, and boundary management: Correlates of policy use and practice, job control, and work-family effectiveness. *Journal of Vocational Behavior, 68*(2), 347–367. https://doi.org/10.1016/j.jvb.2005.07.002.

Kotera, Y., Adhikari, P., & Van Gordon, W. (2018). Motivation types and mental health of UK hospitality workers. *International Journal of Mental Health and Addiction, 16*(3), 751–763. https://doi.org/10.1007/s11469-018-9874-z.

Kotera, Y., Gilbert, P., Asano, K., Ishimura, I. & Sheffield, D. (2018). Self-criticism and self-reassurance as mediators between mental health attitudes and symptoms: Attitudes towards mental health problems in Japanese workers. *Asian Journal of Social Psychology, 22*(2), 183–192. https://doi.org/10.1111/ajsp.12355.

Kotera, Y., Conway, E., & Van Gordon, W. (2019a). Mental health of UK university business students: Relationship with shame, motivation and self-compassion. *Journal of Education for Business, 94*(1), 11–20. https://doi.org/10.1080/08832323.2018.1496898.

Kotera, Y., Gilbert, P., Asano, K., Ishimura, I., & Sheffield, D. (2019b). Self-criticism and self-reassurance as mediators between mental health attitudes and symptoms: Attitudes toward mental health problems in Japanese workers. *Asian Journal of Social Psychology, 22*(2), 183–192. https://doi.org/10.1111/ajsp.12355.

Kotera, Y., Green, P., & Sheffield, D. (2019c). Mental health attitudes, self-criticism, compassion, and role identity among UK social work students. *British Journal of Social Work, 49*(2), 351–370. https://doi.org/10.1093/bjsw/bcy072.

Kotera, Y., Green, P., & Sheffield, D. (2019d). Mental health shame of UK construction workers: Relationship with masculinity, work motivation, and self-compassion. *Revista de Psicología Del Trabajo y de Las Organizaciones, 35*(2), 135–143. https://doi.org/10.5093/jwop2019a15.

Kotera, Y., & Van Gordon, W. (2019). Japanese managers' experiences of neuro-linguistic programming: A qualitative investigation. *Journal of Mental Health Training, Education and Practice, 14*(3), 174–185. https://doi.org/10.1108/JMHTEP-06-2018-0033.

Latkin, C. A., Edwards, C., Davey-Rothwell, M. A., & Tobin, K. E. (2017). The relationship between social desirability bias and self-reports of health, substance use, and social network factors among urban substance users in Baltimore. *Addictive Behaviour, 73*, 133–136. https://doi.org/10.1016/j.addbeh.2017.05.005.

Lickel, B., Kushlev, K., Savalei, V., & Schmader, T. (2014). Shame and motivation to change the self. *Emotion, 14*(6), 1049–1061. https://doi.org/10.1037/a0038235.

Lovibond, P. F., & Lovibond, S. H. (1995). The structure of negative emotional states: Comparison of the depression anxiety stress scales (DASS) with the Beck depression and anxiety inventories. *Behaviour Research and Therapy, 33*(3), 335–343. https://doi.org/10.1016/0005-7967(94)00075-U.

Maekawa, Y., Ramos-Cejudo, J., & Kanai, A. (2016). Help-seeking among male employees in Japan: Influence of workplace climate and distress. *Journal of Occupational Health, 58*(6), 632–639. https://doi.org/10.1539/joh.16-0052-OA.

Markus, H. R., & Kitayama, S. (1991). Culture and the self: Implications for cognition, emotion, and motivation. *Psychological Review, 98*(2), 224–253. https://doi.org/10.1037/0033-295X.98.2.224.

Matos, M., & Pinto-Gouveia, J. (2010). Shame as a traumatic memory. *Clinical Psychology & Psychotherapy, 17*(4), 299–312. https://doi.org/10.1002/cpp.659.

Matos, M., Pinto-Gouveia, J., & Gilbert, P. (2013). The effect of shame and shame memories on paranoid ideation and social anxiety. *Clinical Psychology & Psychotherapy, 20*(4), 334–349. https://doi.org/10.1002/cpp.1766.

Mayer, C. H., & Vanderheiden, E. (2019). *The bright side of shame: Transforming and growing through practical applications in cultural contexts*. Basel: Springer.

Matsumoto, Y., Kunimoto, S., & Ozaki, N. (2013). Developmental risk of depression and gene/environment interaction. *Journal of Mental Health, 59*, 7–15.

Mazmanian, M., Orlikowski, W. J., & Yates, J. A. (2013). The autonomy paradox: The implications of mobile email devices for knowledge professionals. *Organization Science, 24*(5), 1337–1357. https://doi.org/10.1287/orsc.1120.0806.

McGregor, J. (2019). *In overworked Japan, Microsoft tested a four-day workweek. Productivity soared 40 percent.* Retrieved from https://www.washingtonpost.com/business/2019/11/04/overworked-japan-microsoft-tested-four-day-workweek-productivity-soared-percent/?.

Ministry of Health, Labour and Welfare. (2013). *Roudou anzen eisei tokubetsu chousa (Roudousha kenkou joukyou chousa) no gaikyou [Summary of labour safety hygiene special research (workers health status research)]*. Retrieved from http://www.mhlw.go.jp/toukei/list/dl/h24-46-50_05.pdf.

Ministry of Health, Labour and Welfare. (2014). *Revision of the laws about welfare for mental health and people with mental health disorders [Seishinhoken oyobi seishinshougaisha fukushi ni kansuru houritsuno ichibu wo kouseisuru houritsunado no sekoujikouno shousainitsuite]*. Tokyo. Retrieved from https://www.mhlw.go.jp/seisakunitsuite/bunya/hukushi_kaigo/shougaishahukushi/kaisei_seisin/dl/shikou_gaiyo.pdf.

Ministry of Health, Labour and Welfare. (2016). *Karoushitouboushitaisaku hakusho [Karoshi whitepaper]*. Retrieved from http://www.mhlw.go.jp/wp/hakusyo/karoushi/16/dl/16-1.pdf.

Moberly, T. (2015). Two thirds of doctors think NHS has "blame and shame" culture. *BMJ, 350*. https://doi.org/10.1136/bmj.h2272.

Muroi, K. (2019). *More workers are suffering from non-recorded overtime? [Hatarakikatakaikakuhousekou ni hitsuu na koe 'mienai sa-bisu zangyou' ga manen?]*. Retrieved from https://www.excite.co.jp/news/article/Real_Live_46856/.

Nakazawa, T., Okubo, Y., Suwazono, Y., Kobayashi, E., Komine, S., Kato, N., & Nogawa, K. (2002). Association between duration of daily VDT use and subjective symptoms. *American Journal of Industrial Medicine, 42*(5), 421–426. https://doi.org/10.1002/ajim.10133.

Nitobe, I. (1900). *Bushido: The soul of Japan*. Philadelphia: The Leeds and Biddle Company.

Obic Business Consultant (2019). *No effects for 'the initiative to reduce overtime work'? [Sono 'zangyo sakugen no torikumi' kouka nashi?]*. Retrieved from https://www.obc.co.jp/360/list/post66.

O'Connor, J., & Seymour, J. (2003). *Introducing NLP: Neuro-linguistic programming*. London: Harper Collins.

Office of Applied Studies. (2007). *The NSDUH report: Depression among adults employed full-time*. Retrieved from http://www.sprc.org/resources-programs/nsduh-report-depression-among-adults-employed-full-time-occupational-category.

Olson-Buchanan, J. B., & Boswell, W. R. (2006). Blurring boundaries: Correlates of integration and segmentation between work and nonwork. *Journal of Vocational Behavior, 68*(3), 432–445. https://doi.org/10.1016/j.jvb.2005.10.006.

Peakman, J. (2009). Blaming & shaming in whores' memoirs. *History Today, 59*(8), 33–39.

Rao, N., & Kemper, K. J. (2017). Online training in specific meditation practices improves gratitude, well-being, self-compassion, and confidence in providing compassionate care among health professionals. *Journal of Evidence-Based Integrative Medicine, 22*(2), 237–241. https://doi.org/10.1177/2156587216642102.

Saiidi, U. (2018). Japan has some of the longest working hours in the world. It's trying to change. *Consumer News and Business Channel*. Retrieved from https://www.cnbc.com/2018/06/01/japan-has-some-of-the-longest-working-hours-in-the-world-its-trying-to-change.htm.

Sheehy, K., Noureen, A., Khaliq, A., Dhingra, K., Husain, N., Pontin, E., Cawley, R., & Taylord, P. (2019). An examination of the relationship between shame, guilt and self-harm: A systematic review and meta-analysis. *Clinical Psychology Review, 73*. https://doi.org/10.1016/j.cpr.2019.101779.

Skårderud, F. (2007). Shame and pride in anorexia nervosa: A qualitative descriptive study. *European Eating Disorders Review, 15*(2), 81–97. https://doi.org/10.1002/erv.774.

Stevenson, D., & Farmer, P. (2017). *Thriving at work*. London. Retrieved from https://assets.publishing.service.gov.uk/government/uploads/system/uploads/attachment_data/file/658145/thriving-at-work-stevenson-farmer-review.pdf.

Tanaka, G., Ogawa, T., Inadomi, H., Kikuchi, Y., & Ohta, Y. (2003). Effects of an educational program on public attitudes towards mental illness. *Psychiatry and Clinical Neurosciences, 57*(6), 595–602. https://doi.org/10.1046/j.1440-1819.2003.01173.x.

Tangney, J. P., Wagner, P., & Gramzow, R. (1992). Proneness to shame, proneness to guilt, and psychopathology. *Journal of Abnormal Psychology, 101*(3), 469–478. https://doi.org/10.1037/0021-843X.101.3.469.

The Prime Minister of Japan and His Cabinet. (2016). *Hatarakikatakaikaku jitsugenkaigi [Committee for realisation of reform of the working style]*. Retrieved from http://www.kantei.go.jp/jp/singi/hatarakikata/.

Townsend, A. M., DeMarie, S. M., & Hendrickson, A. R. (1998). Virtual teams: Technology and the workplace of the future. *The Academy of Management Executive (1993–2005)*. Academy of Management. https://doi.org/10.2307/4165474.
Tukey, J. W. (1962). The future of data analysis. *Annals of Mathematical Statistics, 33*(1), 1–67.
Voiskounsky, A. E., & Soldatova, G. U. (2019). Epidemic of loneliness in a digital society: Hikikomori as a cultural and psychological phenomenon. *Counseling Psychology and Psychotherapy, 27*(3), 22–43. https://doi.org/10.17759/cpp.2019270303.
von Raumer, K. (1857). *Geschichte der Pädagogik [History of pedagogy]*. ZeitSamuel Liesching.
Welch, B. L. (1947). The generalisation of student's problems when several different population variances are involved. *Biometrika, 34*(1–2), 28–35. https://doi.org/10.1093/biomet/34.1-2.28.

Mr. Yasuhiro Kotera is Academic Lead for Counselling and Psychotherapy and Chair of the Research Ethics Committee at the University of Derby Online Learning. As an Accredited Psychotherapist by the British Association for Counselling and Psychotherapy, he has worked with clients who suffer from diverse problems. He is also a Certified Neurolinguistic Programming (NLP) Trainer by the Society of NLP, having been training NLP and coaching skills mainly to workers in Japan, America, and the UK. He has numerous peer-reviewed academic journal publications and conference presentations regarding work mental health, cross-cultural psychology, compassion, and work motivation.

Dr. David Sheffield is a Registered Health Psychologist and Professor of Psychology at the University of Derby. His research areas include nature connectedness, brief interventions, compassion and mindfulness, mental health, and performance.

Dr. Pauline Green is a Senior Fellow of Advance Higher Education and Course Director for the Inter-professional Portfolio at the University of Derby Online Learning. As a Registered Social Worker, she has been engaged in social work practice for more than 35 years. Her research areas include emotional resilience and social work education.

Dr. Kenichi Asano is a Lecturer in the Department of Psychological Counseling at the Mejiro University and a Visiting Researcher at the National Center for Cognitive Behavioral Therapy and Research in Japan. His research areas include compassion-focused therapy, cognitive behavioural therapy, depression, anxiety disorders, bulimia nervosa, and obsessive compulsive disorders.

Chapter 4
The Meaning of Shame for Malay People in Indonesia and Its Relation to Counterproductive Work Behaviors in the Fourth Industrial Revolution

Hijriyati Cucuani, Marina Sulastiana, Diana Harding, and Hendriati Agustiani

1 Introduction

The deliberate failure to perform job tasks effectively, taking longer breaks at work, corruption, making nasty comments to coworkers, and destroying organizational property are some forms of counterproductive work behavior (CWB) (Spector & Domagalski, 2006). The problem of counterproductive work behavior (CWB) which happens a lot among employees with Malay cultural background at Pekanbaru nowadays is often associated with the absence of shame in the perpetrators. Counterproductive work behavior can happen to employees in other countries, but it is rarely associated with shame, but rather with injustice (Bruk-Lee & Spector, 2006; Izni, 2009; Sackett & Devore, 2005), work stressor (Penney & Spector, 2005; Roxana, 2013; Spector & Fox, 2002, 2005), work dissatisfaction (Mercado, Dilchert, Giordano, & Ones, 2015), leadership types (Bruursema, 2004), etc. This illustrates that shame is important in Malay society. It indicates whether someone knows about what is acceptable and unacceptable and what is expectable and unexpectable and whether someone still holds the traditional, cultural, and religious values.

Shame in Bahasa (Indonesian language) is referred to as *malu*. Shame is a form of emotion, the meaning of which is often associated with culture (Caparas & Hartijasti, 2014; Luyten, Fontaine, & Corveleyn, 2002). How shame is conceptualized depends very much on how a culture sees shame. In general, cultures in the world can be divided into individualist and collectivist cultures (Cohen, Wu, & Miler, 2016).

H. Cucuani (✉)
Psychology Faculty of Islamic State University of Sultan Syarif Kasim, Riau, Indonesia
e-mail: hijriyati18001@mail.unpad.ac.id

M. Sulastiana · D. Harding · H. Agustiani
Faculty of Psychology, Universitas Padjadjaran, Bandung, West Java, Indonesia

C.-H. Mayer et al. (eds.), *Shame 4.0*, https://doi.org/10.1007/978-3-030-59527-2_4

Malay people in Indonesia and surrounding areas as those of collective culture generally see shame more positively (Bagozzi, Verbeke, & Gavino, 2003; Su, 2010).

The results of a study in Pekanbaru (Wulandari & Widyastuti, 2014) showed that positive relationships with other people are the main factors of happiness for Indonesian people because maintaining good relations with others is inherent in collectivist cultures like in Indonesian society. Heine et al. explained that in a collectivist culture, self and others are connected in a social context so that they tend to focus on responsibilities and obligations to others and try to avoid behaviors that can cause interference or disappoint others who are important in their lives (Su, 2010).

Cross-cultural research on shame shows differences in how shame motivates individuals to improve relations with others. Shame in salespersons in the Philippines leads them to make efforts to maintain social ties with colleagues and consumers by increasing their altruistic behavior. As for salespersons in the Netherlands, shame is seen threatening so they make more efforts to maintain their self-concept than maintaining good relations with consumers (Bagozzi et al., 2003).

Because of the important position of shame in Malay society, it is taught to children since early childhood. Children are accustomed to listening to advice and important values taught by their parents. Before sleeping, either their mother, father, grandmother, or grandfather sing them poems that contain advice to become persons who are virtuous and have shame. In the evenings, children are often gathered to listen to stories told by their parents about virtues. Shame is always inserted in the advice of parents to their children (Effendy, 2015).

The emergence of technology in the daily lives of Malay people changes their habits. The Third Industrial Revolution that began around the 1960s was marked by the use of information and technology for automation production (Xu, David, & Kim, 2018) which was felt by people around the world community including in Pekanbaru, Indonesia. Television, gadgets, the Internet, and others keep people busy with activities that make use of technology and the Internet. Children gathering to listen to life advice from their parents and families sharing stories while having a meal together are getting rarely found. Both children and parents are busy in their own rooms. With these problems in mind, the meaning of shame was attempted to be explored again in this present study.

Today, technology development is faster than ever. The use of technology is inevitable. This era is called the "Fourth Industrial Revolution" (4IR) or 4.0. Schwab who popularized this term defines 4IR as "the fusion of technologies that blurs the line between the physical, digital, and biological spheres" (Lee et al., 2018; Menon & Fink, 2019). The Fourth Industrial Revolution brings progress and eases to humans in almost every field, so it can then change human attitudes and behavior for various things including work and relationships. One of the fields that are influenced by technology in 4IR is the human psychological aspects (Ghislieri, Molino, & Cortese, 2018) like organization members' behaviors in the workplace.

The behaviors of members that are contrary to the interests of the organization, which can harm the organization and the people in it, are called counterproductive work behavior (CWB) (Spector & Fox, 2005). According to Sackett and Devore

(2005), at least there are three characteristics that distinguish CWB from other concepts of negative behaviors at the workplaces: (1) CWB places more emphasis on the behavior, not the results; (2) the behavior is contrary to the interests of the organization; and (3) the behavior is done intentionally or can be interpreted to be done on their own volition. Scholars have divided CWB dimensions based on the target of each behavior into interpersonally targeted and organizationally targeted CWB (Fox, Spector, & Miles, 2001; Mercado et al., 2015; Robinson & Bennett, 1995). Interpersonally targeted counterproductive work behaviors (CWB-I) include those behaviors that directly harm people in the organization such as bullying and harm the well-being of organizational members or other stakeholders, while organizationally targeted counterproductive work behaviors (CWB-O) include those behaviors that directly harm the organization such as theft, production deviance, absenteeism, or disloyalty.

Some research on shame in Malay culture proves that shame in Malay people functions as a behavioral control that can prevent a person from committing counterproductive work behaviors. Research on students in Pekanbaru shows shame (for committing acts that break the rules) is negatively related to cyberloafing (Ihsani, Suadana, Muis, Aiyuda, & Nasution, 2018). Rahmah (in press) shows that the shame character of civil servants in Pekanbaru is negatively related to counterproductive work behaviors. Based on this, shame is something that needs to be explored further in order to prevent and overcome counterproductive work behavior which is currently a problem for Malay workers in Pekanbaru.

It turns to be interesting because in many of the previous studies which were mostly carried out on Westerners, negative emotions were seen as a factor in the occurrence of CWB (Bagozzi, Verbeke, & Gavino, 2003; Bauer & Spector, 2015; Fox et al., 2001; Penney & Spector, 2002; Spector & Domagalski, 2006; Spector & Fox, 2002). The stressor-emotion model of counterproductive work behavior explains that negative emotions mediate work stressors and CWB (Spector & Fox, 2005).

The high CWB for workers in Pekanbaru raises a question mark considering that Pekanbaru is a city with Malay culture, the values of which are synonymous with (Islamic) religious values (Suwardi, 2008). Religious teachings are used as a reference in the social norms that govern society in various aspects of life, including in the working life. However, the inclusion of various foreign values and cultures through technology can shift the previous values derived from culture and religion. The shift in values can be seen as a factor of changing one's nature because values can affect one's nature (Roccas, Sagiv, Schwartz, Knafo, & Schwartz, 2002). Schwartz (1992) sees values as criteria by which people choose and justify actions and evaluate people (including oneself) and events. When a value that is felt to be important by someone changes, then the criteria about right and wrong also change so as to form certain behaviors which if continuously carried out will be able to change one's nature. It is likely that people will try to reduce the difference they feel between their values and behavior by changing their behavior (Roccas et al., 2002).

Based on the above problems, the following research questions were sought to answer in this present research: (1) What is the meaning of *malu* in Malay people in

Pekanbaru in the context of work? (2) Is the technology currently developing rapidly in 4IR able to explain counterproductive work behavior in Malay people?

2 Methods

This research used a mixed method. The study was conducted with the indigenous psychological approach, a paradigm that included the context (culture) and its contents (meaning) into the research design (Kim, Yang, & Hwang, 2006). Culture is passed down in members of society so that it becomes so close to human life, therefore affecting human mentality (cognition, affection, and conation) (Fuadhy, Chandrashafira, & Marviani, 2017). Differences in the results of research related to shame in several places are often related to the meaning of shame by respondents who are very dependent on their culture. Therefore, in this research, shame-proneness was explored based on the experience of Malay people in Pekanbaru with Riau Malay culture as the context.

2.1 Samples

The respondents of this study were 120 workers in Pekanbaru, Riau, who are Malay people. Riau is known as the origin of Malay culture in Indonesia; even the Bahasa (Indonesian language) comes from Riau Malay language. Riau Malay people are the largest ethnic group in Riau Province, spread across all regions including Pekanbaru City (Melalatoa, 1995). Pekanbaru is the capital city of the Province which becomes the center of economic growth in Riau so that it is most affected by technology compared to other regions. What is meant by Malay people in Pekanbaru are people (1) living in Pekanbaru, (2) Muslim, (3) applying Malay customs, (and 4) using Malay language (Suwardi, 2008). The selection of research respondents was by means of non-probability sampling. Based on the data obtained, the subject demographics can be described as follows (Table 4.1).

2.2 Data Collection Method

The authors prepared survey sheets for data collection to explore the meaning of shame in the context of work according to employees and the effect of technology in the 4IR on the shame-proneness of Malay people. The survey contains a brief description of the study, informed consent to become a respondent, demographic items, and some open-ended questions, including the following: (1) In your opinion, what is meant by "malu"? (2) How important is the *sifat malu* (shame-proneness) possessed by worker? (3) In your opinion, is there a relationship between rapid

Table 4.1 Demographic descriptions of respondents

Characteristics	Descriptions
Gender	
Male	47.1%
Female	52.9%
Employment status	
Civil servant	32.8%
Non-civil servant	67.2%
Education	
Undergraduates	46.2%
Master graduates	25.2%
High school, diplomas, and doctoral graduates	28.6%
Tenure (in years)	1–35 ($M = 9.94$, $SD = 7.94$)
Age (in years)	18–58 ($M = 33.69$, $SD = 9.8$)

technological advances and its applications at the workplace in the 4IR era and changes in human traits, including shame-proneness? Why is that?

The instrument was first tested with five Malay people who worked as psychology lecturers at a university in Pekanbaru to check the readability of items. The actual data collection was carried out with the assistance of three psychology students who were also volunteers in the Psychology Study Center of UIN Suska Riau. Each volunteer gave survey forms to several people identified as meeting the research subject criteria. The survey forms were also hand-delivered to several government offices. Besides, the survey was also carried out online via email and social media. The data were collected from 4 November to 2 December 2019.

2.3 Data Analysis Technique

The data were analyzed with qualitative and quantitative content analysis techniques. The qualitative content analysis was carried out with an indigenous psychological approach that follows the stages of analysis in the framework grounded theory research which includes open coding, axial coding, and selective coding (Putri & Wicaksono, 2017). In the open coding stage, the researchers identified keywords in the data obtained from the respondents' answers which were then grouped into some categories. This stage was done with the help of three research assistants as proposed by Yuniarti (Arini, Ghazali, Satiti, Kamali, & Yuniarti, 2017). The axial coding was done by elaborating more deeply from the categories that had been identified based on the similarity in the core categories. This process was conducted based on the context of the form of behaviors/emotions derived from the meaning of shame. The selective coding was built from collecting axial categories that have the same construct to be labeled as a representation of shame phenomenon in Malay people. The coding results were validated by two researchers whose focus of research is shame in Malay people. The themes derived from the qualitative content analysis were then summed into percentages using Microsoft Excel 2010.

3 Results

3.1 The Meaning of "Malu" in Malay People

Based on the analysis of the meaning of *malu* according to Malay workers, it was found that *malu* is not only interpreted as shame, as explained in the literature review. Instead, it was also interpreted as shyness and embarrassment by some respondents. Most respondents (69.49%) interpreted *malu* as shame, that is, emotions in which a person feels uncomfortable, discouraged, and guilty for making mistakes or violations of regulations, religious values, and social norms. Based on the subjects' responses, shame is divided into felt shame which is experienced during or after committing a violation or inappropriate behavior and anticipatory shame that arises before someone does something inappropriate and not in accordance with rules and standards. *Malu* as shyness was interpreted by 25.42% of respondents; it is interpreted as emotions and human nature in which a person feels reluctant and hesitant to deal with people who are older or have power due to respect. It is also interpreted as the reluctance and lack of confidence to interact with others and be the center of attention. Some respondents (0.85%) interpreted *malu* as embarrassment, an unpleasant feeling due to an event that makes someone looks bad/careless or loses his/her self-esteem. The remaining responses (4.24%) could not be categorized. The categorization of the respondents' responses in more details can be seen in Table 4.2.

Based on the table above, it appears that the majority of respondents interpret *malu* as shame. The following figures (Fig. 4.1) show the meanings of *malu* by gender and age.

The above figures suggest that most of both male and female Malay workers interpreted *malu* as felt shame. A comparison between genders shows that more male workers interpreted shame as anticipatory shame, while more female workers interpret it as a cognitive component of shyness such as *sungkan* (being reluctant), lack of self-confidence, and fear of being rejected. Besides, the figures also suggest that the older age groups show a greater tendency to interpret *malu* as shame (both felt shame and anticipatory shame) and a lower tendency to interpret it as shyness (both the behavior and cognitive components of shyness).

Furthermore, shame is seen as quite important to workers. Based on respondents' responses to the additional questions of how important shame is to workers, the scores of which ranged from 1 to 7, an average value of 5.78 ($SD = 1.487$) was obtained.

Table 4.2 The categories of shame according to Malay workers ($N = 118$)

	Frequency (%)
I. Shame	
Felt shame	
1. Feelings arising from committing wrongdoings/improper behaviors/violating rules (including the desire to cover up those mistakes)	43.22
2. Feelings that arise from an error or condition that want to be covered but known by others	5.08
Anticipatory shame	
1. Control over behavior and speech that shows attention and awareness of morals and ethics	11.86
2. Maintaining dignity (showing self-esteem and maintaining respect to self and others)	4.24
3. Upholding the teachings of religion (shame as a manifestation form of belief in God and his teachings)	4.24
II. Shyness	
1. Somatic componentSuch as nervous and awkward feelings	2.54
2. Behavioral componentDifficult to express opinions, unwilling to meet other people, dare not to show up, self-covered, respect for respectable people	11.86
3. Cognitive componentFeeling insecure and less competent, feeling inferior	11.86
III. Embarrassment	
Physical pratfalls (e.g., falling down)	0.85
IV. Other/unidentified	4.24

3.2 *The Impacts of Rapid Technological Advances as a Main Feature of the 4IR Culture on "Malu" in Malay People*

Based on the responses, 90.57% of respondents stated that technology influences people's shame, both positively and negatively, as shown in the following table (Table 4.3).

3.3 *Shame-Proneness and Counterproductive Work Behavior*

In general, of the respondents who stated that technology affects *malu* of workers, 51.04% of the changes are negative and 29.17% positive, whereas 4.17% stated that the change could have both positive and negative effects and 15.63% did not provide an explanation. In more details, the respondents' responses about the impacts this technology has on work-life relate to counterproductive work behavior (CWB). In general, CWB is divided into two: CWB-O and CWB-I. The following table (Table 4.4) shows respondents' responses implying CWBs that decrease or shift the shame-proneness of workers in the 4IR:

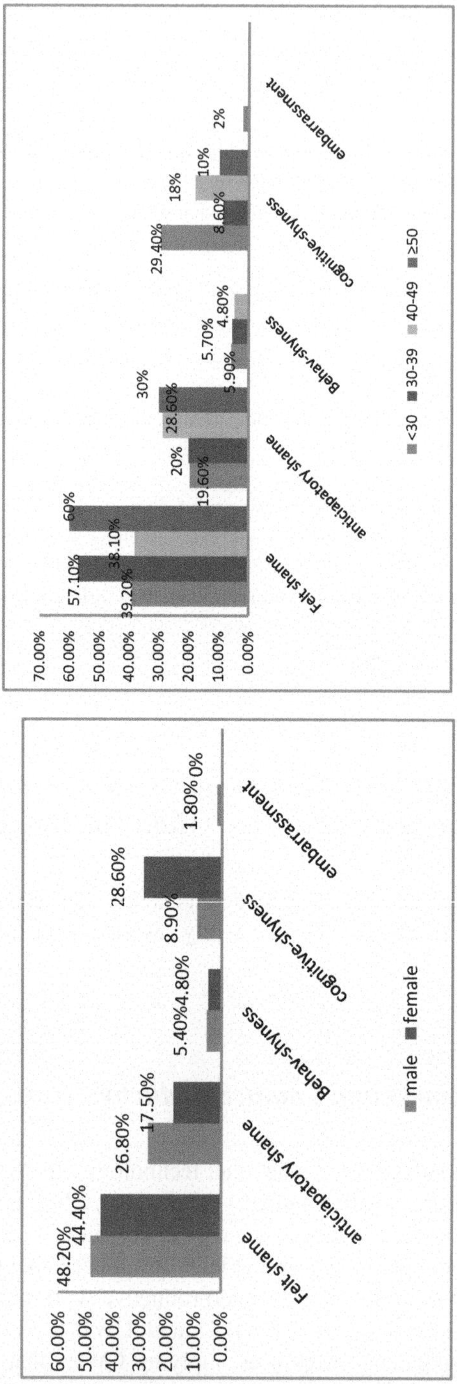

Fig. 4.1 The meanings of *malu* by gender and age

Table 4.3 The impacts of technology on *malu* for Malay people ($N = 106$)

	Frequency (%)
I. Positive impacts	
1. Becoming motivated to master technology	10.42
2. Keeping the integrity	7.29
3. Improving work performance	6.25
4. Facilitating the work	3.13
5. Becoming more confident	2.08
II. Negative impacts	
1. An openness that crosses the line	14.58
2. Less sensitive to the environment	9.38
3. Difficult to filter out inappropriate foreign cultures	8.33
4. Changes in habits and values	6.25
5. Reduced social interaction	5.21
6. Decreased performance	4.17
7. Disclosure of others' flaws to the public	3.13

Table 4.4 CWBs that shift shame-proneness of workers in the 4IR

CWB-O	Cyberloafing Posting nonwork-related activities to social media during work hours Disgracing the company where he/she works Being lazy because of expecting a lot from technology
CWB-I	Various forms of abuses because of anonymity Being indifferent to the environment (apathetic) Being impolite in interactions Posting inappropriate words/pictures/videos about coworkers Discussing colleagues' flaws in social media groups

4 Discussion

For Malay people, shame is still quite important in the context of work. The possession of shame indicates that a person still holds his/her cultural and religious values and thus can tell right from wrong. From the formulation of the meaning of shame, it was found that shame is an emotion in which a person feels uncomfortable, discouraged, and guilty for making mistakes or violations of regulations, religious values, and social norms. The existence of shame indicates an awareness of the rules and expectations of society toward him. Thus, one's behavior becomes more organized and the harmony in the workgroup is maintained. In this case, it is clear that Malay society views shame more positively.

In line with this definition, in general, Poulson (2000) defines shame as a social-emotional force. Shame is learned as we learn about the expectations and standards that other people wear to us and are reinforced with expectations that are developed toward ourselves. Stiles (2008) explains that shame is an emotion that is useful for organizations to motivate individuals to behave at a reasonable level. From an organizational point of view, shame supports company goals, values, encouragement of loyalty and involvement with the team and organization, and compliance with ethics.

As an emotion, shame occurs when someone breaks the rules or standards, either known or unknown to others. This is somewhat different from the previous concept of the difference between shame and guilt from an anthropological perspective where it is explained that shame is more about public emotion (public exposure) while guilt is more on private experience (Tangney & Dearing, 2002). In this study, it was found that a person experiences shame after a violation, even though it is unknown to others, as expressed by the following respondents: "malu is a condition when one feels something that is not right about something he/she has done, for example the shame from doing wrong, or the shame when not completing the task given" *(S67)* and "malu is a feeling that arises from the heart from our own actions" *(S66)*. Only a small proportion of respondents explained that shame arises because the wrongdoing is known by others. This result is in line with previous research which has rejected that perspective, where both shame and guilt can occur because of public exposure and also private experience (Tangney, Miller, Flicker, & Barlow, 1996; Xie & Qian, 2000).

Malay people not only feel shame when they have committed violations but also when they are confronted with situations that have the potential to do so. Thus, shame is not only understood as a felt shame for a violation but also when they hold back so that the situation does not occur. This can be seen from the following subject's answer about the meaning of shame: "the desire to refrain from doing actions that are not in accordance with the norms" *(S46)* and "unwillingness to do something because it is prohibited by norms and regulations" *(S42)*. Shame anticipates that the behavior they value as shameful does not occur so as to cause deeper shame and hurt self-esteem or honor and make them feel guilty or sinful. Therefore, the indications of people who have high anticipatory shame can be seen from their self-control, maintaining the dignity of self and family and upholding the teachings of religious values.

Anticipatory shame is explained by Murphy and Kiffin-Petersen (2017) as personal scripts that are developed based on their past emotional reactions, which helps them to know how to respond to similar future situations in order to avoid experiencing particular emotions. Anticipatory shame is learned by someone from previous experiences of shame. Interestingly, however, Malay people anticipate shame based not only on their own experiences but also on what they learn in their religious teachings, social or family norms, and from others as shameful behavior experience.

Stiles (2008) interprets shame as a signal that social harmony must be restored immediately and that efforts must be made to repair broken relationships. Shame and the threat of exposure to shame are important in highlighting one's behavior. The mechanism of shame becomes important in encouraging the social and moral development of individuals, as long as it is not intended to hurt others. In the world of work, shame is a useful emotion in ensuring that individuals perform at a reasonable level. If the experience of shame arises from underperformance or anticipation from underperformance, then there are three possibilities that may arise: (1) the individual withdraws from the source of shame, so he/she will refrain from engaging in absenteeism, for example, because it will make him ashamed; (2) individuals will express anger and hostility, and (3) individuals try to improve themselves and increase efforts to develop capabilities. At least, two of these possibilities are adaptive actions of shame experienced by workers.

Although most Malay people explain *malu* as shame, several others explain it as shyness and embarrassment. *Malu* in Malay-speaking countries including Indonesia matches some English words such as shame, shyness, and embarrassment (Aknouche & Noor, 2014; Collins & Bahar, 2000; Goddard, 1996). All of these emotions are often used interchangeably in expressing everyday shame. All three are self-conscious emotions, which are a high awareness of what is done or the conditions and events encountered and the great attention of the assessment of others against someone (Tangney et al., 1996). However, many psychological works of literature explain that all three have differences, although sometimes the explanations can vary (Cheek & Watson, 1989; Miller, 1992; Tangney et al., 1996).

Shyness by Leary is explained as an affective-behavioral syndrome characterized by social anxiety and interpersonal barriers resulting from the possibility of interpersonal evaluation (Cheek & Watson, 1989). Based on the results of their research, Cheek and Watson concluded that shyness can be explained from three components: somatic (such as blushing and trembling), behavioral (such as silence, awkward conversation, withdrawal, avoiding social contact), cognitive (such as thought or fear of being rejected, self-awareness), and other symptoms such as saying that he/she is embarrassed and so he/she does not want to do anything.

Although not dominant, there were significant numbers of respondents who explained *malu* as shyness. Malay people as a collective society also prioritize politeness toward older people or people of higher social levels, so they have a sense of *sungkan*, namely, an inhibition that causes shy in the presence of powerful others (Collins & Bahar, 2000). This particular shyness shows someone's respect which is accompanied by a sense of worry to show inappropriate behavior in the eyes of powerful others. The shyness that shows *sungkan* for Malay people is considered more positive than shyness that indicates a lack of confidence while being in public and among new people. Low self-confidence can inhibit someone in developing his/her self and dealing with challenges in the workplace.

As for embarrassment, it is an unpleasant condition of shame and regret that follows a public threat to one's social identity (Miller, 1992). According to Miller, embarrassment occurs when unwanted events communicate undesired information about oneself to others, so to be embarrassed one must be aware of and care about the evaluation of others. Embarrassment by some figures is associated with shame (Tangney et al., 1996). The results of research by Tangney et al. show that embarrassment is the least negative and passes faster than shame, is less painful, has less impact on morale, and is caused by a less serious situation so that telling it is easier and causing laughter. Embarrassment is caused by more shocking and accidental events. Embarrassment cannot be explained much in this present study because of the limited number of relevant responses.

Shame in Malay people is seen more positively and important so that it is taught from an early age to form a character called shame-proneness, namely, the tendency for someone to experience shame in certain situations (Covert, Tangney, Maddux, & Heleno, 2003). Shame-proneness is an honored character of Malay people (Effendy, 2015). However, since the introduction of technology, parents are less likely to give advice to children face to face as they did in the past, so children who have shame-proneness are now rarely found, especially in urban areas such as Pekanbaru. Technology that affects togetherness seems to minimize the role of parents in providing direct teaching to their children.

Xu et al. (2018) explained that the 4IR creates ripples in the community in almost every field. The Fourth Industrial Revolution will change the way humans live, work, and interact with one another. For this reason, understanding the technology and the potential disruption it causes is important, especially for developing countries. Especially in the case of interpersonal relationships, technology in the 4IR that provides convenience in working can minimize the time to settle all matters, thus having plenty of time to interact with others. However, it cannot be denied that the technology in 4IR has the risk of reducing eye contact interactions among humans (Corfe, 2018).

The involvement of humans with technology makes humans exposed to a variety of values and foreign cultures. Actually, Malay parents are wise enough to understand human tendencies to imitate foreign cultures. That is because Riau Malay people are quite open people (Effendy, 2015). Nevertheless, one must be careful so as not to accept or absorb all elements of the foreign culture without preservation. The reduced interaction between children and parents and the easy access to foreign values and cultures make the teaching of shame-proneness decrease. This is actually what to be worried about.

McCrae and Costa explain traits as descriptions of humans in the form of behaviors, thoughts, and emotions that tend to be stable (Parks-leduc, Feldman, & Bardi, 2015); therefore, they are usually sedentary. However, traits can be changed by certain things. Changes in value that occur from what is learned through technology and changes in ways of doing and thinking about something after the existence of technology are very possible. Values will motivate behavior; if the values lead to repetitive behavior, then it can then become a trait because trait includes repetitive behavior patterns (Parks-leduc et al., 2015).

There are several effects of the decline in the shame-proneness of workers in the 4IR related to technology found in this study, including openness that crosses the line, reduced sensitivity to the environment, and difficulty to filter out inappropriate foreign cultures. Technology causes people to no longer be ashamed to share on social media what they think and feel, problems they are facing, complaints, and displeasures about something that otherwise shameful to convey in person. Technology provides space for anyone to give opinions that are intentionally or unintentionally hurt others without showing their true identity. Even with true identity, people become less likely to feel ashamed to do so.

Technology can also cause people to become less sensitive to their environment. Great attention put to the use of technology can sometimes make people ignorant and less concerned about what is around them. Workers become less empathetic to the difficulties faced by their coworkers and consumers when they are preoccupied with doing activities using technology. Politeness is also starting to fade because, for example, sometimes people meet with others without engaging in eye contact communication because each of them is busy doing something with his/her cellphone. Another phenomenon observed in the era of openness is the entry of foreign cultures. Of course, not all foreign cultures are bad, but they need to be filtered because not all are good for Malay people. The exposure to foreign cultures via a variety of technologies causes a decrease in shame. People are not ashamed to imitate foreign cultures including the sexy clothing style of international artists and the way children talk and interact with parents that are not in accordance with Malay culture.

The effects of technology include negative work behaviors called counterproductive work behaviors (CWBs). CWBs due to the lack of shame can be directed to the organization (CWB-O) or other people at work (CWB-I). The Fourth Industrial Revolution can have impacts on CWB-O, including cyberloafing. Computers and Internet connections provided for work are often not only used for work purposes because of so many interesting things people can get from them including various kinds of entertainment, news, shopping, and communication on social media. Even though it does not always have serious impacts, but, in general, it reduces the amount of time supposed to spend for work. Besides, doing activities not related to work during working hours seems no longer to cause shame now because some people even share such actions with others through social media. Disclosing the organization's drawbacks or shortcomings to others, even if only to one person, will embarrass the organization. Today, with technology, people can easily post disgracing news or pictures, including those which concern the organization where they work, on social media. Another form of CWB-O is when a worker becomes lazy because technology enables him/her to do his/her work faster and thus allows a lot of time to finish. Instead of seeing it as an opportunity to do more works, he/she sees it as allowing him/her to work more slowly.

Counterproductive behaviors toward other people are also more likely to occur with technology. People will find it easier to ridicule, insult, or comment negatively on coworkers in social media to make it known by many people or gossip colleagues in social media groups. In addition, the increased intensity in the use of computers at work can cause a decreased attention to the surrounding environment, so that workers become less responsive to the needs and difficulties of others. Workers become less empathetic to what their coworkers would feel when inappropriate pictures, videos, or words about them are shared on social media. If left unchecked, things like this will likely cause inconvenience and conflict which in turn will affect work performance.

However, technology has positive impacts as well. Technology is developing faster and faster, making people feel ashamed if they cannot keep up with it. It can also improve workers' integrity. Automation avoids direct contact between officers and consumers who will make payments; thus, it will be difficult to bribe officers (Menon & Fink, 2019). Transparency in information and data also enables the activities and work of officers to be monitored by the public so workers must have integrity in doing their work.

It was found in this present study that there is a positive effect of the decrease in *malu*, but the *malu* in question is the shy to do good things such as to step forward, learn new things, and question things. There are two kinds of *malu* in Malay culture, namely, shame to do negative things and not to do positive things (Effendy, 2015). This means people should not be shy to improve themselves to enable them to understand and use technology properly.

5 Conclusion

The research shows that shame for most Malay people is still considered adaptive and imperative in the workplace. Felt shame and anticipatory shame of the employees reveal that they understand what is virtuous and not good to do. Meanwhile, the innovations and technologies that characterize 4IR have positive and negative impacts on the shame of employees, who are being motivated to master technology and maintain integrity, but on the contrary also make them open, crossing the line and being less sensitive to the environment. Based on these findings, further research is needed to explore deeper into the issue.

References

Aknouche, N., & Noor, N. M. (2014). The primacy of the self in shame: Can shame be benevolent? *American International Journal of Social Science, 3*(1), 59–79.

Arini, A. T., Ghazali, R. J., Satiti, A., Kamali, m. Y., & Yuniarti, K. W. (2017). Global climate change as perceived by elementary school teachers in Yogyakarta, indigenous psychology approach. *Jurnal Psikologi, 44*(3), 211–222. https://doi.org/10.22146/jpsi.26132.

Bagozzi, R. P., Verbeke, W., & Gavino, J. C. (2003). Culture moderates the self-regulation of shame and its effects on performance: The case of salespersons in the Netherlands and the Philippines. *Journal of Applied Psychology, 88*(2), 219–233. https://doi.org/10.1037/0021-9010.88.2.219.

Bauer, J. A., & Spector, P. E. (2015). Discrete negative emotions and counterproductive work behavior. *Human Performance, 28*(4), 307–331. https://doi.org/10.1080/08959285.2015.1021040.

Bruk-Lee, V., & Spector, P. E. (2006). The social stressors-counterproductive work behaviors link: Are conflicts with supervisors and coworkers the same? *Journal of Occupational Health Psychology, 11*(2), 145–156. https://doi.org/10.1037/1076-8998.11.2.145.

Bruursema, K. (2004). *Leadership style and the link with counterproductive work behavior (cwb): An investigation using the job-stress/cwb model.* College of Arts and Sciences, University of South Florida.

Caparas, M. V. G., & Hartijasti, Y. (2014). *Filipinos and Indonesians' shame: Towards integrity and soundness in organizational performance* (Business and Development Research).

Cheek, J. M., & Watson, A. K. (1989). The definition of shyness: Psychological imperialism or construct validity? *Journal of Social Behavior and Personality, 4*(1), 85–95.

Cohen, A., Wu, M. S., & Miler, J. (2016). Religion and culture: Individualism and collectivism in the east and west. *Journal of Cross-Cultural Psychology, 47*(9), 1236–1249. https://doi.org/10.1177/0022022116667895.

Collins, E. F., & Bahar, E. (2000). To know shame: Malu and its uses in Malay societies. *Journal of Southeast Asian Studies, 14*(1), 35–69.

Corfe, S. (2018). *4IR in the home: Maximising the benefits*. London: The Social Market Foundation.

Covert, M. V., Tangney, J. P., Maddux, J. E., & Heleno, N. M. (2003). Shame-proneness, guilt-proneness, and interpersonal problem solving: A social cognitive analysis. *Journal of Social and Clinical Psychology, 22*. Retrieved from https://e-resources.perpusnas.go.id:2057/docview/224856784/fulltextPDF/A71CFC873F5C47F9PQ/1?accountid=25704

Effendy, T. (2015). *Tunjuk Ajar Melayu*. Pekanbaru: Dinas Pendidikan dan Kebudayaan Pemerintah Propinsi Riau bekerja sama dengan Tenas Effedy Foundation.

Fox, S., Spector, P. E., & Miles, D. (2001). Counterproductive work behavior (CWB) in response to job stressors and organizational justice: Some mediator and moderator tests for autonomy and emotions. *Journal of Vocational Behavior, 59*(3), 291–309. https://doi.org/10.1006/jvbe.2001.1803.

Fuadhy, R. M., Chandrashafira, I. S., & Marviani, V. (2017). Mengenal indigenous psychology. In Faturochman, W. M. Minza, & T. A. Nurjaman (Eds.), Memahami dan Mengembangkan indigenous psychology (I, pp. 3–24). Yogyakarta: Pustaka Pelajar.

Ghislieri, C., Molino, M., & Cortese, C. G. (2018). Work and organizational psychology looks at the fourth industrial revolution: How to support workers and organizations? *Mini Review, 9*, 1–6. https://doi.org/10.3389/fpsyg.2018.02365.

Goddard, C. (1996). The "social emotions " of Malay (Bahasa Melayu). *Ethos, 24*(3), 426–464. https://doi.org/10.1525/eth.1996.24.3.02a00020.

Ihsani, I. N. M., Suadana, S., Muis, I. A., Aiyuda, N., & Nasution, I. N. (2018). Shame and guilt toward cyberloafing of Malay students in Pekanbaru, Riau. In The 1st International conferences on islamic psychology. Yogyakarta.

Izni, D. (2009). *Factors affecting counterproductive work behaviour (CPWB): A case of banking sector*. Universiti Utara Malaysia.

Kim, U., Yang, K.-S., & Hwang, K.-K. (2006). Contributions to indigenous and cultural psychology: Understanding people in context. In U. Kim, K.-S. Yang, & K.-K. Hwang (Eds.), *Indigenous and cultural psychology* (pp. 3–25). Boston, MA: Springer. https://doi.org/10.1007/0-387-28662-4.

Lee, M., Yun, J. J., Pyka, A., Won, D., Kodama, F., Schiuma, G., et al. (2018). How to respond to the fourth industrial revolution, or the second information technology revolution? Dynamic new combinations between technology, market, and society through open innovation. *Journal of Open Innovation: Technology, Market, and Complexity, 4*(21), 1–24. https://doi.org/10.3390/joitmc4030021.

Luyten, P., Fontaine, J. R. J., & Corveleyn, J. (2002). Does the test of self-conscious affect (TOSCA) measure maladaptive aspects of guilt and adaptive aspects of shame? An empirical investigation. *Personality and Individual Differences, 33*, 1373–1387.

Menon, J., & Fink, A. (2019). The fourth industrial revolution and its implications for regional economic integration in ASEAN. *Journal of Asian Economic Integration, 1*(1), 32–47. https://doi.org/10.1177/2631684618821566.

Melalatoa, J. (1995). *Eksiklopedi suku bangsa di Indonesia (L-Z)*. Jakarta: Departemen Pendidikan dan Kebudayaan RI (CV. EKa Putra).

Mercado, B. K., Dilchert, S., Giordano, C., & Ones, D. S. (2015). Counterproductive work behaviors. In *The SAGE handbook of industrial, work and organizational psychology* (pp. 109–211). London: Sage.

Miller, R. S. (1992). The nature and severity of self-reported embarrassing circumstances. *Personality and Social Psychology Bulletin, 18*(2), 190–198.

Murphy, S. A., & Kiffin-Petersen, S. (2017). The exposed self: A multilevel model of shame and ethical behavior. *Journal of Business Ethics, 141*, 657–675. https://doi.org/10.1007/s10551-016-3185-8.

Parks-leduc, L., Feldman, G., & Bardi, A. (2015). Personality traits and personal values: A meta-analysis. *Personality and Social Psychology Review, 19*(1), 3–29. https://doi.org/10.1177/1088868314538548.

Penney, L. M., & Spector, P. E. (2002). Narcissism and counterproductive work behavior: Do bigger egos mean bigger problems? *International Journal of Selection and Assessment, 10* (1&2), 126–134. https://doi.org/10.1111/1468-2389.00199.

Penney, L. M., & Spector, P. E. (2005). Job stress, incivility, and counterproductive work behavior (CWB): The moderating role of negative affectivity. *Journal of Organizational Behavior, 26*(7), 777–796. https://doi.org/10.1002/job.336.

Poulson, C. F., II. (2000). Shame and work. In W. Ashkanazy, N. Hartel, & C. Zerbe (Eds.), *Emotions in the workplace: Research, theory, and practice* (pp. 250–271). Westport, CT: Quorum.

Putri, L. Y. E., & Wicaksono, B. (2017). Contoh operasional penelitian indigenous psychology. In W. M. M. Faturochman & T. A. Nurjaman (Eds.), *Memahami dan Mengembangkan Indigenous Psychology* (pp. 79–110). Pustaka Pelajar: Yogyakarta.

Robinson, S., & Bennett, R. (1995). Mitigating methane production from ruminants; effect of calcium nitrate as modifier of the fermentation in an in vitro incubation using cassava root as the energy source and leaves of cassava or *Mimosa pigra* as source of protein. *The Academy of Management Journal, 38*(2), 555–572. https://doi.org/10.2307/256693.

Roccas, S., Sagiv, L., Schwartz, S. H., Knafo, A., & Schwartz, S. H. (2002). The big five personality factors and personal values. *Personality and Social Psychology Bulletin, 28*(6), 789–801. https://doi.org/10.1177/0146167202289008.

Roxana, A.-C. (2013). Antecedents and mediators of employees' counterproductive work behavior and intentions to quit. *Procedia - Social and Behavioral Sciences, 84*, 219–224. https://doi.org/10.1016/j.sbspro.2013.06.538.

Sackett, P. R., & Devore, C. J. (2005). Counterproductive behaviors at work. In N. Anderson, D. S. Ones, H. K. Sinangil, & C. Viswesvaran (Eds.), *Handbook of industrial, work on organizational psychology* (pp. 145–164). London: Sage.

Schwartz, S. H. (1992). Universals in the content and structure of values: Theoretical advances and empirical tests in 20 countries. *Advances in Experimental Social Psychology, 25*, 1–65.

Spector, P. E., & Domagalski, T. (2006). Emotions, violence, and counterproductive work behavior. In E. K. Kelloway, J. Barling, & J. J. Hurrell (Eds.), *Handbook of workplace violence* (pp. 29–46). Tampa: Sage. https://doi.org/10.4135/9781412976947.n3.

Spector, P. E., & Fox, S. (2002). An emotion-centered model of voluntary work behavior: Some parallels between counterproductive work behavior and organizational citizenship behavior. *Human Resource Management Review, 12*(2), 269–292. https://doi.org/10.1016/S1053-4822(02)00049-9.

Spector, P. E., & Fox, S. (2005). The stressor-emotion model of counterproductive work behavior. In S. Fox & P. E. Spector (Eds.), *Counterproductive work behavior: Investigations of actors and targets* (pp. 151–174). Washington, DC: American Psychological Association. https://doi.org/10.1037/10893-007.

Stiles, P. (2008). *The negative side of motivation: The role of shame*. Cambridge, MA: Cambridge University Press.

Su, C. (2010). *A cross-cultural study on the experience and self-regulation of shame and guilt. Soil science*. Toronto.

Suwardi. (2008). *Dari melayu ke Indonesia: Peranan kebudayaan melayu dalam memperkokoh identitas dan jati diri bangsa*. Pustaka Pelajar: Yogyakarta.

Tangney, J. P., Miller, R. S., Flicker, L., & Barlow, D. H. (1996). Are shame, guilt, and embarrassment distinct emotions? *Journal of Personality and Social Psychology, 70*(6), 1256–1269. https://doi.org/10.1037/0022-3514.70.6.1256.

Tangney, J. P., & Dearing, R. L. (2002). Shame and guilt. In P. Salovey (Ed.). New York: The Guilford Press.

Wulandari, S., & Widyastuti, A. (2014). Faktor-Faktor Kebahagiaan Di Tempat Kerja. *Jurnal Psikologi, 10*(1), 49–60.

Xie, B., & Qian, M. (2000). Phenomenological differences between shame and guilt among Chinese college students. *Chinese Journal of Psychology, 32*(1), 105–109.

Xu, M., David, J. M., & Kim, S. H. (2018). The fourth industrial revolution: Opportunities and challenges. *International Journal of Financial Research, 9*(2), 90–95. https://doi.org/10.5430/ijfr.v9n2p90.

Hijriyati Cucuani is a lecturer of psychology faculty at UIN Sultan Syarif Kasim Riau, Indonesia. Cucuani's concentration is in the field of Industrial and organizational psychology, especially about organizational behavior. Hijriyati obtained a master and psychologist license in education at master program profession of industrial and organizational psychology, Indonesian University, Jakarta. Cucuani is a Ph.D. Student in Padjadjaran University of Bandung, Indonesia. Her Dissertation focuses on counterproductive work behavior and it's correlation with values and shame among Malay people in Indonesia.

Marina Sulastiana is a lecturer of psychology faculty at Padjadjaran University of Bandung. She has a great interest in the industrial and organizational psychology field. She currently serves as the Chair of Science Magister and Doctoral Program Study in psychology faculty at Padjadjaran University. She completed her undergraduate, magister and doctoral program in Padjadjaran University of Bandung.

Diana Harding is a professor in Padjadjaran University. She is active as a lecturer, speaker, researcher and consultant on industrial and organizational psychology. She is also active in every activity initiated by West Java Region of the Industrial and Organization Psychology Association.

Hendriati Agustiani is a professor in Padjajaran University. Agustiani is also a dean (period: 2016–2021) and a lecturer in psychology faculty at Padjadjaran University of Bandung. She is an expert in the field of developmental psychology.

Chapter 5
Shame 4.0: Empirical Evidence of the Importance of Emotions in a Technologising World of Work

Claude-Hélène Mayer

1 Introduction

Industry 4.0—which is part of the Fourth Industrial Revolution—has become an important term in the context of contemporary organisations (Schwab, 2017). However, research has primarily focused on the technological challenges, the change in workspaces, the opportunities which the 4IR might open, and the skills needed with regard to the future workforce (Nankervis, Connell, Cameron, Montague, & Prikshat, 2019). Research has often highlighted negative and disruptive processes, such as job loss, decreasing personal relationships or mismatching skills of employees, new work requirements, and job demands (Kamaruzaman, Hamid, Mutalib, & Rasul, 2019).

Schwab (2016) points out that individuals, as spiritual and emotional beings, need to take emotions into consideration during the 4IR. Karim (2019) emphasises that emotional intelligence in the 4IR is important and can contribute to health and well-being. Previous research has found that individuals communicating mainly through digitalised and technologised devices in 4IR settings need to learn how to deal with negative emotions constructively, in order to develop new meaning and purpose in life and at work (Mayer, 2019). Mayer (2019) argues that a mindful connection to emotions can support creativity in future-orientated workplaces and that negatively experienced emotions, such as shame, need to be transformed towards a constructive and positively experienced emotion to contribute to the organisational climate and culture. However, before negative emotions such as shame can be transformed, empirical research is needed to explore how employees experience emotions within

C.-H. Mayer (✉)
Department of Industrial Psychology and People Management, University of Johannesburg, Auckland Park, Johannesburg, South Africa

Kulturwissenschaftliche Fakultät, Europa Universität Viadrina, Frankfurt (Oder), Germany

C.-H. Mayer et al. (eds.), *Shame 4.0*, https://doi.org/10.1007/978-3-030-59527-2_5

the 4IR, how they deal with their emotions, and how they transform emotions in the organisational context.

At the moment, articles and publications about emotions and their importance in 4IR processes exist on theoretical and conceptual levels (see Karim, 2019; Oosthuizen, 2016; and Schwab, 2016); there is hardly any empirical research published that presents findings on emotions within 4IR transformation organisations. This is particularly true for the exploration of shame in 4IR contexts (see also Mayer, 2019). Therefore, it is argued here that to remain competitive in a globalising 4IR context, organisations need to focus on appropriate skills and mindsets (Kamaruzaman et al., 2019). Often, the focus has been placed on skills and technological know-how while neglecting the importance of emotions in building a positive organisation and future-orientated mindset amid increasing technological change.

New research studies are needed in the context of Industry 4.0 that focus not only on technological change, transformation of workspaces, and challenges which relate to unemployment, technologisation, and digitalisation but also on automation and the use of robots. From an industrial and organisational psychology perspective in particular, it is clear that research studies are needed which do not focus primarily on the technological side, but rather on the emotional impacts which come with the transformation into Industry 4.0.

The chapter reports on qualitative empirical findings on shame within a technological engineering organisation, with reference to the process of Industry 4.0. It refers to the research question: How do managers experience shame during the ongoing transformational process towards Industry 4.0? Conclusions are drawn, and recommendations with regard to future research and practice from an industrial and organisational psychology perspective are given.

2 Emotions and Feelings in Industry 4.0

For many years, organisations and managers did not consider emotions as significant aspects of management, but during the last two decades, research has taken the importance of emotions and emotional processes increasingly into account in organisations (Giardini & Frese, 2004; Rausch, Seifried, & Harteis, 2017).

Emotions occur on different levels, including intrapersonal and interpersonal, as well as organisational and societal, levels which impact on employees (Küpers & Weibler, 2008). Emotions are complex processes and modes of communication (Burkitt, 1997). The differences between emotions and feelings have been discussed extensively in literature, highlighting that feelings are usually anchored in abstract thinking, while emotions are based on psycho-physiological processes (Bigman, Sheppes & Tamir, 2017). Feelings usually manifest consciously, while emotions manifest unconsciously. Further, feelings can develop slowly and are not necessarily intense, while emotions are immediate processes and are particularly powerful (Bigman, Sheppes & Tamir, 2017). These authors emphasise that emotional regulation and reinterpretation of feelings are possible and usually contribute to increased personal health and well-being.

Emotions are socio-culturally embedded and associated with relationships, power and interdependence, meaning, identity formation, and activity (Küpers & Weibler, 2008). Further, they are embodied and include subjectively felt sensations, while they influence thoughts, beliefs, actions, and social relations (Frijda & Mesquita, 1994).

Many aspects of organisational life and culture are co-constituted and influenced by emotions and create emotions (van Maanen & Kunda, 1989). Thereby they affect organisations on all levels, organisational climate conditions, and culture and help employees to thrive in digital workplaces (Coetzee, 2019).

According to a review of previous research on emotions, Küpers and Weibler (2008) conclude that emotions have often been evaluated with regard to their positive and negative impact in organisations and emotions have been mainly researched in connection with performance, motivation and demotivation, stress and conflict, change, transformation, and knowledge management. Already in the 1980s, Hirschhorn (1988) observed that emotions are part of working life and that employees are usually expected to show certain emotions while promoting organisational goals. It has been emphasised that emotions, as well as thoughts, occur during work time and that they affect meaning creation and identity development (Ashforth & Humphrey, 1993).

Emotional labour—referring to the process of managing feelings and expressions to fulfil the emotional requirements of a job—is not negative or positive per se, but it has been pointed out that emotional management in organisations (Zerbe, Ashkanasy, & Hartel, 2006) supports the positive effects of emotional labour. Consequently in the field of management and leadership, it is important to understand the emotions of leaders and how leaders manage their own emotions and the emotions of others (Erickson, 1997), particularly since power can be gained in organisations through mobilising and directing emotions. Further, emotions usually correspond to ambivalences within organisational settings. This means, for example, that change and transformational settings can be experienced as positive (pleasing) or negative (frustrating) (Pratt & Doucet, 2000). Positively experienced emotions usually increase the feeling of self-worth (Palmer & Hardy, 2000); expand the sense of belonging (Collins, 1990), thereby reducing feelings of stress and burnout; and will positively affect job satisfaction, work motivation, and individual performance (Sahu & Srivastava, 2017). Emotional problems, on the other hand, can create mental and physical health issues and lead to distress and burnout (Mayer, 2011). This is why it is argued here that negative emotions experienced in organisations might have a positive effect when they are transformed into more positively experienced emotions.

Emotions in the context of Industry 4.0 have been recently researched with regard to digital workspace and cyberspaces where new and different levels of emotion are experienced in virtual teams through new information technology contexts (Glikson & Erez, 2013; Jonker 2019). In terms of technological but also relationship-orientated changes, Temekova (2018) emphasises that emotional intelligence will play a major role in organisations in Industry 4.0 in supporting managers and leaders to increase their ability to understand and manage their own emotions and feelings, as well as their ability to understand and analyse the feelings of other employees. Oosthuizen and Mayer (2019) point out that often emotions are influenced by unconscious dynamics and that negatively experienced emotions need to be reduced or changed into positively experienced emotions in order to support constructive organisational processes and to make resources available to manage stress, conflict, and anxieties. This is particularly the case since 4IR, in that the future-orientated increases in technology and automation seem to evoke negative rather than positive emotions in the (South African) workplace. Barber (2019) argues that new management and leadership skills are needed to deal with Industry 4.0 changes constructively, highlighting that creative, adaptable, emotionally intelligent, and politically aware individuals are needed to drive Industry 4.0 successfully on all levels.

Therefore, further analysis needs to be conducted on emotions in transformational situations towards Industry 4.0. New strategies need to be developed to tackle and transform negative emotions in the workplace, through emotional labour to support 4IR changes in the best possible way.

3 Shame in Human-Technology Interaction

This chapter focuses on shame as an often negatively experienced emotion. Shame is viewed as a social emotion which regulates social interaction (Gilbert, 2019). As an impactful emotion occurring in organisations, shame has been researched previously (Mayer, Viviers & Tonelli, 2017) and has been defined as a potential resource when it is dealt with constructively (Mayer & Vanderheiden, 2019).

In Industry 4.0 processes, shame and shaming is often used in the virtual and digital realm to exclude individuals and/or members of groups or even whole groups from participation, by designing new boundaries (see also Vanderheiden and Mayer in this book). Wong (2019) asserts that individuals need to act responsibly to shape Industry 4.0 by taking shame and shaming into consideration.

Shame is often interlinked with other emotions such as anxiety or guilt, and when experienced in organisations, it is frequently expressed through withdrawal and avoidance tendencies (Oosthuizen, 2019). This is not least because individuals often accede to the power and judgement of other employees within the organisation (Kets de Vries, 2017).

Jonker (2019) contends that employees may experience shame and shameful situations, as well as frustration, when they experience language barriers; the culture of the organisation will determine how employees and the organisation will react to these kinds of shameful experiences. As pointed out by Wilke (2018), shame is ripe in organisations when people experience failure or when they have to speak about taboo topics, also about the experiences of not belonging to a certain group within the organisation. According to Wilke (2018), experiences of fragmentation within the organisation or "serial disruptions" in connection with leadership also create shameful experiences. Bligh and Ito (2018) emphasise that women leaders in particular are exposed to shame and shameful experiences in organisations and workplaces, while Cohen (2019) notes that shame regarding technology can be experienced in terms of personal and ontological shame. The experience of smart technology can also bring about shame (Müller, 2017). Müller (2017) reflects on the so-called Promethean shame which on one hand relates to identity questions and on the other refers to the power relations which are increased by machine dependence and generational shame. Further, shame can be experienced with regard to the sense of facing old age, illness, and disabilities that come with aging, referring to ideas of the changing body and decreasing health (Brooks Bouson, 2019). Shame can also be experienced in terms of generational changes within organisations, which bring rapid, complex changes which can be difficult to understand.

4 Research Methodology

4.1 Research Paradigm and Approach

The study follows a qualitative research paradigm and uses a hermeneutic-phenomenological research approach (Creswell, 2013). The research methodology is ethnographical and focuses on an organisational ethnographic insight which takes the experiences of the employees and the interpretation of these experiences through the eyes of the researcher into account (Hassan & Ghauri, 2014).

These findings on shame are part of a larger study on Industry 4.0 which was conducted within an organisation. However, for purpose of presenting the data on shame in the context of Industry 4.0, this chapter will only focus on shame without including other findings.

4.2 Research Methods

The research methods that have been used are primarily qualitative semi-structured interviews, as well as notes which were taken during interview sessions and during a 2-day training with one of the top managers within the organisation.

4.3 The Organisation, Access to the Organisation, and the Sample

The research was conducted in a German, world-leading engineering organisation. While the headquarters of this organisation is in Germany, the research was conducted in the South African subsidiary of the organisation which is based in Johannesburg. The company specialises in the area of water and water waste management in the broader sense and develops and produces state-of-the-art industrial applications for different industries, such as the mining, automation, dredging, and building industries. The values and the mission of the organisation in South Africa relate to the German code of conduct and the German corporate values which are anchored in the German organisation. The focus of the organisation is excellence, technology-driven solutions, and reliability as core while transitioning into Industry 4.0.

The researcher conducted a management training in the German organisation with one of the top directors. A need was identified to hear from managers at different levels and in different areas of the South African subsidy, to understand their viewpoints regarding Industry 4.0 and—on the basis of this research—to develop best practices to move forward into the Industry 4.0 transformation.

For the study, a purposeful sampling strategy was used (Shaheen & Pradhan, 2019) which took into account the position of the managers, their leadership role, the different representation of departments within the organisation, and their working years in the organisation (a minimum of 2 years).

The sample comprised 16 managers, of whom 15 were male and 1 female, 15 South Africans, and 1 German, between the ages of 32 and 60 years. The duration of working in the organisation ranged from 2 to 23 years. In terms of first language, eight interviewees spoke English, four Afrikaans, one German, and three were bilingual (Afrikaans and English). All interviewees participated voluntarily.

4.4 Data Collection, Analysis, and Reporting

Data was collected through interviews and notes based on observations and talks during a training session. The researcher spent altogether 3 days in the organisation and took notes when speaking to one of the top organisation managers. The interview sessions were between 60 and 75 minutes long and included these core questions: How do you experience transition into Industry 4.0? How do you feel with the changes happening in the organisation? How are Industry 4.0 and shame connected?

Analysis of the data was based on the five-step model of content analysis of Terre Blanche, Durrheim, and Kelly (2006, pp. 322–326). Accordingly, the following steps for data analysis were used: familiarisation and immersion (getting to know the data and understanding the content), inducing themes (finding the main themes with regard to shame and Industry 4.0), coding (coding of the dataset within the main themes), elaboration (exploring the topic of shame and Industry 4.0 in depth), and interpretation and checking to ensure data quality (exploring interpretation of data and checking the quality of the data and the data analysis).

All 16 interviews were recorded and transcribed verbatim. Written notes were taken electronically. Data was stored electronically and securely for a period of 5 years on a password-encrypted data file.

4.5 Qualitative Quality Criteria and Ethical Considerations

The research study is anchored in applied qualitative quality criteria. Rigour in the data quality was assured through the exploration of rich data material, in-depth analysis, and interpretation (Johnson, Adkins & Chauvin, 2019). The criterion of credibility was adhered to through triangulation of theory and methods (Creswell & Plano Clark, 2011). Confirmability and transferability of data were respected through intra-subjective validation processes and the use of established research theories and methods (Creswell, 2013; Yin, 2009). The study does not aim to provide generalisable findings (Creswell, 2013).

Ethical considerations include the creation of anonymity and transparency. We transparently describe only selected auto-ethnographical experiences and present situations and interactions in an anonymised way. The study was approved by the management of the organisation as well as by a German university. The organisation provided consent to conduct the research and supported access to the organisation and to its employees. Participants gave written consent to participate in the study and to having the findings reported anonymously. All participants were informed about confidentiality and of their rights to withdraw from the participation at any time and to not answer questions if they chose.

5 Findings

Generally, managers in the context of this highly technological engineering company are keenly aware of the transformation of the organisation into Industry 4.0. They associate the shift into Industry 4.0 with concepts of automatisation, implementation and construction of smart systems, technologisation processes, artificial intelligence, robots and robotics, as well as job loss.

The findings show that according to interviewees, emotions play a minor role in the process of Industry 4.0 and are not consciously taken into account. Moving into Industry 4.0 is viewed as a technological process in which human characteristics are not necessarily inherently involved. However, when asked about their views and experiences of shame with regard to the process of transformation, interviewees have a very clear idea about shame as a negative emotion, but also as an emotion with transformational potential and potential for personal growth and development.

5.1 How Are Industry 4.0 and Shame Interconnected?

While 9 of the 16 statements from managers emphasise that shame plays a rather negative role in the change towards Industry 4.0, 4 statements refer to positive connotations of shame in this context (Table 5.1).

In the following, the topics which are connected with shame and Industry 4.0 in a negative and positive way are presented.

Six participants explain that shame is experienced in the 4IR process when individuals see differences of knowledge of technology in the context of age and different generations. Managers expect that the older and highly knowledgeable managers who have worked in the field for many years are also able to drive the technology within the 4IR. However, often members of the older generation need to ask employees of younger generations for help and support in terms of understanding and handling technology. This often leaves them with a feeling of shame. P4 provides an example from a different context to make clear what could also be shameful in the organisational context:

> Let me give you an example. If I take a 56-year-old woman and I give her a piece of technology that she does not know how to use. And I give the same thing to a 10-year-old that can use it, the sense of shame will creep in. I don't care what you tell me. And it's—all you do is just feel that lack of worth. And it doesn't matter that you haven't been exposed to it. The fact that you can't perform the same function as a kid or someone younger than you, actually has that stigma. And it's got nothing to do with intelligence, or anything else. It's just that you haven't been exposed.

P4 explains that nonperformance and not being able to do the same thing as a child can bring shame to an adult. He also refers to the idea that not being able to perform is not necessarily connected to intelligence or ability, but to the fact that one has not had the chance to learn a specific function. However, even if an individual is aware that the non-ability is not connected to intelligence, the person could still feel ashamed since there is a common understanding that an adult, particularly in comparison to someone younger or even a child, should be able to perform at least on the same level as the younger person, if not better.

Besides the interlinkages of shame with age and generational identity, there is an experience of general shame when managers do not know the technology or how to deal with it. Six managers refer to this general shameful experience, independent of age or generational membership. For several of the managers, making mistakes or not being knowledgeable is shameful. However, P16 believes this should not be the case. He highlights that within the same organisation, people can ask questions and point out a gap in knowledge without being shamed or feeling ashamed themselves.

Table 5.1 Shame in the Industry 4.0 workplace

Connection between shame and Industry 4.0 negatively connotated	Connection between shame and Industry 4.0 positively connotated
P1, P3, P4, P5, P8, P11, P12, P13, P16	P1, P3, P5, P9
9 statements	4 statements

This manager emphasises that there is no shame with regard to asking questions or not knowing in this organisation:

> I've got colleagues with me; if they don't know something, they want to ask you how to do it. We've never had problems with people saying or feeling shame about it. If you haven't used it, you haven't used it, you go and ask somebody, and with me it's exactly the same. There's always going to be someone that knows more than you or has worked with the particular program to a greater extent. . . . So, we do help the colleagues that haven't got the experience in IT and that kind of stuff. I'm not aware of any shameful experiences here.

None of the employees should feel ashamed of having a question and learning new aspects which they need on the job.

Five employees report that they experience shame when they make mistakes and/or when they have to ask somebody else for help. P3 refers to this kind of situation: "On a personal level, from making a mistake and someone else laughs at you, that can shame you".

Additionally, shame is related to nonperformance. Managers feel intensely ashamed when they do not perform up to their own standards and to the standards of others or of the organisation. P13 points out that shame is strongly connected to performance:

> I think people think they're stupid; people think they not skilled. Umm. I use, always use my children, if I want anything done on my phone I ask my daughter. Ja of course I feel stupid asking her but I know she can do it because I think they've been brought up in a totally different mindset than what we grew up with. For them, that's the norm. For us, it's another thing we have to adapt to. We as humans are not very prone to changing easily. And it is shameful, if you cannot perform.

Again, here, shame is connected to nonperformance, particularly when compared to other individuals, such as the younger generation.

One manager can relate to shame and shameful experience in the context of social media. He highlights how social media can be a source of shame when people talk about each other on this digital medium. P5 states that he can only see shame within the context of the social media but that he considers social media a term from the 3IR, not even part of the 4IR: "I would say shame only comes in for like social media. But I don't see social media as the IR4".

P8 points out that there is shame when differences in education, educational standards, and backgrounds are seen or experienced. According to this manager, individuals in the organisation can easily feel ashamed when their educational background is lower than that of others and when this low educational standard impacts on their ability to correctly fill in forms, understand, act independently, or manage their work. P8 explains:

> That's when things are rolled out and people are not informed, misinformed or the interpretation of it is not correct. Then we have that way people are like, I'm not interested. Like I give up. I don't want to be involved. People have that, especially if you're in an environment where: "Oh my word. I can't believe you don't know about that!" Or "Oh my word. I can't believe you don't know how to do this." Then you have that, that when people are like, "Ja, thank you but no, thank you". Ja. So that often happens here because our workforce is quite diverse in the sense that we've got people with degrees and masters and doctors, and then

> you have the guy who has Grade 10 his highest grade. So, we do have that where they like, "No we don't talk to those people". We need to breach that.

The experience of shame caused by differences in educational background needs to be addressed in the organisation. Particularly in post-apartheid South Africa, the access to education varies as a consequence of historical and socio-cultural divides concerning where a person grew up and with regard to racial belonging, in terms of structures established during apartheid. The topic of shame with regard to educational standard is therefore very complex and related to culture, race, and socio-economic circumstances which can, again, re-enforce shame on different levels.

Finally, one manager confesses that it is a very shameful experience when a person loses a job because of being replaced by a robot. P11 comments:

> I was a little ashamed, but it wasn't, I wasn't affected too much because of responsibility and stuff. ... But what broke me down was the four years that I was unemployed. And I could have been working so for four years ... Every month I won the award and stuff. At least made a way for me, tried. But I mean they, even at the farewell and stuff, they let you make as if you were never worth it. And I know I was, because my awards tell me all. It was my choice to leave, because I was concerned. They didn't chase me away but I couldn't wait for the last day and pack up and move up.

This manager had lost his previous position owing to automatisation processes in the organisation. He resigned before he was fired, and he felt very ashamed of having lost his job to robots taking over his tasks. This shame was evident during the entire interview, showing the intensity of feelings experienced by this manager.

In parallel to the findings in which shame is described as a force that makes a person stagnate or wish to hide (Fig. 5.1), other managers in the organisational study highlight aspects of shame which impact positively on wanting to learn more and to grow (Fig. 5.2).

A shameful experience can become the motivator to learn or to get training, particularly in the 4IR, where many new things need to be learned. P1 reports that a positive attitude can be developed to overcome shame:

> I think in terms of the 4IR it will be training. I think everyone is open to change. Everyone's open to learning new things. There are people that might feel, okay I'm too old for this or I don't feel that this will benefit from it. But again, it's up to the company to try and motivate these, these, the set of workers to actually open their mind and get trained. I think they will.

In this case, shame can be seen as a motivator to keep an open mind and develop an open mindset based on personal experiences of shame, to ask for training and learning opportunities. This could be a positive and constructive way to deal with shame in the organisation, if shame is anchored in lacking knowledge and/or experience.

Two managers emphasise that being ashamed of not knowing can be painful but at the same time the shame of not knowing needs to be faced and transformed into personal involvement. P3, for example, states:

> Well, get involved, learn more. I like to get involved with developments, know what's going on. If there's something new, I want to know how to use it. Know how it works, do not be ashamed of not knowing it yet.... I need to know. Ja.

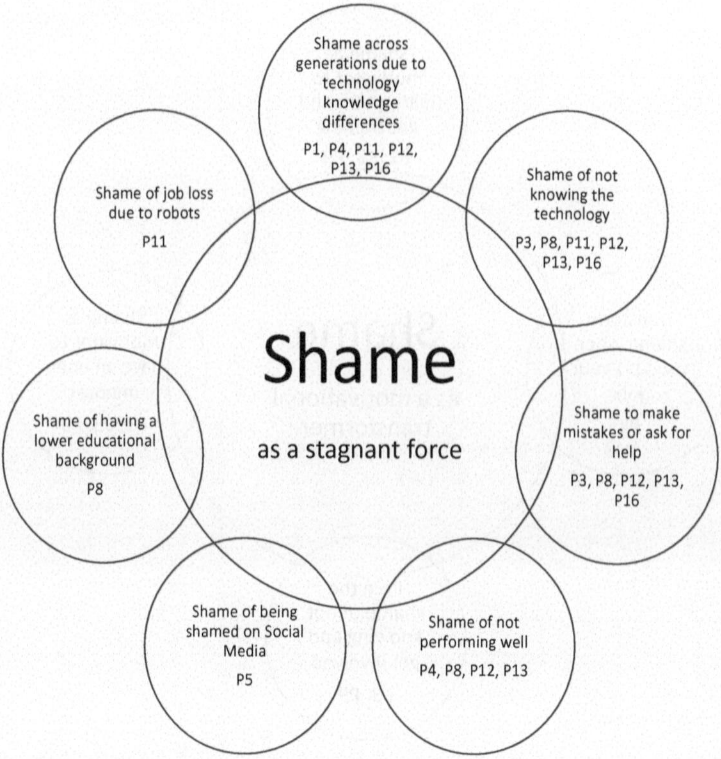

Fig. 5.1 Shame as a stagnant force

Finally, shame needs to be addressed and changed when individuals lose their jobs. The shame of job loss needs to be transformed into a feeling that can activate resources and help the individual to cope better (see Fig. 5.2).

6 Discussion

As suggested by Schwab (2017), managers in the organisation are emotionally affected by the transformation into Industry 4.0. On one hand, these processes are experienced as disruptive, while on the other, they are seen as an opportunity to change, develop, and grow. In the study, the question arose of how to deal with negatively experienced emotions to allow them to develop new meaning, positive aspects, and purpose in work (see Mayer, 2019). This study deepens the body of research on emotions in Industry 4.0, with special focus on shame. It supports previous studies which emphasise that emotions play a highly important role (Giardini & Frese, 2004; Rausch et al., 2017) and that they are connected to relationships, power, interdependence, meaning, identity formation, and activity

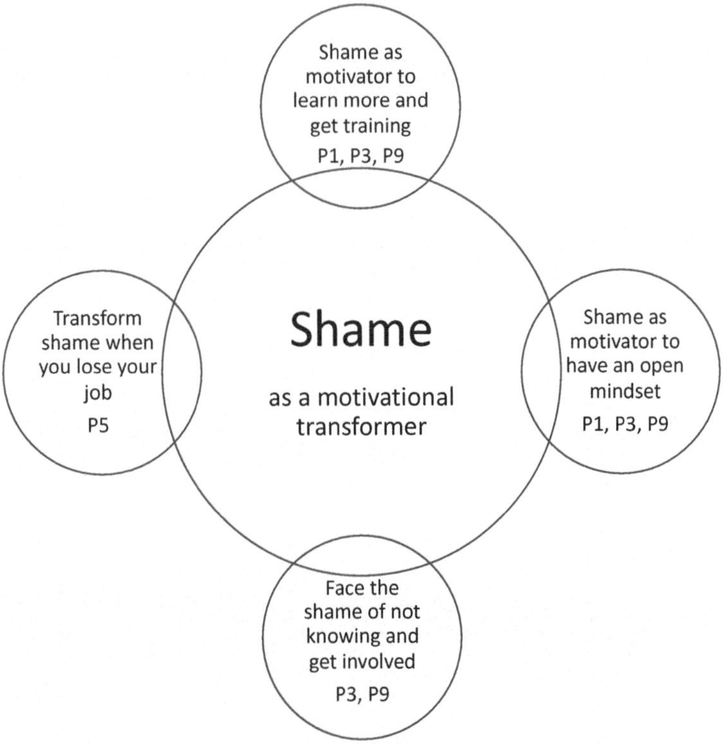
Shame as
motivator to
learn more and
get training
P1, P3, P9
Transform
shame when
you lose your
job
P5
Shame
as a motivational
transformer
Shame as
motivator to
have an open
mindset
P1, P3, P9
Face the
shame of not
knowing and
get involved
P3, P9

Fig. 5.2 Shame as a motivational transformer

(Küpers & Weibler, 2008). This study further supports the conclusion of Küpers and Weibler (2008) that emotions are defined as either negative or positive.

While emotions are supposed to contribute to organisational goals (Hirschhorn, 1988), it is questionable, based on the dataset on shame, whether experienced shame in the organisation contributes to the goals of the organisation.

Since managers identify shame, created by a generational split in terms of knowledge of technology, as well as shame with regard to a lack of knowledge in technology management, it might be assumed that the goals of shifting smoothly into Industry 4.0 are not fully supported. Further, the shame experienced when making mistakes, asking for help, or not performing well enough might not contribute to transforming the organisation with regard to its goals. It might instead hamper the achievement of these goals. Shame in the organisation also seems to be interlinked with managers' fears of not being able to work according to the new technological standards or of experiencing a lack of knowledge and ability. They also fear being shamed on social media, being judged according to differences in educational background, or of job loss to robots. Thereby, meaning and identity are created and developed along the lines of experiencing shame which defines the borders of in-group and out-group identities: the young and the old generations, the technological knowledgeable and the technological unknowledgeable, the educated and the uneducated, performers and nonperformers, those working with machines and those replaced by machines, the ones ashamed by mistakes and questions, and the ones who use questions and mistakes to move beyond. Obviously, shame creates boundaries to define identity within the organisation, as well as meaning (see Ashforth and Humphrey, 1993).

As demonstrated by Pratt and Doucet (2000), findings show that emotions can be experienced as positive and negative, while the data shows that shame is experienced as negative rather than as positive in the organisation studied. That means that not all the positive ripple effects of emotional labour are being used in the organisational transformation process. From the data analysis, it is obvious that the managers do not generally focus on emotions, emotional labour, or the impact of emotions within the organisation. The focus is on technological know-how and strategic management processes rather than on emotional and relationship-orientated social interaction. Therefore, it is understood that shame and the conversation about shame as a force for regulating social interaction (Gilbert, 2019) are not a very common topic within the organisation. The contention of Kets de Vries (2017), however, can be supported, in that shame shows to which power and judgement employees in the organisation adhere to. In this research, shame about language barriers in the organisation (see Jonker, 2019) is not expressed. However, the findings concur with those of Wilke (2018) that shame is experienced when managers make mistakes. The findings provide no information with regard to shame and gender, in view of the fact that most of the workforce is male and the interviewees, except one, were also only male. However, the findings support Cohen's (2019) proposition that shame can be experienced in the context of technology and that of Müller (2017) which is that shame impacts on identity and power relations within the organisation. In this case, power—through shameful experiences—is given to the younger generation by the older generation and to the technologically knowledgeable. This interlinks with the fact that when shame is experienced as a motivational transformer, it can encourage the desires to learn and be trained, to develop personally, to keep an open mind, and to face the shame of a lack of knowledge by getting involved and treating crises as a new starting point in life and career. A strong focus in this study is on shame in the context of generational divides and technological knowledge, taking age into consideration (see Brooks Bouson, 2019). However, there appears to be a lack in the literature since hardly any research could be found that highlights the shameful experiences of male, technologically orientated leaders and their shameful experiences in the context of rapid technological change, and the experience of failing to keep up with the latest trends in technology in their professional field.

The in-depth exploration of shame in particular can reveal fragile aspects of the organisation and highlight where to support employees to increase self-worth, a common, positive, and future-orientated mindset and meaningful identity.

7 Limitations

This study is limited to organisational ethnographical views and presents the voices of managers commenting on Industry 4.0 and shame in the context of their organisation. Findings only provide insight into 16 interviews and notes taken by one researcher during a limited amount of time spent in the organisation. Therefore, the data and findings of the study are limited and not generalisable. They only provide limited insight in the specific views of the managers interviewed with regard to the single organisation. Further, the data was analysed and interpreted by one single researcher, and this might lead to a researcher's bias which cannot be completely avoided in a qualitative study with regard to the individual choice of theory and methodology chosen as well as the interpretation of findings.

8 Conclusion

Emotions and feelings within the technologically orientated organisation impact strongly on employees. In the context of Industry 4.0, most of the managers in this study experience shame as negative emotion; however, a few also emphasise positive, transformational, and motivational aspects of shame in the context of the organisation. Shame defines boundaries in terms of generational divides, technological knowledge, identity creation, educational background, and the ability either to suffer through the pain of shame and stay within the negative aspects experienced through the emotion or to transform it into a resource for personal and organisational growth and development.

9 Recommendations from an Industrial and Organisational Psychology Perspective

Further research is needed which not only focuses on shame within the organisation but which also explores shame in depth, through mixed-method approaches and across industries in different cultures and countries. Further exploration is required to understand how Industry 4.0 is experienced by employees on different levels. Accordingly, negatively and positively experienced emotions can be taken into account; strategies to transform negative into positive, resourceful emotions need to be developed. In so doing, the boundaries which are created in organisations—based on emotional boundaries and experiences—can be taken into conscious consideration.

In particular it is recommended that shame in technological and engineering contexts is researched by industrial and organisational psychologists with regard to gender (female/male perceptions), along age and generational lines (younger and older generations) and in terms of technological knowledge and education (organisational impact). An understanding of shame can contribute to future critical research on identity, meaning, and power.

On a practical note, the organisation should focus on making processes more conscious with regard to emotional labour within the organisation. Industrial and organisational psychologists can support the processes of working with emotions in the organisation positively connotated and transformed emotions and to use the changes in the organisation towards Industry 4.0, as a position from which to grow and develop.

To expand self-worth, sense of belonging, conscious identity, and meaning creation in the organisation, the leadership of the organisation could provide managers and employees and the emotional labour involved with training in change management for Industry 4.0, so that negatively experienced emotions such as shame and anxiety can be transformed into creative and positive processes.

Boundary shifts within the workforce can then be implemented according to the organisational goals, once the emotional lines within the organisation are clearly explored and defined and the direction of change is agreed upon.

Acknowledgements Thanks to the organisation, to its employees and managers, and in particular to the CEO who provided the access and made it possible to run this research project.

References

Ashforth, B. E., & Humphrey, R. H. (1993). Emotional labor in service roles: The influence of identity. *Academy of Management Review, 18*(1), 88–115.

Barber, S. (2019). *A truly 'transformative' MBA: Executive education for the fourth industrial revolution*. University of Bedfordshire. UK. Retrieved from http://hdl.handle.net/10547/622822

Bigman, Y. E., Sheppes, G., & Tamir, M. (2017). When less is more: Effects of the availability of strategic options on regulating negative emotions. *Emotion, 17*(6), 993–1006.

Bligh, M., & Ito, A. (2018). Chapter 18. Organizational processes and systems that affect women in leadership. In S. R. Madsen (Ed.), *Handbook of research on gender and leadership*. Cheltenham, UK: Elgar Online.

Brooks Bouson, J. (2019). *Shame and the aging woman. Confronting and resisting ageism in contemporary women's writing*. Cham, Switzerland: Springer.

Burkitt, I. (1997). Social relationships and emotions. *Sociology, 31*(1), 37–55.

Coetzee, M. (2019). Organisational climate conditions of psychological safety as thriving mechanism in digital workspaces. In M. Coetzee (Ed.), *Thriving in digital workspaces* (pp. 311–327). Cham, Switzerland: Springer.

Cohen, B. (2019). A contemporary Jungian Lense o temporality and shame. *Jung Journal. Culture & Psyche, 13*(2), 106–114.

Collins, R. (1990). Stratification, emotional energy, and the transient emotions. In T. D. Kemper (Ed.), *Research agendas in the sociology of emotions* (pp. 27–57). Albany, NY: State University of New York Press.

Creswell, J. W. (2013). *Qualitative inquiry & research: Choosing among five approaches* (3rd ed.). London: Sage.

Creswell, J. W., & Plano Clark, V. I. (2011). *Designing and conducting mixed methods research* (2nd ed.). London: Sage.

Erickson, R. J. (1997). Putting emotions to work (or, coming to terms with a contradiction in terms). In R. J. Erickson & B. Cuthbertson-Johnson (Eds.), *Social perspectives on emotion* (pp. 3–18). Greenwich, CT: JAI Press.

Frijda, N. H., & Mesquita, B. (1994). The social roles and functions of emotions. Emotion and culture. In S. Kitayama & H. Markus (Eds.), *Emotion and culture: Empirical studies of mutual influence* (pp. 51–87). Washington, DC: Springer.

Giardini, A., & Frese, M. (2004). Emotionen in organisationen. In G. Schreyögg & A. von Werder (Eds.), *Handwörterbuch Unternehmensführung und Organisation* (pp. 205–214). Stuttgart: Schaeffer-Poeschel.

Gilbert, P. (2019). Distinguishing shame, humiliation and guilt: An evolutionary functional analysis and compassion focused interventions. In C.-H. Mayer & E. Vanderheiden (Eds.), *The bright side of shame. Transforming and growing through practical applications in cultural contexts* (pp. 413–431). Cham: Springer.

Glikson, E., & Erez, M. (2013). Emotion display norms in virtual teams. *Journal of Personnel Psychology, 12*(1), 22–32.

Hassan, I., & Ghauri, P. N. (2014). Evaluating companies for mergers and acquisitions. *Book Series: International Business and Management, 40*, 75–89.

Hirschhorn, L. (1988). *The workplace within: Psychodynamics of organizational life*. Cambridge, MA: MIT Press.

Johnson, J. L., Adkins, D. & Chauvin, S. (2019). Quality indicators of rigor in qualitative research. *American Journal of Pharmaceutical Education, 84*(2), 1–22. Retrieved from https://www.ajpe.org/content/ajpe/early/2019/12/10/ajpe7120.full.pdf

Jonker, C. (2019). Emotion experiences and management within digital work contexts. In M. Coetzee (Ed.), *Thriving in digital workspaces* (pp. 131–144). Cham, Switzerland: Springer.

Kamaruzaman, F. M., Hamid, R., Mutalib, A. A., & Rasul, M. S. (2019). Conceptual framework for the development of 4IR skills for engineering graduates. *Global Journal of Engineering Education, 21*(1), 54–61.

Karim, N. K. A. (2019). Doing emotional labour in the fourth industrial revolution (4IR): Is religious television a humanized workplace? *Jurnal Komunikasi: Malaysian Journal of Communication, Jilid, 35*(2), 379–396.

Kets de Vries, M. F. R. (2017). *Riding the leadership rollercoaster*. London: Palgrave McMillian.

Küpers, W., & Weibler, J. (2008). Emotions in organization: An integral perspective. *International Journal of Work Organizations and Emotions, 2*(3), 256–287.

Mayer, C.-H. (2011). *The meaning of sense of coherence in transcultural management. Internationale Hochschulschriften Series*. Münster: Waxmann.

Mayer, C.-H. (2019). Key factors of creativity and the art of collaboration in twenty-first-century workspaces. In M. Coetzee (Ed.), *Thriving in digital workplaces: Innovations in theory, research and practice* (pp. 147–166). Cham, Switzerland: Springer.

Mayer, C.-H., & Vanderheiden, E. (2019). *The bright side of shame. Transforming and growing through practical applications in cultural contexts*. Cham, Switzerland: Springer.

Mayer, C.-H., Viviers, R., & Tonelli, L. (2017). 'The fact that she just looked at me…' Narrations on shame in South African workplaces. *South African Journal of Industrial Psychology SA Tydskrif vir Bedryfsielkunde, 43*(0), a1385. https://doi.org/10.4102/sajip.v43i0.1385.

Müller, C. J. (2017). *Günther Anders, smart technology and the rise of promethean shame*. Rowman & Littlefield International Blog.

Nankervis, A., Connell, J., Cameron, R., Montague, A., & Prikshat, V. (2019). 'Are we there yet?' Australian HR professionals and the Fourth Industrial Revolution. *Asia Pacific Journal of Human Resources*.

Oosthuizen, J. H. (2016). Entrepreneurial intelligence: Expanding Schwab's four-type intelligence proposition to meaningfully address the challenges of the fourth industrial revolution. In *Proceedings of the 28th Annual Conference of the Southern African Institute of Management Scientists*. Retrieved from http://mediachef.co.za/saims-2016/papers/SME4_Full.pdf

Oosthuizen, J. H. (2019). Managing shame in organizations: Don't let shame become a self-destructive spiral. In C.-H. Mayer & E. Vanderheiden (Eds.), *The bright side of shame: Transforming and growing through practical applications in cultural contexts* (pp. 217–234). Cham, Switzerland: Springer.

Oosthuizen, R. M., & Mayer, C.-H. (2019). At the edge of the fourth industrial revolution: Employees' perceptions of employment equity from a CIBART perspective. *SA Journal of Industrial Psychology/SA Tydskrif vir Bedryfsielkunde, 45*(0), a1695. https://doi.org/10.4102/sajip.v45i0.1695.

Palmer, I., & Hardy, C. (2000). *Thinking about management: Implications of organizational debates for practice*. London: Sage.

Pratt, M. G., & Doucet, L. (2000). Ambivalent feelings in organizational relationships'. In *Emotion in organizations* (2nd ed., pp. 204–226). London: Sage.

Rausch, A., Seifried, J., & Harteis, C. (2017). Emotions, coping and learning in error situations in the workplace. *Journal of Workplace Learning, 29*(5), 370–389.

Sahu, A., & Srivastava, K. B. (2017). Antecendents and consequencesof positive emotions in the workplace. *International Journal of Work Organisation and Emotion, 8*(2), 99–217.

Schwab, K. (2016). *Welcoming faith in the fourth industrial revolution: Responding to globalization, governance, and norms*. Berkley, Georgetown University. Retrieved August 20, 2018, from https://berkleycenter.georgetown.edu/responses/welcoming-faith-in-thefourth-industrial-revolution

Schwab, K. (2017). The Fourth Industrial Revolution: What it means, how to respond. In *World Economic Forum.*

Shaheen, M., & Pradhan, S. (2019). Sampling in qualitative research. In *Qualitative techniques for workplace data analysis* (pp. 25–51). Pennsylvania: IGI Global.

Temekova, M. (2018). Studying the leadership style of business organizations' management under the conditions of the Fourth Industrial Revolution. *Asia Pacific Journal of Research and Business Management, 9*(2), 1–15.

Terre Blanche, M., Durrheim, K., & Kelly, K. (2006). First steps in qualitative data analysis. In M. Terre Blanche, K. Durrheim, & D. Painter (Eds.), *Research in practice: Applied methods for the social sciences* (pp. 321–344). Cape Town, SA: University of Cape Town.

van Maanen, J., & Kunda, G. (1989). Real feelings: Emotional expression and organizational culture. *Research in Organizational Behavior, 11*, 43–103.

Wilke, G. (2018). The art of group analysis in organizations. In *The use of intuitive and experiential knowledge*. New York, NJ: Routledge.

Wong, P. T. P. (2019). Foreword: from shame to wholeness: An existential positive psychology perspective. In C.-H. Mayer & E. Vanderheiden (Eds.), *The bright side of shame. Transforming and growing through practical applications in cultural contexts* (pp. v–xi). Cham, Switzerland: Springer.

Yin, R. K. (2009). *Case study research: Design and methods* (4th ed.). London: Sage.

Zerbe, W. J., Ashkanasy, N., & Hartel, C. (Eds.). (2006). *Overview: Individual and organizational perspectives on emotion management and display. Research on emotions in organizations: Individual and organizational perspectives on emotion management and display* (Vol. 2, pp. xv–xxiii). Oxford, UK: Elsevier JAI.

Claude-Hélène Mayer (Dr. habil., Ph.D., Ph.D.) is a Professor in Industrial and Organisational Psychology in the Department of Industrial Psychology and People Management at the University of Johannesburg; an Adjunct Professor at the European University Viadrina in Frankfurt (Oder), Germany; and a Senior Research Associate at Rhodes University, Grahamstown, South Africa. She holds a Ph.D. in Psychology (University of Pretoria, South Africa), a Ph.D. in Management (Rhodes University, South Africa), a Doctorate (Georg-August University, Germany) in Political Sciences (socio-cultural anthropology and intercultural didactics), and a Habilitation (European University Viadrina, Germany) in Psychology with focus on work, organisational, and cultural psychology. She has published several monographs, text collections, accredited journal articles, and special issues on transcultural mental health and well-being, sense of coherence, shame, transcultural conflict management and mediation, women in leadership in culturally diverse work contexts, constellation work, coaching, and psychobiography.

Chapter 6
Bias, Prejudice and Shame in Predictive Policing: State-of-the-Art and Potential Interventions for Professionals

Claude-Hélène Mayer

> *The interpretation of our reality*
> *through patterns not our own*
> *only makes us ever more unknown,*
> *ever less free,*
> *ever more solitary.*
> —Gabriel Garcia Marquez

1 Introduction

How to deal with prejudice and bias is a question that has long been addressed by social psychologists, not only with regard to individuals but also with regard to groups (Correll, Judd, Park, & Wittenbrink, 2010). A new aspect of this question which has impacted on the discourse during the past years is how to address prejudice (Bryne, Rosenblat, & Boyd, 2015) and bias (Garcia, 2017) when it is technologised and automated through the use of computerised programs, algorithms, and in the collection, analysis and use of big data.

This is particularly relevant to the new predictive policing programs which are implemented in crime prevention, as well as early offender and victim detection, particularly in the USA, Australia and Europe (Brantingham, Valasik & Mohler, 2018). Brantingham et al. (2018) have pointed out that these programs make use of and even strengthen prejudice and bias, particularly targeting minority groups and individuals belonging to these groups. Their study shows that arrests of criminals in Los Angeles, for example, were numerically higher at the algorithmically predicted locations, while convictions were lower or remained unchanged. Other recent reports from Los Angeles (Ahmed, 2018) recalculate "hot spots" of criminal acts within

C.-H. Mayer (✉)
Department of Industrial Psychology and People Management, University of Johannesburg, Auckland Park, Johannesburg, South Africa

Kulturwissenschaftliche Fakultät, Europa Universität Viadrina, Frankfurt (Oder), Germany

C.-H. Mayer et al. (eds.), *Shame 4.0*, https://doi.org/10.1007/978-3-030-59527-2_6

metropolitan areas by adapting models which predict earthquake aftershocks. According to the author, these models continue "pathologising" individuals and specific neighbourhoods. They proceed with historical discriminatory practices and racist policing practices while they claim computer-based objectivity (Ahmed, 2018). Human rights activists claim that "justice should be blind, right?" However, US-developed predictive policing tools use programs—called HunchLab, ComStat or PredPol—which have bias, prejudices and misunderstanding built into their programming (O'Neil, 2017). This is particularly the case in the USA, where "geography is a highly effective proxy for race" (O'Neil 2017). O'Neil (2017) argues that big data in predictive policing increases inequality and threatens democracy.

Besides the cognitive and behavioural impacts, bias and prejudice in predictive policing also impact emotionally. According to Zarsky (2012, p. 247), predictive policing produces transparency which "facilitates shaming". The author emphasises that expected transparency and surveillance affect behavioural performance and conformity to avoid shame. At the same time, it can be expected that individuals and groups feel ashamed when they are predicted to be offenders or victims of future crime, based on computerised programs that use information about friendships, networks, territory, social media activity and drug use (Schnelle, 2015). However, the way in which shame will manifest differently in potential offenders and victims needs to be researched empirically in future studies.

In this chapter, prejudice and bias in the context of predictive policing are discussed, and predictive policing, as a new way of predicting criminal activity, offenders and victims in times of Industry 4.0, is introduced. Perspectives on interlinkages of prejudice, bias on the side of program developers, analysts and policing officers, together with shame potentially experienced by perpetrators and victims, are reflected. Shame becomes Shame 4.0—an emotion that might be evoked through computerised predictive categorisation, bias and prejudice imposed on individuals and group members who are categorised as potential offenders or victims (see also Mayer and Vanderheiden on Investigating an Emotion in Digital Worlds and the Fourth Industrial Revolution in this book).

In this theoretical and reflective chapter, the author explores the topic from a social psychology perspective and responds to the theoretical question of how prejudice, bias and shame are connected in the predictive policing context which uses the Fourth Industrial Revolution technology to combat crime more effectively. Not only does the chapter refer to situations where these techniques are currently used, but it also touches on other cultural contexts, such as South Africa, in which politicians and criminal scientists aim to introduce predictive policing to find smart solutions to the overwhelming impact of crime on the society (see also Vanderheiden and Mayer on "Who Could Breathe Without Hope"—Some Theses on Shame and Shaming in the Age of Corona Pandemic in this book).

2 Social Psychology Perspectives on Prejudice, Bias and Emotion

In the history of social psychology, numerous researchers have studied prejudice and have come up with manifold definitions (Allport, 1954; Dovidio & Gaertner, 1986; Correll et al., 2010). The definition most often used refers to a negative attitude held by an individual or a group towards a particular social group and its members (Correll et al., 2010). Prejudices are divided into three components (cognitive, affective and behavioural) and are often associated with stereotypes, which are category-based generalisations that connect members of the social group to typical attitudes and discrimination (Correll et al., 2010).

Social psychologists have addressed the topic of prejudice over the past century from different theoretical and conceptual directions, such as essentialist and constructivist approaches, evolutionary and intergroup explanations, ideological systems and developmental theories, as well as cognitive theory and social neuroscience (Jackson, 2011). Fiske (2019) explains that prejudice is usually defined as affective bias, stereotyping as cognitive bias and discrimination as behavioural bias which are often unconsciously directed against members of other social groups, then leading to discriminative practices. Prejudice and bias are not always directed against members of other groups; it can also be held against members of the own group (Fiske, 2019).

The focus on forms of prejudice (such as implicit and explicit forms) has developed according to context, socio-cultural and temporal epochs and has changed over time (Ferguson, Branscombe & Reynolds, 2019). At the beginning of social psychology research in the 1920s, psychologists researched white superiority and were often guided by open racism against other groups and minorities. This changed in the 1930s when social and cultural biases were in focus, and since then, prejudice and bias in research are questioned. Research on prejudice has been classified as research reflecting social change and reformations of group membership based on categorisations of in-group and out-group memberships (Ferguson et al., 2019). According to research conducted by Haslam, Reicher, and Reynolds (2012), there is evidence that in-group members—when viewed as prototypical—gain more support than when seen as peripherals, even when they seem to be harmful to others in their prototypical roles.

Emotions play a crucial role in research on prejudice and biases. Fiske (in Chamberlin, 2004), who is based at Princeton University and has conducted a relevant meta-study on prejudice and emotions, indicates that emotions play an important role in the context of prejudice and bias across cultures. Thereby, the amygdala described as the part of the brain responsible for the prejudice, as well as explicit and implicit bias (Lu, 2016).

Strategies to combat prejudices, to counteract them or even to transform them have been adjusted spatiotemporally, always depending on the contextual determinants of prejudice (Correll et al., 2010; Mayer, 2004). Lu (2016) concludes that emotions are a key component in terms of aiming at reducing prejudice and bias based on the evaluation of self and others. Consequently, social emotions such as shame play a particularly important role as social influence which shapes the thoughts, decision-making and broader behaviour of individuals (Damasio, 2010). Further, Damasio (2010) indicates that the emotional aspect of prejudice is strongly connected to the idea of what is socially acceptable and what is not. Implicit bias, in particular, is deeply rooted in emotional processing and learning, based on individual learning processes, but also influenced by implicit and unconscious social conditioning. In later research, Damasio (2010) observes that conscious willpower can influence the conscious emotional reaction based on prejudice and bias. It cannot, however, influence the emotional processing which leads to unconscious emotional reactions such as body language. An example of body language which is beyond conscious emotional control is the frequency of blinking the eyes. It has been shown that the frequency of blinking is an element of discriminatory expression of unconscious prejudice and bias. This implicit socio-emotional behaviour forms part of unconscious behaviour within a society; it is deep-rooted and change-resistant since emotions are linked with implicit bias, socio-collective behaviour and racial stimuli (Lu, 2016). Focusing on prejudice and bias should therefore also include gaining deeper insight into shame as a social emotion which interlinks with concepts such as ethics, fairness and morals.

3 Shame in the Context of Policing, Prejudice and Bias

Shame can be considered a prosocial emotion—which means that when people experience shame concerning a specific behaviour, they are willing to amend their own behaviour. However, individuals do not usually welcome the experience of self-critical emotions and therefore tend to avoid them. Ideally, shame could consciously be transformed to contribute to personal and collective growth and development (Mayer, 2019c, d). If shame is experienced by an individual, it can lead to a change in action, although positively experienced feelings may lead to more positive intergroup relationships and positive human-orientated values than negative emotions (Abrams, 2010). So, shame—as an emotion that is usually avoided—can, according to Sullivan (2017), even be used consciously in organisations to evoke changes of behaviour in individuals who tend to be prejudiced or biased. However, Abrams (2010) believes that individuals should not be shamed with the aim of changing their behaviour into a more acceptable form. Jacquet (2015) emphasises that using shaming as a tactic of socialisation can prevent corporate misconduct, institutional abuse and also impact on politics and other collectives. The author describes different ways in which shaming can contribute positively to the well-being of a collective and also suggests that shame used in the online virtual world could potentially minimise misbehaviour and misconduct. Shame might therefore be an emotion that regulates behaviour but is also an emotion which is viewed as a stepping stone in seeking help and being willing to take on help (Efrati, 2018).

Shame has generally been believed to promote positive behavioural change by improving the self-image of people when they experience shame and change towards the better (De Hooge, Zeelenberg, & Breugelmans, 2011). Jacquet, Hauert, Traulsen, and Milinski (2011) argue that shame promotes motivation to contribute to a common good. At the same time, shame can also evoke a flight or escape mechanism and lead to even more problematic behaviour (Tangney & Dearing, 2002). Therefore, shame might, according to Efrati (2018, p. 30), be "more a risk factor than a deterrent" (see also Vanderheiden on The Terror of Being Judged: Public Shaming as Resource and Strategic Tool in this book).

Previous research has concluded that individuals with drug abuse behaviour who display shame when talking about their addiction tend to relapse and decline in health faster than those who do not evince shame. Based on this observation, it might be counterproductive to use shaming punishment against certain kind of individuals and groups in crime prevention and criminal justice procedures (Efrati, 2018). Efrati (2018) comments on the discourse which was first started by Braithwaite (1989) who argued that shaming punishment can support crime prevention when offenders are shamed by community members and when they are then actively reintegrated. Shaming in criminal justice in terms of the so-called disintegrative shaming—which aims at the stigmatisation of individuals—is viewed critically, since the individual is focused on, shamed, isolated and humiliated, while in reintegrative shaming (Braithwaite, 1989), the person is respected, and the crime, not the person, is identified as the problem. The person is reaccepted into the community or society and can make reparation for the criminal act. Research has shown that when stigmatisation practices are used, instead of reintegrative shaming, higher rates of re-offence occur (Murphy & Harris, 2007).

Tangney, Stuewig and Hafez (2011) report that experiences of shame often evoke hiding, denial or escape and that shame disrupts the ability to be empathic with others. They have further found that shame is generally associated with the externalisation of blame, anger and aggression, as well as with hostility. In earlier research, Tangney (1990) pointed out that feelings of shame might lead to externalised, uncontrolled and rage towards any person, irrespective of their connection with the shameful event. Tangney et al. (2011) also observe that shame can be linked to different symptoms of psychological problems, such as low self-esteem, depression, anxiety, eating disorders or suicide. Further, although different studies highlight that shame in childhood and shame-proneness in general might predict criminal behaviour later in life, it has also been shown that studies are contradictory and shame may also not predict criminal behaviour (Tangney, Stuewig, & Hafez, 2011).

Mayer (2019a, b, c, d) proposes that the relationships between shame, shaming and crime, as well as between shame, individuals and their cultural background, need to be explored further before applying general statements to whether shaming can support minimising crime and criminal behaviour. Studies may not provide a holistic and comprehensive view on shame and crime and might relate only to specific socio-cultural groups (e.g. white and African-American inmates in prison in Hosser, Windzio and Greve's 2008 study). Additionally, it has been highlighted that shame can be viewed in a positive light as being able to transform a negatively experienced emotion towards personal growth and well-being (Mayer & Vanderheiden, 2019; Vanderheiden & Mayer, 2017).

Harris (2017) points out that there is scant research on shame within criminological theory in terms of its benefits and its positive effects. There are also hardly any studies of shame in the context of crime, prejudice and bias (Mayer, 2019a). However, those that exist touch on crime, the experience of stigmatisation and shame (Benson, Alerid, Burtn, & Cullen, 2011; Schwarcz, 2003). Shame in potential offenders and victims, as classified by predictive policing processes, might differ according to the socio-cultural value sets of the social groups and the judgement behaviour of predictors and victims within the social communities besides the individual scope of reaction.

In the following paragraphs, the author draws attention to prejudice and bias in the technological age, before focusing on prejudice and bias in the context of predictive policing.

4 Prejudice and Bias in the Technological Age

Prejudice and bias are no longer regarded only as social phenomena but as widespread socio-technological phenomena, fostered, in predictive policing contexts, by historical data bias and decisions on how to analyse and interpret big data collections (Meijer & Wessels, 2019). The impact of prejudice has become a technologised phenomenon in a world that relies increasingly on technology, digitalisation, artificial intelligence programs and algorithms (Hvistendahl, 2016).

In this context, prejudice research has gained particular interest in studies focusing on technology and technological bias, including predictive policing (Spencer, Charbonneau, & Glaser, 2018). The technological innovation often refers to artificial intelligence and algorithms which are contemporarily used in policing and law enforcement, the combat of criminal offence and victimisation, to minimise crime and predict potential crime scenes, crime offenders and victims (Uchida, 2014). Related topics which are often discussed in the context of technologised crime prevention are privacy, transparency, fairness, accountability and ethical considerations (Asaro, 2018). Additionally, bias, discrimination of minorities and prejudices (Weitzer & Tuch, 2005) as well as critical evaluations and requests for further systematic research on benefits and drawbacks (Meijer & Wessels, 2019) have been made public.

From a positive perspective, Lu (2016) points out that technological evolution can support the change in bias and prejudice by controlling emotional responses to the self and others more effectively, since emotional reactions might be more neutral when technologised. Accordingly, Lu (2016) reasons that online chatrooms might support controlling chat and communication spaces regarding prejudice and bias and guide discourses into a more neutral or even more positive direction. This may be the case since subtle discriminatory behaviour and clues are reduced and mediated through technology when communicating with others. White, Abu-Rayya, Bliuc and Faulkner (2015) confirm that technologically structured internet interactions can support the optimal managing of intergroup biases when individuals act online and through computerised technology. However, when dealing with algorithms in artificial intelligence and machine learning, Devlin (2017) emphasises that programs and algorithms are ingrained with racial and gender prejudices and biases which are implicitly inherited in the language use patterns. Since machines lack moral ideas, logic and common sense, they are not equipped to deal with biases. Counteraction of biases and prejudices lies in the hands of programmers, analysts and decision-makers. Therefore, it is argued here that individuals in key predictive policing positions need to become aware of the potential social implications of their roles in terms of prejudices and biases.

5 Predictive Policing, Prejudice and Bias

This chapter focuses on shame with regard to prejudices and bias in predictive policing which is mediated through programming, predictive police data collection and its use in decision-making regarding potential crime scenes and its connection to shame. Predictive policing is defined as "the use of analytical techniques by law enforcement to make statistical predictions about potential criminal activity" (Perry, McInnis, Price, Smith, & Hollywood, 2013). It is argued here that human bias is no longer a socio-cultural problem only but also a socio-cultural-technologised problem which is based on defined algorithmic patterns, as well as the collection and analysis of big data (Weitzer & Tuch, 2005). These patterns and programs often seem to prejudice against race, gender, culture, language, neighbourhood or other minority-related groups (see Brantingham et al. 2018; Devlin, 2017; and Schnelle, 2015).

During the past years, bias and prejudice have come into focus in policing in the USA, Europe and Australia, not only in face-to-face policing interactions but also in predictive policing programs (Hvistendahl, 2016; Schnelle, 2015; Siegel, 2018). Bauer (2019) points out that predictive policing in Germany is particularly successful in selected contexts and is supposed to be based on the use of computerised technical data in combination with a clear and defined ethical understanding to protect individuals and minority group members in particular from being misjudged. For specific crimes, such as domestic burglaries in the German context, Gerstner (2017) highlights that predictive policing can assist with prevention. The South African president has also recently highlighted the potential value of predictive policing for the crime-ridden South African context (SAPS, 2019).

Ahmad Malik (2016) comments that predictive policing aims to cater for crime reduction and to address the challenges of a growing range of criminal offences, shifting ethnological and demographic environments and urbanisation trends, which increase crime in certain areas of developed and developing countries. Further, it has been emphasised that machine-based policing predictions cannot stand on their own and should only function to provide system advice to reinforce human advice (Joh, 2015). Often, crime mapping tools and data mining techniques are combined to create adequate predictive policing. And Egbert (2019) points out that predictive policing tools build primarily on location-based policing, rational choice theory, problem-orientated policing and environmental criminology, all of which are well-known concepts in classical policing theory.

The application of predictive policing seeks to predict "where and when crime is likely to occur or (it) identifies people most at risk of becoming perpetrators or victims" (Hvistendahl, 2016). However, depending on the contextual deterrents, prejudice and bias need to be monitored and controlled in predictive policing systems and their contexts. Therefore, for example, Germany uses mainly an algorithmic-mediated analysis approach (Kitchin, 2014).

Researchers have pointed out that a major cause of prejudiced and biased policing is that of the so-called implicit bias which often operates outside conscious knowledge and awareness (Spencer et al., 2018). Implicit prejudices are described as being problematic, since they unconsciously influence decisions and behaviours, often negative ascriptions, towards members of a specific group (Spencer et al., 2018; Wittenbrink, Correll & Ma, 2019). The implicit bias might be caused by different factors and is found in computerised programs and algorithms, depending on the foci of the programs and the way data is collected, analysed and finally interpreted. However, Završnik (2017) contends that the automated criminal justice system through algorithmic pattern analysis should eliminate bias, being based on mathematical concepts without prejudice while assisting with predicting, investigating and solving crimes. Ioimo (2018) affirms that these programs can support decision-making and provide tactical and strategic recommendations to combat crime.

Focusing on the reason for the development of biases, Wittenbrink et al. (2019) argue that implicit bias might develop particularly in response to limited motivation to make free and conscious decisions, missing awareness and a different (e.g. technologised) focus or as a consequence of generalisations of personal or collective experiences with members of specific groups. Spencer et al. (2018) suggest, for example, that black people might be unconsciously associated with crime, hostility and violence in different socio-cultural settings. Others have supported the view that algorithms increase particularly racial bias and are a threat to data privacy, because the programs use computer-generated predications based on big data sets which predict that individuals as members of certain groups are more likely to be involved in crime (as either offenders or victims) than others (Bryne et al., 2015). Bauer (2019) highlights that crime is predicted, on one hand, in terms of individual crime and people involved in crime, while it can also be predicted, on the other hand, in terms of territory and location of crimes. Boyd, Levy and Marwick (2014) conclude that algorithmic discrimination is usually based on the social network nature of the individual, using digital and computerised information about individuals' social networks. Consequently, the individual is identified based on personal social network connections (Boyd et al., 2014). These connections lead to biases against in-group or out-group members (Bryne et al., 2015; Malone, 2018) but often against members of specific groups, such as urban refugees (Nyaoro, 2010), racial minorities (Weitzer & Tuch, 2005), LGBT+ group members (Pickles, 2019) or specific cultural groups (Murphy et al., 2017). Social group socialisation and projection impact on the experience and perception of prejudices against individuals with different ethnic group memberships (Gatto & Dambrun, 2012). Greene (2019) even calls predictive policing "a scam that perpetuates systemic bias" for covering up unlawful policing and spreading misinformation. Individuals affected by predictive policing—as either potential perpetrators or victims—might experience shame.

Research has shown that prejudice is not linked to only one specific attitude towards certain membership criteria such as race, ethnicity, sex or age, but rather to a combination of different intersectionalities (meaning a combination of prejudice and discriminative attitudes towards more than one attribution). In this regard, it has been observed that intersectionalities impact in complex ways on perception and prejudice in the policing context, as is the case, for example, with regard to policing and black women (Chigwada, 2013). Sidanius, Hudson, Davis and Bergh (2018) emphasise that in policing, categories such as race and gender cannot be viewed as independent, but rather as intersectional. Race and gender intersect with one another, often to maintain group-based hierarchies and oppression (Sidanius et al., 2018). Fiske (2019) even highlights that the world of the twenty-first century becomes so complex, uncertain and volatile that previous prejudices, stereotypes and categories are no longer valuable or plausible and that people need to recognise the individual characters of other people, rather than creating superficial and outside-based (social and power-related) categories of historically ascribed social group membership. However, the idea of intersectionalities and their impact on social group relationships has been underestimated in social psychology as well as in crime science and has therefore been underutilised to explain group behaviour (Bowleg, 2017).

Experiencing prejudice and bias through machine learning, algorithms and predictive policing can lead to feelings of shame. Fox (2007) emphasises that the power of shame only affects those who experience shame, not those who are "shameless". Taking Brayne's (2018) differentiation regarding place-based predictive policing and person-based predictive policing into consideration, it might be assumed that person-based predictive policing—which focuses on the individual's criminal history, social networks, contacts and their classification as "highest-risk individuals" (Brayne, 2018, p. 297)—is experienced as prejudiced and biased in terms of policing strategies. This might further create shame with regard to potential person-or placed-based policing predictions. However, this issue has scarcely been addressed in the research on predictive policing, prejudice and bias.

6 Social Identity Theory and Its Impact on Predictive Policing

In policing studies and with regard to the historical contexts of prejudice, attitude and criminal behaviour, the individual, as a social group member, plays an important role in the development of criminal behaviour and crime science (Viki & Abrams, 2012). Social group membership is considered highly significant in terms of cultural deviance, social disorganisation and the impact of social force theories which are well known in criminal sciences (Viki & Abrams, 2012). From a social psychology perspective, social identity theory (Tajfel & Turner, 1986) has emphasised that individuals usually define their own group as positive, while they classify members of other social groups as negative. The motivation to define the own group as positive includes the wish for a meaningful social belonging, positive self-enhancement and stability (Tajfel, 1972).

In the context of social identity theory, much research has been conducted in the field of group identity and polarisation, highlighting that in-group discussions lead to radical divergence of attitudes within and across groups, when group members seek support for their own ideas (Isenberg, 1986). They then strengthen the ideas of other in-group members through new arguments (called persuasive argument theory). Social comparison theory posits that individuals usually want to be seen in a favourable light, even more favourable than other members of the group, and they therefore shift towards an extreme and contrasting position within the in-group (Viki & Abrams, 2012). Multiple research has supported the theoretical reflections on in- and out-group separation and emphasised that these social dynamics within groups and the experience of opposing viewpoints lead to shifts in norms within in-group cultures (see Hogg & Reid, 2006).

With regard to predictive policing, it might be assumed that these theoretical stances influence the programming and analysis of socio-cultural, ethnic, racial and neighbourhood patterns which are used in algorithmic searches for future offenders and crime victims. Often, predictive policing programs appear to take an extreme and divisive stance, reflecting a specific mindset and definition of potential future offenders and victims. As in the above described theories on social identity creation, predictive policing programs polarise mindsets, shifting the norms regarding potential victims and offenders and might lead to shameful experiences in out-group members.

Together with this change in mindset and norms through predictive policing, the meaning of social identities, predicted crimes, offenders and victims shifts as well, as described in social identity theory (Hogg & Reid, 2006). However, (Meijer & Wessels, 2019) asserts that the patterns used in predictive policing have scarcely drawn on empirical evidence or systematic analysis, but rather on social and anecdotal evidence selected from big data sets and selected intersectional social networks which then are predicted as creating potential offenders or victims. Surely these selections of patterns impact on socio-cultural meanings related to social identity creations and re-enforce power relationships on a large scale, since prototypes of socio-cultural identities of individuals and groups are redefined in terms of classifications of offenders and victims of predicted crime scenes (Ferguson, 2017). These offender and victim classifications may evoke feelings of shame in the context of group identification and assessing the social self—particularly when the underlying tone connects to power relations and historically grown hierarchies. The effect of these feelings should not be underestimated in terms of defining one's social identity within a social group's context or outside of a social group's context.

The use of big data and technology in the development of predictive policing programs is prone to bias and prejudice because of the potential discrimination data collection and analysis, as well as algorithmic decision-making which might reinforce discrimination, particularly of historically disadvantaged group members. These discriminations are connected to power and power relations in policing based on social identity constructions and their dynamics (Bryne et al., 2015). The power relations, which are strongly connected to social identity categories, might induce shame. This is particularly the case when a person is categorised as a potential offender or victim of crime through predictive policing, as described by (Meijer & Wessels, 2019). Predictive policing—which usually claims to be an objective method of predefining offenders and victims—then appears to be even more shameful and detrimental to the individual who is classified as either perpetrator or victim. As highlighted above, shamed individuals either tend to develop based on the shaming experience or might lean towards a riskier and more problematic behaviour (Efrati, 2018; Tangney & Dearing, 2002). Since the outcome of shaming behaviour is not easy to predict and might have a problematic impact—particularly when it is associated with minority-orientated prejudice, bias and polarised social identity formation—interventions to address implicit and explicit bias, and thereby potential shame, should be applied.

In the following pages, two selected interventions which could be used in different cultural contexts are discussed. These are presented as possible training interventions to assist predictive policing officials in preventing shame altogether or else in transforming their predictions to enable shame to be experienced as restorative or as a resource-orientated emotion.

7 Interventions to Address Prejudice and Bias and Potential Shame

It might be assumed that programmers, system developers, administrators and system analysts who have defined, created and selected data and manufactured programs and algorithms in predictive policing, as well as isolated computerised patterns, might carry explicit and implicit biases and prejudices (*The Guardian*, 2019). Recent research (FitzGerald et al., 2019) particularly stresses that implicit biases and stereotypes, as discussed above, need to be explored and addressed within real-world scenarios, because they foster discrimination in an unconscious and automated manner and are alive in many professional contexts, such that of computerised predictive policing.

Social psychologists need to present and implement interventions that can support the minimisation of both explicit and implicit bias and prejudice which are active in the predictive policing context (Baeza-Yates, 2018). Creating a basic awareness in this context can support the experience of bias and prejudice in potential offenders and victims and transform shame, shaming and its potential negative effect and identity formation, self-image, social networks and negative emotions.

A systematic review by FitzGerald et al. (2019) shows that implicit bias and prejudice research is growing based on increasing general awareness in research. The authors highlight recent research efforts regarding implicit bias and prejudice interventions and related behaviour and discrimination. However, the "evidence for the effectiveness of different interventions to reduce implicit bias" lacks systematic evaluation and conclusions (FitzGerald et al., 2019). This is problematic since "interventions that are not designed based on empirical evidence have the potential to do more harm than good" (FitzGerald et al., 2019). The authors present interventions which are often used to address implicit bias in Australia, the USA, the UK, Pakistan, New Zealand, Belgium and Taiwan, the Netherlands, Hungary, Spain and Italy. Examples of these interventions are reflecting biases, avoiding implicit biases (often leading to an increase in implicit bias and stereotyping) and reflecting on positively managing implicit biases or presumed failures to contain implicit bias.

Interventions to address bias and prejudice range from a change of perspective and consciousness-raising and imaginary interventions to self-identification, counter-stereotypical exemplars, egalitarian value trainings, evaluative conditioning, inducing emotions and intentional strategies to overcome bias (FitzGerald et al., 2019). Most effective are the interventions which refer to intentional strategies to overcome bias, and those which involve individuals emotionally, with associated sets of concepts and include addressing motivations, sets of goals and mental resources. This is supported by the research of Case (2013). However, the complexity of success of interventions, the influence of socio-cultural and religious background and the impact of exposure to repeated stereotypic associations are still not fully understood. The way in which the transformation of bias and prejudice relate to shame and how these constructs are influenced through interventions are questions which, until now, have received very little attention and need further empirical study. Findings of the meta-study by FitzGerald et al. (2019) lead to the proposed interventions in this chapter to tackle implicit bias and prejudice in predictive policing. It is argued that interventions need to address individual, organisational and societal levels as well as specific target groups (such as data analysts or members of minorities) and can be short-term (discussion rounds, reflective circles, coaching) or long-term orientated (self-development coaching, courses or training, therapeutic interventions, resource-orientated long-term group interventions). Interventions should be resource-orientated and transformational (Baeza-Yates, 2018), and, if possible, they not only need to address prejudices and biases but also should create awareness of the negative emotions which might be stimulated through prejudice and bias, such as shame.

8 Social Psychology Interventions for the South African Predictive Policing Context

As one of the countries most riddled by crime in the world (Bhorat, Thornton, & van der Zee, 2017), South Africa has recently called for the introduction of predictive policing tools in the combat of crime (Matlala, 2018) as well as wildlife crime (Mayer, 2019a, b, c, d). Focusing on predictive policing and implicit prejudice and bias in post-apartheid South Africa, historical bias and prejudice in terms of intersectionalities of race, gender, age, first language in police services, data analysts and decision-makers, as well as living and crime areas, need to be taken into account.

Two potential interventions are taken into consideration for the described context: the empowerment confrontation approach and the guided Buddhist mediation. The combination of these interventions is expected to create awareness of bias and prejudice in individuals who are developing and using predictive policing tools, thereby reducing potential shame experiences on the side of predicted offenders and victims.

Cox and Devine (2019) suggest an *empowerment confrontation approach* to transform implicit bias in a Western context. This approach is intended to break the habit of prejudices by creating an awareness of bias and prejudice, raising concern and motivation to address unintentional biases. It is a long-term intervention, addressing individual and socio-cultural bias through discussions and exercises in group settings. However, this intervention only focuses on egalitarian individuals with the openness to address their biases (Cox & Devine, 2019). It aims to fill the current void in effective interventions to transform implicit bias and can be used as a positive psychology and empowerment intervention in the policing sector. It has been evaluated in randomised controlled studies.

For the South African context specifically, research has shown that a *guided Buddhist mediation intervention* can tackle racial bias and prejudice (Harding, 2017). By using the Implicit Association Test (IAT) measurement on day 1, 3 and 5 of the 5-day guided meditation sessions (1 h/day), Harding (2017) found that participants' sensitivity levels increased significantly across race groups (comparing the experimental group with the control group). The data revealed a stronger change in reduction of implicit biases (however, nonsignificant) in black than in white participants (Harding, 2017).

It is argued here that a combination of the two interventions will deal with implicit bias and prejudice at different levels of consciousness by using alternative methodological approaches, thereby aiming to cater for a diverse police staff unit. Participants should be diverse and intersectional in background (race, gender, age, socio-culture, language), with professional positions in predictive policing (such as analysts, programmers and decision-makers) to become aware of individual and collective biases and their potential impact on the predictive policing context.

Twice each month, a 3-hour empowerment confrontation group training should take place, for a duration of 3 months. The intervention will address individual but also socio-cultural bias and prejudice in a group setting and should include critical discussions, self-reflections and exercises (individual and group), confronting implicit bias and prejudice with regard to the above-mentioned intersectionalities.

Guided Buddhist meditations should be conducted twice per week for 30 minutes, for the duration of 3 months. This intervention helps to enhance loving kindness and mindfulness, as well as general mental health, well-being, inner peace and spiritual connection. It has been reported that Buddhist mediation encompasses cognitive, emotional, social and ethical perspectives (Harding, 2017), thereby creating inner harmony and a holistic, integrated worldview (Brito, 2013) which will support the counteracting of biases and prejudices and strengthens the perception of a common human race, as described by Shonin, van Gordon and Griffiths (2014).

The interventions and their effects on bias and prejudice should be researched using a qualitative research approach, by conducting semi-structured interviews on the topic of implicit and explicit bias and prejudice before the start of the interventions, after 6 weeks and following the 3-month period of interventions. The three interview sessions of 30 min (recorded and transcribed verbatim) will provide deep insight into the development of views on biases and prejudices. Changes of mindset might be detected through the long-term, multiple method assessment. Any changes of implicit biases recognised in the qualitative interviews will count as success. In the interviews, questions will address both interventions and aim at exploring their in-depth impact on the participants.

The IAT questionnaire should be used to measure implicit bias and prejudice from a quantitative perspective with measurements at the time of the interviews, in the beginning, in the middle and at the end of the interventions (three test periods). Success with regard to the IAT is defined in the way that an increase in sensitivity and a reduction of implicit bias will be recognised during data analysis and interpretation.

The strengths of the interventions lie in their well-researched, theory-based and validated history, in their easy implementation and monitoring and in their combinations to tackle bias and prejudice. Potential limitations include the need for voluntarily openness and for self-motivation to reflect, develop and change through training and meditation in professional contexts. Individuals working within highly technologised professions might be sceptical or critical and consequently biased against attending such interventions. Facilitators and researchers need to cater for potential phases of demotivation during the interventions and the research study, and participants need to attend on a regular basis. Psychological guidance might be a good solution for participants in creating awareness with regard to individual and collective shifts of prejudice and bias.

These training interventions might support professionals to reduce their bias and prejudice and to develop strategies to counteract bias and prejudice in predictive policing interventions. The growing awareness should bring a change of perspective with regard to the experience of potential perpetrators or victims of being categorised and ashamed when addressed, based on algorithmic patterns. Strategies how to address the potential perpetrators and victims should also be changed and adjusted, in ways that make use of the concept of Braithwaite's (1989) reintegrative shaming which takes the community into account, does not focus on the stigmatisation of individuals as in disintegrative shaming approaches and instead takes the problem of crime into account while the person is respected.

9 Conclusions and Recommendations

The aim of this chapter was to reflect on the interlinkages of bias, prejudice and shame in predictive policing, to present the state of the art of predictive policing and potential interventions and to reflect on possible ways forward based on provided conclusions.

It can be concluded that bias and prejudice affect different levels of predictive policing and the development of computerised programs, algorithms and intersectional categorisation clusters. A need has been detected to create awareness of implicit bias in professionals working in this area, to discover bias and prejudice in these programs and to protect individuals who are members of minorities from stigmatisation and shame when being predicted as either offenders or victims of crime, according to person-based and place-based predictive policing. Predictive police measures which include contacting potential offenders and victims of crime alike and increasing patrols in certain high-risk crime areas, as well as increased identity checks, increase the experience of stigmatisation and shame as disintegrative rather than as reintegrative shaming. This again increases the potential for negative reactions and could evoke flight or fight mechanisms and increased problematic behaviour. Professionals in predictive policing need to increase awareness of their own biases to adjust their programs and algorithmic patterns and reduce bias and prejudice as much as possible. They should also adjust their intervention strategies to address potential offenders and victims and take into consideration that predictive policing based on persons and locations might cause extreme shame in individuals, which in turn might counteract policing intentions and become self-fulfilling prophecies. This risk needs to be anticipated by professionals in predictive policing.

Future research should explore thoughts, emotions and experiences of individuals who have experienced the impact of being categorised in terms of person-based and place-based predictive policing and study their reactions to the potential stigmatisation.

Additionally, professionals who work in predictive policing need to be encouraged to take account of their own biases and prejudices. Technological and computerised programs should be evaluated with regard to the problem of potential implicit and explicit bias.

On a practical note, regulatory impact could be gained through anti-discriminatory policies. Further, trainings to tackle these problems should be offered in professional organisations and scientifically evaluated to minimise bias and prejudice in designing algorithms and decision-making in strategic action.

Civil society should also be better informed about predictive policing measures and strategies to combat crime in contemporary societies. Community centres and community key players could be involved in preparing communities for predictive policing measures in their areas and the critical as well as positive implications.

References

Abrams, D. (2010). Processes of prejudice: Theory, evidence and intervention. Equality and human rights commission. *Research Report* 56. University of Kent, UK. Retrieved from https://www.equalityhumanrights.com/sites/default/files/research-report-56-processes-of-prejudice-theory-evidence-and-intervention.pdf

Ahmad Malik, A. (2016). Urbanization and crime: A relational analysis, *21*(1), 6. Retrieved from https://pdfs.semanticscholar.org/a090/6d4d7fb65f135b6c28d6dcba9a2bfed52759.pdf

Ahmed, M. (2018, May 11). Aided by Palantir, the LAPD uses predictive policing to monitor specific people and neighborhoods. *The Intercept*. 11. Retrieved from https://theintercept.com/2018/05/11/predictive-policing-surveillance-los-angeles/?comments=1

Allport, G. W. (1954). *The nature of prejudice*. Reading, MA: Addison-Wesley.

Asaro, P. M. (2018, March 15). *AI ethics in predictive policing: From models of threat to an ethics of care*. Retrieved from https://peterasaro.org/writing/Asaro_PredictivePolicing.pdf

Baeza-Yates, R. (2018). Bias on the web. *Communication of the ACM, 61*(8), 54–61.

Bauer, V. (2019) *Predictive policing in Germany. Opportunities and challenges of data-analytical forecasting technology in order to prevent crime*. Master thesis. Management Center Innsbruk. Retrieved from https://www.researchgate.net/publication/338411808_Predictive_Policing_in_Germany_Opportunities_and_challenges_of_data-analytical_forecasting_technology_in_order_to_prevent_crime

Benson, M. L., Alerid, L. F., Burtn, V. S., & Cullen, F. T. (2011). Reintegration or stigmatization? Offenders' expectations of community re-entry. *Journal of Criminal Justice, 39*(5), 385–303.

Bhorat, H., Thornton, A., & van der Zee, K. (2017). *Socio-economic determinants of crime in South Africa: An empirical assessment*. AfricaPortal. Development Policy Research Unit Center for International Governance Innovation. Retrieved from https://www.africaportal.org/publications/socio-economic-determinants-crime-south-africa-empirical-assessment/

Bowleg, L. (2017). Intersectionality: An underutilized but essential theoretical framework for social psychology. In B. Gough (Ed.), *The Palgrave handbook of critical social psychology* (pp. 507–529). London: Palgrave Macmillan.

Boyd, D., Levy, K., & Marwick, A. (2014). *The networked nature of algorithmic discrimination*. Open Technology Institute, New America, Data & Discrimination. Retrieved from http://www.danah.org/papers/2014/DataDiscrimination.pdf

Braithwaite, J. (1989). *Crime, shame and reintegration*. Cambridge: Cambridge University Press.

Brantingham, P. J., Valasik, M., & Mohler, G. O. (2018). Does predictive policing lead to biased arrests? Results from a randomized controlled trial. *Statistics and Public Policy, 5*(1), 1–6.

Brayne, S. (2018). The criminal law and law enforcement implications of big data. *The Annual Review of Law and Social Science, 14*, 293–308.

Brito, G. (2013). Rethinking mindfulness in the therapeutic relationship. *Mindfulness, 5*(4), 351–359.

Bryne, S., Rosenblat, A., & Boyd, D. (2015). Predictive policing. Data & civil rights: A new era of policing and justice. *The leadership conference*. Retrieved from http://www.datacivilrights.org/pubs/2015-1027/Predictive_Policing.pdf

Case, K. (2013). *Deconstructing privilege. Teaching and learning as allies in the classroom*. New York: Routledge.

Chamberlin, J. (2004). What's behind prejudice? *Monitor Staff, 35*(9), 34.

Chigwada, R. (2013). The policing of black women. In E. Cashmore & E. McLaughlin (Eds.), *Out of order? Policing black people* (pp. 134–150). Routledge Revivals: Oxon, OX.

Correll, J., Judd, C. M., Park, B., & Wittenbrink, B. (2010). Measuring prejudice, stereotypes and discrimination. In J. F. Dovidio, M. Hewstone, P. Glick, & V. M. Esses (Eds.), *The SAGE handbook of prejudices, stereotyping and discrimination* (pp. 45–62). Thousand Oaks, CA: Sage.

Cox, W. T. L., & Devine, P. G. (2019). The prejudice habit-breaking intervention: An empowerment-based confrontation approach. In R. Mallett & M. Monteith (Eds.), *Confronting prejudice and discrimination. The science of changing minds and behaviours* (pp. 249–274). New York: Academic Press.

Damasio, A. (2010). *Self comes to mind: Constructing the conscious brain*. New York: Vintage Books.

De Hooge, I. E., Zeelenberg, M., & Breugelmans, S. M. (2011). A functionalist account of shame-induced behavior. *Cognition & Emotion, 25*, 939–946.

Devlin, H. (2017, April 13). AI programs exhibit racial and gender biases, research reveals. *The Guardian*. Retrieved from https://www.theguardian.com/technology/2017/apr/13/ai-programs-exhibit-racist-and-sexist-biases-research-reveals

Dovidio, J. F., & Gaertner, S. L. (1986). Prejudice, discrimination, and racism: Historical trends and contemporary approaches. In J. Dovidio & S. Gaertner (Eds.), *Prejudice, discrimination, and racism* (pp. 1–34). New York: Academic Press.

Efrati, Y. (2018). Adolescents with a disposition toward compulsive sexual behavior: The role of shame in willingness to seek help and treatment. *Sexual Addiction & Compulsivity, 25*(1), 28–45.

Egbert, S. (2019). Predictive policing and the platformization of police work. *Surveillance & Society, 17*(1/2), 83–88. https://doi.org/10.24908/ss.v17i1/2.12920.

Ferguson, A. G. (2017). Policing predictive policing. *Washington University Law Review, 94*(6), 1109–1111.

Ferguson, M. A., Branscombe, N. R., & Reynolds, K. J. (2019). Social psychological research on prejudice as collective action supporting emergent ingroup members. *Applied Psychology: An International Review, 58*(1), 1–32.

Fiske, S. T. (2019). *Prejudice, discrimination, and stereotyping*. Introduction to psychology. Retrieved from https://openpress.usask.ca/introductiontopsychology/chapter/prejudice-discrimination-and-stereotyping/

FitzGerald, C., Martin, A., Berner, D., & Hurst, S. (2019). Interventions designed to reduce implicit prejudices and implicit stereotypes in real world contexts: A systematic review. *BMC Psychol, 7*, 29. https://doi.org/10.1186/s40359-019-0299-7.

Fox, J. (2007). The uncertain relationship between transparency and accountability. *Development in Practice, 17*, 663–671. https://doi.org/10.1080/09614520701469955.

Garcia, M. (2017). Racist in the machine: The disturbing implications of algorithmic bias. *World Policy Journal, 33*(4), 111–117.

Gatto, J., & Dambrun, M. (2012). Authoritarianism, social dominance, and prejudice among junior police officers. *Social Psychology, 43*, 61–66.

Gerstner, D. (2017). *Predictive Policing als Instrument zur Prävention von Wohnungseinbruchdiebstahl [Predictive policing as an instrument for crime prevention]. Research brief* (p. 50). Max-Planck-Institut für ausländisches und internationales Strafrecht: Freiburg im Breisgau.

Greene, T. (2019). Predictive policing is a scam that perpetuates systemic bias. *Artificial Intelligence*. Retrieved from https://thenextweb.com/artificial-intelligence/2019/02/21/predictive-policing-is-a-scam-that-perpetuates-systemic-bias/

Grierson, J. (2019, September 16). Predictive policing poses discrimination risk, thinktank warns. *The Guardian*. Retrieved from https://www.theguardian.com/uk-news/2019/sep/16/predictive-policing-poses-discrimination-risk-thinktank-warns

Harding, T. (2017). *Penetrating the illusion of our separateness: Buddhist meditation and implicit racial prejudice*. Master's thesis, Department of Psychology, University of Cape Town, Cape

Town, South Africa. Retrieved from http://www.psychology.uct.ac.za/sites/default/files/image_tool/images/117/Logos/thesis/Tarryn%20Harding.pdf

Harris, N. (2017). Shame in regulatory systems. In P. Drahos (Ed.), *Regulatory theory. Foundations and applications*. Acton: Australian National University Press.

Haslam, S. A., Reicher, S. D., & Reynolds, K. J. (2012). Identity, influence, and change: Rediscovering John Turner's vision for social psychology. *British Journal of Social Psychology, 51*, 201–218.

Hogg, M. A., & Reid, S. A. (2006). Social identity, self-categorization, and the communication of group norms. *Communication Theory, 16*, 7–30.

Hosser, D., Windzio, M., & Greve, W. (2008). Guilt and shame as predictors of recidivism: A longitudinal study with young prisoners. *Criminal Justice and Behavior, 35*, 138–152.

Hvistendahl, M. (2016). Crime forecasters. *Science, 353*(6307), 1484–1487.

Ioimo, R. (2018). Crime analysis and crime mapping. In R. Ioimo (Ed.), *Introduction to criminal justice information systems* (pp. 181–206). Cleveland, OH: CRC Press.

Isenberg, D. J. (1986). Group polarization: A critical review and meta-analysis. *Journal of Personality and Social Psychology, 50*(6), 1141–1151.

Jackson, L. M. (2011). *The psychology of prejudice: From attitudes to social action*. Washington: American Psychological Association. https://doi.org/10.1037/12317-000.

Jacquet, J. (2015). *Scham: Die politische Kraft eines unterschätzten Gefühls*. Berlin: Fischer.

Jacquet, J., Hauert, C., Traulsen, A., & Milinski, M. (2011). Shame and honor drive cooperation. *Biology Letters, 7*, 899–901.

Joh, E. (2015). The new surveillance discretion: Automated suspicion, big data, and policing. *Harvard Law & Policy Review, 10*, 15–42.

Kitchin, R. (2014). *The data revolution: Big data, open data, data infrastructures and their consequences*. London: Sage.

Lu, L. (2016). Emotional insight: Discovering the nature of prejudice development and reduction through emotional mechanisms. *Exposé Magazin*. Retrieved from https://projects.iq.harvard.edu/expose/book/emotional-insight-discovering-nature-prejudice-development-and-reduction-through

Malone, S.C. (2018). *Intra-racial prejudice amongst African-Americas when policing members of their own racial background*. Doctoral Dissertation, Union Institute and University Ann Habor, USA. Retrieved from https://media.proquest.com/media/pq/classic/doc/4327164149/fmt/ai/rep/NPDF?_s=q0%2Fg3ZcOkCbyRMLgvXkYTZ0aZcE%3D

Matlala, R. L. G. (2018). Defining e-policing and smart policing for law enforcement agencies in Gauteng Province. *Acta Criminologica: African Journal of Criminology Victimology, 31*(1), 136–148.

Mayer, C.-H. (2004). *Mauern aus Glass*. Münster: Waxmann.

Mayer, C.-H. (2019a). Crime and shame. Crime and shame: Reflections and culture-specific insights. In C.-H. Mayer & E. Vanderheiden (Eds.), *The bright side of shame. Transforming and growing through practical applications in cultural contexts* (pp. 117–130). Cham, Switzerland: Springer.

Mayer, C.-H. (2019b). *Combating wildlife crime in South Africa. Using gelatin lifters for forensic trace recovery. Springer briefs in criminology*. Cham, Switzerland: Springer.

Mayer, C.-H. (2019c). Opening the black box part 1: On collective shame in the German society. In C.-H. Mayer & E. Vanderheiden (Eds.), *The bright side of shame. Transforming and growing through practical applications in cultural contexts* (pp. 3–20). Cham, Switzerland: Springer.

Mayer, C.-H. (2019d). Opening the black box part 2: Exploring individual shame in German research. In C.-H. Mayer & E. Vanderheiden (Eds.), *The bright side of shame. Transforming and growing through practical applications in cultural contexts* (pp. 21–34). Cham, Switzerland: Springer.

Mayer, C., & Vanderheiden, E. (2019). *The bright side of shame. Transforming and growing through practical applications in cultural contexts*. Cham: Springer.

Meijer, A., & Wessels, M. (2019). Predictive policing: Review of benefits and drawbacks. *International Journal of Public Administration, 42*(12), 1031–1039.

Murphy, K., Cramer, R. J., Waymire, K. A., & Barkworth, J. (2017). Police bias, social identity, and minority groups: A social psychological understanding of cooperation with police. *Justice Quarterly, 35*(6), 1105–1130.

Murphy, K., & Harris, N. (2007). Shaming, shame and recidivism. *British Journal of Criminology, 47*, 900–917.

Nyaoro, D. (2010). Policing with prejudice: How policing exacerbates poverty among urban refugees. *The International Journal of Human Rights, 14*, 126–145.

O'Neil, C. (2017, April 6). *Justice in the age of big data.* TECH. Retrieved from https://ideas.ted.com/justice-in-the-age-of-big-data/

Perry, W. L., McInnis, B., Price, C. C., Smith, S. C., & Hollywood, J. S. (2013). Predictive policing: The role of crime forecasting in law enforcement operations. *RAND safety and justice program.* Retrieved from http://www.rand.org/content/dam/rand/pubs/research_reports/RR200/RR233/RAND_RR233.pdf

Pickles, J. (2019). Policing hate and bridging communities: A qualitative evaluation of relations between LGBT+ people and the police within the north east of England. Policing and society. *An International Journal of Research and Policy.*

SAPS. (2019). Protecting our youth. Protecting our future. On a journey to a safer South Africa. Retrieved March 16, 2020, from https://www.saps.gov.za/resource_centre/publications/police_mag/pol_june_2019_final.pdf

Schnelle, N. (2015, September 25). Police departments embracing pre-crime strategy: Program aims to pinpoint those most likely to offend. *National Post.* Retrieved from https://nationalpost.com/news/world/u-s-predictive-policing-program-uses-computer-analytics-to-pinpoint-those-most-likely-to-commit-crimes-before-they-happen

Schwarcz, D. (2003). Shame, stigma, and crime: Evaluating the efficacy of shaming sanctions in criminal law. *Harvard Law Review, 116*, 2186.

Shonin, E., Van Gordon, W., & Griffiths, M. D. (2014). The emerging role of Buddhism in clinical psychology: Toward effective integration. *Psychology of Religion and Spirituality, 6*(2), 123–137.

Sidanius, J., Hudson, S.T.J., Davis, G., & Bergh, R. (2018). The theory of gendered prejudice: A social dominance and intersectionalist perspective. *The Oxford handbook of Behavioural politics.* Retrieved from https://www.oxfordhandbooks.com/view/10.1093/oxfordhb/9780190634131.001.0001/oxfordhb-9780190634131-e-11

Siegel, E. (2018, February 19). How to fight bias with predictive policing. *Scientific American.* Retrieved from https://blogs.scientificamerican.com/voices/how-to-fight-bias-with-predictive-policing/

Spencer, K.B., Charbonneau, A.K., & Glaser, J. (2018). Implicit bias and policing. Social and Personality Psychology Compass, 10(1), 50–63

Sullivan, J. (2017, November 20). *Corporate shame - why doesn't your firm predict and prevent sexual harassment? Talent Management & HR.* Retrieved from https://www.tlnt.com/how-to-use-predictive-analytics-to-prevent-workplace-sexual-harassment/

Tajfel, H. (1972). Some development in European social psychology. *European Journal of Social Psychology, 2*(3), 307–322.

Tajfel, H., & Turner, J. (1986). *The social identity theory of intergroup behavior.* Chicago, IL: Nelson-Hall.

Tangney, J. P. (1990). Assessing individual differences in proneness to shame and guilt: Development of the self-conscious affect and attribution inventory. *Journal of Personality and Social Psychology, 59*, 102–111.

Tangney, J. P., & Dearing, R. L. (2002). *Shame and guilt.* New York, NY: Guilford.

Tangney, J. P., Stuewig, J., & Hafez, L. (2011). Shame, guilt and remorse: Implications for offender populations. *Journal of Forensic Psychiatry and Psychology, 22*(5), 706–723.

Uchida, C. D. (2014). Predictive policing. In G. Bruinsma & D. Weisbund (Eds.), *Encyclopedia of criminology and criminal justice*. New York: Springer.

Vanderheiden, E., & Mayer, C.-H. (2017). *The value of shame. Exploring a health resource in cultural contexts*. Cham, Switzerland: Springer.

Viki, G. T., & Abrams, D. (2012). The social influence of groups on individuals. In J. L. Wood & T. A. Gannon (Eds.), *Crime and crime reduction: The importance of group processes* (pp. 3–33). New York: Routledge.

Weitzer, R., & Tuch, S. A. (2005). Racially biased policing. Determinants of citizen perceptions. *Social Forces, 83*(3), 1009–1030.

White, F., Abu-Rayya, H., Bliuc, A., & Faulkner, N. (2015). Emotion expression and intergroup bias reduction between Muslims and Christians: Long-term internet contact. *Computers in Human Behavior, 53*, 435–442.

Wittenbrink, B., Correll, J., & Ma, D. S. (2019). Implicit prejudice. In K. Sassenberg & M. L. W. Vliek (Eds.), *Social psychology in action. Evidence-based interventions from theory to practice* (pp. 163–177). Cham, Switzerland: Springer.

Zarsky, T. Z. (2012). Governmental data mining and its alternatives. *Penn State Law Review, 116* (2), 285–330.

Završnik, A. (2017). *Big data, crime and social control. Routledge Frontiers of criminal justice* (p. 50). New York: Abington.

Claude-Hélène Mayer (Dr. habil., Ph.D., Ph.D.) is a Professor in Industrial and Organisational Psychology in the Department of Industrial Psychology and People Management at the University of Johannesburg; an Adjunct Professor at the European University Viadrina in Frankfurt (Oder), Germany; and a Senior Research Associate at Rhodes University, Grahamstown, South Africa. She holds an M.A. (hist-phil) degree in Socio-cultural Anthropology, Intercultural Didactics and Socio-economics of rural development (Georg-August University, Germany) and an MSc degree in Crime Science, Investigation and Intelligence (University of Portsmouth, UK). She further holds a Ph.D. in Psychology (University of Pretoria, South Africa), a Ph.D. in Management (Rhodes University, South Africa), a Doctorate (Georg-August University, Germany) in Political Sciences (socio-cultural anthropology and intercultural didactics) and a Habilitation (European University Viadrina, Germany) in Psychology with focus on work, organisational and cultural psychology. In Crime Science, she has focused on wildlife crime combat, as well as on concepts and interventions in positive criminology/positive victimology as well as crime and shaming.

Part II
Shame 4.0 in Therapy, Counselling and Health

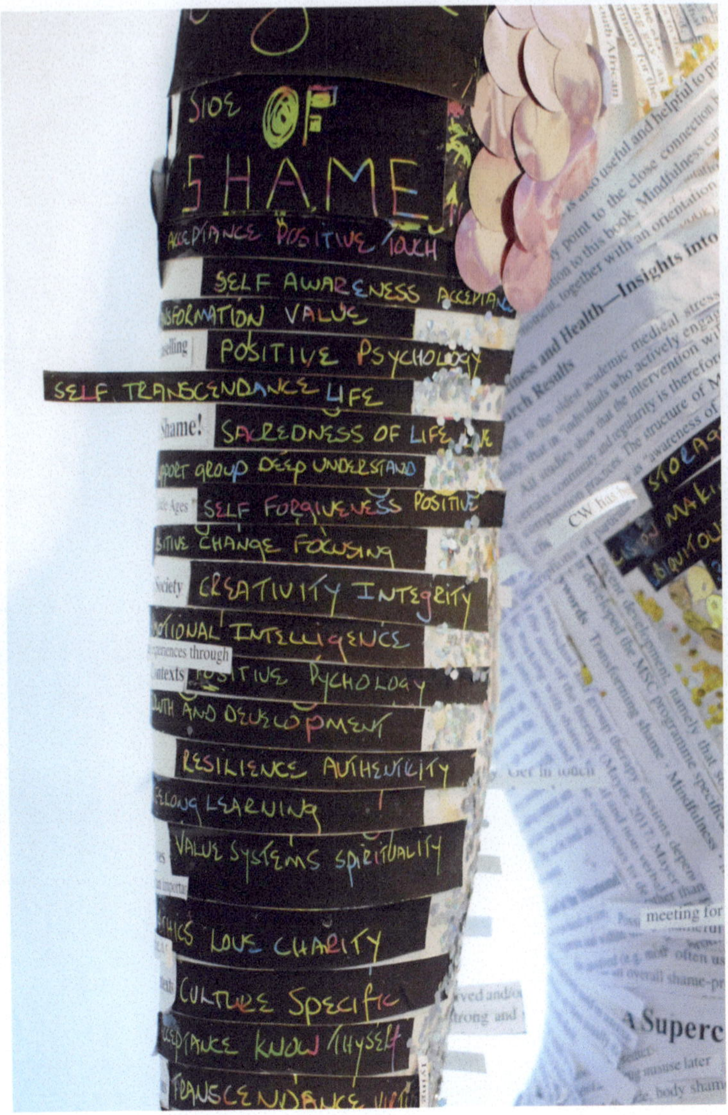

Chapter 7
The Second Wave Positive Psychology of Shame in East and West in the Age of the 4IR

Paul T. P. Wong and Kwang-Kuo Hwang

1 Introduction

Mayer and Vanderheiden's *The Bright Side of Shame: Transforming and Growing Through Practical Applications in Cultural Contexts* (2019) represents a landmark publication on shame from different theoretical and cultural perspective; it is encyclopedic in its breath, covering almost every aspect of shame research. However, shame, as one of the most ancient emotions, along with guilt and fear, is extremely complex both in its nature and effects; it is possible that that we may never get to the bottom of this emotion, no matter how deep we dig in our research. In this chapter, we want to explore the second wave positive psychology (PP 2.0) perspective of shame in the East and West within the context of the Fourth Industrial Revolution (4IR). We hope that this paper will lead to better ways of curtailing public shaming and channeling shame into positive transformation.

The framework of PP 2.0 emphasizes the existential and indigenous dimensions of positive psychology (Wong, 2019a, 2020). This approach is much needed because it recognizes shame as a core universal emotion for all people, but experienced, expressed, and managed differently in different cultures. For example, we are more affected by relative rankings in performance- and guilt-based shame in Western culture, but more affected by concerns about other people's opinions and possible violations of social norms in Asian societies.

PP 2.0 also calls for more research on both the negative and positive sides of shame and other unpleasant emotions such as guilt, fear, and anger as the foundation of emotional intelligence and well-being. COVID-19 shows the need for this

P. T. P. Wong (✉)
Trent University, Toronto, ON, Canada

K.-K. Hwang
Department of Psychology, National Taiwan University, Taipei, Taiwan, Republic of China
e-mail: kkhwang@ntu.edu.tw

C.-H. Mayer et al. (eds.), *Shame 4.0*, https://doi.org/10.1007/978-3-030-59527-2_7

emphasis. For example, shame has everything to do with the global spread of COVID-19. China leaders' fear of losing face (i.e., the presence of a sense of shame) led to their decision to cover up the first signs of COVID-19 when it first broke out in Wuhan in November 2019 (Sky News Australia, 2020). Shameless lying and misinformation led to the spread of COVID-19 (Boxwell, 2020). This delay allowed thousands of infected people from Wuhan to travel to other cities on China and other countries. Only public shaming of such irresponsible behavior from all the world leaders could pressure the CCP to be more truthful in reporting infectious diseases in order to prevent future pandemics like COVID-19.

Thus, research on shame in the East and West can increase our emotional intelligence to understand each other's feeling and behaviors related to shame. More importantly, it could show how we can reduce the need to lie about things we are ashamed of by cultivating the virtues of humility, honesty, and courage to confess, make amends, and improve one's behavior. This chapter will discuss some of the exercises of positive transformation of shame.

2 The Challenges of COVID-19

With the death toll approaching one million globally, COVID-19 has shown that the basic tenets of PP 2.0 (Wong, 2019a) are undeniable aspects of the human condition: (1) We all live in a dangerous world full of evil and suffering. (2) All human being have inherent limitations and vulnerability. (3) Flourishing is impossible without overcoming the frailty and the dark side of life (Fowers, Richardson & Slife, 2017; Wong, 2020; see also Vanderheiden and Mayer "Who Could Breathe Without Hope"—Some Theses on Shame and Shaming in the Age of Corona Pandemic in this book). In spite of all their might in science, technology, and wealth, so many powerful countries have been brought to their knees, not knowing how to find a cure at this point. COVID-19 has demonstrated in a convincing manner that human beings are defenseless against an airborne steadily evolving micro-pathogen that is capable of killing millions of people. One good thing that comes out from this global catastrophe is that COVID-19 reminds us that we are fallible and fragile beings. We need to humble ourselves and learn to work with each other, as well as live in harmony with nature. Such an attitude of humility may have saved humanity from the COVID-19 disaster. In addition to making cover-up unnecessary, it would also prevent Western leaders from over-confidence because of their "positive illusion" (Taylor & Brown, 1988)—a cognitive bias toward the illusion of control and optimism.

Communication is vital in containing infectious diseases. A critical ingredient for preventing future pandemics is to restore public trust in governments and international communication. Scientific research and education may increase general acceptance of the imperative of speaking the truth. When it comes to highly contagious infectious diseases, every county is responsible for every other country because infectious disease knows no political borders. Leaders and researcher need to work together to ensure truthful communications. Saving lives is more important than saving face. Truth could save lives, whereas cover-ups to save face could kill millions of people. Another challenge has to do with climate change. Deforestation and other environmental disruptions may result in novel diseases due to increased human-animal interactions and wildlife markets for human consumption, according to Harvey (2020). It is important to remember that we are part of the ecosystem and we need to learn how to protect the environment.

In other words, COVID-19 was a disaster waiting to happen, because we have ignored the fundamental truth that there are inherent limitations. When we play God and entertain the false confidence that with science, wealth, and power we can do anything, there will be a global catastrophe soon or later. Now COVID-19 teaches us that there is a "forbidden fruit" (Genesis 3) after all and there are serious consequences for violating this basic rule, such as eating wild animals (which may cause novel diseases). COVID-19 awakens us to the truth that we need to live within human limitations and we are morally accountable to a higher power, whether you call it God, Jesus, Buddha, or Nature, for things beyond human understanding and control. There is no shame in our humility, but ironically, the desire to be like God would lead to disaster and shame.

For psychologists, there is a greater challenge of how to cope with the psychological impact of COVID-19, even when the crisis is over. Yong (2020) observed that:

> At a moment of profound dread and uncertainty, people are being cut off from soothing human contact. Hugs, handshakes, and other social rituals are now tinged with danger. People with anxiety or obsessive-compulsive disorder are struggling. Elderly people, who are already excluded from much of public life, are being asked to distance themselves even further, deepening their loneliness.

One good thing from the widespread mental health problems may be the decline of the stigma surrounding mental illness, because we are all negatively impacted psychologically by COVID-19. Finally, the coronavirus is a good metaphor for shame, which is also ubiquitous, insidious, and destructive. We all have experienced its effects and tried to live with it in the best way we can. We may try to hide some embarrassing mistakes in the past or some family secret, but we pay the price for building up defenses, isolating ourselves, and constantly worrying about being exposed. We may avoid expressing our opinions or doing something differently because of the fear of rejection and humiliation by others. Worse still, we keep on revising our life story, trying to mitigate against our sense of shame by blaming others or distorting our memories. In one or another, we try to avoid or tolerate it as an ever-present threat to our pride and self-esteem.

Yet, we often have difficulty articulating our shame, even when we can feel its presence everyday. We cannot pinpoint its cause or source. We don't know where it is lurking under. All we can do is to avoid being shamed by others. But in a meritocratic society, it is inevitable that we have to compete for status and access to limited resources. The age of COVID-19 also reveals the power of IT technology in controlling the pandemic and monitoring people's daily movement (Tidy, 2020).

For example, drones from the sky can monitor people's every move (Pietsch, 2020). Such universal surveillance may be here to stay and may also extend to other less-affected countries, even after COVID-19. This is a scary vision because it means that people will be increasingly concerned about their privacy and fearful that their secrets may be exposed, leading to public shaming.

3 The Digital Culture, 4IR, and Shame

In this uncertain and scary time, the power of surveillance by Big Brother and the public shaming on social media have become a serious issue. *The New York Times* article "The Industrial Revolution of Shame" said it all (Scibona, 2019). New technologies have given both individuals enormous power to shame others and authoritarian governments the ability to socially control citizens on an unthinkable scale. Such social and political forces released by information technologies also challenge us to act responsibly to shape the Fourth Industrial Revolution for the common good (Schwab & Davis, 2018). *Shame Nation: The Global Epidemic of Online Hate* (Scheff & Schorr, 2017) is the first book to examine the phenomenon of online shaming and cyberbullying and offer practical guidance and inspiring advice on how to prevent and protect against cyber blunders and faceless bullies. Any troll could bring down a business or ruin a celebrity, causing public humiliation and real psychological damage.

The callout or outrage culture (Susaria, 2020) is a form of public shaming to keep certain individuals accountable for their behaviors that may offend some individuals or groups. Such outrage can go viral on the social media, because some platforms write algorithms that maximize engagement to amplify the outrage through a snowball effect. On a personal level, shame is commonly experienced when one's self-identity or self-esteem is damaged because of mistakes, failures, or defeats. It is a self-conscious emotion involving a negative evaluation of one's moral self. But shame is also commonly experienced through a process of group identification and the negative evaluation of one's social self (Salice & Sánchez, 2016).

These shameful feelings can be greatly amplified because of the prospect for public shaming and punishment through new technologies. This chapter focuses on cultural differences between the East and the West in two major types of shame: relational shame and moral shame. The East is a shame-based culture, while the West is a guilt-based culture (Wong & Tsai, 2007). The East emphasizes relational shame as necessary for maintaining interpersonal relationships and group harmony. In contrast, the West views shame more negatively as a moral failure worse than guilt—guilt means I have done something bad, while shame means that I am a bad person (Brown, 2012; Lewis, 1998; Van Norden, 2002).

According to the Pew Research Center (Duggan, 2017), roughly 4 in 10 Americans have personally experienced online harassment and 62 percent consider it to be a major problem. Cyberbullying or online harassment of scientific and health professionals could have a damping effect on academic freedom or free speech to express unpopular views. Therefore, people are afraid to express independent thoughts in an age of tyranny where everyone has to conform to some ideology, political correctness, or groupthink (Blackford, 2018). This is what John Stuart Mill would call "the tyranny of the prevailing opinion and feeling." Social media and callout culture make it possible to ruin any person's career or any business through shaming and ostracize anyone who has the courage to express their unique ideas, which may offend someone.

Another major concern in the age of 4IR is the rise of AI and robotic-processing automation (RPA; Galer, 2020). By 2022, International Data Corporation (IDC; Jyoti & Schubmehl, 2019) predicted that 75 percent of enterprises will embed intelligent automation into technology and process development (see also Oosthuizen in this book). A 2020 EdelmanTrust Survey (Purtill, 2020) showed increasing worries about job losses and a looming recession due to automation. Nearly two in three people felt that the technological changes are too fast and they had no control over the robotic revolution. Carrying the logic of the computer model to its extreme would be Yuval Noah Harari's controversial book *Homo Deus: A Brief History of Tomorrow* (2018); it gives us a chilling future when dataism becomes our new God and our faith will be placed in the power of data processing and algorithms. "Having raised humanity above the beastly level of survival struggles, we will now aim to upgrade humans into gods and turn Home sapiens into Homo Deus," Harari boldly declared.

3.1 Shame and Meritocracy

Paradoxically, in our efforts to become out best and climb the dominance hierarchy in order to overcome our own sense of inadequacy and shame, we set ourselves up for more failures and more shame in the ruthless global competition. The age of the 4IR only magnifies the digital inequality and the income gap between people. There are no winners in a meritocratic society (Markovits, 2019). Markovits argued that a meritocracy produces radical inequality in any society with inherent social economic inequality. Roger Karma (2019) explains why a meritocracy makes everybody miserable. Meritocracy turns life into an endless competition. The race begins in early childhood (competing to enter the best preschools), continues into the teenage years (competing for admissions into top schools), and then extends into the workplace (competing for good paying jobs).

According to Paul Gilbert's (2000) social rank theory, our emotions and moods are significantly influenced by the perceptions of our social status or rank. Shame, social anxiety, and depression are all related to defensive submissive strategies when individuals find themselves placed in inferior ranks. But winners do not fare much better. Meritocracies constantly feed a sense of shame to the losers in this endless competition and fear of failure to the winners, who are worried about losing. Thus, shame permeates through society and imprisons all of us. How can we be liberated from this bondage of shame so that we can freely pursue an ideal life and engage in creative work for the greater good? We are suggesting that the answer may be more existential-spiritual and political, as Thompson (2015) pointed out.

The future for a great life is not promising, even before the current COVID-19 pandemic. According to Shum (2020):

> All manner of Great Life Plans for houses, cars, and families, most goals tend to gravitate towards some form of self-preservation and stability. But in a world where natural disaster is the order of the day and artificial intelligence (the ubiquitous AI!) is charted to surpass our own, it's often tough to figure out what we can do that really helps us get there.

Now, the prospect of over 200,000 deaths in American alone (according to the White House; see Zapotosky, Wagner, and Iati, 2020) casts a dark cloud on all of us. The widespread lockdowns and self-isolation have resulted in the economic shutdown of many business sectors. The economic fallout from COVID-19 is staggering and incalculable at this point (Monderer, 2020). In short, the old meritocracy is no longer working in the age of COVID-19. We need to reimagine a new world order, and we need to collectively awaken to some enduring values that can save humanity. In other words, we need to consider Thompson's view of shame seriously.

3.2 *Shame from an Existential Spiritual Perspective*

In an earlier article, Wong (2019b) mentioned that the biblical narrative of the fall of Adam and Eve shed much light on the human condition. "Then the eyes of both of them were opened, and they realized they were naked; so they sewed fig leaves together and made coverings for themselves" (Genesis 3:7, NIV). Thompson (2015) elaborated on the theme that we were made for happiness but were banished from paradise with the burden of shame, guilt, and fear for disobeying God's command and wanting to be as wise as God:

> We walk on the earth burdened with the ancient code that we received from our first parents. We hide behind our rhetoric and have come to depend on our various garments to protect us not so much from the other but from ourselves. (p. 109)

In other words, shame, guilt, and fear (anxiety) are the core emotions that have plagued us from antiquity since our ancestors ate the forbidden fruit to become as wise as God. The metaphorical truth in this ancient narrative is still relevant today. While we owe much of our physical well-being to scientific progress, at the same time, we still bear the burden of being, conscious of our own nothingness, aloneness, and insignificance in this vast cosmos as helpless orphans. By spiritual, Thompson meant that we were made for happiness through relationships and creative work. We can heal shame and restore joy by restoring our relationships with ourselves, others, and the Creator. This existential spiritual understanding of shame as part of the dark side of the human condition explains that we can only be healed through returning to the purpose for which we were created; namely, to glorify God and enjoy Him forever by living in harmony and attunement. Even for unreligious people or unbelievers, it is still helpful to hold a high view of human beings that we were wired for happiness through good relationships and creative work. The main reason for our unhappiness is that not only have we allowed shame, guilt, and fear to enter into our lives; we also are pretending that they do not exist or they would just go away, if we only focus on happiness.

The main lesson from COVID-19 is that toxic thoughts and emotions do not just go away if we focus on the positive. We need to realize that we can be infected with the virus of shame, even as a baby without any language. Shame weaves its way into our lives simply through "an emotional sharing," without the necessary language "through the brainstem, limbic shame and right hemisphere" (Thompson, 2015, p. 82). All through our life, we have been wounded by a thousand needles through shame, the silent killer. The emotion of shame is always part of our daily experience especially in the important domains of achievements and relationships. Shame is also the emotion we often anticipate as we look into an uncertain future because of past experiences. Thompson pointed out that shame, if allowed to do its destructive wok, will not only ruin our life, but the world in which we live:

> The way of life is the way of shame. Shame, as evil's vector would like it to be, keeps itself hidden among life's e everyday events. It wants to be known as an artifact...However, it intends to dismantle a world that was destined for goodness and beauty. (p. 131)
>
> But honest vulnerability is the key to both healing shame–and its inevitably anticipated hellish outcome of abandonment–and preventing it from taking further roots in our relationships and culture. (pp. 104–105)

That is why Wong (2019a) has long argued that the science of sustainable positive psychology can only be established by embracing our vulnerability to shame and other negative emotions and situations, similar to how we cannot maintain good physical health without dealing with negative pathogens:

> But naked vulnerability is not merely a representation of our having been created to be in relationship. God desires us to live like he lives. Thus, to be created in God's image also refers to our having creative dominion within the world. And to be maximally creative also requires that we are vulnerable. (Thompson, 2015, p. 122)

Here is another important insight regarding creative work. We must be willing to be vulnerable to failures, rejections, obstacles, and the painful emotions of shame, guilt, and fear that accompany such endeavors. To engage in meaningful work is not simply a matter of goal-setting and being committed to achieve it. It is better to view the pursuit of meaningful work as an existential struggle to endure suffering in order to create meaning and a world of goodness, beauty, and happiness. That is the main tenet of second wave positive psychology. Citing Romans 5:1–5, Thompson observed: "Note the progression from suffering to perseverance to character to hope, and hope of this sort does not put us to shame" (p. 179). Thus, hope is not magic. Hope is not wishful think, nor magical thinking. Hope does not depend on miracles most of the time. It calls for perseverance toward the idea while ignoring the shame that accompanies such efforts until we no longer feel the sting and see a "hopeful future" emerging.

Contrary to the prevailing view that existential psychology focuses on the dark side of life, existential positive psychology actually focuses on the positive view. For instance, pain, shame, and guilt could serve adaptive functions—they are existential givens that inform us that we need to change collectively and individually, so that we can become what we were meant to be. COVID-19 changes our lives in a fundamental way and calls for a global awakening of our need for transformation. As long as there is ego, pride, and the desire to be appreciated, we are vulnerable to the destructive power of shaming, which can be transmitted by the tone of one's voice or the look in one's eyes. It can also be transmitted by judging others or excluding them. COVID-19 has taught us that we are responsible to not transmit the virus of shame. The interpersonal dark side of existence includes the accumulated toxic experiences of rejection, bullying, marginalization, and alienation. A sense of shame because of one's language and cultural handicap is a big part of acculturation stress, which happens to all people transplanted to a different country, whether as refugees, immigrants, or returnees.

3.3 Shame in the Asian Culture

According to the Analects (Watson, 2009), Confucius held that using punishment to influence ordinary citizens will do little to develop a sense of shame (chi 恥) in them. This term is usually understood as a predisposition to feel ashamed when one does something wrong because it seems wrong to oneself, and not because others regard it as wrong or shameful. Mencius, who was said to have studied under Confucius's grandson Zisi, went even further than Confucius. Mencius believed that every person has some things that he or she would be ashamed to do and these are expressions of innate virtue of righteousness. He even declared that individuals without a sense of shame were no longer human (Stanford Encyclopedia of Philosophy, 2004). Shame may have been a factor that contributed to the longevity of China's civilization. The Chinese are much more sensitive to relational shame, and they have many shades of shame. Li, Wang, and Fischer (2004) started with a list of 83 words that were related to 羞 xiu "shame/shyness," 耻 chi "disgrace," and 辱 ru "humiliation/shame" from the dictionary; the list was then expanded to 113 shame-related words and phrases, most of which are relationally related shame and are not translatable to English. Even when there are equivalent translations, the emotional content encoded in the words might be different (Bai, 2015; Lin & Yao, 2016) (see also Kotera et al., Cucuani et al., Bhawuk, Puttaraju and D'souza, Wang et al. and Jochan and Banerjee in this book).

Guilt cultures in the West rely on an internalized conviction of sin as the enforcer of good behavior, emphasizing punishment and forgiveness as ways of restoring the moral order, whereas shame cultures in the East depend on external sanctions, emphasizing self-denial and humility as ways of restoring the social order (Hiebert, 1985). For both cultures, the violation of personal identity leads to shame. However, for shame cultures, personal identity is dependent on continued relations with the group, since shame is a more effective way of social control rather than guilt (Bedford & Hwang, 2003).

Shame is understood in the Chinese culture as related to "face." The most complete definition of face was offered by Ho (1976):

> Face is the respectability and/or deference which a person can claim for himself from others, by virtue of the relative position he occupies in his social network and the degree to which he is judged to have functioned adequately in that position as well as acceptably in his general conduct; the face extended to a person by others is a function of the degree of congruence between judgments of his total condition in life, including his actions as well as those of people closely associated with him, and the social expectations the others have placed upon him.

In a similar vein, Hwang and Han (2010) also emphasized the vital role of face-saving (zuo mianzi) and fighting for one's face or honor (zheng mianzi) in all social interactions. They further pointed out that the Chinese usage of face can be divided into two broad categories: namely, moral face and social face; both are related to the Confucian concepts of morality. With respect to mental health, moral guilt is more related to mental health problems, and forgiveness and self-compassion are antidotes, whereas relational shame is more related to the virtue of humility and self-improvement, in order to regain group acceptance or social status. The best way to understand current Chinese nationalism is to remember the 100 years of painful humiliation in the hands of foreign invaders starting from the Opium Wars. The government can harness this collective shame as a rallying point against Western countries.

Let us examine China's fight against the coronavirus as an example to illustrate the positive and negative function of shame in Chinese society. On December 8, 2019, collective pneumonia broke out in a wholesale wet market of Wuhan. Several medical workers reported the incident and sounded the alarm in their WeChat groups. They were subsequently arrested by the local public security unit for spreading rumors and forced to write self-criticisms for their professional misconduct. One of the whistleblowers, Dr. Li Wenliang (李文亮), had also been admonished but was still allowed to work in the medical frontline.

Dr. Li declared himself a confirmed case of COVID-19 as early as January 8, 2020, when the epidemic situation became uncontrollable. By January 23, 2020, Wuhan was put into lockdown in order to contain the spread. Dr. Li died of pneumonia on February 1, 2020.

His death transformed him into a national hero, who had sacrificed his life for the public good. Meanwhile, his death also transformed people's dissatisfaction into anger. The turbulent force of public opinion asked for the freedom of speech along with a fair investigation into the cover-up of this event. This public criticism of the Chinese government amounted to the shaming of officials.

Moreover, *The Wall Street Journal* published an article titled "China is the Real Sick Man of Asia" on February 3, 2020 (see Mead, 2020). For a while, terms as "Yellow alert" and "Yellow peril" became prevailing winds in Western major medias and social networks; *Der Spiegel*, a German news magazine, even added "Corona virus: Made in China" on its cover!

The international criticisms of the Chinese government over their initial handling of the COVID-19 outbreak reminded many Chinese people of the shame of being invaded by Western imperial powers during the century of humiliation, resulting in a rise in patriotism. The loss of national face (Chen & Hwang, 2016) prompted the government to take immediate action to save their face. On February 11, both the chairperson and party secretary who were in charge of the Hygiene and Health Committee in Hubei were dismissed by the provincial standing committee of the CPC. Dismissal from a high-ranked position may not mean that one is guilty, but it at least implies that one is incompetent to make appropriate decisions for good governance. In other words, one may suffer from the shame of losing social face, but not moral face (Hwang, 2006).

On February 13, 2020, the Chinese Center for Disease Control (China CDC) issued the "Order of Control for Wartime" to activate its first-level public health emergency response to control the outbreak. The local government was ordered to bring the situation under control, and therefore, no one was exempt from screening and testing (掌握情況，不漏一人).

In addition to the implementation of disinfection and ventilation procedures, and body temperature monitoring in public areas, while in lockdown, the local government had to take effective measures to curb pollution, to cancel public gatherings, to suspend tourism group tours, to close scenic areas, etc. Special reimbursement rules were also issued by the local government to resolve the shortage of medical supplies and daily necessities. Price gouging and hoarding could now be subjected to the maximum penalty.

Meanwhile, the "Leading Group of the CPC Committee for Novel Coronavirus Prevention and Control" was organized and led by Prime Minister Li Keqiang (李克強) under the supervision of President Xi Jinping (習近平) and the Political Bureau of the CPC to formulate the "whip system" of administration (一條鞭式管理體制) from central to local government. Thus, the major leaders of the nation became responsible for the successes or failures of their policies, which have been linked with their social face (臉面) as well as the stability of their positions. The Chinese CDC on their part, learning from the SARS experience, had requested all medical institutions to report individual case of infectious diseases. The National Health Committee began to announce the up-to-date statistics and the related policies for epidemic control on a daily basis.

Four thousand soldiers of the People's Liberation Army (PLA) were sent to help workers in Wuhan build two hospitals (Houshenshan 火神山 and Leishenshan 雷神山) with 813 and 1600 beds, respectively, to accommodate severe COVID-19 cases. In addition, 14 mobile cabin hospitals were built for general patients. More than 40,000 medical staff and healthcare workers were mobilized from other provinces to support Wuhan. Eventually, the epidemic situation was under control at the beginning of March 2020. Nobody knows what will happen in the future, but this story may help us to understand the functioning of Confucian culture in contemporary China.

3.4 The Positive Side of Shame

According to biological evolution, shame evolved to encourage group collaboration through following social norms because survival depended on it. Even when one person did not live by the rules (such as stealing or murdering another), the cohesiveness of the whole group was threatened. This is especially true in any collectivist society; group interpersonal harmony is valued. Even in an individualist society, there are still some social norms to facilitate social interaction or political correctness to avoid unnecessary offences against minority. Jennifer Jacquet's *Is Shame Necessary? New Uses for an Old Tool* (2015) examined how shaming—exposing a transgressor to public disapproval—could be used in a productive way. In other words, we can use shaming as a deterrent of a bad behavior without destroying anyone's reputation or life (see Vanderheiden on The Terror of Being Judged: Public Shaming as Resource and Strategic Tool in this book).

At a personal level, we often suffer from our unconscious defense mechanisms against shame (Michaelson, 2015; Thompson, 2015). Many psychological problems have their roots in hidden shame. Acceptance and transformation of shame are important in facilitating recovery from psychological disorders and transforming negative experiences into emotional resilience, character strengths, and human flourishing. In overcoming the self-deceptions and emotional lies, we become mentally healthier, stronger, and happier (see Mayer and Vanderheiden on The Meaning of Shame in Cultures of the Fourth Industrial Revolution and Mayer on Transforming Shame Through Love: Envisioning Positive Transcultural Leadership in Contemporary and Future Workplaces).

An Introduction According to Benau (2012), therapists should help their clients accept and transform shame, rather than trying to avoid or reduce it in order to develop "shame resilience." This is the position advocated by Wong (2019b).

What follows are a few paragraphs from a monograph titled *Shame as the Master Emotion of Everyday Life* by Drs. Sheff and Retzinger, summarized by Kimberley Nichols (2013):

1. Shame is a key component of conscience, responsible for our moral behavior. Listening to the voice of conscience will enable us to do the right thing.
2. Shame signals trouble in a relationship and motivates us to restore intimacy and trust to the source in shared ideals.
3. Finally, shame plays a central role in regulating the expression of emotions. It helps us guard our innermost feelings which may embarrass us, if they are disclosed or revealed inappropriately.

Additional benefits of shame include learning to not set up unrealistic measures of one's value of self-worth, as we have discussed in the meritocracy section. We need to focus more on our intrinsic values as growth and making a unique useful contribution to society. We also need to develop the courage to not be afraid of being disliked or criticized by others, as long as we are following our conscience and best judgment. The pain of shame also alerts us to the problem of shaming others unintentionally when we make unreasonable demands or frequently judge and criticize others simply because they do things differently. PP 2.0 advocates the adaptive benefits of confronting rather than avoiding painful emotions.

Awareness of all the problems related to shame opens the gateway to healing and transformation, so that we will not do things that we will be ashamed of and we can die well without major regrets. Self-reflection and examination of one's beliefs and values may lead to self-restructuring. Finally, there is also the spiritual message for us to recognize our limitations and frailty and the need to hold ourselves accountable to higher power or moral authority.

4 Conclusion

Most human emotions are complex. The human quest for personal growth and wholeness necessarily involves struggling with ambivalent feelings through the dialectical process as proposed by PP 2.0 (Wong, 2011). This struggle makes us both stronger and wiser. Shame can both stymie and motivate learning and personal growth. Unfortunately, there is not enough public discourse on the positive side of shame:

> As Dirkx implored us over a decade ago, we need to stop shying away from emotions in adult learning and to begin to courageously engage that which lies in the unconscious but which drives our everyday actions and interactions. Shame is at the core of who we are—and who we can become—as adult learners and educators. (Walker, 2017)

We need to cultivate the virtue of humility as the antidote to both relational and moral shame. We humbly acknowledge that we can never as good as other people in some areas and we are never good enough to be above criticisms or corrections in our work and relationships. Therefore, in humility, we accept our limitations and failure and are determined to improve ourselves each day. Humility also delivers us from our self-righteousness and arrogance which blind our eyes to our moral failure and from the misguided need to cover up failures.

Existential competency in therapy deals with both the negative and positive aspects of shame. We can readily distill several basic skills in existential competency from various chapters. These clinical skills include:

- Self-awareness, acceptance, and acknowledgment of one's failures and limitations
- Self-forgiveness and self-compassion
- Self-affirmation through re-authoring and reframing
- Self-affirming the intrinsic value and sacredness of life
- Taking personal responsibility for positive change
- Seeking a support group
- Focusing on the meaning people attach to events
- Seeking deeper meaning and self-transcendence
- Seeking deeper understanding through verbalizing one's emotions and dreams

We want to conclude this chapter by citing Ron Farmer (2013):

> The path of self-transformation demands that we return to accepting ourselves for who we are; that we make our feelings of self-worth impregnable against unexpected errors and misfortunes. What follows are some guidelines for achieving this aim.

The world would be better if we pay more attention to shame. May the force of shame be with you all—to prevent us from doing anything we may be ashamed of and spur us to improve ourselves daily to be better and stronger people.

References

Bai, L. (2015). *Emotion categorization and early bilinguals: A study of Chinese-English bilinguals' understanding of the* shame *category* (Doctoral dissertation, Nanyang Technological University, Singapore). Retrieved from https://pdfs.semanticscholar.org/7903/8b8181db083274bb930c3e3ef14d36f6b28f.pdf?_ga=2.111065285.1750197583.1564586688-610348782.1563216195

Bedford, O., & Hwang, K. K. (2003). Guilt and shame in Chinese culture: A cross-cultural framework from the perspective of morality and identity. *Journal for the Theory of Social Behaviour, 33*(2), 127–144. https://doi.org/10.1111/1468-5914.00210.

Benau, K. S. (2012). A review of shame in the therapy hour by Ronda L. Dearing and June Price Tangney (Eds.). *PsycCRITIQUES, 57*(6). https://doi.org/10.1037/a0026226.

Blackford, R. (2018). *The tyranny of opinion*. London, UK: Bloomsbury Academic.

Boxwell, R. (2020). How China's fake news machine is rewriting the history of Covid-19, even as the pandemic unfolds. *South China Morning Post.* Retrieved from https://www.politico.com/news/magazine/2020/04/04/china-fake-news-coronavirus-164652

Brown, B. (Keynote speaker). (2012). *Listening to shame* [online video]. Retrieved from https://www.ted.com/talks/brene_brown_listening_to_shame?language=en

Chen, R., & Hwang, K. K. (2016). Nation, face, and identity: An initial investigation of national face in East Asia. *Frontiers in Psychology, 7*, 1557. https://doi.org/10.3389/fpsyg.2016.01557.

Duggan, M. (2017). *Online harassment 2017*. Pew Research Center. Retrieved from https://www.cybersmile.org/wp-content/uploads/PI_2017.07.11_Online-Harassment_FINAL.pdf

Farmer, R. (2013). Self-transformation: From shame to self-worth. *Wellbeing.* Retrieved from https://www.wellbeing.com.au/mind-spirit/mind/self-transformation-shame-self-worth.html

Fowers, B. J., Richardson, F. C., & Slife, B. D. (2017). *Frailty, suffering, and vice: Flourishing in the face of human limitations*. Washington, DC: American Psychological Association.

Galer, S. (2020). Intelligent robotic process automation is not your average top 2020 trend. *Forbes.* Retrieved from https://www.forbes.com/sites/sap/2020/02/06/intelligent-robotic-process-automation-is-not-your-average-top-2020-trend/#3e86ed561cc9

Gilbert, P. (2000). The relationship of shame, social anxiety and depression: The role of the evaluation of social rank. *Clinical Psychology & Psychotherapy, 7*(3), 174–189. https://doi.org/10.1002/1099-0879(200007)7:33.0.CO;2-U.

Harvey, C. (2020). What would warming mean for pathogens like coronavirus? *Scientific American.* Retrieved from https://www.scientificamerican.com/article/what-could-warming-mean-for-pathogens-like-coronavirus/

Hiebert, P. G. (1985). *Anthropological insights for missionaries*. Grand Rapids, MI: Baker Book House.

Ho, D. Y. F. (1976). On the concept of face. *American Journal of Sociology, 81*(4), 867–884. https://doi.org/10.1086/226145.

Hwang, K. K. (2006). Moral face and social face: Contingent self-esteem in Confucian society. *International Journal of Psychology, 41*(4), 276–281.

Hwang, K. K., & Han, K. H. (2010). Face and morality in Confucian society. In M. H. Bond (Ed.), *Oxford handbook of Chinese psychology* (pp. 479–498). Oxford, UK: Oxford University Press.

Jacquet, J. (2015). Is shame necessary? In *New uses for an old tool*. New York, NY: Vintage Books.

Jyoti, R., & Schubmehl, D. (2019). IDC FutureScape webcast: Worldwide Artificial Intelligence 2020 Predictions. *IDC*. Retrieved from https://www.idc.com/getdoc.jsp?containerId=WC20191118

Karma, R. (2019). The meritocracy trap, explained. *Vox*. Retrieved from https://www.vox.com/policy-and-politics/2019/10/24/20919030/meritocracy-book-daniel-markovits-inequality-rich

Lewis, M. (1998). Shame and stigma. In P. Gilbert & B. Andrews (Eds.), *Shame: Interpersonal behavior, psychopathology, and culture* (pp. 126–140). New York, NY: Oxford University.

Li, J., Wang, L., & Fischer, K. (2004). The organisation of Chinese shame concepts? *Cognition and Emotion, 18*(6), 767–797. https://doi.org/10.1080/02699930341000202.

Lin, J., & Yao, Y. (2016). Encoding emotion in Chinese: A database of Chinese emotion words with information of emotion type, intensity, and valence. *Lingua Sinica, 2*, 6. https://doi.org/10.1186/s40655-016-0015-y.

Markovits, D. (2019). *The meritocracy trap: How America's foundational myth feeds inequality, dismantles the middle class, and devours the elite*. London, UK: Penguin Press.

Mayer, C. H., & Vanderheiden, E. (Eds.). (2019). *The bright side of shame: Transforming and growing through practical applications in cultural contexts*. Cham, Switzerland: Springer.

Mead, W. R. (2020). China is the real sick man of Asia. *WSJ*. Retrieved from https://www.wsj.com/articles/china-is-the-real-sick-man-of-asia-11580773677

Michaelson, P. (2015). *Why we suffer: A Western way to understand and let go of unhappiness*. London, UK: Prospect Books.

Monderer, M. (2020). Reassessing the global economic fallout from COVID-19. *Stratfor*. Retrieved from https://worldview.stratfor.com/article/reassessing-global-economic-fallout-covid-19-coronavirus-pandemic-economy

Nichols, K. (2013). Tools of transformation # 18: The Master Emotions: Shame, Guilt and Fear. *Newtopia Magazine*. Retrieved from https://newtopiamagazine.wordpress.com/2013/05/15/tools-of-transformation-18-the-master-emotions-shame-guilt-and-fear

Pietsch, B. (2020). China is using drones to scold people for going outside and not wearing masks amid the coronavirus outbreak. *Business Insider*. Retrieved from https://www.businessinsider.com/china-uses-drones-to-patrol-citizens-during-wuhan-coronavirus-outbreak-2020-1

Purtill, J. (2020). People no longer believe working hard will lead to better life, survey shows. *ABC.net*. Retrieved from https://www.abc.net.au/triplej/programs/hack/2020-edelman-trust-barometer-shows-growing-sense-of-inequality/11883788?fbclid=IwAR0k9AGBXutKULaFIYMrwKc52-yxqQqe0302hQAbpv62q8auYFPVthrc9Uc

Salice, A., & Sánchez, A. M. (2016). Pride, shame, and group identification. *Frontiers in Psychology, 7*(557). https://doi.org/10.3389/fpsyg.2016.00557.

Scheff, S., & Schorr, M. (2017). *Shame nation: The global epidemic of online hate*. Chicago, IL: Sourcebooks.

Schwab, K., & Davis, N. (2018). *Shaping the future of the fourth Industrial Revolution*. New York, NY: Penguin Random House.

Scibona, S. (2019). The industrial revolution of shame. *The New York Times*. Retrieved from https://www.nytimes.com/2019/03/09/opinion/sunday/internet-shaming.html

Shum, S. (2020). The trick to succeeding in life? Just be human. *Vice*. Retrieved from https://www.vice.com/en_asia/article/qjdvpw/trick-succeeding-life-be-human-stress-management?utm_source=viceasiatw

Sky News Australia. (2020). *Special report: China's deadly coronavirus cover-up*. Retrieved from https://www.youtube.com/watch?v=pKmUxSlOoUE

Stanford Encyclopedia of Philosophy. (2004). *Mencius*. Retrieved from https://plato.stanford.edu/entries/mencius/

Susaria, A. (2020). Hate cancel culture? Blame algorithms. *PHYSORG*. Retrieved from https://phys.org/news/2020-01-cancel-culture-blame-algorithms.amp

Taylor, S. E., & Brown, J. D. (1988). Illusion and well-being: A social psychological perspective on mental health. *Psychological Bulletin, 103*(2), 193–210. https://doi.org/10.1037/0033-2909.103.2.193.

Thompson, C. (2015). *The soul of shame: Retelling the stories we believe about ourselves*. London, UK: Inter-Varsity Press.

Tidy, J. (2020). Coronavirus: How China's using surveillance to tackle outbreak. *BBC News*. Retrieved from https://www.bbc.com/news/av/world-asia-52104798/coronavirus-how-china-s-using-surveillance-to-tackle-outbreak

Van Norden, B. W. (2002). The emotion of shame and the virtue of righteousness in Mencius. *Dao (A Journal of Comparative Philosophy), 2*(1), 45–77. https://doi.org/10.1007/BF02856995.

Walker, J. (2017). Shame and transformation in the theory and practice of adult learning and education. *Journal of Transformative Education, 15*(4). https://doi.org/10.1177/1541344617699591.

Watson, B. (2009). *The analects of Confucius*. New York, NY: Columbia University Press.

Wong, P. T. P. (2011). Positive psychology 2.0: Towards a balanced interactive model of the good life. *Canadian Psychology, 52*(2), 69–81. https://doi.org/10.1037/a0022511.

Wong, P. T. P. (2019a). Second wave positive psychology's (PP 2.0) contribution to counselling psychology. *Counselling Psychology Quarterly*. https://doi.org/10.1080/09515070.2019.1671320.

Wong, P. T. P. (2019b). Foreword: From shame to wholeness: An existential positive psychology perspective. In C. H. Mayer & E. Vanderheiden (Eds.), *The bright side of shame: Transforming and growing through practical applications in cultural contexts* (pp. v–ix). Cham, Switzerland: Springer.

Wong, P. T. P. (2020). The maturing of positive psychology and the emerging PP 2.0 [Book review of Positive psychology (3rd ed.) by William Compton and Edward Hoffman]. *International Journal on WellBeing, 10*(1). https://doi.org/10.5502/ijw.v10i1.885.

Wong, Y., & Tsai, J. (2007). Cultural models of shame and guilt. In J. L. Tracy, R. W. Robins, & J. P. Tangney (Eds.), *The self-conscious emotions: Theory and research* (pp. 209–223). New York, NY: Guilford Press.

Yong, E. (2020). How the pandemic will end. *The Atlantic*. Retrieved from https://www.theatlantic.com/health/archive/2020/03/how-will-coronavirus-end/608719

Yuval, N. H. (2018). *Homo Deus: A brief history of tomorrow*. New York, NY: Harper Perennial.

Zapotosky, M., Wagner, J., & Iati, M. (2020). Coronavirus pandemic could kill as many as 200,000 in U.S., White House Warns. *The Washington Post*. Retrieved from https://www.washingtonpost.com/national/coronavirus-deaths-warning-america/2020/03/30/522221ce-72a6-11ea-87da-77a8136c1a6d_story.html

Paul T. P. Wong, Ph.D., C.Psych., is Professor Emeritus of Trent University and Adjunct Professor at Saybrook University. He is a Fellow of APA and CPA and President of the International Network on Personal Meaning (www.meaning.ca) and the Meaning-Centered Counselling Institute. Editor of the *International Journal of Existential Psychology and Psychotherapy*, he has also edited two influential volumes on *The Human Quest for Meaning*. A prolific Writer, he is one of the most cited existential and positive psychologists. The Originator of Meaning Therapy and International Meaning Conferences, he has been invited to give keynotes and meaning therapy workshops worldwide. He is the recent recipient of the Carl Rogers Award from the Society for Humanistic Psychology (Div. 32 of the APA).

Kwang-Kuo Hwang, Ph.D., is Professor Emeritus of the National Taiwan University. His primary research focuses on the field of Personality and Social Psychology. He received his Ph. D. at the University of Hawaii and is the recipient of many awards and honors since 1977. Most recently, he received the Dr. Son yet-sen's Awards for Academic Work.

Chapter 8
Deterritorialization of Shame in Japan During the Fourth Industrial Revolution (4IR)

Yoshiyuki Takano and Paul T. P. Wong

1 The 4IR and Social Issues of Shame in Japan

Technological advancements and globalization—as a result of the Fourth Industrial Revolution (4IR)—have contributed to the well-being of many people's lives in Japan. The issue of shame in the 4IR is not just caused by the advancement of technology. Tensions also exist as Japan moves toward multinational capitalism; the advancement of modern culture co-exists with the need to preserve traditional Japanese culture. However, the 4IR has also brought challenges to the traditional collective culture, which values respect and honor of others, the harmony of relationships over individuals' rights, and the achievement of goals (see Kotera, Sheffield, Green, and Asano in this book).

The 4IR affects the human-to-human connection in numerous ways. Heavy reliance on virtual communication through emails, social media, Skype, or Zoom has severely reduced person-to-person contacts in real-life situations, thus reducing the opportunities of full-fledged communications that involve human touch, body language, deep sharing, and the joy of doing things together.

The big data from powerful corporations such as Google and Facebook have stored the private and confidential information of millions of people. Hackers and marketers can tap into such information. The lack of adequate protection of confidential information means that familial and individual secrets could be exposed from unintended sharing. The power of instant communication though social medial can be abused too, as in the case of cyberbullying. Depending only on virtual platforms to contact others also created the phenomenon of *hikikomori* in Japanese culture.

Y. Takano (✉)
University of Prince Edward Island, Charlottetown, Canada
e-mail: takanoy@alumni.ubc.ca

P. T. P. Wong
Trent University, Toronto, ON, Canada

C.-H. Mayer et al. (eds.), *Shame 4.0*, https://doi.org/10.1007/978-3-030-59527-2_8

2 Hikikomori Is a Recent Social Phenomenon

This is a phenomenon whereby Japanese youth physically withdraw from society and isolate themselves for extended periods of time, sometimes for many years. Rather than interacting with others face-to-face, they stay in touch with the outside world through cyberspace (Furlong, 2008; Koyama et al., 2010; Tateno et al., 2019).

A study done by Tateno et al. (2019) indicates that, out of 478 college/university students in Japan, 22.2% display symptoms of *hikikomori* and 39.8% show smartphone addiction. The cause of *hikikomori* is not entirely clear, but many theorists suggest that the decrease in direct communication between individuals and their families, alongside rapidly changing societal and familial relationship dynamics—due to the modernization of Japanese daily life—may be contributing to the development and prolonged duration of *hikikomori* (Koyama et al., 2010; Saito, 1998).

One of the more problematic symptoms experienced by people with *hikikomori* is an increased likelihood to be perpetrators of domestic violence. Saito (1998) states that sufferers often engage in violent behavior and express hatred toward their parents; they feel rejected and judged for not meeting their parents' and society's expectations of success. In Saito's research, among 80 participants (66 males and 14 females of average age 19.6 with 39 months of social withdrawn at the time of study), all diagnosed with *hikikomori*, roughly 62% had engaged in some form of violent behavior at home (e.g., breaking things, punching walls, and yelling), and 51% had displayed violent behavior toward family members (Saito, 1998).

Sufferers of *hikikomori* appear to have underlying deep-rooted emotional issues. In Saito's study, 53% of subjects experienced a sense of hopelessness and guilt, and 88% experienced a sense of loneliness, boredom, and emptiness. However, contrary to what people might imagine, over 70% came from middle-class families; their parents were married, and they came from stable socioeconomic backgrounds.

Hikikomori—with its symptomatic violent behavior—appears to be rooted in a sense of shame that is unique to current Japanese society. The source of this shame may be the sufferers' sense that they have failed to meet societal and parental expectations, as well as a loss of dignity due to being unable to accept who they are. In Japanese culture, psychological and behavioral issues are perceived as resulting from a lack of willpower, self-control, and self-discipline; discussing personal issues with those who are outside of their kinship creates a sense of shame (Tamura & Lau, 1992). In view of the stigma of mental problems, Japanese people generally prefer to deal with their issues within their immediate families and only get help from extended family if necessary; mental health and family issues create a strong sense of humiliation.

A similar phenomenon can also be found in Chinese families. Wong (this chapter's co-author) has worked with young Chinese people who had left their university education or work and stayed in their room for weeks or months. Their only companion was their computer. They seldom met people or went out to socialize. They spent most of their time surfing the Internet, playing electronic games, or indulging in pornography. They also developed symptoms of depression, anxiety, and poor self-esteem. They suffered from a sense of shame because they knew that they had failed their parents' expectations and they had to depend on their parents for financial support. China is a Confucian society where saving "face" is very important (see Wong & Hwang, 2020) (see Wong and Hwang in this book).

The inevitable by-product of such isolation means boredom. Humans are wired for relationships, which are critical for meaning and well-being (Baumeister & Leary, 1995; McDonald, Wong, & Gingras, 2012). The lack of interpersonal and group activities leads to boredom and unhappiness. Another related problem is the lack of necessary social skill development, which leads to social anxiety and fear of social failure.

Shame is one of the strongest stigmas in Japanese culture. Interestingly, as a result, it can also increase the drive for excellence, as people try to avoid it at all costs. Ethical codes of conduct, such as *bushidō* (the way of life of traditional Japanese samurai warriors) (Nitobe, 1899/2019), have been strongly rooted in Japanese culture for centuries. *Bushidō* is "the unwritten code of laws governing the lives and conduct of the nobles of Japan, equivalent in many ways to the European chivalry" (Nitobe, 1899/2019, p. 5). The samurais, knights, and aristocratic warriors of medieval Japan who were prevalent from the twelfth to the fifteenth century followed the *bushidō's* seven core ethical codes of conduct: rectitude/justice, courage, benevolence, politeness, veracity and sincerity, honor, and loyalty. These codes are based on Buddhist, Shintoist, and Confucius beliefs, and they form the principles of *bushidō* (honorable living).

In Japan, a sense of shame is often caused by the gaze of others, and the shame is internalized, i.e., directed toward the self (Doi, 1973). This sense of shame is created by one's thoughts, behavior, and emotions as they compare themselves to Japanese society's moral and ethical standards (Sakuta, 1964). Shame is often experienced before others, especially mentors and elders, but it can also emerge when individuals compare their thoughts, actions, and feelings to their internalized criteria or frames of reference (Sakuta, 1964).

Thus, in Japan, people have a strong sense of obligation to avoid creating disharmony and to follow societal norms. In Japan, people concern themselves with *sekentei*, which refers to individuals' perceptions of how society/others view them (Tatara, 1998). *Sekentei* is closely linked to individuals' perceptions of their own faces, reputations, appearances, and sense of who they are. This often becomes a strong frame of reference and can lead to stigma in terms of judging one's own social worthiness; thus, it promotes conformity in group settings.

In Japanese culture, it is a common practice for people to address one another by their family names. The family names to which people belong—*kamei*—are not simply their names but also the representations of their entire genealogies and their responsibility to honor their commitments; thus, shame follows if they fail. Japanese people are extremely careful not to bring any disgrace or shame to their family names.

Japanese culture has clear boundaries between individuals' perceptions inside and outside of their family systems (Doi, 1973). The word for people considered "outsiders" is *tannin*, which means "persons with no blood relationship to oneself" or "persons unconnected with oneself" (Doi, 1973, p. 36). Doi (1973) states that it takes time and effort to build authentic and close relationships that can become as close as those within one's own family; until that time, those relationships remain *tannin*, i.e., acquaintances, not in the realm of kinship. In the relationship with *tannin*, a boundary between individuals—*enryo*—often exists to protect individuals from being overly intrusive with overbearing on one another.

Holding a sense of honor and dignity and avoiding shame are important to the Japanese way of life. If one member of a family is shamed—otherwise known as "loss of face"—the respect and status of the entire family in a community are diminished (Hsu, 1970). It is not simply a sense of embarrassment but a disgrace against ethical codes of conduct that brings shame to the entire family.

Therapy for sufferers of *hikikomori* involves working with them on their sense of shame. Shame is a core issue for violence, and those who resort to violence cannot change without facing their own shame (Hydén, Gadd, & Wade, 2016; Jenkins, 2009). The relationship between shame, violence, and aggression has been reported by various researchers (e.g., Gilligan, 2009; Simon, 2002; Teyber & Teyber, 2017).

Although facing shame is an important part of the change process, challenging people to simply take responsibility and own their shame may push them further away. Facing shame is a painful experience because "shame always speaks about our inner self rather than our actions" (Nathanson, 1992, p. 19). Moreover, "shame often follows a moment of exposure; what has been exposed is something that we would have preferred kept hidden, usually something of an intimate and personal nature" (Nathanson, 1992, p. 19). Thus, denial, minimization, and blame for another person's behavior—as well as denial, minimization, and displacement for one's own responsibility to alleviate shame—may provide a protective function for a perpetrator's self-esteem (Maruna & Mann, 2006).

Meaning therapy (Wong, 2016, 2019) is another kind of therapy that could help clients overcome their shame. Simply put, this therapy firstly emphasizes the importance of providing a safe and trusting therapeutic relationship for clients to face their painful memories. Secondly, clients would learn to name their painful emotions, such as shame or fear, so that they can tame it. Thirdly, they would reconstruct a more positive narrative about the shameful feelings. Finally, they would learn to take responsibility to pursue some meaningful and satisfying goal in small, realistic steps.

3 Therapeutic Application of Deterritorialization of Shame

Traditionally, in the field of psychology, shame has been understood as a multifaceted experience that includes feelings of anxiety, anger, disgust, and/or sadness, with a variety of negative cognitive appraisals of self, such as feelings of helplessness, resentment toward others, self-hatred, a sense of inferiority, and a sense of exposure. These feelings are related to unpleasant physiological arousal, which can in turn cause shamed individuals to hide and avoid others (Bradshaw, 2005; Dearing & Tangney, 2011; Gilbert, Pehl, & Allan, 1994; Tracy, Robings, & Tangney, 2007).

Shame is often thought to be caused by traumatic experiences, and, therefore, therapists look for causes and then go about attempting to find solutions to "cure" the shame. However, this common and current worldview—the dominant narrative—can territorialize experiences of shame and can serve as a constraint on exploring other possibilities of meaning. Territorialization refers to numerous forms of preconceived definitions or boundaries of human phenomena that provide a series of vocabulary to identify and categorize such phenomena (Patton, 2006). Such preconceived definitions can be constraining; they serve to keep meanings stuck within particular—and perhaps unhealthy—realms. This strict boundary of meaning also defines the functions of what phenomena should do. Territorialization can create toxic shame, as well as its persistent nature. To work on shame, we must deconstruct the meanings we have assigned to it and look beyond the traditional "cause and effect" relationship. The process of "[d]eterritorialisation occurs when an event of becoming escapes or detaches from its original territory" (Colebrook, 2002, p. 59). Livesey (2010) points out that deterritorialization is an emergent, innovative, and productive process that creates a new reality.

Shame is often considered to be a by-product of the events of one's life, such as abuse, divorce, and negative emotional experiences. We often treat history as fact; as a result, therapists often attempt to investigate the "roots" of shame and use history as a succession of facts that creates a cohesive story of "cause and effect." However, there is a distinction between history and facts. Parr (2006) challenges the historical understanding of collective experience (absolute) and pits it against the unique individual experiences in time (relative). Parr (2006) summarizes this point by invoking Libeskind's (2000) comment on the Holocaust: "[H]istory is not the statistics of the six million Jews, but a unique Jewish individual multiplied six million times" (pp. 132–133). In other words, the meaning of collective experiences of historical events may not capture everyone's distinct and in-depth understanding of them.

Deleuze and Guattari's concept of becoming is essential. It refers to pursuing opportunities for new possibilities (Colebrook, 2002). When facing shame, it is critical to explore the unique meaning that each individual has created and not to categorize the meaning of shame based on a preconceived "cause and effect" relationship narrative; such territorialization prevents shame from "becoming." This is similar to Wong's meaning therapy described earlier.

When working with shame by using certain types of therapeutic approaches (e.g., psychodynamic, objective relations theory), therapists often focus on an interpretive process, and they consider the therapeutic relationship to be a vehicle for change through perspective as projection, countertransference, and attachment rebuilding. However, in the deterritorialization process of facing shame, the therapeutic relationship is not an interpretive relationship but rather a dialogic one (Shotter, 2008). It is a different epistemological understanding of "intersubjectivity" and "mutuality."

In this dialogical relationship—unlike the psychoanalytic and relational approaches—the client is not an object of consciousness or subjectivity; as the relationship develops, "another form of life emerges between us, a collective or shared form of life with *its own unique character* and *its own unique world*" (Shotter, 2011, p. 1). Similarly, Kvale (1996) explains dialogical interaction as "a situation of knowledge production in which knowledge is created between the views of the two partners in the conversation" (p. 296). Kvale points out the importance of co-construction of knowledge through interaction.

Therefore, instead of pursuing a "cause and effect" relationship in an attempt to "fix" and "heal" shame, the goal is to deterritorialize it, which refers to the process of "becoming other than itself" (Colebrook, 2002, p. 56). The goal is to create new territories that do not concur with those organized by the dominant narrative (Parr, 2006). Deterritorialization is not just a cognitive restructuring process but an experiential process of deconstructing a territorialized meaning of shame and co-constructing new territory by implementing one's own desire and yearning to break away from restrained territorialized meanings of shame and to explore new possibilities.

The critical process helps those who suffer from shame to have a dialogue with shame in their own current territory of meaning, because such a dialogical process constructs new meaning. The concept of "singular memory" in the deterritorialization process is key. Singular memory "enervates the majoritarian system of history" (Parr, 2006, p. 126). Singular memory rejects the dominant narrative of shame; instead, exploration of singular memory can create narratives that have previously been unavailable (Jenkins, 2011).

"[S]ingular memory is where deterritorialisation and reterritorialisation meet (Deleuze & Guattari, 1994, p. 110)" (Parr, 2006, p. 129); it breaks down territorialized ideas and creates new and reterritorialized concepts. Deterritorialization and reterritorialization occur at a "moment when history becomes other than what it once was, that moment when singular memory breaks through the colonising and re-territorialising movement of memory" (Parr, 2006, p. 133). Therefore, the aim of working on shame is not to "heal" or "cure" it, but instead to break it away from such constrained territory and reclaim it with a reterritorialization by inviting other singular memories that were not previously included in one's narrative.

The experience of going inside the territories of shame can also lead individuals to new territories and thus deterritorialize the shame. Having a dialogue with shame in a different and unique way—where one faces the shame head-on and breaks down the secrecy—may immediately create new meaning, i.e., integrity, strength, and commitment. Such actively created meaning may become one's own lived experience. Gergen (1999) calls attention to this process where meaning is "located in either my actions or in yours, but within the action-supplement conjunction, or essentially, in the form of coordination we achieve" (Gergen, 1999, p. 146). This is a process of re-positioning shame by deconstructing its meaning, exploring singular memory, and aligning it with forces of deterritorialization (Jenkins, 2015).

When we fail to live up to the ethical codes we believe in, for example, the *bushidō*, we experience shame. Morita therapy (Morita 1928/1974)—Japanese traditional psychotherapy—acknowledges that human beings are motivated to seek self-preservation and self-actualization, which is a universal constructive desire called the "desire for life" (*sei no yokubo*) (Ishiyama, 1990; Morita, 1928/1974, 1998). This desire for life is compatible with the forces of shame, fear, and anxiety (Ishiyama, 1990; Morita, 1928/1974, 1998; Takano & Ishiyama, 2013). People wish to live well and excel in their social activities and relationships, so much so that they often experience "inconvenient feelings" (Ishiyama, 1990), which are negative feelings such as shame, anxiety, fear, and anger. However, it is a natural reaction for people to feel anxious and even fearful when they face important life events, such as examinations and job interviews, because they naturally want to excel.

Morita therapy appreciates the positive value of such "inconvenient feelings" as a reflection of clients' constructive desires. Focusing on such a desire for life without being preoccupied with "inconvenient feelings" allows people to engage in purpose-oriented action (Takano & Ishiyama, 2008, 2009, 2010, 2013). Putting feelings into action is where real change occurs, regardless of one's emotional state. According to Ishiyama (1990), "They (people) may realize that they *can* engage in productive activities *nervously*" (p. 569). Similarly, Satir also acknowledges the role of human yearning—the universal longing that all human beings have to be loved, accepted, validated, and confirmed—and the fact that human beings are driven to positive directional goals (Satir, Banmen, Geber, & Gomori, 1991).

However, the concept of desire should not be limited to a commonly understood sense of desire that is based on a lack (Bignall, 2010; Carter & Jackson, 2004; Colebrook, 2002); Carter and Jackson (2004) deny the concept of desire "that all motivation ... is rooted in the unachievable desire to fill this lack" (p. 108). Conceptualizing desire based on a deprivation can create constraints. For instance, using a traditional conception of desire when working with people who suffer from attachment issues could cause them to get stuck, because the "desire" is to fill what is lacking. In a way, the desire in this sense can remain unfillable because one's process of growth is differentiation, which is needed to create a unique identity of self (Carter & Jackson, 2004). In this conceptualization of desire, the goal becomes how to "fill" what is missing (lacking), and thus people often end up feeling stuck, as the process leads to the pursuit of what is missing.

Similarly, yearning can be perceived as something that is missing in one's life. Unmet yearning creates higher expectations on self and others, and unmet expectations can create a sense of being stuck (Satir et al., 1991). As Pipher (2016) explains, "The opposite of yearning is savoring the exquisite now" (p. 172). People may seek and yearn for what is missing and may not be fully present in the here and now (Pipher, 2016).

Deleuze and Guattari discuss an ontological shift in the concept of the meanings of desire and yearning. They "reject the notion that desire is a secondary function to lack, arguing that desire is the primary, that desire does not lack anything, it just is" (Carter & Jackson, 2004, p. 116). In Deleuzian and Guattarian terms, desire is a power of expansion (Colebrook, 2002). Desire is a connection, and connecting with other desires can preserve and enhance life and eventually creates communities and societies as a whole (Colebrook, 2002). Deleuze and Guattari conceptualize desire as more of an energy of creation, proliferation, expansion, and dispersion (Linstead & Pullen, 2006).

Living according to the dominant narrative of shame can create constraints as well as a sense of being stuck; if our sense of shame suppresses us, we might struggle with constant unfulfilled desire. To deterritorialize shame is to refuse to "participate in limiting and disabling historical narratives of self" (Jenkins, 2011, p. 41); deterritorializing shame challenges the deconstruction of conventional knowledge and creates new possibilities. Moreover, such dialogical interaction can disrupt dominant meaning systems and resist the dominant narrative of self (Jenkins, 2011), and thus it can construct meanings that transcend shame.

The therapeutic process involves facilitating active dialogue within the self and between therapists and clients in a way that explores possibilities for singular memories that have not previously been investigated. This breaks down the meanings of shame and constructs new ones.

4 Conclusion

Although the 4IR has brought profound material benefits to people's lives, it has also created tension between the desire to preserve traditional Japanese culture while moving toward multinational capitalism and the advancement of modernism. Shame remains a critical component of Japanese culture; traditional Japanese codes of ethics and morals remain ubiquitous in Japan.

The tension between the old ways of doing things and the newer ways of life has caused the meaning of shame to become more complex in present-day Japan, as exemplified by the recent phenomenon of *hikikomori*. Traditionally, in the field of psychology, therapists have searched for "causes" and have tried to provide "healing," but this chapter instead proposes the radical process of deterritorialization of shame, which promotes a dialogue with shame that works as an invitation to explore different dimensions of shame and one's vast desires.

These possibilities of expansive meaning can be demonstrated in people who violate their own values and integrity, as they often feel stuck in their lives and unsatisfied with what they have or have not done. Having a dialogue with one's own shame can be an overwhelming and painful experience because it comes up against one's own expansive desires and yearning (Takano, 2014). As a result, people may try to blame, rationalize, and minimize their responsibility, and then they emotionally withdraw. However, individuals who attempt to rationalize their violent behavior are in fact demonstrating that they recognize that their behavior is wrong (Todd, 2010; Todd, Weaver-Dunlop, & Ogden, 2014). Deterritorialization of shame is a process of inviting new possibilities of meaning through dialogue and by implementing singular memory into the dominant narrative. This process can create reterritorialization, i.e., new meaning of shame. As a result, the new possibilities in meaning can create transformation in individuals' experiences with shame.

Regarding future directions for research, to implement into a therapeutic approach, first, it is critical to investigate qualitatively the concept of shame and desire, as well as the therapeutic effectiveness of using the deterritorialization approach. Shame has been commonly conceptualized in neuropsychological and attachment perspectives (e.g., Nathanson, 1992; Ogden, Minton, & Pain, 2006), but it can be useful to investigate it through deconstruction. The purpose is to add another dimension to the phenomenon of shame in order to comprehend it in a more holistic manner, as some theorists and researchers suggest (i.e., Frankl, 1988; Takano, 2014; Wong, 2016).

Second, future research should investigate evidence-based ways of inviting the therapeutic narrative that can lead to the deterritorialization of shame and to expand one's desire and yearning. The therapeutic narrative should not be a random, non-purposeful conversation, but instead should be a precise dialogue with purpose and intention. Arvay (2002) writes, "Narrative is the linguistic form that we employ to make lived experience accessible and meaningful. It is through our narrative descriptions of personal experience that we make ourselves and others known to us" (p. 114). Narrative allows us to access other people's worlds, i.e., how they make sense of their experiences, actions, and events (Riessman, 1993). Narratives are our ways of sharing our worldviews and unique personal experiences, and such dialogues can lead us to new meanings that we may not have previously envisioned.

Clinically, the lack of opportunity of developing deep and authentic relationship during the 4IR is worrisome, when people increasingly depend on the Internet as a means of communications. The virtual world can never fully satisfy the human need for intimacy, physical contact, and body language to fully convey one's feelings and thoughts. Authentic relationships usually require mutual trust with honest and sincere communication. Sincerity or insincerity cannot be easily detected in virtual communication. Failing to meet the basic human need for love and intimacy may lead to mental illness, such as shame and depression. Therefore, meaning therapy emphasizes the need to develop meaningful work and meaningful relationship as a way to overcome shame or other toxic emotions.

References

Arvay, M. J. (2002). Talk as action: A narrative approach to action theory. *Canadian Journal of Counselling, 36*(2), 113–120.

Baumeister, R. F., & Leary, M. R. (1995). The need to belong: Desire for interpersonal attachments as a fundamental human motivation. *Psychological Bulletin, 117*(3), 497–529. https://doi.org/10.1037/0033-2909.117.3.497.

Bignall, S. (2010). Deleuze and political activism. In M. Svirsky (Ed.), *Desire, apathy and activism* (pp. 7–27). Edinburgh, UK: Edinburgh University.

Bradshaw, J. (2005). *Healing the shame that binds you.* Deerfield Beach, FL: Health Communications.

Carter, P., & Jackson, N. (2004). Gilles Deleuze and Félix Guattari. In S. Linstead (Ed.), *Organization theory and postmodern thought* (pp. 105–126). London: Sage.

Colebrook, C. (2002). *Gilles Deleuze*. New York, NY: Routledge.

Dearing, R., & Tangney, J. (2011). *Shame in the therapy hour.* Washington, DC: American Psychological Association.

Deleuze, G., & Guattari, F. (1994). *What is philosophy*? (G. Burchell & H. Tomlinson, trans.). London: Verso. (Original work published 1991).

Doi, T. (1973). *The anatomy of dependence*. Tokyo: Kodansha.
Frankl, V. E. (1988). *The will to meaning: Foundations and applications of logotherapy*. New York, NY: Meridian.
Furlong, A. (2008). The Japanese hikikomori phenomenon: Acute social withdrawal among young people. *The Sociological Review, 56*(2), 309–325. https://doi.org/10.1111/j.1467-954X.2008.00790.x.
Gergen, K. J. (1999). *An invitation to social construction*. Thousand Oaks, CA: Sage.
Gilbert, P., Pehl, J., & Allan, S. (1994). The phenomenology of shame and guilt: An empirical investigation. *British Journal of Medical Psychology, 67*(1), 23–36. https://doi.org/10.1111/j.2044-8341.1994.tb01768.x.
Gilligan, J. (2009). Sex, gender, & violence: Estela Weldon's contribution to our understanding of the psychopathology of violence. *British Journal of Psychotherapy, 25*(2), 239–256.
Hsu, F. L. K. (1970). *Americans and Chinese*. New York: Doubleday.
Hydén, M., Gadd, D., & Wade, A. (2016). Introduction to response based approaches to the study of interpersonal violence. In M. Hydén, D. Gadd, & A. Wade (Eds.), *Response based approaches to the study of interpersonal violence* (pp. 1–16). New York, NY: Palgrave Macmillan.
Ishiyama, F. I. (1990). A Japanese perspective on client inaction: Removing attitudinal blocks through Morita therapy. *Journal of Counseling and Development, 68*(5), 566–570. https://doi.org/10.1002/j.1556-6676.1990.tb01412.x.
Jenkins, A. (2009). Becoming ethical: A parallel. In *Political journey with men who have abused*. Dorset, UK: Russell House.
Jenkins, A. (2011). Becoming resilient: Overturning common sense—Part 1. *The Australian and New Zealand Journal of Family Therapy, 32*(1), 33–42. https://doi.org/10.1375/anft.32.1.33.
Jenkins, A. (2015). *Becoming ethical: A parallel, political journey with men who have abused. Two-day training for service providers for domestic violence*. Tokyo, Japan: Hakuyosha.
Koyama, A., Miyake, Y., Kawakami, N., Tsuchiya, M., Tachimori, H., & Takeshima, T. (2010). Lifetime prevalence, psychiatric comorbidity and demographic correlates of "hikikomori" in a community population in Japan. *Psychiatry Research, 176*(1), 69–74. https://doi.org/10.1016/j.psychres.2008.10.019.
Kvale, S. (1996). *InterViews: An introduction to qualitative research interviewing*. Thousand Oaks: Sage.
Libeskind, D. (2000). *The space of encounter*. New York, NY: Universe.
Linstead, S., & Pullen, A. (2006). Gender as multiplicity: Desire, displacement, difference and dispersion. *Human Relations, 59*(9), 1287–1310. https://doi.org/10.1177/0018726706069772.
Livesey, G. (2010). Assemblage. In A. Parr (Ed.), *The Deleuze dictionary: Revised edition* (pp. 18–19). Edinburg, UK: Edinburgh University.
Maruna, S., & Mann, R. E. (2006). A fundamental attribution error? Rethinking cognitive distortions. *Legal and Criminological Psychology, 11*(2), 155–177. https://doi.org/10.1348/135532506X114608.
McDonald, M. J., Wong, P. T. P., & Gingras, D. T. (2012). Meaning-in-life measures and development of a brief version of the personal meaning profile. In P. T. P. Wong (Ed.), *The human quest for meaning: Theories, research, and applications* (2nd ed., pp. 357–382). New York, NY: Routledge.
Morita, S. (1928/1974). *Shinkeishitsu-no hontai-to ryoho [Nature and treatment of nervosity]*. Tokyo, Japan: Hakuyosha.
Morita, S. (1998). *Morita therapy and the true nature of anxiety-based disorders (Shinkeishitsu)* (A. Kondo & P. LeVine, trans.). New York, NY: State University of New York.
Nathanson, D. L. (1992). *Shame and pride: Affect, sex, and the birth of the self*. New York: W.W. Norton & Company.
Nitobe, I. (1899/2019). *Bushido: The samurai code of Japan*. Tokyo, Japan: Tuttle.
Ogden, P., Minton, K., & Pain, C. (2006). *Trauma and the body: A sensorimotor approach to psychotherapy*. New York: W. W. Norton.
Parr, A. (2006). Deterritorializing the holocaust. In I. Buchanan & A. Parr (Eds.), *Deleuze and the contemporary world* (pp. 125–145). Edinburg, UK: Edinburgh University.

Patton, P. (2006). Deleuze's practical philosophy. *Symposium: Canadian Journal of Continental Philosophy/Revue canadienne de philosophie continentale, 10*(1), 285–303.

Pipher, M. (2016). *Letters to a young therapist: Stories of hope and healing*. New York, NY: Basic.

Riessman, C. K. (1993). *Narrative analysis*. New York, NY: Sage.

Saito, T. (1998). *Shakaiteki Hikikomori [Social Withdrawal]*. Tokyo: PHP Kenkyuujo.

Sakuta, K. (1964). *Haji no bunkasaiko [Reflecting cultural perspective on shame]*. Tokyo: Chikuma Shobou.

Satir, V., Banmen, J., Geber, J., & Gomori, M. (1991). *The Satir model: Family therapy and beyond*. Palo Alto, CA: Science and Behavior.

Shotter, J. (2008). *Conversational realities revisited: Life, language, body and world*. Chagrin Falls, OH: A Taos Institute.

Shotter, J. (2011). *Language, joint action, and the ethical domain: The importance of the relations between our living bodies and their surroundings*. Plenary paper at III Congreso de Psicologia y Responsabilidad Social, 5–9 March, Campus San Alberto Magno.

Simon, J. L. (2002). Analysis of the relationship between shame, guilt and empathy in intimate relationship violence. *Dissertation Abstracts International: Section B: The Sciences and Engineering, 63*(6-B), 3026.

Takano, Y. (2014). *Stories of change in men who were violent and abusive to their partners: A collaborative narrative inquiry*. (Unpublished doctoral dissertation). University of British Columbia, Vancouver, BC.

Takano, Y., & Ishiyama, F. I. (2008, October). *Application of Morita therapy in abusive men's treatment program*. In Paper presented at the 26th annual meeting of the Japanese Society for Morita Therapy, Japan.

Takano, Y., & Ishiyama, F. I. (2009, October). *Application of Morita therapy in abusive men's treatment on denial and minimization*. In Paper presented at the 27th annual meeting of the Japanese Society for Morita Therapy, Japan.

Takano, Y., & Ishiyama, F. I. (2010, October). *Application of Morita therapy in abusive men's treatment*. In Paper presented at the 28th annual meeting of Japanese Society for Morita Therapy, Japan.

Takano, Y., & Ishiyama, F. I. (2013, November). *Process of change in men who were violent and abusive to their partners: From a Moritian perspective*. In Paper session presented at the meeting of the 32nd annual meeting of the Japanese Society for Morita Therapy, Japan.

Tamura, T., & Lau, A. (1992). Connectedness versus separateness: Applicability of family therapy to Japanese families. *Family Process, 31*(4), 319–340. https://doi.org/10.1111/j.1545-5300.1992.00319.x.

Tatara, M. (1998). *Haji to iji [Shame and determination]*. Tokyo: Kohdansha.

Tateno, M., Teo, A. R., Ukai, W., Kanazawa, J., Katsuki, R., Kubo, H., & Kato, T. A. (2019). Internet addiction, smartphone addiction, and hikikomori trait in Japanese young adult: Social isolation and social network. *Frontiers in Psychiatry, 10*(455), 1–11. https://doi.org/10.3389/fpsyt.2019.00455.

Teyber, E., & Teyber, F. H. (2017). *Interpersonal process in therapy: An integrative model*. Boston, MA: Cengage Learning.

Todd, N. (2010). The invitations of irresponsibility: Utilizing excuses in counselling with men who have been abusive. *Journal of Systemic Therapies, 29*(3), 65–81. https://doi.org/10.1521/jsyt.2010.29.3.65.

Todd, N., Weaver-Dunlop, G., & Ogden, C. (2014). Approaching the subject of violence: A response-based approach to working with men who have abused others. *Violence Against Women, 20*(9), 1–21. https://doi.org/10.1177/1077801214549638.

Tracy, J., Robings, R., & Tangney, J. (2007). *The self-conscious emotions: Theory and research*. New York: Guilford.

Wong, P. T. P. (2016). Integrative meaning therapy: From logotherapy to existential positive interventions. In P. Russo-Netzer, S. E. Schulenberg, & A. Batthyány (Eds.), *Clinical perspectives on meaning: Positive and existential psychotherapy* (pp. 323–342). New York, NY: Springer.

Wong, P. T. P. (2019). Foreword: From shame to wholeness: An existential positive psychology perspective. In C.-H. Mayer & E. Vanderheiden (Eds.), *The bright side of shame: Transforming and growing through practical applications in cultural contexts* (pp. v–ix). Cham, Switzerland: Springer.

Wong, P. T. P., & Hwang, K. K. (2020). The second wave positive psychology of shame in east and west in the age of the 4IR. In C. H. Mayer, E. Vanderheiden, & P. T. P. Wong (Eds.), *From shame to well-being in Industry 4.0* (pp. 1–23). Cham, Switzerland: Springer.

Yoshiyuki Takano, Ph.D., is originally from Japan and currently works in the field of forensic and cross-cultural psychology in Canada. He has worked in post-secondary education, forensic mental hospitals, and court-mandated domestic violence intervention programs. He has expertise in various psychological assessments, including violence risk, personality, and cognitive assessments. He is widely published in Japan and Canada, and his publications include "Coping with domestic violence by Japanese Canadian women" in the Handbook of Multicultural Perspectives on Stress and Coping (2006) and "Co-constructing meaning: Women and men define taking responsibility and making amends" in Innovations in Interventions to Address Intimate Partner Violence: Research and Practice (2017).

Paul T. P. Wong, Ph.D., C.Psych., is Professor Emeritus of Trent University. He is a Fellow of APA and CPA and President of the International Network on Personal Meaning (www.meaning.ca) and the Meaning-Centered Counselling Institute Inc. Editor of the *International Journal of Existential Positive Psychology*; he has also edited two influential volumes on *The Human Quest for Meaning*. A prolific writer, he is one of the most cited existential and positive psychologists. The originator of Meaning Therapy and International Meaning Conferences, he has been invited to give keynotes and meaning therapy workshops worldwide. He is the recent recipient of the Carl Rogers Award from the Society for Humanistic Psychology (Div. 32 of the APA).

Chapter 9
A Re-conceptualisation of Erikson's Life Cycle: A Proposed Process to Address Individual Experiences of 'Shame'

Piers Worth

1 Introduction

The intention of this book is too be a primary reference source on 'shame' from a trans-disciplinary, cultural and trans-cultural perspective in the context of employment changes of the Fourth Industrial Revolution. This is a creative and insightful goal and perspective that focuses on the potential influence on individuals of the 4IR and changes that may have to be faced. Yet as well as considering the individual, there is also an implication that we must also look outwards to our societal context and consider the 4IR there as well.

Towards this end, this chapter will:

- Orientate the reader to what is called the 4IR, its potential impact within society and its capacity to negatively emotionally impact those who lose jobs because of it, in a manner that may bring and cause shame.
- Define the experience of 'shame' and its origins and affect by considering it in the context of Erikson's life cycle of human development (1950).
- Offer a potentially new description of how Erikson's life cycle could be used in the circumstances of 4IR job losses as an addition to the one he proposed in the original model.
- Extend and contextualise the proposed revised model in what is called 'Second Wave Positive Psychology' (Ivtzan,Lomas, Hefferon, & Worth, 2016; Wong, 2011) or Wong's (2010) existential positive psychology. In doing so the author argues 'shame' related to the 4IR is not unique, and a psychological framework exists from which to mitigate and work with its impact as well as offering a context and process for personal growth.

P. Worth (✉)
Buckinghamshire New University, Bucks, UK
e-mail: piers.worth@bucks.ac.uk

C.-H. Mayer et al. (eds.), *Shame 4.0*, https://doi.org/10.1007/978-3-030-59527-2_9

– Consider some of the research that these changes and the proposed intervention may need as the 4IR continues to unfold.

2 The 4IR and Its Risk of the By-Product of 'Shame'

The 4IR is described as a phase of new industrial activity, a name given to widespread changes already in process that will profoundly affect the world economy at macro and micro levels. It has been defined as industrial development "characterised by a much more ubiquitous and mobile internet, by smaller and more powerful sensors that have become cheaper and by artificial intelligence and machine learning" (Schwab, 2016: cited in Prisecaru, 2016, p. 58). The World Economic Forum (2016) proposes that previously unconnected developments and advances in the areas of genetics, biotechnology, artificial intelligence, robotics and machine learning are now building on and becoming connected with each other in staggeringly diverse ways that are increasing the volume and speed of change. These changes are altering the ways in which industries may operate and the regulatory frameworks used for industry and finance and presenting activity geographically in previously unseen ways (World Economic Forum, 2019). The factors and an indication of these connections are illustrated in the diagram below (Fig. 9.1).

Carney (2018) portrays these changes as making industrial and commercial activity faster, more direct, simpler, and driven by the Internet as a primary means of communication and transaction. He describes this as 'revolutionising how people consume, work and communicate' (p. 3).

The World Economic Forum believes that the challenges and possibilities presented by these changes require proactive adaptation by governments, societies, corporations and individuals (p. 8). In the findings of an international survey (2016) presented in their report, changing employment and work environments were the biggest single factors and 'driver of change' already being experienced (p. 6).

Opinions on the consequences of the 4IR are potentially as polarised as could be, suggesting, positively, it could bring about a 'cultural renaissance', one that could create 'a more inclusive, sustainable and harmonious society' (Schwab, 2015) to a balanced view believing there will be a transitionary period of adjustment for employment levels and patterns that could take many years, to a negative extreme, one where unemployment levels could be catastrophically high thereby dramatically affecting the capacity of governments to function financially (Prisecaru, 2016, citing Borg, 2016; Carney, 2018).

Carney (2018) offers what could be seen as a more balanced view of likely outcomes. He acknowledged that 10%–15% of the jobs in the UK and Ireland economy may be subject to at least partial automation. He acknowledged there will be a mix of job losses, the nature of jobs changing, job creation and the stimulation of new demand that will in turn create further and new forms of work. However he is blunt in his description that change will be disruptive and widespread, there will be a 'destruction effect' in this change, and new productivity and job gains

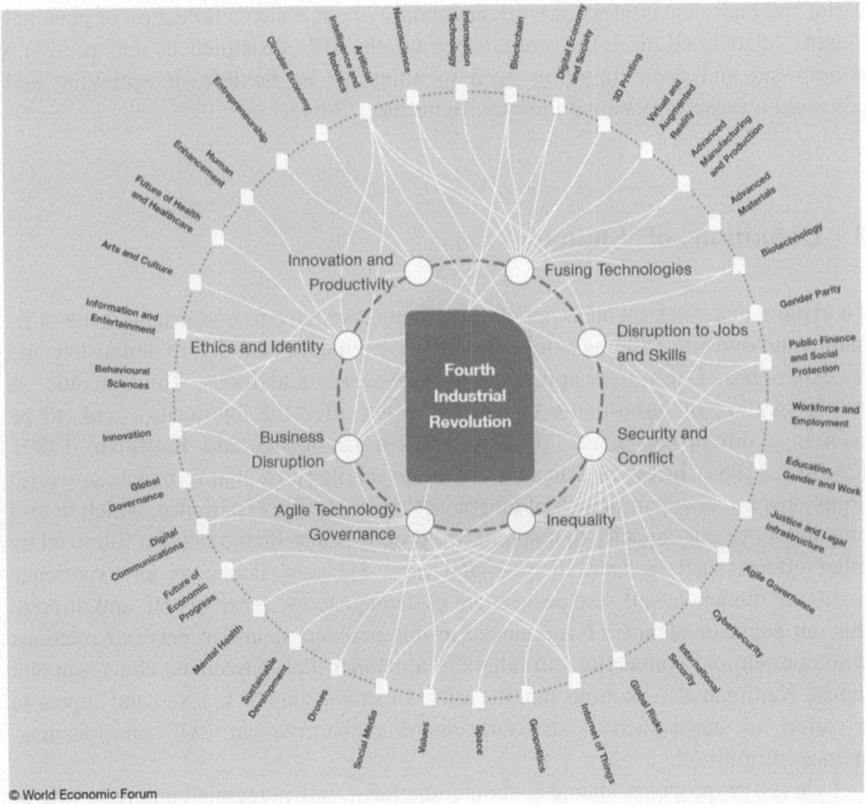

Fig. 9.1 Fourth Industrial Revolution (diagram used with permission of the World Economic Forum)

will lag behind these changes; '...every technological revolution mercilessly destroys jobs and livelihoods, and therefore identities, well before the new ones emerge' (p. 3). Taking this view, from the position of national and international responsibility he held at that time,[1] Carney acknowledged an impact on and increase in inequality would occur and public and private institutions could and need to take steps to shorten the duration of the change and support the transitionary impact on individuals, in such areas as institutionalising support for re-training mid-careers. Schwab (2016) suggested that this resultant inequality and its impact represented the greatest societal concern connected with the 4IR. It is in this backdrop and context that the proposed insight on shame outlined in this chapter may fit and positively contribute.

Looking at these dynamics, there has to be an assumption that job losses and changed employment circumstances will involve a range of psychological impacts on individuals, including a potential experience of shame at their situation. Given the

[1]Governor of the Bank of England.

social and historical context of work and employment is also a reflection of personal identity (elaborated on in the sections below), the 4IR consequences may present a widespread and even on-going need to adjust or be flexible in achieving and adjusting a sense of personal identity (Schachter, 2004).

3 Definitions of 'Shame'

To explore and work on an experience of shame, we have to understand some of its nature and dynamic. Shame can be considered both a noun and verb and a state and an experience. Definitions appear to vary in words and focus. They include 'A painful feeling of humiliation or distress'; 'An affect of interiority'; and 'to be seen in a diminished sense' (Oxford English Dictionary and Kaufman, 1989). Kaufman (1989) in his classic text on the psychology of shame makes powerful arguments for an apparent lack of language to describe the experience, which in turn may influence our capacity to respond. He proposes that shame may be followed by other effects such as fear, distress and rage. He sees shame as an experience involving the whole self, and as a source of damage to the sense of self, and through this our sense of identity. Experienced in this manner, shame affects our relations with our self and connections to others in a manner that may create alienation and defeat. Kaufman also cautions that the affect of shame may be masked and appear in a variety of states such as discouragement, embarrassment, self-consciousness, shyness or guilt.

Lyle (2019) proposes shame is about judgement, self-judgement and receiving or being subject to the judgement of others. Shame can change depending on factors such as social context, distance from the event and the involvement of group shame. It arouses negative emotions, so therefore links to our 'negativity biases'. Yet whilst this is customarily being defined via emotions and emotional processes, can we feel shame without also going through a cognitive process? We have to judge our experience and reaction before deciding whether we 'choose' to feel shame. Described in this manner Lyle is emphasising the social experience and interaction creating shame. Therefore, exploring shame via Erikson's life cycle allows us to look at the psycho-social nature of these experiences.

Shame is being defined and articulated in this manner and detail due to its potential impact and lasting consequence within job losses brought about by the 4IR (see also Kotera, Sheffield, Green and Asano's chapter in this book; see Mayer on Shame 4.0—Empirical Evidence of the Importance of Emotions in a Technologising World of Work).

4 'Shame' Within the Life Cycle of Human Development

Whilst accepting all of these as possible experiences and consequences of shame, the author proposes there is value and utility and a scope for influencing by returning to consider and explore shame in Erikson's theory of the life cycle of human development. This theory suggests that 'shame' exists in a polarity with positive emotions and experiences. The dynamic of this wider context of human development must be considered to allow the impact of shame to be fully understood. Further, how, in turn, there may also be a positive experience in this encounter—how shame may be, as the book editors propose, a trans-formational experience, one that leads to further change.

This chapter proposes that if the experience of shame generated by loss of employment, skills or work can be understood more broadly in the context of and impact on human development, this creates the means to explore and work with what occurs as a result of the 4IR through a psychological intervention or exercise described later in this chapter that offers a means for reframing life experience in the context of shame.

The context proposed is that of Erik Erikson's theory of the life cycle. Erikson's (e.g. 1958, 1980, 1988) theory was a turning point in psychoanalysis and psychology in its offering of a perspective of the whole lifespan, in addition to proposing development was not just psychological but psycho-social in its nature, that our 'psychology' exists within the social context. The findings of the Harvard Grant Study of Adult Development have found Erikson's structure empirically as existing within its own data (Vaillant, 1977, 2002) albeit their own work offering more detail of what occurs within the actual adult life stages. This theory may be considered dated given its emergence 70 years ago. However the author proposes it represents a 'broad brush canvas' against which other theories may be placed. The journey of growth and change the life cycle illustrates is the gradual formation of the 'ego' and then a personal identity and its further development and revision through time. Social context will influence the ego and identity (Welchman, 2000), hence the implication of this book, the impact of the 4IR on working lives and in potentially creating shame and other affects.

Erikson's theory was developed through his psychoanalytic work, his work with healthy adolescents and ethnographic work with the Sioux and Yurok American Indian tribes (Kivnick & Wells, 2013; Welchman, 2000). It is a theory that is meant both to encompass both sexes and to be cross-cultural in its nature.

Erikson proposed the life cycle contained eight sequential stages through which eight basic developmental strengths may emerge coming from a developmental confrontation occurring at specific times, one that illustrated what may go right, or not (Erikson, 1968) (see Mayer and Fouché on Lessons Learned From Baruch Spinoza: Shame and Faith Development in the Light of Challenges in Contemporary Society). Each developmental stage is characterised as a 'crisis' by Erikson that comes through the polarity of two possible experiences specific to that time of life, one positive and one negative (see also Vanderheiden on "In the depths of winter, I finally learned that within me there lay an invincible summer."—Life Crises, Shame and Digitalisation in this book). This illustrates in the author's view one of the key contributions of Erikson that life experience involves polarities that we encounter throughout life and struggle with. Erikson saw the polarity of experience at each stage as a form of struggle or crisis. Erikson recognised that outcomes were not 'either or', one end of the polarity or the other, but an outcome on balance that led to a developmental strength or virtue if positive (Kivnick & Wells, 2013; Roazen, 1976). This positions development as psychological *and* social, in the family, culture and time (Kivnick & Wells, 2013; Sokol, 2009). This immediately offers a link to more recent theories of human strength in positive psychology (e.g. Peterson & Seligman, 2004) and also reflects Wong's (2011) proposal that the discipline of positive psychology must involve a dialogue between positive and negative experiences.

Erikson's use of the word 'crisis' was intended to illustrate a developmental turning point, an opportunity at points and periods of time, and that the experience of the two sides of each polarity could influence individual development in either positive or negative directions. The nature of the resolution achieved within the polarity would influence each following life cycle stage (Perlmutter & Hall, 1992). In a perspective that could be considered profound even in more recent times, and within the intention of this book, Erikson believed growth and development occurred through integration or balancing of the polarity's conflicting forces at each stage and cumulatively over time. He believed that each person would interpret and experience this pattern through their own particular traits and character, a style unique to them (Roazen, 1976). A reflection of the emerging sophistication of this theory is that in Erikson's view the individual faces holding the presence and tension of each polarity and stage that is traversed *from that point on through life*, with the implication that this may need to be revisited and revised over time. The goal or aim is to achieve a tendency towards the positive, 'on balance' rather than 'either or'. Joan Erikson, writing in parallel to her husband, made explicit her belief that a failure to achieve a positive outcome on balance to a developmental stage could be readdressed at a later time and stage (Erikson, 1988).

Erik Erikson portrayed the eight stages described in the paragraph above in the following chart (Fig. 9.2).

Stage titles are taken from Erikson (1968, p. 599).

This illustrates that Erikson considered the experience of 'shame' to emerge in early childhood. His definition of the experience will be described in the summaries of the stages below. The diagram below summarises the stage names and the emerging developmental strength (Fig. 9.3).

Erikson saw each stage as emerging from, connected to, and dependent on the one before. As such, each developmental stage is seen as grounded or rooted in all the ones preceding it. The achievement of the emerging strength from the polarity is believed to give new experiences, perspectives and insights for all preceding strengths that have been experienced so far (Erikson & Erikson, 1997; Stevens, 1983). This reflects a process that may be seen in Vaillant's (2002) findings: we

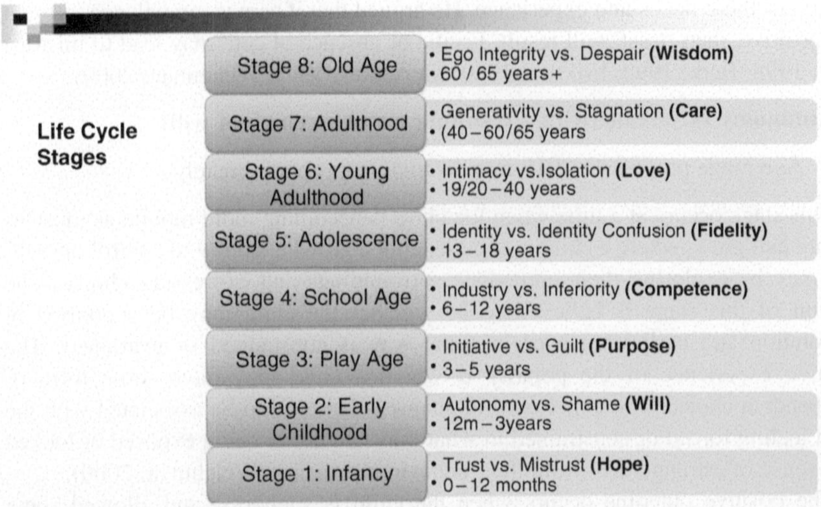

Fig. 9.2 Life cycle stages (Erikson, 1968, p. 599)

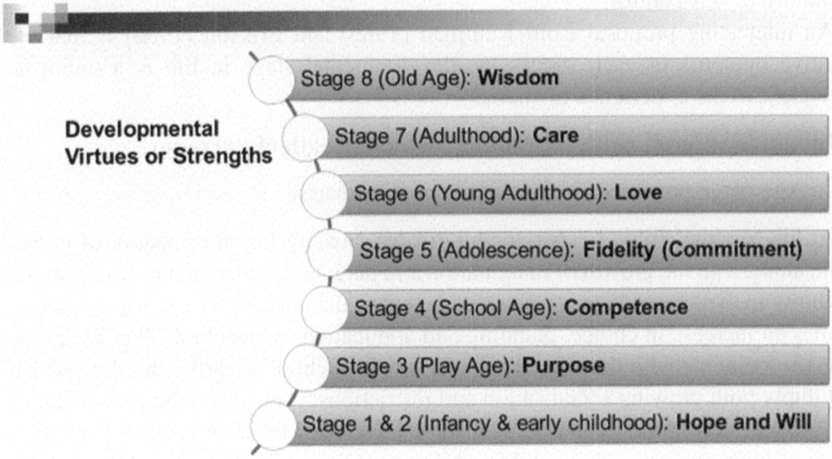

Fig. 9.3 Developmental virtues or strengths (Erikson)

continue to process and re-understand our experiences in conscious awareness and unconsciously over time.

The proposed nature and content of each developmental stage are summarised below.

- **Basic trust vs. basic mistrust (with a resulting virtue/strength of hope)**
  - Age range proposed: 0–12/18 months approximately

This stage involves a child's experiences of basic, critical needs of food and support being met in the early time of life. Will the needs be met and in what way? Erikson also proposed this stage involved the child's own ability to cope with the tension of these needs and experience. He argued that if care is, on balance, present and positive, then 'trust' will result. Erratic or absence of care may lead to mistrust (Bee, 1998; Berk, 1998; Erikson, 1980; McAdams, 1993; Welchman, 2000).

- **Autonomy vs. shame (with a resulting virtue/strength of will)**
  - Age range proposed: 12/18 months to 3 years approximately

This stage occurs at a time when the child is becoming more mobile as muscles mature and grow, where a child is experiencing a growing ability to control oneself, and may be exploring their immediate surroundings and expressing choice. The tension of this stage is believed to be whether the child may be supported in exploration and early choice or in some way is constrained or restrained. The positive experience of the polarity is where a child may have some form of independent choice. The experience of shame is believed to be associated with the child feeling forced or constrained in what they can do, or being exposed or looked at, a sense of estrangement from their behaviour or being (Welchman, 2000).

The positive outcome occurs when the child is supported and allowed some independent choice and action. In the negative, the child is thought to feel forced, shamed or doubting what he or she can or can't do and to question his or her own autonomy or self-control.

An interesting proposal from Kaufman (1989) and Erikson (1980) is that the negative outcome of each successive developmental stage in life is a linguistic equivalent to the experience of shame.

- **Initiative vs. guilt (with a resulting virtue/strength of purpose)**
  - Age range proposed: 3–5 years old approximately

At this age the child is experiencing greater capacity for and freedom of movement, along with the growth of imagination and language, which in turn brings about an ability to explore and experience a wider space than before. The word 'initiative' implies an increase in choice, planning and application by the child. This age range may also coincide with the experience of a nursery school or early schooling which will imply both growing socialisation and restrictions. Initiative is the expression of this growth, and 'guilt' proposed as a sense of learned badness occurs. The emergence of 'purpose' reflects the child's ability to choose and direct their focus (Berk, 1998; Erikson, 1980; Welchman, 2000).

- **Industry vs. inferiority (with a resulting virtue/strength of competence)**
  - Age range proposed is 6–12 years old.

In the early school years, a child is focusing on an 'industry' that occurs with a gradual learning and developing ability associated with knowledge and skills and the social and cultural norms in their context. The child will receive forms of recognition for what they learn, tasks and outcomes that are accomplished, plus communication and cooperation that may be associated with them. A sense of 'inferiority' may emerge from experiences of failures to learn and a questioning of their personal capacity. The sense of 'competence' develops with the experiences of learning over time (Bee, 1998; Berk, 1998; Erikson, 1980; McAdams, 1993; Welchman, 2000).

Kerpelman and Pittman (2018) offer the reminder that all preceding stages of the life cycle will reflect qualities of psychological 'attachment theory' and in its sense of safety and support (or lack of it) set the stage for emerging identity.

- **Identity vs. identity confusion (with a resulting virtue/strength of fidelity)**
  - Age range proposed is 13–18 years old, the period of adolescence.

This is a period of time where it is proposed the young person is experiencing the inadequacy of their childhood sense of self and identification with the family. The need emerges to move to something that is beyond it. This move may be built upon or developed from a relationship to knowledge, skills and tools being gained. The change might involve questions like 'who am I?' The period may involve reflections on experiences, relationships and beliefs from the past and present, along with considering how these may suggest who they wish to be in the future. The individual will be seeking a sense of who they are within the social context and what principles and beliefs they would stand up for in the future. The arrival at a sense of identity represents how the individual would 'fit' within the social world. McAdams (1993) proposed that this would have qualities of ideology (beliefs), relational and occupational choices. The strength of 'fidelity' may be more readily understood as a sense of 'commitment', and with the length of this stage, this may take years to reach.

The inability or failure to reach this sense of self is described as 'identity confusion'. This may result from a search or struggle that has not resulted in an outcome, has been postponed, or alternatively is an acceptance of the norms of others, such as parents or the cultural context. Arnett (2000) proposes that the exploration goes well beyond this age range, into the 20s, as a distinct period of 'emerging adulthood' that is likely to occur experientially in parallel to the phase described below and also that the emerging adulthood exploration is culturally and demographically situated. However, Erikson acknowledged that the sense of self would be forever revised (Bee, 1998; Erikson, 1988; McAdams, 1993; Perlmutter & Hall, 1992; Schwartz, 2002; Schwartz, Zamboanga, Meca, & Ritchie, 2012; Welchman, 2000). This stage is in some way the pinnacle of Erikson's structure because it represents a person becoming individual, likely to be self-directed and choosing and who will engage with the social world in an adult manner.

- **Intimacy vs. isolation (with a resulting virtue/strength of love)**
  - Age range proposed varies with authors, yet is approximately 19/20 to 40 years old.

The length of Erikson's stages in this period of life is increasing in time and the content becoming broader. This is a period of relational and occupational choices beyond the context of family. Most interpretations of Erikson's ideas tend to reflect that of relating and the capacity to commit to an intimate partner and finding or involving love. The relationship reflects surrendering, sacrificing or compromising some aspects of independence to become a partnership, and mutual, whilst also maintaining a sense of self, a dynamic balance and self-expression. More recent interpretations imply the commitment, and 'love' may also involve a relationship with a form of work. These relationships are believed to form a security from which the young adult moves safely into the adult world. If this is not achieved, Erikson proposed a tendency to isolate and that an isolation of loneliness or self-absorption may result.

The achievement of 'intimacy', personal or occupational, may also be seen as the foundation of the stage that follows, involving 'generativity' and a link between the generations (Bee, 1998; Berk, 1998; Erikson, 1988; Perlmutter & Hall, 1992; Welchman, 2000).

- **Generativity vs. stagnation (with a resulting virtue/strength of care)**
  - Age range proposed is 40 to approximately 60/65 years old.

Commitment, care and love expressed or offered in this period of life are believed to now extend beyond the family, the biological and into the social, the wider group of society. Generativity is a care, concern and guiding of the wider context that will outlive the individual, into the next generation. It may also involve broader creative contributions to society. This is a period of life where there is a realisation that time is limited and the reality of mortality is believed to surface and be more clearly felt. This form of care may be seen to be a form of influence on that which survives after our own lives.

The negative outcome of this stage of the life cycle is believed to be a form of stagnation or impoverishment reflected in self-centredness (Bee, 1998; Berk, 1998; Erikson, 1988; Welchman, 2000).

- **Integrity vs. despair (with a resulting virtue/strength of wisdom)**
  - Age range from 60/65 years old

This stage is described as implying a coming to terms with our individual life as it is, with a capacity to see our life events and experiences as part of a larger whole, and where we take responsibility for the life we have lived. It is a time where we adapt or adjust ourselves to successes and disappointments that have occurred in life. This stage could be seen as the 'fruit' or output of the previous seven stages and a crucial point where a sense of meaning is found.

Despair is described as a fear of death, a realisation that time is running out and a wish or chance for another opportunity to live life or change what has occurred (Bee, 1998; Berk, 1998; Erikson, 1980; Erikson, Erikson, & Kivnick, 1986; Kivnick & Wells, 2013; Welchman, 2000).

(Please note that age ranges are approximate. Erikson was unclear in some cases, and this has led to some differences between authors on what ages apply, particularly to the adult stages.)

These stages are generalisations that are culturally and contextually specific. As such reinterpretation may be relevant. Erikson's theories are hard to evaluate and have been criticised. The complexity and time encompassed by Erikson's theory make it very hard to test; however Vaillant (1977) considered the data of the Harvard

Grant Study of Adult Development confirmed Erikson's proposals for the adult lifespan. The breadth of particularly Erikson's adult stages has been added to via the work of Levinson, Darrow, Klein, Levinson and McKee (1978), Levinson and Levinson (1996), Gould (1978) and Vaillant (2002). The early non-verbal stages of life are probably beyond verification or refutation (Bee, 1998; Perlmutter & Hall, 1992; Roazen, 1976).

Erikson puts forwards his theory as cross-cultural and universal; yet others (e.g. Perlmutter & Hall, 1992; Stevens, 1983) acknowledge that its focus on individualism makes it oriented to Western culture and the generality of the research which originated these theories makes such claims at best still unproven.

5 The Implications of Erikson's Life Cycle to Concerns of the 4IR

If we accept that a sense of identity involves an individual seeking a sense of who they are within the social context, the arrival at a sense of identity represents how the individual would 'fit' within the social world. McAdams (1993) proposed that this would have qualities of ideology (beliefs), relational and occupational choices. Therefore the 4IR, with inherent changes to education needed, work content and speed of changes, along with a possibility of multiple employers (Hirschi, 2018), presents a clear likelihood that these experiences will require on-going adjustment to the sense of identity of those affected, e.g. this will involve a repudiation or loss of certain identifications that shape identity and a need to locate and absorb new configurations of a sense of self (Schachter, 2004). The adjustments will involve Erikson's stages and polarities, in addition to the sense of safety and support found or not found in adult attachment theory (Kerpelman & Pittman, 2018).

The author proposes that one of the great focusing gifts of Erikson's theory is highlighting that our lives are not one side of these life cycle stage polarities or the other. Life is a dynamic balance of both aspects of the polarity and one we must seek, ideally consciously, to balance (Ivtzan, Lomas, Hefferon, & Worth, 2016; Kivnick & Wells, 2013). Erikson wrote that in his view we could not exist without learning to be ashamed, allowing us an existence that involves our navigation of the outer world, but the key issue for him is that, on balance, we have the sense of personal autonomy. Erikson proposed that the experience of each polarity is revisited and extended in each stage of life. This may involve a deepening of our experience of the polarity and a reorientation to its nature (Bee, 1998; Erikson, 1988; McAdams, 1993; Perlmutter & Hall, 1992; Schwartz, 2002; Schwartz et al., 2012; Welchman, 2000).

The chapter moves at this point to propose what the author believes is a revised conceptualisation of Erikson's model. The social and historical context from which his model emerged (the 1950s and 1960s) was one of relative economic stability and growth, and from which employment was stable and generally increasing. The changes seen in the last generation[2] characterised by employment structures such as fixed term contracts, 'zero hour' contracts, outsourcing, 'gig' occupations and now the automation of work argue that human development and in particular the achievement and growth of a sense of identity involving employment occur against a volatile and changing workplace context that may influence the success, or otherwise, of this aspect of development.

Erikson (1980) and McAdams (1993) propose that 'identity' has to be formed and re-formed over time based on changing experiences. The fact that this happens offers us a means to respond and adjust to 4IR experiences. An implication of this chapter is that the need to revise and adjust in the context of the 4IR may become a recurring feature of our lives. Stages of development that were once seen as foundational have to be revisited and adjusted against a backdrop of social change. A concept of what this might mean dynamically in the life cycle emerged from the author's undergraduate students. The students proposed that in the face of significant life changes, in considering a 'stage theory' model, earlier life stages and needs had to be revisited, re-checked and re-established, even if briefly in the face of the change, to continue building upon personal and life development. The author proposes that this is a re-orientation that has to happen here as well in the face of 4IR changes. Kaufman (1989) articulated this more precisely: When desire or goals outrun fulfilment, shame occurs. Employment, work, and expression through work are an interpersonal bridge between the person and the employer. In the face of loss and implied inadequacy of the individual in contrast to that offered by work automation, the interpersonal bridge is fractured, broken. Kaufman argues further that the personal impact is higher still; individuals identify with an event and impact and cause and view themselves 'I' as the cause or fault. This in turn leads to a personal sense of belittlement, humiliation and powerlessness. Future purposes and dreams have been frustrated. The potential for this affect becomes a driving need for a process of psychological support in the face of 4IR change (implied in Carney, 2018) and the reason for proposing the development of the intervention below.

Converting this idea and need to Erikson's life cycle, progression or movement through time may become a life cycle of spiral development, moving between and revisiting stages at different ages (rather than sequentially upwards with age).

What is being proposed by the chapter author is when confronted with a major life change, which within life cycle theory will also confront our sense of identity, the individual will undergo a re-orientation to the life cycle perceptions and developmental strengths they draw upon, which is summarised in Fig. 9.3. Erikson et al. (1986) imply that this would happen in some way, inside or outside awareness regardless of external intervention by 'reviewing, re-experiencing and re-solving' (p. 44) each of the polarities. If we consider the strengths Erikson proposed for each stage, which imply a cumulative growth of capability, when we face a major life change or crisis (such as 4IR loss of employment), we have to re-check and re-establish each strength in turn again as a means of adjusting to this change. Knight (2017) points towards this possibility in another discipline and use by

[2]Presumed to be approximately 30 years.

suggesting that the life stages may form a structure of psychodynamic psychotherapy and that each stage of life may offer different gifts of understanding if used reflectively.

The author proposes this re-orientation for the first six stages be brought about in a structured and supportive manner. If an individual, for example, loses work and occupation; in a period of re-adjustment, they are seeking to readjust their sense of previously achieved identity. A possible focus for stage-by-stage exploration and changed perception is summarised below:

- Stage 1: Strength of 'hope'. Re-establish 'basic trust'—that their needs may on balance be met?
- Stage 2: Strength of 'will'. Find a new 'autonomy' of their own. What can they influence? What decisions are open?
- Stage 3: Strength of 'purpose'. Take the initiative. What would the individual wish to choose? What choices are available? What opportunity is there to seek variety and flexibility in the available choices?
- Stage 4: 'Industry'. In what ways can the individual's skills be seen in a new way or used in a new way? Are there new skills that can be developed? Seek new work opportunities?
- Stage 5: 'Identity': In what ways might we perceive of our identity now to be different? Whilst this may naturally be phrased at this time as a form of 'loss', can a realistic 'positive' be established?
- Stage 6: 'Commitment': What can we now commit to? What would we choose to commit to now?

The author suggests that these steps could be written into a reflective self-help structure or form a basis for coaching, outplacement or counselling support in a manner reflective of Erikson et al.'s (1986) key findings of engaging with life as it is in present time, revisiting the dynamic balance of the stage polarities or opposites, and through a personal vital involvement in life circumstances (Kivnick & Wells, 2013).

The reflective structure would potentially support the re-establishment of an appropriate dynamic balance of polarities found in each stage opposites in changed circumstances such as job and employment losses in the 4IR.

This structure for re-experiencing and consolidating polarities in changed circumstances mirrors developments in positive psychology. A concept and structure for 'Positive Psychotherapy' (Rashid & Seligman, 2019) has been offered in that context via a sequence of exercises that ground us, connect us, to positive and broader aspects of our lives at the individual and behavioural level. The structure proposed above might be considered a reflection of Second Wave Positive Psychology (Ivtzan et al., 2016) or existential positive psychology (Wong, 2019b) whereby polarities in life can be encountered, recognised and respected and that we can constructively seek change and ways to move forward. This might represent a form of 'existential positive psychotherapy or coaching', alongside such resources as Wong's Meaning Therapy (e.g. Wong, 2012).

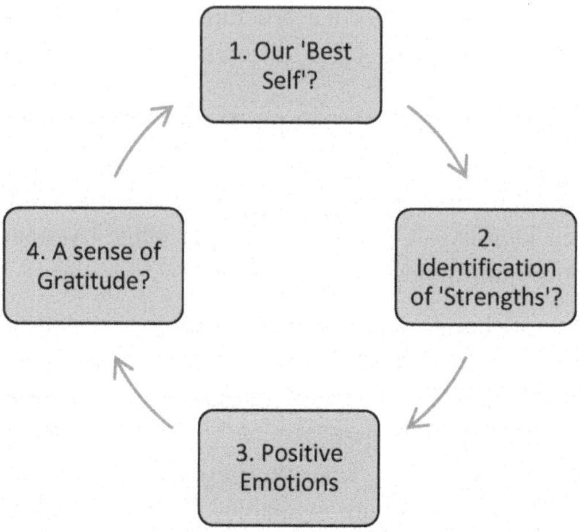

Fig. 9.4 Four steps of reflection in each re-visited stage above

Drawing on research and processes established in positive psychology (Rashid & Seligman, 2019), might a structure and process of reflection for this work within each developmental stage comprise four possible steps, illustrated and diagrammed below (Fig. 9.4), for exploration within each developmental stage outlined to connect with positive experiences as a means of re-orientating ourselves to the developmental virtue or strength? For example:

Example references for the four elements of this model are:

- Best self: Roberts, Dutton, Spreeitzer, Heaphy and Quinn (2005)
- Strengths: Peterson and Seligman (2004)
- Positive emotions: Fredrickson (2009)
- Gratitude: Watkins (2014)

Whilst there is a research evidence for the therapeutic and cross-cultural use of positive psychotherapy, if the suggested form of exploration is developed, then research is also needed to establish its functional and cross-cultural efficacy.

From the perspective of Erikson's developmental model, the capacity for a negative personal outcome in the face of these 4IR changes is real. Wong (2019a) suggests this is already underway.

6 Reflections and Questions About This Proposal in the Context of the 4IR

The intervention proposed within this chapter above has been written with the goal of understanding and support of individuals in mind. Carney (2018) argued that support for individuals to adjust skills, concepts of careers and their ability to cope would be a core need institutionally and governmentally as a response to the 4IR. Hirschi (2018) offers an articulate and detailed exploration of changed perceptions of careers and how individuals may face an inevitability of repeated adjustments and change to work contexts in the 4IR. Descriptions of the 4IR impact (e.g. Carney, 2018; World Economic Forum, 2016) suggest that these are already widespread with more unfolding; this means coping responses for individuals affected are needed and will become more urgent. The intervention proposed in this chapter is a concise possibility mirrored in positive psychology research-based achievements (e.g. Rashid & Seligman, 2019). Hill and Burrow (2012), drawing on extensive research on the psychological impact of the presence of purpose in individual lives, imply that this re-orientation of the individual towards their life stage experience, in supporting a changed sense of identity, may also promote a revision to a sense of purpose. This, too, would represent a possible intervention to support individuals in change. Therefore even within the theoretical backdrop of this chapter, some changes are proposed and possible.

The literature and exploration in this chapter are written from a UK and Western culture focus. Erikson argued that his theories were culturally sensitive and developed in the context of different cultures. This is mirrored in his writing and there is recognition of his efforts in this respect. However, criticism also exists about how accurate that may be in current times, and further research is needed to establish this (Syed & Fish, 2018). Therefore this framework for contribution and action would need research to confirm its efficacy, along with that of the proposed intervention.

Yet recognising that the 4IR changes are happening and gathering speed (Carney, 2018; World Economic Forum, 2016), a repertoire of supportive responses are needed, and indeed research to explore both needs and the contribution of interventions intended to support.

References

Arnett, J. J. (2000). Emerging adulthood: A theory of development from the late teens through the twenties. *American Psychologist, 55*(5), 469–480.

Bee, H. (1998). *Lifespan development* (2nd ed.). Harlow: Longman.

Berk, L. E. (1998). *Development through the lifespan*. London: Allyn and Bacon.

Borg, A. (2016, January 28). *How will the Fourth Industrial Revolution affect economic policy? Talk given at World Economic Forum*, Davos.

Carney, M. (2018, September 14). *The future of work. Speech given by Mark Carney, Governor of the Bank of England, at the 2018 Whitaker Lecture*, Central Bank of Ireland.

Erikson, E. H. (1958 & 1980). *Identity and the life cycle*. New York: Norton.
Erikson, E. H. (1968) *The human life cycle*. New York: International Encyclopedia of the Social Sciences. Crowell-Collier, pp. 286–292. Reprinted in: Schlien, S. (Ed.) (1987). A way of looking at things: selected papers from 1930 – 1980.
Erikson, E. H. (1980). On the generational cycle: An address. *International Journal of Psychoanalysis, 61*, 213–223.
Erikson, J. M. (1988). *Wisdom and the senses: The way of creativity*. New York: Norton.
Erikson, E. H., & Erikson, J. (1997). *The life cycle completed – Revised and extended Version*. New York, W.W. Norton & Company Inc.
Erikson, E. H., Erikson, J. H., & Kivnick, H. Q. (1986). *Vital involvement in old age*. New York: W.W. Norton.
Fredrickson, B. L. (2009). *Positivity*. New York: Crown Publishers.
Gould, R. (1978). *Transformations: Growth and change in adult life*. New York: Simon and Schuster Ltd.
Hill, P., & Burrow, A. (2012). Viewing purpose through an Eriksonian Lens. *An International Journal of Theory and Research, 12*(1:1), 74–91.
Hirschi, A. (2018). The fourth industrial revolution: Issues and implications for career research and practice. *The Career Development Quarterly, 66*. https://doi.org/10.1002/cdq.12142.
Ivtzan, I., Lomas, T., Hefferon, K., & Worth, P. (2016). *Second wave positive psychology*. London: Routledge.
Kaufman, G. (1989). *The psychology of shame*. London: Routledge.
Kerpelman, J. L., & Pittman, J. F. (2018). Erikson and the relational context of identity: Strengthening connections with attachment theory. *International Journal of Theory and Research, 18* (4), 306–314.
Kivnick, H. Q., & Wells, C. K. (2013). Special issue: Remembering our roots - Untapped richness in Erik H. Erikson's Rootstock. *The Gerontologist, 54*(1), 40–50.
Knight, Z. G. (2017). A proposed model of psychodynamic psychotherapy linked to Erik Erikson's eight stages of psychosocial development. *Clinical Psychology Psychotherapy, 24*, 1047–1058.
Levinson, D. J., Darrow, C. N., Klein, E. B., Levinson, M. H., & McKee, B. (1978). *The seasons of a man's life*. New York: Ballantine Books.
Levinson, D. J., & Levinson, J. D. (1996). *The seasons of a woman's life*. New York: Alfred Knopf.
Lyle, L. (2019). *Personal communication with the author*.
McAdams, D. P. (1993). *The stories we live by: Personal myths and the making of the self*. London: Guildford Press.
Perlmutter, M., & Hall, E. (1992). *Adult development and aging* (2nd ed.). Chichester: Wiley.
Peterson, C., & Seligman, M. E. P. (2004). *Character strengths and virtues*. Oxford: Oxford University Press.
Prisecaru, P. (2016). Challenges of the fourth industrial revolution. *Knowledge Horizons: Economics, 8*(1), 57–62.
Rashid, T., & Seligman, M. E. P. (2019). *Positive psychotherapy: Clinicians manual*. Oxford: Oxford University Press.
Roazen, P. (1976). *Erik H. Erikson: The power and limits of a vision*. New York: Free Press.
Roberts, L. M., Dutton, J. E., Spreeitzer, G. M., Heaphy, E. D., & Quinn, R. E. (2005). Composing the reflected best-self portrait: Building pathways for becoming extraordinary in work organizations. *Academy of Management Review, 30*(4), 712–736.
Schachter, E. P. (2004). Identity configurations: A new perspective on identity formation in contemporary society. *Journal of Personality, 72*(1), 167–199.
Schwab, K. (2015). *Will the Fourth Industrial Revolution have a human heart*. Article from the World Economic Forum Web site.
Schwab, K. (2016, January 14). *The fourth industrial revolution: What it means, how to respond. Talk given at World Economic Forum*, Davos.

Schwartz, S. J. (2002). In search of mechanisms of change in identity development: Integrating the constructivist and discovery perspectives on identity. *International Journal of Theory and Research, 2*(4), 317–339.

Schwartz, S. J., Zamboanga, B. L., Meca, A., & Ritchie, R. (2012). Identity around the world: An overview. *New Directions for Child and Adult Development, 138*, 1–18.

Sokol, J. T. (2009). Identity development throughout the lifetime: An examination of Eriksonian Theory. *Graduate Journal of Counselling Psychology, 1*(2), 14.

Stevens, R. (1983). *Erik Erikson*. Milton Keynes: The Open University Press.

Syed, M., & Fish, J. (2018). Revisiting Erik Erikson's legacy on culture, race and ethnicity. *International Journal of Theory and Research*. https://doi.org/10.1080/15283488.2018.1523729.

Vaillant, G. E. (1977). *Adaptation to life*. Boston: Little, Brown and Company.

Vaillant, G. E. (2002). *Aging well*. Boston: Little Brown.

Watkins, P. C. (2014). *Gratitude and the good life: Toward a psychology of appreciation*. London: Springer.

Welchman, K. (2000). *Erik Erikson: His life, work and significance*. Buckingham: Open University Press.

Wong, P. T. P. (2010, July). What is existential positive psychology? *International Journal of Existential Psychology and Psychotherapy, 3*(1).

Wong, P. T. P. (2011). Positive Psychology 2.0: Towards a balanced interactive model of the good life. *Canadian Psychology, 52*(2), 69–81.

Wong, P. T. P. (2012). Toward a dual system model of what makes life worth living. In P. T. P. Wong (Ed.), *The human quest for meaning: Theories, research and applications* (2nd ed.). London: Routledge.

Wong, P. T. P. (2019a). A cross cultural perspective of shame and its implications for mental health and social control. *International Network for Personal Meaning*.

Wong, P. T. P. (2019b). *The maturing of positive psychology and the emerging PP 2.0: A book review of positive psychology*, (3rd ed.). William Compton and Edward Hoffman. Retrieved from http://www.drpaulwong.com/the-maturing-of-positive-psychology-and-theemerging-pp20-a-book-review-of-positive-psychology-3rd-ed-by-william-compton-andedward-hoffman/

World Economic Forum. (2016). *The future of jobs: Employment, skills and workforce strategy for the fourth industrial revolution*. A 'Global Challenge Insight Report' published by the World Economic Forum in January 2016.

World Economic Forum. (2019). *Centre for the Fourth Industrial Revolution network for global technology governance*. Report produced in May 2019.

Piers Worth, PhD is a 'Visiting Professor' in Psychology at Bucks New University. He is a Charted Psychologist and accredited psychotherapist. Piers' PhD research focused on how creativity changes as we age and how it may support positive ageing. Piers was a co-course leader of the University's MSc Applied Positive Psychology programme. He co-authored the *Second Wave Positive Psychology: Embracing the Dark Side of Life* book that was published in November 2015. His research and writing focus at the present time is on subjects and applications that may broaden the base of positive psychology. Prior to this part of his career, Piers worked for over 35 years in human resources in industry and blue chip companies and for 20 years as an organisation development consultant. He has work and project experience in 17 countries.

Chapter 10
Overcoming Shame: A Positive Psychology Perspective

Athira Alex and A. T. P. Farisha

1 Introduction

Shame is a universal emotion which may end up in a negative sequel if left unnoticed. This fundamental emotion within us will grab ourselves from being exposed to many life experiences and social interactions. It usually arises in social situations in which an individual perceives a drop of personal status or feelings of rejection. Shame seems to drive several other negative emotions and thereby express certain violence like war and other aberrant behaviours. This self-conscious emotion evokes in situations where a person's behaviours are considered discrepant from social as well as ethical standards (Kim, 2016).

As cited by Poulson (2000), Lewis (1992) describes that shame is the product of a complex set of cognitive states such as the evaluation of an individual's action in regard to his/her standards, rules and goals and one's global evaluations of the self. When a person experiences shame, he or she wishes to disappear or even to die. Shame is a highly negative state that can also result in the disruption of ongoing behaviour, confusion in thought and the ability to speak. The physical behaviours associated with shame include a shrinking of the body in a way to disappear from the eye of the other. This emotional state is sometimes even acute and has such a destructive effect on the self that individuals presented with such a feeling must attempt to hide themselves from it. However, since shame results in a global threat on the self, people have a huge difficulty coming out of this emotion. Individuals act particularly when shamed, by which they try to undo the shame feeling.

Shame is defined as the negative side of an individual's motivational scheme by Gidden (1991) (c.f., Stiles, 2008). Hence a study examining the relationship between

A. Alex (✉)
Department of Psychology, Don Bosco Arts and Science College, Kannur, India

A. T. P. Farisha
Ramana Vidyalaya, Sholinganallur, Chennai, India

C.-H. Mayer et al. (eds.), *Shame 4.0*, https://doi.org/10.1007/978-3-030-59527-2_10

shame and motivation has been done by Stiles (2008). According to the author, shame is being related to our self-regulation where it is influenced by our capacity to modify an individual's behaviour and thoughts. They came up with the findings that more intense feelings are elicited by negative emotions rather than positive emotions. That is, more intensive feelings are elicited by shame, and it has a significant role in affecting the motivation of an individual to act in any particular situation.

1.1 Factors Contributing to Shame

Shame is the output of many psychological states and situations. The feeling of shame is contributed by several factors according to Heshmat (2015) which is summarised as follows:

- Self-awareness: Self-awareness is one of the crucial factors which contribute to shame. If we are aware of ourselves completely, we experience shame when we couldn't meet up to the standards we set for ourselves.
- Standard: All of us have a certain set of acceptable standards concerning thoughts, actions and feelings. Any kind of violation of these standards ends up in shame.
- Personal trait: People high on this trait of public self-consciousness are likely to be shame prone.
- Fragile self-esteem: People with a fragile self-esteem also experience shame more frequently than people with stable self-esteem.

1.2 Existential Positive Psychology (EPP) and Shame

According to Seligman (2000), positive psychology is the study of human strengths and virtues and nurturing what is best within us. Thus, it helps human beings develop those qualities that lead to self-fulfilment and also for others. It aims to discover and promote factors that allow individuals, communities and societies to thrive and flourish. Existential psychology can learn from positive psychology, its scientific methods and its clarity in communication. Therefore, existential positive psychology represents a natural amalgam between positive psychology (PP) and existential psychology (EP). Wong (2009) states that what qualifies existential positive psychology as a positive psychology is its emphasis on the human capacities for positive change and growth (Narayanan, 2014) (see Wang and Hwang's chapter in this book).

Positive and existential psychology on its own is lacking in a number of aspects. Combining the two domains can result in a field with intense depth, wisdom and youthful vitality. Modern positive psychology has realised that its root has always been deeply embedded in the existential-humanistic approach, which has helped to rediscover the richness of lived experience and the pathways to meaning in life. Existential-humanistic psychology is dependent on positive psychology as well. Existential positive psychology represents the natural balance between the two fields. Existential positive psychology is open to information from all sources making research richer. Hence existential positive psychology broadens the definition of positive psychology as "the qualitative and quantitative study of what enables people to survive and flourish individually and collectively in the totality of life circumstances".

EPP is intended for all people, with its emphasis on integrating negative experiences with positive ones. EPP stresses that it is only through struggle and fortitude that we grow psychologically and spiritually. It is only through embracing life in its totality and wrestling with ultimate concerns that we can uplift humanity and improve the human condition.

Even though shame is considered as a negative emotion, proponents of existential theory consider shame as a powerful social emotion which strongly predicts the motivation for positive self-change. Existential theorists even name this feeling as existential shame (Pattison, 2000). Wong (2018) described the three advantages when explaining from an existential viewpoint. First, it recognizes shame as a universal condition of human existence; therefore, all therapies need to address this fundamental existential issue. Second, it recognizes the common humanity and human frailty of all human beings; therefore, this consciousness should contribute to our empathy and compassion for all people, regardless of their race, culture, socioeconomic status or physical condition. Third, it also makes us aware of the existential-spiritual core that exists in all individuals; therefore, it behoves us to tap into this spiritual resource to address mental health issues (c.f. Wong, 2018).

2 Managing Shame

There are various strategies through which the feeling of shame can be intervened. Few of them are described below as explained by various theorists.

2.1 *Shame Resilience Theory (SRT)*

Shame creates the feeling of fear, blame and disconnect. It is a strong painful feeling or experience believing that we are not good enough to be accepted by or belong to the family, community, causing the individual to isolate themselves from family, friends and society (Brown, 2007). It is Brown (2007), who came up with the strategies to deal with the shame, which he explained through her theory named shame resilience theory. In the theory, she explained what is shame and what are its consequences. According to the theory, there are four steps to deal with shame. First is to recognize the vulnerability, second is to recognize the external factors involved, third is to connect with others for getting and giving empathy, and finally fourth is to discuss and deconstruct the feelings themselves. Moreover, experiencing intense shame leads to mental health issues such as depression, suicide, addiction and low self-esteem. Shame resilience theory (SRT) is based on building resilience to shame. It is a grounded theory, wherein it works by connecting one's shame feeling with our authentic selves and enriching meaningful relationships with others. Shame resilience means moving towards empathy (compassion, courage and connection) when we are experiencing shame and away from shame (blame, fear and disconnection).

The shame resilience has four elements crucial to describe:

1. *Recognizing shame and understanding triggers:* Brown (2007) has identified 14 common triggers of shame. They are appearance, body image, mental health, physical health, sexuality, family, motherhood, parenting, professional identity, work, ageing, religion, speaking out and surviving trauma.
2. *Practising critical awareness:* This element means why something exists and how it works, in addition, how our society is impacted or impacting on that something and who benefits from it.
3. *Reaching out and telling our story:* This element indicates reaching out to our support network and sharing our story; we can increase our resilience and create change.
4. *Speaking about our shameful experiences with those who have earned the right to listen to them is so important:* that is through secrecy and silence.

Subsequently, if we recognize and understand our triggers, practise critical awareness and reach out to others, and we can grow our resilience as we practise communicating about our shame with our most trusted advisors who use their own compassion and courage whilst listening and supporting us (Selva, 2019).

As a reaction to shame, people use a defence mechanism to protect ourselves; Brown (2007) called it as shame screen, and we use this shame screen in one of the three ways:

- Moving against shame by trying to gain control or power over others or being aggressive
- Moving away from shame by withdrawing, hiding, keeping secret or staying silent
- Moving towards shame by seeking approval and belonging

In her research, Brown (2007) proves that by developing empathy through practising shame resilience, an individual can create things in life that he or she wants the most as a worthwhile person. Because developing empathy always builds connection, courage and compassion.

2.2 Internal Shame and External Shame

Another perspective in shame management is introduced by Gilbert and Procter (2006). According to them, managing shame has to be done addressing both internal and external shame. He explains internal shame as thoughts emerging from criticizing and evaluating our own, whereas external shame refers to our thoughts and beliefs on other people's opinion about us. This article will explain shame and the means to manage it from a positive psychology and following existential principles.

To manage the experience of shame, the individual can apply the following ways:

(a) *Being aware about feeling shame when we experience it rather than ignoring or escaping from it.*

Because when we are hiding this feeling, it becomes dominant over us. But if we acknowledge it and share our experience with trusted people in our lives, their empathy will allow us to keep our sense of shame in perspective. And also, their suggestions make us get rid of the feeling.

(b) *Unhitch what you do from what you are.*

Never let our self-worth be lost in the face of shame. Always remember that mistakes, imperfections and flaws are part of the human experience and something we all share. When we start to accept ourselves with all that we are, the experience of shame just passes as it is, and we move on. Always remember that we have never been defined by our one action or mistakes. Learn to look at both praise and condemnation with the perspective they deserve, absorb any helpful critiques, and move on.

(c) *Identify triggers of shame.*

By recognizing our shame triggers, we can nip this process in the budding stage itself. According to Brown (2007), the major shame trigger is physical appearance for women, and for men, it's the fear of being perceived as weak. By realizing and accepting who you are instead of trying to fulfil an outside notion of who you should be, the individual can manage shame.

(d) *Make connections.*

Our fear of social devaluation causes shame to a certain extent. By reaching out to family and friends, to our communities, to society, or to our idea of a higher power, we can make connections that allow us to learn to accept ourselves and other people as well. The social connectedness also boosts our compassion for ourselves, meaning we are more likely to handle our shame without resorting to measures such as masking the feeling with addiction or lashing out at those around us or giving in to shame's message that we are indeed bad. In sum, developing compassion and empathy will help us to get rid of it (Sack, 2015).

2.3 *Meaning Therapy*

Meaning therapy is a form of modern integrative psychotherapy which ultimately aims to help the individual to reach a state of self-transcendence. This therapy basically builds upon principles of logotherapy and positive psychotherapy, and also it incorporates some other therapeutic modalities like cognitive as well as existential-humanistic therapeutic approaches. The basic assumption of MT is "meaning is all we have and relationship is all we need". We all know that as humans we all go through a wide variety of experiences and all those experiences have an emotional content. Some of them may be pleasant; others may be shameful and disappointing, etc. (INPM, 2020).

There is a saying that every experience teaches us something new, and the new learning is always the result of the meaning we derive from the particular experience. The thing is that we cannot always find the meaning of a particular experience at that moment. We get the real meaning of that experience only through self-reflection. If we learn to reflect on those experiences even for shameful one, rationally and wisely, that can help us to get to the heart of what really matters or the real meaning of the events. And this new meaning in turn enriches the quality of our lives and alters the way we look at situations. This makes us more confident, stress free, enthusiastic and revitalized. Since shame is considered as the master of all negative emotions, finding meaning through reflection is always helpful to view the particular experience from a logical sense.

Meaning therapy, also known as meaning-centred counselling and therapy, is an integrative, positive existential approach to counselling and psychotherapy (Wong, 2010). Originated from logotherapy, meaning therapy employs personal meaning as its central organizing precepts and incorporates various schools of psychotherapy to obtain its therapeutic goal. Meaning therapy pays attention to the positive psychology of making life worth living in spite of sufferings and limitations. There are two strategies under meaning therapy, PURE strategy and ABCDE strategy, which are explained below.

2.3.1 The PURE Strategy of Life Expansion

In the PURE strategy, "P" stands for purpose, which is the motivational component. It consists of goals, direction and values of the individual. The letter "U" stands for understanding, which is the cognitive component of meaning, encompassing a sense of coherence, making sense of situations, understanding self-identity and identity of others and effective communications. "R" stands for responsible action; the behavioural component includes the reactions and actions, doing what is right and taking actions that are congruent with highest values. The "E" indicates evaluation, which is associated with the affective component. This component consists of assessing the levels of contentment or disappointment with the situation or life as a whole.

All of these components need a set of interventions that manage negative and positive areas of life in an adaptive and healthy manner. These four components work together. With each successful completion, one's level of positivity moves up. Some of the commonly used techniques include challenging unrealistic or irrational thoughts, clarifying values, goal-setting, prioritizing, reality check, fast-forwarding of consequences of choices and Socratic questioning (Wong, 2018).

2.3.2 The ABCDE Strategy of Life Protection

The ABCDE intervention strategy is the main device in dealing with prolonged negative life experiences. The ABCDE strategy gives prominence to action and commitment to values. Here, A stands for acceptance, B for belief and affirmation, C for commitment to action and specific goals, D for discovering new meaning and understanding and E for evaluation of the outcome and enjoying positive results. This strategy involves following psychological principles: (a) Accept and confront the reality based on the reality principle. (b) Believe that life is worth living based on the faith principle. (c) Commit to goals and actions based on the action principle. (d) Discover the meaning and significance based on the AHA principle. (e) Evaluate the above based on the self-regulation principle.

2.4 Compassion-Focused Therapy and Shame

In an intervention study by Harris (2017), he reports that compassion-focused therapy may reduce trait shame and intimacy fears and increase relationship functioning and self-compassion in shame-prone individuals. Gilbert (2003) defined compassion from a Buddhist perspective. According to the Dalai Lama (1995), compassion is defined as a sensitivity to suffering in self and others, with a commitment to try to alleviate and prevent it (Harris, 2017). The major aspects and attributes of compassion in CFT are well-being, sensitivity, distress tolerance, empathy and non-judgement.

Compassion-focused therapy (CFT) is a relatively novel form of psychotherapy that was developed by the British clinical psychologist Dr. Paul Gilbert for people who have mental health problems primarily linked to high shame and self-criticism (Leaviss & Uttley, 2015). Recently compassion gets a lot of attention in positive psychology. In addition, research has shown that compassion can have amazing benefits. Compassion is considered a vital quality and now it has its own therapy. This therapy emphasizes the importance of applying compassion—for the self and others for living a healthy and happy life.

According to Gilbert and Procter (2006), individuals who experienced extreme shame are low in expressing self-compassion and receiving compassion from others, and thus CFT aims to teach these skills. CFT helps the shame-prone individuals to reduce self-directed hostility and assist them to develop a more compassionate view on the self, so that associated feelings of shame are alleviated and psychological well-being is enhanced.

Whilst compassion-focused therapy is the underpinning theory and process of applying a compassion model to therapy, compassionate mind training (CMT) refers to the specific activities designed to develop compassionate attributes and skills (Gilbert & Procter, 2006). Compassionate mind training refers to the specific/techniques that can be used to help the client to experience compassion and develop the various aspects of compassion for self and others.

The strategies include mindful breathing, compassion-focused imagery, compassionate chair work, compassionate letter writing and practising compassionate behaviour and thinking (Harris, 2017).

CMT has two fundamental components:

(a) Identification of safety strategies and functional analysis of self-criticism

In CMT, self-criticism is framed as a safety behaviour. That is, self-criticism is the result of shame-prone individuals to do the best they can, to cope with painful situations, memories and emotions. According to Gilbert and Procter (2006), a key element of therapy involves developing one's ability to "stand back" and see these safety behaviours as automatic defences since many individual who experienced extreme shame believe that they are fundamentally bad or incompetent and this is crucial to a de-centring process, which aids empathy and understanding of one's shame and self-criticism. Without this understanding, CMT can be difficult for individuals, who are reluctant to give up self-criticism. During therapy, a functional analysis of self-criticism takes place. The therapist helps the clients to be more in tune with the feelings associated with their memories, understand the development of safety strategies, learn compassionate acceptance and empathy for the origins and use of safety strategies and develop compassionate imagery and mindful ways of responding to fears and safety strategies (Harris, 2017).

(b) Development of compassionate images and warmth using imagery

A key aspect of CMT is assisting individuals to create their own images of warmth using imagery. According to Gilbert and Procter (2006), this can be done in two ways. The first one is aimed to help people with unpleasant ruminations. For this, individuals are asked to recall their own compassionate motives and feelings flowing outwards to others (e.g. imagine compassion and warmth for someone one cares about).

Secondly, individuals are asked to choose their own image. Instead than the therapist providing individuals with a universal, compassionate image (e.g. a Buddha image), for generating feelings of compassion flowing into the self, individuals are asked to imagine their own ideal of caring. Ideal is defined as what is best for the individual. However, this ideal image must have the qualities of wisdom, strength, warmth and non-judgement. Imagery is focusing on creating particular feelings and states of mind in order to enhance individuals' ability to engage with shame. The key to the image is that it has a "mind" that can understand the individual, and can communicate with them, and has the qualities of warmth, understanding and compassion. According to Gilbert and Procter (2006), the more unique and personal the person feels their image to be, the better it may work for them (Harris, 2017).

2.5 *Mindfulness Empathy*

Mindfulness empathy is a five-step practice through which it can be helped to get out of shame memories, integrating mindfulness practice with empathy feelings (Graham, 2010).

1. Resourcing
   Resourcing means re-sourcing. This is the starting step during which an individual begins to feel or sense the shame memories from the person from whom he/she feels to be safe. When someone is imaging the face of a loved one, there occurs the release of oxytocin in the brain, which is the hormone of safety and trust, of calm and connection. This resource helps the clients to cover the effects of shame which is unpleasant.
2. Regulating
   Even before an individual experiences the toxicity of shame, there comes the first foundation of mindfulness of the body. All memories including trauma of shame are stored within us as body sensation, posture and movement. The second one, mindfulness of feeling tone, catches the initial response to any experience as positive, negative or neutral. Later is the third one, noticing and naming thoughts, feelings and beliefs. We notice what is happening and we name it. Mindfulness is the primary tool we have to stay in and expand the windows of tolerance. When we are too anxious or hyperaroused, we go up out of tolerance; if we are too ashamed, we collapse down outside the window.
3. Self-compassion/self-empathy
   We should learn to hold any experience that arises with compassion including the moments of shame, failure, etc. It contains the implicit memory of shame. Beyond trusting that others find us lovable, we need to claim ourselves as lovable. We should ourselves receive love, care and empathy.
4. Reflection
   When we step back from the experience of moments, we are strengthening our capacity of mentalizing. We should step back from the experience that makes us feel ashamed and be aware and should hold that experience so we can begin to work with these states to rewrite them in ways that are more adaptive.
5. Re-pairing
   In this step, the old shame memory is repaired with novel experiences of self-empathy and self-compassion. It was found that repairing is essential for rewriting the old brain networks related to shame. This flexibility in the way brain processes lets us relate ourselves with new ease and love with acceptance.

2.6 *Other Strategies to Manage Shame*

Apart from these strategies, the feeling of shame can be intervened by cognitive behaviour therapies (CBT), prolonged exposure (PE), stress inoculation training (SIT) and cognitive processing therapy (CPT) (Good therapy, 2020). These lists are based on the assumptions that shame comes from a traumatic life event. CBT deals with the connections between thoughts, behaviour and feelings associated with shame response, whereas PE works in a way that exposing the affected individual with intense stimuli to which he/she associates a trauma will help the individual to come out of it. The same can be applied to guilt feelings and anxiety as well. A variant of CBT is SIT where an individual is trained to respond to stress before it overwhelms. It can be through muscle relaxations, systematic breathing techniques, addressing automatic thoughts and even role plays.

Finally, CPT is a long step process during which the individual can talk about the trauma and have a self-understanding and insight on how it is affecting one's emotions and behaviours and then implementing strategies for managing them. If shame is not associated with any traumatic incidents, another group of therapies which can be practised to address the shame includes compassionate mind training (CMT) and emotionally focused couples therapy (EFCT). In CMT, the therapist encourages the people who are highly self-critical to be more self-compassionate. On the contrary, EFCT takes a different route that a therapist following this approach fosters feelings of connection and intimacy among couples. It benefits if the shame is associated with relationships and if it interferes with the closeness among couples (Good therapy, 2020).

3 Shame in Fourth Industrial Revolution

According to Dombrowski and Wagner (2014), the Fourth Industrial Revolution (4IR) is the change of the technological economic and social system in the industry. This revolution has changed the life circumstances as a whole. This is considered as one of the crucial societal and economic as well as digital trends in the world. The fourth industrialization is entirely different from previous industrial revolutions since the present technology is mainly focusing on replacing cognitive operations and human work altogether. But in previous revolutions, the focus was on replacing physical labour and supporting humans in their work.

The Fourth Industrial Revolution is changing our lifestyle, work life and the way we communicate. It's reshaping almost every aspect of life. The digital platform functions as a cultural socialization agent. As a socialization agent, the mass-mediated images that appear on televisions and social media can have a tremendous impact on the way people view themselves and others. According to Schwab "The Fourth Industrial Revolution, finally, will change not only what we do, but also who we are. It will affect our identity and all the issues associated with it: our sense of privacy, our attitudes and beliefs, the time we devote to work and leisure, and how we develop our careers, cultivate our skills, enhance the way we manage our emotions, and nurture relationships and living up-to our values" (Dombrowski & Wagner, 2014).

Emotions have become increasingly important of late, in all realms of social reality. Emotions linked to the use of technology and, secondly, the Internet as a space in which emotions are activated and expressed. The technology not only arouses emotions in users and serves as a channel for the expression of affection but also influences the way in which this affection is exhibited.

In the wake of digitalization, shame spreads faster and is more wide-reaching. Shamings today happen fast, with most often devastating consequences. The major reason behind this is Internet anonymity, in essence the lack of physical presence and face-to-face communication. People who use social media keep their identity fake or anonymous. They have no accountability for their actions via social media.

In this 4IR, generally we can view shame from two different points of view. On one hand, people experience less shame, since they are not physically present via social media. Hence, they are trying to open up more. Moreover, the majority of the population has learned an attitude of "Nothing to be ashamed of". On the other hand, there are a lot of people who just use the media as a platform for self-presentation. Such people have a fear of loss of status and social exclusion and lack a realistic view on life.

Another significant factor is the importance of having an optimal level of emotional intelligence (EQ) in the present scenario. The 4IR is highly demanding individuals to have emotional intelligence. Houston (2020) says that EQ has an enormous impact in all of our relationships, how we make decisions and identify opportunities as well as the way we perceive failures and learn from it and how to recover from its impact.

According to Bar-On and Parker (2000), advancement in EI is becoming a vital prerequisite in intense areas of "emotional work" especially in works such as the service industry and management roles. High EI enhances the physical and emotional health of people. When people experience intense shame, they can easily manage those experiences by viewing those experiences and feelings from another perspective or thinking about them unemotionally or logically, because being capable of viewing the shame-triggering incidents unemotionally helps the individual to see the connection between current feelings and the wounds caused by shame (Pollak, 2017).

Emotional intelligence is an integral part of forming and developing meaningful human relationships. Schutte et al. (2001) found that, over a series of studies, there were significant links between high EI and more successful interpersonal relations. Those participants who exhibited higher levels of EI also showed a greater propensity for empathic perspective taking, cooperation with others, developing affectionate and more satisfying relationships as well as greater social skills in general.

Digital technology is central to how we live in the 4IR. Of late, digital technology presents us with new opportunities to deliver mental health services. As all realms of medicine and science, the field of behavioural and mental health is also now fully entering the world of technology-enhanced services. The review report by Mohr et al. (2013) reveals that technology-driven mental health supporting systems are very simple yet highly effective. It was concluded that web-based intervention standard telephone technologies have shown efficacy across a broad range of mental health outcomes. It was also found that video technology has become less expensive and these technologies provide options for both telehealth and remote supervision that help people to get directly connected with efficient mental health consultants (Mangnavita, 2018).

According to Mangnavita (2018) various treatment strategies are emerging hand in hand with mobile applications as an alternative to traditional treatment strategies like pharmacotherapy and psychotherapy. These are very affordable and easily accessible. It is important to note that all these technological advancements have the potential to move the clinical research ahead (Mangnavita, 2018).

The Fourth IR is highly recognized by integrating information technology and electronic media in the enhancement of mental well-being. According to Velotti, Garofalo, Bottazzi and Caretti (2016), shame feelings were associated with low self-esteem. Low self-esteem is propelled by shame, and feelings of shame trigger thoughts that say we are unworthy and not enough in any aspects, and it stops us from coming out of our comfort zone (Velotti et al., 2016).

Nowadays, we can use technology to pay attention to our surroundings, to really look, to really listen to our everyday. And, ultimately, we can use technology to reconnect to ourselves. Mindfulness teaches us how to feel emotions in our bodies. Feelings, like shame, can be felt somewhere in the body; emotion is not just an intellectual thing. Mindful self-compassion (MSC) is a best strategy to comfort a person who experiences shame. With MSC, an individual treats himself/herself like a dearest friend. When individuals comfort themselves whilst they feel shame, that's self-compassion—self-love. That's a countermeasure to shame (Potiker, 2019). According to Gunatillake (2017), since we are surrounded by technology in all realms of our lives today, a new perspective of mobile mindfulness meets us where we are and enfolds the realities of our modern lifestyle (Tartakovsky, 2018). There are various mindful applications available, promising to assist the users combat their shame and anxiety, increase their focus, and more. Aura, Calm, Buddhify, breathe, headspace, ten percent happier and mindfulness daily are some of the popular apps (Developgoodhabits, 2019).

According to Robson and Robson, the emergence and explosion of cyber counselling have had a stupendous impact in the field of psychology. Enhanced information technology efficiency has allowed cyber counselling services to be offered using various tools like email, text messaging, real-time chat, Internet phone, videoconferencing and mobile device apps. Researchers reveal that cyber counselling was effective in the treatment of emotional distress (Zainudin & Yusop, 2018).

4 Conclusion

Shame is a painful emotion arising from public exposure and denunciation. People who experience shame do worry about how others might evaluate them. The feelings of shame involve a painful scrutiny of the entire self, a feeling that "I am an unworthy or incompetent individual". People who experience shame often report a sense of shrinking or being small. Denial and a desire for concealment are also part of the experience of extreme shame. Shame begins to be toxic when the innate yearning and the inborn need seen to be big and masterful are not met positively. When these yearnings are ignored and dismissed or when we are shamed, criticized or judged on a regular basis, this state becomes ingrained. Existential positive psychology emphasizes the uniquely human capacities for resilience and positive change. The existential perspective of therapy views shame as a universal condition of human existence. It recognizes common humanity and human frailty and makes us aware of the existential-spiritual core that exists in all individuals.

There are various positive psychological strategies through which shame can be intervened. Few of them mentioned in this article are meaning therapy, compassion-focused therapy specifically and mindfulness empathy which is proved to be effective on reducing shame feeling. For instance, Westerman, McCann and Sparkes (2020) suggest from their study that mindfulness- and compassion-based therapies are promising approaches for reducing psychological distress developed from shame among adult populations.

Even though shame is a universal feeling, if it's intervened in an effective way, it can be rerouted for a better sequel. Feldman (2013) says that the research shows promise on the effectiveness of technological advancements in psychotherapies. Based on several research results, the effectiveness of the online interventions seemed to be in the same range as in-person interventions. But still, the outcome depends on factors such as the age of the client and other physical ability (Feldman, 2013). Ultimately, we can use technology to reconnect to ourselves, which indeed helps to overcome various forms of social anxiety and shame, in presenting or conveying what is there in our mind. Online platforms and social network websites are turning to be a great opportunity to communicate regardless of shyness and anxiety. Moreover, the increased statistics of people depending on online counselling websites indicates that at least some of us don't want others to know what is happening in our lives and we wish to address our personal constraints within the four walls. Anyhow, cyber counselling and other technological advancements aimed at enhancing the well-being of the visitors are getting widespread acceptance and popularity, which indicates that 4IR greatly benefited the people all over the world to maintain their mental health.

References

Brown, B. (2007). Shame resilience theory: A grounded theory study on women and shame. *Families in Society-The Journal of Contemporary Social Services, 87*(1), 43–52.

Developgoodhabits. (2019). *15 best meditation and mindfulness apps for 2020*. Retrieved March 20, 2020, from https://www.developgoodhabits.com/best-mindfulness-apps/

Dombrowski, U & Wagner, T. (2014). *Mental strain as a field of action in the 4th industrial revolution*. Retrieved February 13, 2020, from http://core.ac.uk/download/pdf/82084599.pdf

Feldman, D. B (2013). *Will technology replace traditional psychotherapy?* Retrieved March 14, 2020, from https://www.psychologytoday.com/us/blog/supersurvivors/201309/will-technology-replace-traditional-psychotherapy?amp

Gilbert, P & Procter, S. (2006). Compassionate mind training for people with high shame and self-criticism: Overview and pilot study of a group therapy approach. *Clinical Psychology and Psychotherapy, 13*, 353–379. Retrieved February 12, 2020, from https://self-compassion.org/wp-content/uploads/publications/Gilbert.Procter.pdf

Good therapy. (2020). Retrieved January 27, 2020, from https://www.goodtherapy.org/learn-about-therapy/issues/shame/healing

Graham. L. (2010). *The power of mindful empathy to heal toxic shame*. Retrieved November 26, 2019, from https://lindagraham-mft.net/the-power-of-mindful-empathy-to-heal-toxic-shame/

Harris, K. L. (2017). *Compassion focused therapy for shame-prone individuals: An eight-week group therapy investigation*. Retrieved January 31, 2020, from https://pdfs.semanticscholar.org

Heshmat, S. (2015). *Five factors that make you feel shame*. Retrieved December 27, 2019, from https://www.psychologytoday.com/us/blog/science-choice/201510/5-factors-make-you-feel-shame

International Network on Personal Meaning (INPM). (2020). Retrieved May 3, 2020, from https://www.meaning.ca/meaning-centred-interventions/meaning-therapy/

Kim, Y. (2016). *Antecedents and consequences of self-conscious emotions in the workplace: Guilt, shame and pride*. Retrieved May 13, 2020, from https://conservancy.umn.edu/bitstream/handle/11299/200320/Kim_umn_0130E_17214.pdf?sequence=1&isAllowed=y

Leaviss, J., & Uttley, L. (2015). Psychotherapeutic benefits of compassion-focused therapy: An early systematic review. *Psychological Medicine, 45*(5), 927–945.

Mangnavita, J. J. (2018). *Using technology in mental health practice*. Retrieved February 17, 2020, from https://www.apa.org/pubs/books/Using-Technology-in-Mental-Health-Practice-Intro-Sample.pdf&ved=2ahUK

Narayanan, J. (2014). *Existentialism echoes in the works of R K Narayan*. Retrieved December 29, 2019, from https://shodhganga.inflibnet.ac.in/bitstream/10603/27326/8/08_chapter_2_existential%20positive%20physchological%20perspectives.pdf

Pattison, S. (2000). *Shame - theory, therapy, theology*. Cambridge, UK: Cambridge University Press. Retrieved February 12, 2020, from https://books.google.co.in/books?id=CIhEhpLR6qEC&dq=pettersen%2B+existential+shame&source=gbs_navlinks_s

Pollak, R. (2017). *Emotional intelligence can protect you from shame*. Retrieved February 13, 2020, from http://renapollak.com/emotional-intelligence-helps/

Potiker, J. (2019). *Using mindfulness to overcome shame and guilt*. Retrieved March 2, 2020, from https://mindfulmethodsforlife.com/using-mindfulness-to-overcome-shame-and-guilt/#iLightbox

Poulson, C. (2000). *Shame: The master emotion?* Retrieved February 12, 2020, from https://eprints.utas.edu.au/1471/1/Shame_the_Master_Emotion_.pdf

Sack, D. (2015). *Five ways to silence shame*. Retrieved December 23, 2019, from https://www.psychologytoday.com/us/blog/where-science-meets-the-steps/201501/5-ways-silence-shame

Seligman, M. E., & Csikszentmihalyi, M. (2000). Positive psychology. An introduction. *American Psychological Association, 55*(1), 5–14.

Selva, J. (2019). *Shame resilience theory: How to respond to feelings of shame*. Retrieved November 20, 2019, from https://positivepsychology.com/shame-resilience-theory/

Stiles, P. (2008). *The negative side of motivation: The role of shame*. University of Cambridge. Retrieved January 27, 2020, from https://www.jbs.cam.ac.uk/fileadmin/user_upload/research/workingpapers/wp0807.pdf

Tartakovsky, M. (2018). *Using technology to help us practice mindfulness*. Retrieved March 20, 2020, from https://psychcentral.com/blog/using-technology-to-help-us-practice-mindfulnes

Velotti, P., Garofalo, C., Bottazzi, F., & Caretti, V. (2016). Faces of shame: Implications for self-esteem, emotion regulation, aggression, and well-being. *The Journal of Psychology – Interdisciplinary and Applied, 151*, 171–184. Retrieved March 15, 2020, from https://www.tandfonline.com/doi/full/10.1080/00223980.2016.1248809#

Westerman, G., McCann, E., & Sparkes, E. (2020). Evaluating the effectiveness of mindfulness and compassion-based programs on shame and associated psychological distress with potential issues of salience for adult survivors of childhood sexual abuse: A systematic review. *Mindfulness*. Retrieved May 13, 2020, from https://link.springer.com/article/10.1007%2Fs12671-020-01340-7

Wong, P. T. P. (2010). *Meaning therapy: An integrative and positive existential psychotherapy*. Retrieved November 20, 2019, from http://www.drpaulwong.com/meaning-therapy-an-integrative-and-positive-existential-psychotherapy/

Wong, P. T. P. (2018). *From shame to wholeness: An existential positive psychology perspective*. Retrieved November 20, 2019, from http://www.drpaulwong.com/from-shame-to-wholeness-an-existential-positive-psychology-perspective/

Zainudin, Z. N. & Yusop, Y. M. (2018). Cyber counselling: Is it really new? *International Journal of Science and Education, 2*, 13–24. Retrieved from https://www.researchgate.net/publication/329735840_Cyber-Counseling_Is_It_Really_New

Athira Alex (MSc Clinical and Counselling Psychology) is currently working as Assistant Professor in the Department of Psychology Don Bosco Arts and Science College, Kerala. Both the authors are interested in positive psychology interventions applied to various fields.

A T P Farisha (MSc Clinical and Counselling Psychology, NET) is currently working as Student Wellness Manager in a reputed school in Chennai. She has 5 years of teaching experience as Assistant Professor in Kannur University of Kerala. She worked as consultant psychologist as well.

Chapter 11
Making the Cut: Mass Media and the Growing Desire for Genital Cosmetic Surgery by Young Women and Girls

Thula U. Koops, Catherine Wilkinson, Grace Perry, Samantha Wilkinson, and Sergio A. Silverio

1 Introduction

Women and girls have long been confronted with unrealistic, unattainable body image norms. Additionally, the 'ideal feminine' body has been subject to constant change over the last centuries and decades. With the proliferation of the Internet, women and girls are continuously exposed to advice from heteronormative discourses of womanhood. Demand for cosmetic surgery has dramatically increased and is still expanding. Recently, women's and girls' awareness has shifted towards how they should 'improve' the aesthetic appeal of their labia, 'optimise' their vaginas, and generally make their vulva 'healthier', leading to a growing popularity

T. U. Koops
Institut für Sexualforschung, Sexualmedizin und Forensische Psychiatrie, Universitätsklinikum Hamburg-Eppendorf, Hamburg, Germany
e-mail: T.Koops@uke.de

C. Wilkinson
School of Education, Liverpool John Moores University, Liverpool, UK
e-mail: C.Wilkinson@ljmu.ac.uk

G. Perry
Division of Epidemiology, University of Utah, Salt Lake City, UT, USA
e-mail: Grace.Perry@hsc.utah.edu

S. Wilkinson
School of Childhood, Youth and Education Studies, Manchester Metropolitan University, Manchester, UK
e-mail: Samantha.Wilkinson@mmu.ac.uk

S. A. Silverio (✉)
Department of Women & Children's Health, King's College London, London, UK
e-mail: Sergio.Silverio@kcl.ac.uk

C.-H. Mayer et al. (eds.), *Shame 4.0*, https://doi.org/10.1007/978-3-030-59527-2_11

of female genital cosmetic surgery. Proponents of surgical interventions (falsely) claim them as agentic methods of self-expression and promise 'improvement' beyond the individual's control. The marketing of these procedures is predicated on shame and has been described as aggressive. Our postmodern era brings new visions of desired body image, and a rise of Internet-based digital connections between people. This means new body image 'norms' are instantly circulated and changed, and body image is continuously scrutinised and shamed. Coupled with increased accessibility of Internet-based nudity and pornographic material, and prevailing associations of shame and taboo about female genitalia, consequences particularly for young women's perceptions of body image are drastic. This chapter discusses the Internet's role in the recent desire by young women and girls to seek genital cosmetic surgery.

Body modification and cosmetic surgery have gained notable public awareness with the advent of mass media through the Internet, together with the marketisation of new 'feminine ideals'. 'Failure' to meet these bodily norms can distance women away from society's 'ideal feminine' and lead to an internalisation of body image-oriented shame. We note this chapter is written from a Western perspective and therefore might be limited in its transferability to other cultural contexts. We further accept that the following discussions of female genital cosmetic surgery [FGCS] in this chapter centre on cisgender women and girls and thus necessarily omit trans, non-binary and intersex individuals, who face unique challenges surrounding genital surgery and modifications. We write in the knowledge and understanding that the experiences and discourses which affect non-Western and non-cisgendered women and girls are diverse, complex, and worth exploring in their own right, hence are not tackled here directly. This chapter will interrogate the Internet's role in the recent desire by young women and girls to seek genital cosmetic surgery. We have decided to focus particularly on 'young' women (18–29-year-olds) and girls due to their high usage rates of social media (Primack & Escobar-Viera, 2017), through which we know new body image 'norms', including those of new genital aesthetic 'norms', are being propagated (Iglesia, Yurteri-Kaplan & Alinsod, 2013). We unpack this relationship between young women and girls and FGCS by foregrounding literature which writes on the intersections between the Internet, mass media and body image and the links between shame and cosmetic surgery. Following these sections, we provide an analysis of conditions promoting the uptake of FGCS, culminating in implications for clinical practice and concluding thoughts.

1.1 The Ever-Oscillating Nature of Female Body Ideals

The society has continually propagated unrealistic—and ever-changing—standards and so-called norms of what it means for women and girls to be feminine and therefore beautiful. The variation of feminine beauty norms demonstrates that they are both temporally and culturally situated, meaning changes in sociocultural opinion can enforce profound changes to what is classed as desirable and what no longer meets the 'feminine ideal'. This ideology has been documented by Wolf (1991), who claims imagery of women's so-called beauty has been used against women in a move to commodify women's bodies and keep women occupied by shame about their bodies not meeting the new 'beauty' standard. For example, the Ancient Egyptians and Ancient Chinese dynasties preferred a slender figure, demure in posture and quaint in poise, associated with modesty (see Silverio, 2019 for a detailed discussion of postural aspects of women and shame). On the contrary, denizens of Ancient Greece, the Italian Renaissance and Victorian Britain favoured fuller-figured women, with larger breasts and shapely hips—taken as visual synonyms for enhanced fertility (Magli, 2007; Rice, 1981). Moving to more modern casts of the 'ideal feminine', Western society during the 1920s desired an androgynous 'flapper girl' build, in what was a dramatic shift away from the portly Victorian figure of the previous century. Before long, the three subsequent decades (1930s–1950s) once again saw new trends in femininity with the dawn of the Golden Age of Hollywood, which brought with it the hourglass figure as the most desirable. A further change to what was deemed feminine, and therefore beautiful in the Western world, came to fruition in the 1960s, with tall and thin becoming the exemplar for feminine beauty. Eventually, the desire for the 'stick-thin' feminine vanished, only to be replaced by a societal desire for a version of femininity which came to be known as the 'supermodel'. This era, which dominated the 1980s, saw 'slim, but still buxom' as the new feminine standard filling the spotlight previously held by those mentioned above. The 1990s gave way to 'heroin chic', where *thin* was once again *in.* Women were again considered to be the embodiment of feminine beauty if they were waifish and gaunt, effectively equating *sexy* with *skinny*, and deviations from this attracted disdain and shame.

This fluctuation between often polar opposites supposed *feminine* traits (i.e. from voluptuous to willowy and back again) illustrates beauty standards and desired forms of femininity are arbitrary, capricious, and fragile. It shows that throughout history, certain bodies are not *naturally* more beautiful or attractive than others, but rather the social desirability of some body types has waxed and waned according to sociocultural, patriarchal, masculinist desires and discourse. Moreover, hegemonic heteronormative discourses have long dictated which bodies are favourable and therefore valued whilst simultaneously and implicitly deciding which ones are made invisible, erased from favour, or worse *shamed.*

One way women and girls are seen to be circumventing this issue is by seeking cosmetic surgery. As the new millennium brought with it the advent of the desire for the *healthy curvy* woman, cosmetic surgery became increasingly more accessible to the average person, and pioneering efforts in the field of plastics and reconstructive surgeries were adapted for *'the aesthetic improvement on otherwise healthy bodies'* (Davis, 1995, p. 16).

2 Society, Body Image, and Cosmetic Surgery

Social media use amongst adolescents continues to increase annually, with early adolescents now actively using social media, whilst simultaneously undergoing physical changes and identity development, forming attitudes about their bodies, and trying to establish themselves as an individual. Sociocultural theories of body image argue individuals internalise the largely unattainable cultural body norms projected on social media, which pressure young people, and particularly young women, to try to change their bodies (see Salamon & Spears Brown, 2019). This is largely due to a preoccupation with body surveillance (the excessive monitoring of the outer appearance) and self-objectification behaviours or commodification (when people view themselves as objects for use instead of as human beings) as explained by Salamon and Spears Brown (2019). Moreover, Manago, Ward, Lemm, Reed and Seabrook (2015) have contended that social networking websites are popular avenues for young people to curate flattering images of themselves, post provocative photographs and gain both attention and validation. Anyone posting on these websites is vulnerable to the dark side of social media (Craker & March, 2016), including cyberbullying, trolling (the act of leaving an insulting message on someone else's social media post), and online harassment, with many instances linking to body image. It is on such platforms that Manago et al. (2015) argue that young people learn what is considered sexy and attractive, and we argue that for women an important tertiary factor is that they learn what is the current feminine 'norm'.

2.1 *The Internet and Body Image*

The role of the Internet in body image projection and consumption has been a hot topic in the mass media in what has become known as the *complicated truth* about social media and body image (see Chap. 18 in this book). Women users of social media have reported they tend to compare their own appearance negatively with their peer group and with celebrities, but not with family members (see Fardouly & Vartanian, 2015). Social media and its impact on body image have also been the subject of academic debate internationally. For instance, in Australia, Tiggeman and Slater (2013) examined the relationship between Internet exposure and body image concern in adolescent girls. The authors found that time spent by participants on the Internet and social media was significantly related to internalisation of the thin 'ideal', body surveillance and a drive for thinness. Moreover, in a study engaging with American students, Manago et al. (2015) found that social media fosters a heightened experience of the self from an observer's perspective, which has consequences for body image and sexual agency amongst both women and men. Further, Vandenbosch and Eggermonth (2012) note more adolescent girls in Belgium report observing sexually objectifying content on their social media newsfeeds, which led to increased endorsement of Western beauty ideals, increased surveillance of their own bodies, and increased prioritisation of appearance with regard to self-worth.

We live in an age where there is an increasing emphasis on the body and its perfection. Whilst television and its role in the domestication and normalisation of cosmetic surgery and the risks associated with it through reality television programmes have been well documented (Ashikali, Dittmar & Ayers, 2016; Crockett, Pruzinsky & Persing, 2007; Tait, 2007), the rapid proliferation of Internet technologies and smart phone applications have much to answer for. Recent estimates suggest approximately 90% of 18–29-year-olds use social media, with most visiting such sites at least once daily (Primack & Escobar-Viera, 2017). Alongside the rise in social media applications focused on photographs and videos, there has been an increase in teenagers *sexting* (*sex*ual-tex*ting*) images to one another, which has seen associations with sexual shame (Ringrose & Harvey, 2015) and social grooming (Won Kim & Chock, 2015). Further, there has been a widely documented correlation between exposure to appearance-related social media websites, in what Salamon and Spears Brown (2019, p. 539) term the *'selfie generation'* and what has been linked to body image dissatisfaction (see Fardouly & Vartanian, 2015; Ghaznavi & Taylor, 2015; Pepin & Endresz, 2015), particularly amongst females (Tiggeman & Slater, 2013).

Another way the Internet has influenced the marketing of new 'feminine ideals' has been the increased access to the sexualised body and pornography. The Internet has also revolutionised how individuals access pornographic materials, and there has been a subtle seeping of pornography-influenced imagery used in mainstream mass media, through the use of overtly and overly sexualised images, especially of women, in what could be described as *pornography-lite*. Given pornography is known for dramatic, unrealistic and sometimes falsified sexual imagery, consumers of pornography are often exposed to bodies and genitalia which are unattainable to the majority of viewers, in what Barbara, Facchin, Meschia and Vercellini (2015; p. 916) argue is *'a new vulvovaginal standard'* women *must* meet and their partners *should* expect and what we refer to as the 'ideal' genital aesthetic.

2.2 *Shame and the Desire for Cosmetic Surgery*

Whilst changing a part of one's physical appearance is often a harmless desire, for some the desire to change their body lies in the shame they hold in relation to their bodies and its so-called imperfections (see Feder, 2011; Northrop, 2012). The phrase 'the beauty myth' was coined by Wolf (1991), to highlight the power of the media, particularly through the beauty industry and its advertising, in provoking women a destructive obsession with unrealistic beauty ideals, and how the myth of female beauty can in the actual fact be oppressive. Some individuals, faced with unrealistic body ideals in the media, undergo cosmetic procedures, and it is therefore right to explore cosmetic surgery in the context of shame.

Duarte, Pinto-Gouveia, Ferriera and Batista (2015, p. 657) define shame as a *'multifaceted, self-conscious and socially shaped emotion that emerges in the context of competition for social attractiveness'*. For Salamon and Spears Brown (2019, p. 541), shame is simply *'when individuals feel particularly negative about their bodies'*, whereas Feder (2011) talks of shame as having the ability to provoke disgust. For some with the confidence, financial means, and peer support, cosmetic surgery is thus seen as a solution to internalised and societally governed shame and associated disgust. However, the modification of women's bodies through cosmetic surgery has faced critique from feminist scholars who believe that succumbing to cosmetic surgery positions women as victims of a construction of femininity and beauty standards which exist in our patriarchal society (Taylor, 2012). This has been discussed by scholars such as Jones (2008, p. 12) as *'the never-ending renovation of the self'*. However, Alsop and Lennon (2018, p. 95) attempt to push back against the negative feminist stance towards cosmetic surgery, arguing it enables *'the expressive body'*, which allows for a modicum of possibilities for intersubjective relations with others.

Body modification has become part of the postmodern self, and appropriation of the body in this sense is intertwined with fashion and identity (Sweetman, 1999). Sociological and cultural studies help place the rise of cosmetic surgical practices and industries within a historical, social, and cultural context. They do so by locating cosmetic surgery within post-Enlightenment projects of individualisation, self-transformation and self-improvement for the betterment of both the individual, and in turn society (see Tanner, Maher & Fraser, 2014). Stemming from this is a fascination in self-making and self-reinvention, and the perception of beauty as a commodity (see Gimlin, 2000).

Normalisation of cosmetic surgery has been attempted by disentangling aesthetic procedures from shame, arguing that confidence and self-esteem should be a priority. The taboo around undergoing cosmetic surgery is, however, still so prevalent that many women who have a cosmetic surgical procedure 'take it to the grave' as they feel ashamed due to societal scorn. Cosmetic surgery is understood to be part of the individual's reflexive construction of self-identity (Askegaard, Gertsen & Langer, 2002). The rhetoric narrative that *'The women are doing it for themselves'* to borrow from Braun (2009, p. 233) is a common discourse in cosmetic surgery (Morgan, 1991). It constructs a reflexive, but individualised, acultural subject—someone who is aware of the motivations for their desires and practices. However, motivations behind cosmetic surgery sometimes move beyond the self, in a step towards appeasing others or to meet the new societal standards. For instance, Atari, Barbaro, Sela, Shackelford and Chengeni (2017) present a consideration of cosmetic surgery as part of women's mate retention strategy to minimise the risk of partner infidelity and relationship dissolution. The authors conclude that women consider plastic surgery as part of a strategy to retain a long-term mate. Considering whether gender differences exist in young people's attitudes towards cosmetic surgery, Wen, Chia and Xiaomin (2017) found that young people of both sexes generally held positive attitudes towards cosmetic surgery and that no significant gender disparities exist.

However, the authors contend that female audiences are more likely than their male counterparts to identify with cosmetic surgery-related media.

Whilst many forms of cosmetic surgery are visible (for instance, rhinoplasty, botox, and arguably 'tummy tucks' and liposuction), others are hidden from the public view. Dobson, McDonald, Kirkman, Souter and Fisher (2017) discuss tensions and ambiguities which exist in modifying the *private* body, with specific reference to FGCS (something which is only seen by the self or intimate others). Lloyd, Crouch, Minto, Liao and Creighton (2005) argue although representations of female nudity are common, detailed accurate representations of female genitals are rare and there is a lack of awareness of the diversity of female genital appearances. Perhaps due to this lack of awareness, in recent years, an increased number of healthy girls and young women have been seeking female genital cosmetic surgery in a bid to get what is often colloquially referred to as a *designer vagina* (see Braun, 2005, 2009; Green, 2005; Holliday, 2018; Jones, 2017). This is a controversial topic, with questions surrounding legality arising since comparisons emerge between female genital cosmetic surgery and 'traditional' forms of genital cutting—often referred to as female genital mutilation (Braun, 2009; Dyer, 2019; Essén & Johnsdotter, 2004). But away from all controversy, the demand for FGCS is booming.

3 Shame and Female Genital Cosmetic Surgery

Women often claim to undergo FGCS because they are unhappy with the function and/or appearance of their vulva/vagina. Regarding functional aspects, women request FGCS when feeling sustained discomfort in their clothing, or during sports or sexual activities, or if they appear to lack sensation during sexual intercourse due to vaginal *looseness* (Goodman, 2009). A judgement of genital appearance is often based on qualities of the labia minora. In a Dutch survey, 42% of female respondents stated the appearance of the labia minora was important (Koning, Zeijlmans, Bouman & van der Lei, 2009). A vulva without visible labia minora is predominantly considered the visual ideal (Clerico, Lari, Mojallal & Boucher, 2017; Howarth, Hayes, Simonis & Temple-Smith, 2016), with variations in shape, colour, or asymmetry of the labia viewed as undesirable (Braun, 2010). Whereas genital appearance is mentioned as the main driver for FGCS in interviews and online communities (Howarth et al., 2016; Zwier, 2014), physical discomfort is noticeably more often given as a reason in clinical contexts, which has been interpreted as women supposing the latter to be more of a guarantor to be accepted for surgery (Bramwell, Morland & Garden, 2007; Zwier, 2014). Women's anxiety to show their vulva to their sexual partner and the resulting negative impact of genital appearance on one's sex life has been mentioned as another motivation for surgery (Bramwell et al., 2007), though as Barbara et al. (2015, p. 915) point out: '*surgery is not a definitive solution to treat psychologically based pain or dysfunction. Moreover, there is no robust evidence supporting the effectiveness of female genital cosmetic surgery, especially regarding sexual enhancement'*. However, the questions of why women's distress about their genital aesthetic reaches an intensity which leads to surgical interventions and why more and more young women and girls decide to follow this path are more complex and require unpacking.

3.1 The 'Ideal' Female Genital Aesthetic and Shame

Generally, negative sentiments towards female genitalia are by far no novelty. The lack of non-vulgar, non-derogatory words for them in everyday use, let alone the words used for female masturbation, in comparison to the male versions of both speaks to the age-old tradition of female sexuality being taboo (Silverio, 2019; see also Stevenson, 2016). Correspondingly, girls are brought up in Western society where visual media has made female genitalia invisible (Bramwell, 2002), effectively asking women and girls to live up to the 'barbie doll' role model where *smooth and hairless* and *neat and tidy* is desirable (see Epperlein & Anderson, 2016). It is therefore unsurprising that 'vagina' is still commonly used for female genitalia as a whole, despite it being biologically incorrect, whereby 'vagina' refers to the muscular tract which connects the vulva (the visible external part of the female sex organs) to the cervix (the lower part of the uterus, which is internal). The linguistic and attentional neglect of the clitoris by caretakers add to this obscuration of the vulva and are considered as momentous for female development (Lerner, 1976).

Next to the vagina's 'absence' from social discourse, Braun and Wilkinson (2001) identified six other negative representations of it, in which the vagina is positioned, for example, as 'disgusting' or 'dangerous'. An interview study (Fahs, 2014) exploring women's narratives on their genital identified seven themes: 'dirty' or 'gross', needing maintenance, unknown or frustrating, unnatural, comparative, ambivalent, and affirmative. Anxiety, excess and need for control were dominant references in women's narratives. On this basis, it is no wonder that Western discourses of the female body have evolved without explicit reference to female genitalia. The effects on women's self-perception are mirrored in the data: In a qualitative analysis of US American, British, and Dutch women's posts in on-line communities and international surgery providers' websites about labial reduction (Zwier, 2014), 71% of women mentioned emotional discomfort regarding their genital appearance, meaning they felt 'freakish', ashamed or scared of a negative reaction by a partner. Another key aspect is the desire for being 'normal' in a heteronormative society that only allows for two distinct and mutually exclusive sexes and, accordingly, two types of genitalia. Female genital cosmetic surgery offers means to counter shame and fear of 'abnormality' by creating prototypical genitalia and thereby shrouding genital plurality (see Liao & Creighton, 2019; Nurka, 2018).

3.2 Shame and the Rise of Female Genital Cosmetic Surgery

Aesthetic surgeons have expanded their repertoire, and the relative ease of access to these surgeries coupled with their increasing affordability has seen rising uptake amongst women across the world. Today's postmodern world of the gym-going social media influencer venerates women who are 'strong, not skinny' and 'fit, not thin', and now, more than ever, we see cosmetic 'enhancement' and surgery being utilised as a way of reaching current 'feminine ideals'. In particular, facial aesthetic surgery had become an increasingly common part of a woman's lifecourse, to—at least visually—*defy* the signs of ageing. The trend for cosmetic surgery in younger women, however, has often been intrinsically linked to a sexualisation of the female body (see Kinnunen, 2008). Women influenced by Western celebrity culture and visual media are more frequently opting for breast enlargement, buttock enhancement, liposuction and fat transfer surgeries, amongst others (Markey & Markey, 2009), under the guise of self-care and self-improvement (Selwyn Delinsky, 2005), though procedure preference is said to differ by race (Prendergast et al., 2011) and generational age (see Placik & Arkins, 2014).

What has come to concern scholars, activists and those in the medical profession more recently is the rise in popularity of, and requests for, genital cosmetic surgery, in particular amongst young girls (see Shaw et al., 2013). Female genital cosmetic surgery can include a variety of procedures which are undertaken to improve appearance and occasionally functionality but in the absence of clinical indication (Braun, 2015). The binary notion of gender and the lack of reflection on it in FGCS scholarship—attributing 'female' genitalia exclusively to ciswomen's bodies—are problematic (see Braun, 2019) but are, as discussed above, inherent to a phenomenon in which the creation of 'prototypical' genitalia is pursued. According to the British Association of Aesthetic Plastic Surgeons (BAAPS, 2017), FGCS procedures range from 'labial reduction' (reduction of the skin on either side of the vaginal opening) to 'liposculpture' (fat transfer from one area of the body into the mons pubis) and 'vaginal tightening' (where the vaginal opening is either sutured or where the 'excess' vaginal mucosa is excised and the vaginal wall muscles are 'tightened'). Other, more experimental FGCS procedures include the 'hoodectomy' (exposure of the clitoris via removal of the clitoral hood) and 'hymenoplasty' ('reconstruction' of the hymen), and with the advancement of experimental cosmetic surgery, the list is becoming seemingly endless (see Braun, 2009, who provides an extensive listing). Interventions which can be found listed under the FGCS label often vary between publications, as does the nomenclature. Indeed, some terms used by providers have been considered misleading and proprietary (Goodman, 2009). The fact that cosmetic surgery is not a medical speciality with recognised training and accreditation conditions in many countries is likely to contribute to these inconsistencies (Liao & Creighton, 2019).

The Western world has been at the forefront of much of this genital modification work (Braun, 2010), and although it is steeped in controversy (see Essén & Johnsdotter, 2004; Kelly & Foster, 2012; Liao, Taghinejadi & Creighton, 2012) and robust data on successful treatments and complications of FGCS are scarce (Michala, 2019), the number of women seeking these surgeries is set to continue to rise. The American Society for Aesthetic Plastic Surgery (ASAPS, 2018) reported 12,746 labiaplasties performed in the United States of America in 2018, an increase of 18.3% compared to 2017 and of 52.9% compared to 2014. Results from the annual Global Aesthetic Survey indicate the number of performed labiaplasties worldwide increased by 1% from 2016 to 2017 and that 22% more 'vaginal rejuvenations' had been conducted over that period (ISAPS, 2018a). Taken together their increase of 23% was the largest amongst all procedures surveyed (ISAPS, 2018b). It has been noted that those data presumably even underestimate the actual number of FGCS, given that they are based on voluntary self-report and collected by organisations of providers (Braun, 2010; Liao & Creighton, 2019). The spike in the FGCS trend has been attributed to aggressive marketing on behalf of the cosmetic surgeons who offer and perform these surgeries (Braun, 2010). The increase has also been attributed to the associations being made by surgeons and the media that FGCS can improve female sexual pleasure, specifically the ability to reliably and repeatedly achieve orgasm after the procedure has healed (Braun, 2005; Goodman, 2011; Simonis, Manocha & Ong, 2016). However, perhaps the most influential has been the perpetuation of new 'ideal feminine' norms which now extend to the visual and tactile aesthetic of the female genitals (Koning et al., 2009; Liao et al., 2012; Swami et al., 2008).

4 Normalising Female Genital Cosmetic Surgery: The Influence of the Fourth Industrial Revolution

The feelings of shame and experience of taboo with regard to female genitalia have only been emboldened by the proliferation of new 'feminine ideals' by the mass media. The Fourth Industrial Revolution [4IR] and advent of almost universal, quick and easy access to the internet have made it possible to share images to a large audience almost instantaneously.

4.1 Body Talk... Bodies Talk

Bodies, specifically those which are female, are often the central focus of these visual media. More specifically, research has found that nude imagery has significantly shifted focus from the breast in the mid-twentieth century to the vaginal area in the post-millennium era which could account for the increase in the desire for FGCS (Placik & Arkins, 2014). Above we have seen the linking of female genitalia to shame through inadequate social discourses; however it can now be argued that the 4IR has utilised these feelings of shame to drive forwards the aggressive marketisation of FGCS, which has—in some Western contexts—normalised the idea that one *can* and perhaps *should* change the female genital aesthetic if it is deemed by oneself, by one's intimate partner, or by one's healthcare professional, to not conform to the socially desired 'norm'.

Evidence that the Internet has facilitated the normalisation of FGCS in response to internalised feelings of shame related to one's genitalia has been derived from pockets of research from across the world. In their analysis of published research, Mowat, McDonald, Dobson, Fisher and Kirkman (2015) draw on five studies which have either analysed the content of FGCS providers' websites (Ashong & Batta, 2013; Liao et al., 2012; Moran & Lee, 2013) or were mixed analyses of provider websites, pornographic websites, and other publications (Howarth, Sommer & Jordan, 2010; Zwier, 2014). Their review identified five dominant and interrelated patterns which have assisted in FGCS becoming normalised in modern society: *'pathologisation of genital diversity; female genital appearance as important to wellbeing; characteristics of women's genitals are important for sex life; female body as degenerative and improvable through surgery; and FGCS as safe, easy, and effective'* (Mowat et al., 2015, p. 1). The authors further explain that the Internet has a key role in informing, promoting and normalising FGCS. The claim that the Internet has *a*, if not *the* key role in perpetuating a certain vaginal aesthetic and normalising FGCS in order to achieve it, is unsurprising. There is a growing body of literature which has stated that the Internet has facilitated greater exposure to the female genitalia through easy access to pornography (Barbara et al., 2015), has encouraged the view that FGCS is a *treat* and not a *treatment* (Tiefer, 2008), and has aggressively marketed FGCS as sexually liberating and relationship enhancing (Braun, 2005, 2009; Goodman, 2011), despite there being a lack of evidence and even some to the contrary (see Cartwright & Cardozo, 2008; Iglesia et al., 2013).

4.2 Pathologising the Female Body

Throughout this chapter, we have drawn on literature which has demonstrated how the female body has been an object of both desire and of shame and how the societal discourse which exists around women's bodies has often been used to control women's aesthetic. Shame is commonly considered a toxic rather than an adaptive emotion. To fully grasp the role shame plays with regard to FGCS, it is important to recognise its functional aspects for the human psyche, for example, concerning the regulation of boundaries and bounded bodies. Azoulay (2011) characterises shame as a vital constituting factor of psychosexual identity. It is excessive shame, leading individuals to avoid shameful issues instead of actively addressing and coping with them, which becomes detrimental. As we have seen from the above debate, advertising of FGCS not only fuels shame, but also encourages avoidance by 'making the problem disappear' through FGCS.

This has, perhaps shockingly, made its way into clinical practice as well, where women after childbirth have presented as anxious about having a 'loose' vagina

(Goodman, 2009). The idea that one's vagina is not 'tight' enough is bounded and intertwined with the concept of shame about not having the same genital aesthetic as pre-childbirth and adopting the assumption that sexual intercourse will not feel the same or elicit the same pleasure for either partner, with the post-childbirth vaginal form. Again, to 'make the problem disappear', obstetric surgeons and nurses over the last few decades in the Western world have been found to introduce what has come to be known as 'the husband stitch' (Dobbeleir, Van Landuyt & Monstrey, 2011; Green, 2005). 'The husband stitch' is a non-clinically indicated procedure where a(n) (extra) stitch is placed in the woman's post-natal vaginal wall often without consent or even knowledge of the woman receiving it. It is either administered on its own or—where sutures are required for a perineal tear—in combination with clinically indicated perineal repair. Here, the patriarchal society in which Western women live has enforced a non-existent pathology on postpartum women, which the culture in which they work has made it possible to believe that it is their right and duty to 'fix'. The moniker it has been assigned is a flagrant reminder that this procedure is not to benefit the woman who has endured this procedure, but her male partner—and the wider hegemonic, masculinist society—who through advertisement, perpetual social discourse and stereotyped cultural narratives have been conditioned to expect one kind of female genital aesthetic as a key factor in the desired 'feminine ideal'.

5 Implications, Considerations, and Conclusions

Non-clinically indicated cosmetic surgery has almost always been associated with being a financially driven endeavour by those who perform it. Moreover, surgeons performing procedures on otherwise healthy beings are predicated on the fact there is a constantly shifting body image 'ideal' being designed and propagated. Women have usually been the target of such social discourses, and where once the cosmetic surgeon was visited to enhance what was visible to the public (i.e. face lifts, rhinoplasty, or breast augmentation), the expansion to FGCS has been argued by some as unprecedented and others as inevitable (see Tiefer, 2008). Alongside the development of aesthetic surgery has been the advent of the use of visual media to market anything which can be sold. At the forefront of visual media mass marketisation in the age of the 4IR has been the Internet. The boundary of these two phenomena becomes the point of rupture at which *the body* can be sexualised and marketised through *the Internet* to an audience who indulge themselves in mass media and assimilate those messages into their own everyday discourse. As Kinnunen (2008, p. 38) argues, *'Media images are discursive condensations of gender and sexuality, and they powerfully set the models for body discipline. As part of the pornographisation of culture, the female body is excessively sexualised in the media'.*

5.1 Psychological and Social Implications

Whilst the Internet has arguably helped engender positive social change, when used to market the new 'feminine ideal', new myths about 'beauty', and now seemingly, newly desired genital aesthetics, the Internet allows such content to be widely circulated within seconds, meaning body image 'norms' are continually and continuously consumed. With this increased exposure also comes more opportunity for bodily scrutiny, surveillance and shame (Swami, 2009). And with evermore avenues to target the population through mass media on the Internet, it is no wonder FGCS and the surgeons who make a living performing them are advertised in the same way. Sexualisation of the female body is not new (see Silverio, 2019), but what we see in terms of body image issues is an intrinsic link to mental wellbeing. With the focus of these body image issues, Barbara et al. (2015, pp. 916–917) describe a *'dictatorship of beauty ideals'* which portrays unique variations in genital aesthetics *'as a limit and not as a value'* and go on to argue *'FGCS interventions performed on perfectly normal women may confirm and even strengthen this idea'* whereby the root causes of women's insecurities are being cosmetically ameliorated, but not psychologically alleviated.

5.2 Clinical and Ethical Considerations

The above commentary on the psychological and social impacts of FGCS really focuses on the body as a site of personal scrutiny and surveillance. However, as has been evident in this chapter, the body often is the site of wider surveillance by clinicians and also by academic commentary (see Cartwright & Cardozo, 2008). Here we are beginning to see a growing literature base comparing FGCS to female genital mutilation/cutting [FGM/C] with poignant questions being asked about how scholars, activists, clinicians, and the general public are meant to understand the difference between the two procedures (see Dyer, 2019; Liao & Creighton, 2007; Rodrigues, 2012; Sheldon & Wilkinson, 1998). These questions have become especially prevalent given one category—FGM/C—has seen widespread legislation brought in against it across the Western world and the other—FGCS—is openly marketed to women of all ages (see Kelly & Foster, 2012). Further, although there is some anecdotal knowledge of lifecourse risks FGCS might pose, the relative novelty of aesthetically inclined FGCS does not have a sound evidence base for its safety. The lifecourse risks discussed has pondered whether the obstetric complications associated with FGM/C (e.g. sexual dysfunction, prolonged labour, perinatal mortality) could translate to women who undergo FGCS procedures, particularly those who seek FGCS before giving birth (see Johnsdotter & Essén, 2010; see also Braun, 2010). In response to these debates, some have called for greater regulation, where currently there is none (Essén & Johnsdotter, 2004; Liao & Creighton, 2011) and others have chosen to adopt a 'women-centred' approach of advocating choice aided by education and counselling when the FGCS is 'medically indicated' (Shaw et al., 2013).

5.3 Concluding Comment

The aim of this chapter was to discuss the role of the Internet in the trend which has seen an increasing number of young women and girls desire FGCS procedures. This area of research is currently predominantly derived from evidence-based medicine, and whilst this work has been critical, there has been an overwhelming lack of theoretical criticality as the world awaits the path FGCS will take. This chapter has drawn on the available scholarship to help build on the work by others (specifically see Barbara et al., 2015; Braun, 2005, 2009, 2010, 2015, 2019; Tiefer, 2008) in an attempt to establish a theoretical critique of FGCS. We note the work of Nurka (2018, p. 207), who stakes the claim: *'If I am critical of FGCS, it is not because I think that it is a violation of nature, but because the fantasy of proper sex is offered to women as the cure for their suffering when it is in fact the cause'*. This eloquently sums up the growing opinion that if FGCS was disaggregated from the marketised narrative of *sexual pleasure* and women were fully informed about FGCS procedures and their risks, a regulated FGCS branch of specialised medicine might be somewhat more acceptable. The intrinsic issue which we, in this chapter, have also raised is that the Internet allows these messages of overly sexualised women's bodies to be shared and altered with an immediate effect, meaning the social desirability of one body image 'norm' is precarious and fragile in our heteronormative patriarchal society. The principle of FGCS being agentic cannot yet be accepted as true, whilst the marketed discourse of FGCS is tainted by the shaming of variation amongst the genital aesthetic.

References

Alsop, R., & Lennon, K. (2018). Aesthetic surgery and the expressive body. *Feminist Theory, 19*(1), 95–112.

Ashikali, E. M., Dittmar, H., & Ayers, S. (2016). Adolescent girls' views on cosmetic surgery: A focus group study. *Journal of Health Psychology, 21*(1), 112–121.

Ashong, A. C., & Batta, H. E. (2013). Sensationalising the female pudenda: An examination of public communication of aesthetic genital surgery. *Global Journal of Health Science, 5*(2), 153–165.

Askegaard, S., Gertsen, M. C., & Langer, R. (2002). The body consumed: Reflexivity and cosmetic surgery. *Psychology & Marketing, 19*(10), 793–812.

Atari, M., Barbaro, N., Sela, Y., Shackelford, T. K., & Chengeni, R. (2017). Consideration of cosmetic surgery as part of women's benefit-provisioning mate retention strategy. *Frontiers in Psychology, 8*, 1–7.

Azoulay, I. (2011). Rettet die scham! *Zeitschrift für Sexualforschung, 24*(3), 272–278.

Barbara, G., Facchin, F., Meschia, M., & Vercellini, P. (2015). "The first cut is the deepest": A psychological, sexological and gynecological perspective on female genital cosmetic surgery. *Acta Obstetricia et Gynecologica Scandinavica, 94*(9), 915–920.

Bramwell, R. (2002). Invisible labia: The representation of female external genitals in women's magazines. *Sexual and Relationship Therapy, 17*(2), 187–190.

Bramwell, R., Morland, C., & Garden, A. S. (2007). Expectations and experience of labial reduction: A qualitative study. *BJOG: An International Journal of Obstetrics & Gynaecology, 114*(12), 1493–1499.

Braun, V. (2005). In search of (better) sexual pleasure: Female genital 'cosmetic' surgery. *Sexualities, 8*(4), 407–424.

Braun, V. (2009). The women are doing it for themselves': The rhetoric of choice and agency around female genital 'cosmetic surgery'. *Australian Feminist Studies, 24*(60), 233–249.

Braun, V. (2010). Female genital cosmetic surgery: A critical review of current knowledge and contemporary debates. *Journal of Women's Health, 19*(7), 1393–1407.

Braun, V. (2015). Female genital cosmetic surgery. In A. Bolin & P. Whelehan (Eds.), *The international encyclopedia of human sexuality* (pp. 372–373). Hoboken, NJ: Wiley.

Braun, V. (2019). Selling a perfect vulva? Selling a 'normal' vulva! In S. M. Creighton & L.-M. Liao (Eds.), *Female genital cosmetic surgery: Solution to what problem?* (pp. 23–32). Cambridge, United Kingdom: Cambridge University Press.

Braun, V., & Wilkinson, S. (2001). Socio-cultural representations of the vagina. *Journal of Reproductive and Infant Psychology, 19*(1), 17–32.

Cartwright, R., & Cardozo, L. (2008). Cosmetic vulvovaginal surgery. *Obstetrics, Gynaecology & Reproductive Medicine, 18*(10), 285–286.

Clerico, C., Lari, A., Mojallal, A., & Boucher, F. (2017). Anatomy and aesthetics of the labia minora: The ideal vulva? *Aesthetic Plastic Surgery, 41*(3), 714–719.

Craker, N., & March, E. (2016). The dark side of Facebook®: The dark tetrad, negative social potency, and trolling behaviours. *Personality and Individual Differences, 102*, 79–84.

Crockett, R. J., Pruzinsky, T., & Persing, J. A. (2007). The influence of plastic surgery "reality TV" on cosmetic surgery patient expectations and decision making. *Plastic and Reconstructive Surgery, 120*(1), 316–324.

Davis, K. (1995). *Reshaping the female body: The dilemma of cosmetic surgery*. New York: Routledge.

Dobbeleir, J. M. L. C. L., Van Landuyt, K., & Monstrey, S. J. (2011). Aesthetic surgery of the female genitalia. *Seminars in Plastic Surgery, 25*(2), 130–141.

Dobson, A. S., McDonald, K., Kirkman, M., Souter, K., & Fisher, J. (2017). Invisible labour? Tensions and ambiguities of modifying the 'private' body: The case of female genital cosmetic surgery. In A. S. Elias, R. Gill, & C. Scharff (Eds.), *Aesthetic labour: Rethinking beauty politics in neoliberalism* (pp. 351–367). London: Palgrave.

Duarte, C., Pinto-Gouveia, J., Ferriera, C., & Batista, D. (2015). Body image as a source of shame: A new measure for the assessment of the multifaceted nature of body image shame. *Clinical Psychology and Psychotherapy, 22*(6), 656–666.

Dyer, C. (2019). FGM: Surgeons who do cosmetic genital surgery may risk prosecution. *BMJ, 367* (16094), 1.

Epperlein, E., & Anderson, I. (2016). Man vs. Vagina—A Foucauldian analysis of men's discourses about the perfect vagina and female genital grooming. *Psychology of Women Section Review, 18* (1), 5–12.

Essén, B., & Johnsdotter, S. (2004). Female genital mutilation in the West: Traditional circumcision versus genital cosmetic surgery. *Acta Obstetricia et Gynecologica Scandinavica, 83*(7), 611–613.

Fahs, B. (2014). Genital panics: Constructing the vagina in women's qualitative narratives about pubic hair, menstrual sex, and vaginal self-image. *Body Image, 11*(3), 210–218.

Fardouly, J., & Vartanian, L. R. (2015). Negative comparisons about one's appearance mediate the relationship between Facebook usage and body image concerns. *Body Image, 12*, 82–88.
Feder, E. K. (2011). Tilting the ethical lens: Shame, disgust, and the body in question. *Hypatia, 26* (3), 633–650.
Ghaznavi, H., & Taylor, L. D. (2015). Bones, body parts, and sex appeal: An analysis of #thinspiration images on popular social media. *Body Image, 14*, 54–61.
Gimlin, D. (2000). Cosmetic surgery: Beauty as commodity. *Qualitative Sociology, 23*(1), 77–98.
Goodman, M. P. (2009). Female cosmetic genital surgery. *Obstetrics & Gynecology, 113*(1), 154–159.
Goodman, M. P. (2011). Female genital cosmetic and plastic surgery: A review. *The Journal of Sexual Medicine, 8*(6), 1813–1825.
Green, F. J. (2005). From clitoridectomies to 'designer vaginas': The medical construction of heteronormative female bodies and sexuality through female genital cutting. *Sexualities, Evolution & Gender, 7*(2), 153–187.
Holliday, R. (2018). Vagina dialogues: Theorizing the 'designer vagina'. In G. Griffin & M. Jordal (Eds.), *Body, migration, re/constructive surgeries* (pp. 192–208). New York: Routledge.
Howarth, C., Hayes, J., Simonis, M., & Temple-Smith, M. (2016). 'Everything's neatly tucked away': Young women's views on desirable vulval anatomy. *Culture, Health & Sexuality, 18* (12), 1363–1378.
Howarth, H., Sommer, V., & Jordan, F. M. (2010). Visual depictions of female genitalia differ depending on source. *Medical Humanities, 36*(2), 75–79.
Iglesia, C. B., Yurteri-Kaplan, L., & Alinsod, R. (2013). Female genital cosmetic surgery: A review of techniques and outcomes. *International Urogynecology Journal, 24*(12), 1997–2009.
International Society of Aesthetic Plastic Surgery. (2018a). *Latest international study shows global rise in cosmetic surgery*. New York: ISAPS Press Office.
International Society of Aesthetic Plastic Surgery. (2018b). *ISAPS year-to-year comparisons: 2017 vs. 2016*. New York: ISAPS Press Office.
Johnsdotter, S., & Essén, B. (2010). Genitals and ethnicity: The politics of genital modifications. *Reproductive Health Matters, 18*(35), 29–37.
Jones, M. (2008). *Skintight: An anatomy of cosmetic surgery*. New York: Berg.
Jones, M. (2017). Expressive surfaces: The case of the designer vagina. *Theory, Culture & Society, 34*(7–8), 29–50.
Kelly, B., & Foster, C. (2012). Should female genital cosmetic surgery and genital piercing be regarded ethically and legally as female genital mutilation? *BJOG: An International Journal of Obstetrics & Gynaecology, 119*(4), 389–392.
Kinnunen, T. (2008). Breast augmentation surgery: Carving the flesh as female. In V. Burr & J. Hearn (Eds.), *Sex, violence and the body* (pp. 34–52). London: Palgrave Macmillan.
Koning, M., Zeijlmans, I. A., Bouman, T. K., & van der Lei, B. (2009). Female attitudes regarding labia minora appearance and reduction with consideration of media influence. *Aesthetic Surgery Journal, 29*(1), 65–71.
Lerner, H. E. (1976). Parental mislabeling of female genitals as a determinant of penis envy and learning inhibitions in women. *Journal of the American Psychoanalytic Association, 24*, 269–283.
Liao, L. M., & Creighton, S. M. (2007). Requests for cosmetic genitoplasty: How should healthcare providers respond? *BMJ, 334*(7603), 1090–1092.
Liao, L. M., & Creighton, S. M. (2011). Female genital cosmetic surgery: A new dilemma for GPs. *British Journal of General Practice, 61*(582), 7–8.
Liao, L. M., & Creighton, S. M. (2019). Female genital cosmetic surgery: Solution in pursuit of problem. In S. M. Creighton & L. M. Liao (Eds.), *Female genital cosmetic surgery: Solution to what problem?* (pp. 1–10). Cambridge, UK: Cambridge University Press.
Liao, L. M., Taghinejadi, N., & Creighton, S. M. (2012). An analysis of the content and clinical implications of online advertisements for female genital cosmetic surgery. *BMJ Open, 2*(6), 1–6.

Lloyd, J., Crouch, N. S., Minto, C. L., Liao, L.-M., & Creighton, S. M. (2005). Female genital appearance: 'Normality' unfolds. *BJOG: An International Journal of Obstetrics & Gynaecology, 112*(5), 643–646.

Magli, I. (2007). *Il mulino di Ofelia: Uomini e Dei [The mill of Ophelia: Men and God]*. Milan, Italy: Biblioteca Universale Rizzoli—Alta Fedeltà.

Manago, A. M., Ward, M. L., Lemm, K. M., Reed, L., & Seabrook, R. (2015). Facebook involvement, objectified body consciousness, body shame, and sexual assertiveness in college women and men. *Sex Roles, 72*(1–2), 1–14.

Markey, C. N., & Markey, P. M. (2009). Correlates of young women's interest in obtaining cosmetic surgery. *Sex Roles, 61*(3–4), 158–166.

Michala, L. (2019). Clinical evidence of the effects of female genital cosmetic surgery. In L.-M. Liao & S. M. Creighton (Eds.), *Female genital cosmetic surgery: Solution to what problem?* (pp. 51–57). Cambridge, UK: Cambridge University Press.

Moran, C., & Lee, C. (2013). Selling genital cosmetic surgery to healthy women: A multimodal discourse analysis of Australian surgical websites. *Critical Discourse Studies, 10*(4), 373–391.

Morgan, K. (1991). Woman and the knife: Cosmetic surgery and the colonization of women's bodies. *Hypatia, 6*(3), 25–53.

Mowat, H., McDonald, K., Dobson, A. S., Fisher, J., & Kirkman, M. (2015). The contribution of online content to the promotion and normalisation of female genital cosmetic surgery: A systematic review of the literature. *BMC Women's Health, 15*(110), 1–10.

Northrop, J. M. (2012). *Reflecting on cosmetic surgery: Body image, shame and narcissism*. New York: Routledge.

Nurka, C. (2018). *Female genital cosmetic surgery: Deviance, desire and the pursuit of perfection*. London: Palgrave Macmillan.

Pepin, G., & Endresz, N. (2015). Facebook, Instagram, Pinterest and co.: Body image and social media. *Journal of Eating Disorders, 3*(1), 1.

Placik, O. J., & Arkins, J. P. (2014). Plastic surgery trends parallel Playboy magazine: The pudenda preoccupation. *Aesthetic Surgery Journal, 34*(7), 1083–1090.

Prendergast, T. I., Ong'uti, S. K., Ortega, G., Khoury, A. L., Onwuka, E., Bolorunduro, O. B., et al. (2011). Differential trends in racial preferences for cosmetic surgery procedures. *The American Surgeon, 77*(8), 1081–1085.

Primack, B. A., & Escobar-Viera, C. G. (2017). Social media as it interfaces with psychosocial development and mental illness in transitional age youth. *Child and Adolescent Psychiatric Clinics, 26*(2), 217–233.

Rice, P. C. (1981). Prehistoric Venuses: Symbols of motherhood or womanhood? *Journal of Anthropological Research, 37*(4), 402–414.

Ringrose, J., & Harvey, L. (2015). Boobs, back-off, six packs and bits: Mediated body parts, gendered reward, and sexual shame in teens' sexting images. *Continuum: Journal of Media & Cultural Studies, 29*(2), 205–217.

Rodrigues, S. (2012). From vaginal exception to exceptional vagina: The biopolitics of female genital cosmetic surgery. *Sexualities, 15*(7), 778–794.

Salamon, I., & Spears Brown, C. (2019). The selfie generation: Examining the relationship between social media use and early adolescent body image. *Journal of Early Adolescence, 39*(4), 539–560.

Selwyn Delinsky, S. (2005). Cosmetic surgery: A common and accepted form of self-improvement? *Journal of Applied Social Psychology, 35*(10), 2012–2028.

Shaw, D., Lefebvre, G., Bouchard, C., Shapiro, J., Blake, J., Allen, L., et al., on behalf of the Clinical Practice Gynaecology Committee and the Ethics Committee of the Society of Obstetricians and Gynaecologists of Canada. (2013). Female genital cosmetic surgery. *Journal of Obstetrics and Gynaecology Canada, 35*(12), 1108–1112.

Sheldon, S., & Wilkinson, S. (1998). Female genital mutilation and cosmetic surgery: Regulating non-therapeutic body modification. *Bioethics, 12*(4), 263–285.

Silverio, S. A. (2019). Reconstructing gender to transcend shame: Embracing human functionality to enable agentic and desexualised bodies. In C.-H. Mayer & E. Vanderheiden (Eds.), *The bright side of shame: Transforming and growing through practical applications in cultural contexts* (pp. 149–165). Cham, Switzerland: Springer.

Simonis, M., Manocha, R., & Ong, J. (2016). Female genital cosmetic surgery: A cross-sectional survey exploring knowledge, attitude and practice of general practitioners. *BMJ Open, 6*(9), e013010.

Stevenson, J.H. (2016). *"You start to think you're the only woman that must do it": An interpretive phenomenological analysis of female pornography use within a heterosexual relationship.* Unpublished dissertation. Nottingham: Nottingham Trent University.

Swami, V. (2009). Body appreciation, media influence, and weight status predict consideration of cosmetic surgery among female undergraduates. *Body Image, 6*(4), 315–317.

Swami, V., Arteche, A., Chamorro-Premuzic, T., Furnham, A., Stieger, S., Haubner, T., & Voracek, M. (2008). Looking good: Factors affecting the likelihood of having cosmetic surgery. *European Journal of Plastic Surgery, 30*(5), 211–218.

Sweetman, P. (1999). Anchoring the (postmodern) self? Body modification, fashion and identity. *Body & Society, 5*(2–3), 51–76.

Tait, S. (2007). Television and the domestication of cosmetic surgery. *Feminist Media Studies, 7*(2), 119–135.

Tanner, C., Maher, J. M., & Fraser, S. (2014). *Vanity: 21st century selves.* New York: Palgrave Macmillan.

Taylor, S. J. (2012). Buying and selling breasts: Cosmetic surgery, beauty treatments and risk. *The Sociological Review, 60*(4), 635–653.

The American Society for Aesthetic Plastic Surgery. (2018). *Cosmetic (aesthetic) surgery national data bank.* New York: The Aesthetic Society.

The British Association of Aesthetic Plastic Surgeons. (2017). *Aesthetic genital surgery: Female genital aesthetic surgery.* London: The Royal College Surgeons of England.

Tiefer, L. (2008). Female genital cosmetic surgery: Freakish or inevitable? Analysis from medical marketing, bioethics, and feminist theory. *Feminism & Psychology, 18*(4), 466–479.

Tiggeman, M., & Slater, A. (2013). Netgirls: The internet, Facebook, and body image concern in adolescent girls. *International Journal of Eating Disorders, 45*(6), 630–633.

Vandenbosch, L., & Eggermonth, E. (2012). Understanding sexual objectification: A comprehensive approach toward media exposure and girls' internalisation of beauty ideals, self-objectification, and body surveillance. *Journal of Communication, 62*(5), 869–887.

Wen, N., Chia, S. C., & Xiaomin, H. (2017). Does gender matter? Testing the influence of presumed media influence on young people's attitudes towards cosmetic surgery. *Sex Roles, 76*(7–8), 436–447.

Wolf, N. (1991). *The beauty myth: How images of beauty are used against women.* London: Vintage.

Won Kim, J., & Chock, T. M. (2015). Body image 2.0: Associations between social grooming on Facebook and body image concerns. *Computers in Human Behaviour, 48*, 331–339.

Zwier, S. (2014). "What motivates her": Motivations for considering labial reduction surgery as recounted on women's online communities and surgeons' websites. *Sexual Medicine, 2*(1), 16–23.

Thula U. Koops is a Psychologist with a clinical and academic background. Taking a general interest in women's sexualities, her research focusses on women's sexual problems, particularly with regard to sexual pain. Her aim is to further knowledge on women's experiences of sexual problems and the conditions giving rise to them, adopting both individual and societal perspectives. Other ambitions are the reflection on implications for sex therapy and diagnostics on the role of the body and the application of qualitative research methods. Looking into the expression of sexuality in a changing society, she has also published on sexual activities in the online sphere. After graduating from the University of Hamburg in 2013 with a Master's Degree in Psychology, she started her training in Psychodynamic Psychotherapy. She joined the Institute for Sex Research and Forensic Psychiatry at the University Medical Center Hamburg-Eppendorf a year later to work both clinically and in a research capacity. Since then, she has published in internationally peer-reviewed journals, given conference presentations and talks, as well as having taught sexuality-related classes to medical students. Her engagement reaches beyond the scope of her academic career: As secretary-treasurer of the German Society for Social-Scientific Sexuality Research, she has published statements relevant to the current public debate, for example, on the abortion law in Germany.

Catherine Wilkinson is a Senior Lecturer in Education based at the School of Education at Liverpool John Moores University. Catherine has a creative interdisciplinary background with a BA (Hons) in Fashion Brand Management, an MSc in Marketing Management, and a PhD in Environmental Sciences. She has a recognised research achievement in researching 'with' children, young people and their families via creative and/or participatory approaches, including mixed-methods, ethnographic and field-based qualitative research. Catherine completed her PhD in Environmental Sciences at the University of Liverpool, funded by an ESRC CASE award. Undertaking 18 months of ethnographic research, Catherine adopted a participatory mixed-methods approach to explore the ways in which young people use community radio as a platform to find and realise their voices, build stocks of social capital and create their own communities and senses of self. Catherine previously explored the portrayal of mothering a child with complex healthcare needs, considering the competing identities of mother, nurse, carer and advocate that these mothers fulfil as part of their daily regimes in 'being mum'. This paper was presented at the American Association of Geographers annual meeting, New Orleans, 2018, where Catherine was awarded funding from the AAG Enrichment Fund for her attendance as a 'distinguished non-geographer'. Though researching on diverse topics including youth voice, disfigurement and eyebrows, Catherine's research is united under the theme of identity. Catherine is committed to culturally credible means of disseminating research, including the creation of audio artefacts, poetry, comic strips and YouTube videos.

Grace Perry is a Qualitative Research Analyst at the Division of Epidemiology at the University of Utah. Grace graduated *magna cum laude* from Colorado College with a degree in Sociology and an emphasis on community-based, participatory action research. As a member of the LGBTQIA+ community, Grace has been especially interested in pursuing research surrounding (trans)gender equity and queer justice. During her senior year of college, Grace completed an award-winning thesis exploring the daily, lived experiences of trans and gender nonconforming students on her campus, which resulted in several trans-affirming policy changes at her undergraduate institution. Furthermore, over the summer of 2018, Grace completed her journalism capstone unpacking intersex 'corrective' surgeries and their harmful physiological and psychological repercussions. In her current position at the University of Utah, Grace works on a variety of qualitative research projects, from the ones seeking to understand the impact of childhood traumas—including physical and mental abuse—to the ones evaluating current opioid addiction programmes. As a researcher, Grace is committed to ethical and agentic practices which centre on and foreground members of marginalised communities and engender positive social change, whilst facilitating the unpacking of dominant discourses.

Samantha Wilkinson is a Senior Lecturer in Childhood and Youth Studies at Manchester Metropolitan University. Prior to this, she was a Lecturer in Human Geography at the same institution. She holds a BA (Hons) in Human Geography, an MSc in Environmental Governance and a PhD in Human Geography, all obtained from the University of Manchester. Samantha's PhD was funded by the ESRC CASE award and Alcohol Research UK and explored atmospheres of drinking, alcohol-related im-/mobilities, the role of friendship and care in drinking practices and intergenerational drinking experiences. Samantha currently works on a number of interdisciplinary, multi-institution, research projects. Her diverse research interests include young people and identity, hair, home care for people with dementia, Airbnb, animal geographies, and alcohol consumption practices and experiences. Samantha is also interested in utilising innovative qualitative methods when researching 'with' participants, including drawing-elicitation interviews, mobile phone methods, team ethnography, diaries and video methodologies. Samantha has published extensively around these diverse themes in a number of high-impact, peer-reviewed, journal articles and has presented her research at a number of international conferences.

Sergio A. Silverio is an academic Psychologist whose work can be best described as falling within the field of 'Medical Psychology', that is, the application of psychological knowledge to both health and healthcare services. His work in this area aims to understand both personal experiences of psychopathology and health system policy and practice regarding public health priorities. Specifically, the main focus of Sergio's work has been women's mental health and psychological wellbeing over the lifecourse and through key life transitions (i.e. pregnancy, birth, ageing and widowhood). His early work which explored older never married women's gender identity and social networks attracted critical acclaim from The British Psychological Society. Later work, using hospital ethnography to explore anxiety relating to early pregnancy and antenatal clinic visits, received international acclaim from The Society for Reproductive and Infant Psychology. Methodologically, Sergio specialises in qualitative methods and analysis, and he has a particular expertise in conducting in-depth interviews on sensitive topics. This has led to the development of a theoretical interest into the ethics of qualitative inquiry. Sergio's work involves—at one end—embracing critical psychology perspectives to contribute new theoretical bases for research and—at the other—adopting formal evaluative frameworks to influence, adapt, and transform policy. He is currently employed at the Department of Women & Children's Health, King's College London, and holds Honorary Fellowships at the Elizabeth Garrett Anderson Institute for Women's Health, University College London, and the Department of Psychological Sciences, University of Liverpool. He is an Associate Fellow of The British Psychological Society, a Life Fellow of The Royal Anthropological Institute, and a Fellow of the Royal Society for Public Health.

Chapter 12
"In the depths of winter, I finally learned that within me there lay an invincible summer". Life Crises, Shame Experience and Coping with the Support of Digital Media

Elisabeth Vanderheiden

It's a long way to come to own your ego (Es ist ein weiter Weg, bis man sich in den Besitz des eigenen Ichs gebracht hat.).

Roger Willemsen (translated by the author)

1 Introduction

This chapter aims to improve the understanding of the connection between life crises and shame experiences and to gain new insights into the relevance of digital media in coping with life crises. This chapter presents the results of a recent ongoing international online survey with 39 participants. The goal of this chapter is to investigate how the interviewees describe a life crisis, what special connections exist for them between a life crisis and shame on the one hand and on the other hand to describe whether and what significance digital media have in coping with these life crises. Diverse cultural backgrounds and perspectives are taken into account as well as gender differences between participants. The chapter contributes to the existing literature on life crises in cultural and transcultural contexts by asking people from different cultural backgrounds to provide answers to different questions, for instance: "What event in your biography can you remember that you perceived as a life crisis?", "What exactly was this crisis?", "What was the meaning of shame in the context of this crisis?", "What meaning did digital resources have for you in this context?" and "What digital resources were they and for what reasons were they

Albert Camus as translated in *Lyrical and Critical Essays* (1968), p. 169; also in *The Unquiet Vision : Mirrors of Man in Existentialism* (1969) by Nathan A. Scott, p. 116

E. Vanderheiden (✉)
Global Institute for Transcultural Research, Römerberg, Germany
e-mail: ev@keb-rheinland-pfalz.de

C.-H. Mayer et al. (eds.), *Shame 4.0*, https://doi.org/10.1007/978-3-030-59527-2_12

important?" By examining the answers to these questions, the chapter offers in-depth insights into the life crises of selected individuals with different cultural backgrounds, their experiences with shame in this context and their coping strategies using digital sources.

2 Life Crises

Life crises mark individual turning points and upheavals and describe phases of standstill as well as explosive changes. Life crises are events that usually lead to serious changes in the life situation of an individual and have an uncertain outcome. As a rule, they interrupt habitual courses of action and usually force reflection and changes in previous behaviour patterns (Hoffmann & Hofmann, 2017). They are often experienced as a traumatic stress event, as an acute and sudden clash of one's own convictions with reality (Tavrovetska, 2020). Often the events that trigger a life crisis lie outside the normal horizon of expectations and experiences and beyond everyday realities. They are usually accompanied by strong emotions (Filipp & Aymanns, 2018, p. 31) and can lead to excessive demands (Hofer-Moser, Hintenberger, Schwarzmann, Dominicis & Brunner, 2020). They are often described as adjustment disorders, in which people are confronted with a situation that requires reorientation and positioning because living conditions have changed fundamentally or no longer prove to be functional (Hoffmann & Hofmann, 2017, p. 15). Similarly, Hofer-Moser and his colleagues (Hofer-Moser et al., 2020) describe crises as "instabilities of a system" that are not compensated for by existing resources and coping strategies and can therefore lead to a "threat to the continued existence of the system" (Hofer-Moser et al., 2020, p. 13). This can be accompanied by far-reaching upheavals of the world view and self-image and lead to final alienation phenomena. Life crises can lead not only to impairments of physical and psychological integrity (Filipp & Aymanns, 2018, p. 38) but also to concrete losses of resources at other levels, such as income, jobs or restrictions at the level of the social network.

In the literature, **critical life events** and **life crises** are not strictly distinguished from each other and are used synonymously (Vanderheiden, 2020a). Critical life events are defined by the fact that they are perceived as stressful. Stressors can arise not only, for example, from novelty, intensity, difficulty level, time pressure, work overload or underload, but also from the fact that they are events that upset people (Filipp & Aymanns, 2018, p. 57), cause their self-image to falter and limit their scope to take goal-orientated action (Filipp & Aymanns, 2018, p. 64). Wettstein (Gesundheitsförderung Schweiz, 2016, p. 22) recommends making a distinction between normative and non-normative critical life events, whereby normative events are understood to be those which, in a particular cultural group, are closely tied to an age group or a foreseeable period of life. They are socially desirable and to a certain extent predictable (marriage, leaving home, starting a family of one's own), while non-normative critical life events are mostly undesirable and usually hit people unprepared. In principle, they can occur throughout life, for instance, as an accident, serious illness, winning the lottery, resignation, death of a relative, war or an escape experience. Whether they are normative or non-normative, critical life events are experienced as "tense" and in many cases irrespective of whether they are events that at first glance appear "positive" (e.g. marriage) or "negative" (e.g. loss of job) and change one's life (Filipp & Aymanns, 2018). Nevertheless, such events differ greatly in their affective quality. The consequences they have, and how well and by what means they can be managed, depend to a large extent on the level of affect involved. Events that are undesirable, such as the loss of a partner or a serious material loss, lead far more often to personal crises than those that occur in the "normal" course of life, such as moving house or changing jobs.

Dealing with critical life events in crisis can lead to a crisis if attempts to reorganise the person-environment adaptation do not seem to succeed and options for action and problem-solving skills are perceived as increasingly limited (Filipp & Aymanns, 2018, p. 28). Filipp and Aymanns (2018, pp. 43–44) point out that from a developmental psychological perspective, life crises can be interpreted in three different ways: They serve to describe developmental and life courses, they represent a marker in the reconstruction of one's own biography and they serve to explain why certain changes in one's own life occurred.

Filipp and Aymanns (2018, p. 28) stress that the confrontation with a critical life event can potentially lead to a life crisis if all attempts to reorganise one's environmental adaptation seem to fail and even the negative effects occurring cannot be regulated.

2.1 *Life Crises and Gender*

Clear gender differences can be observed in the perception and handling of life crises. Filipp and Aymanns (2018), for example, point to gender differences in relation to life crises in terms of **autobiographical memory** (2018, p. 385). They refer to the fact that women can generate more autobiographical memories of their childhood than men and can also recall them more quickly. They are able to date them more precisely and include them more often in conversations with others. Events remembered by women relate significantly more often to emotionally significant events, especially in interpersonal contexts. This is confirmed by Riecher-Rössler (2016) who also emphasises that women generally differ from men with regard to their emotional expression, as they are more willing to talk about their emotions, articulate themselves more intensively and are more likely to recall emotional situations (Riecher-Rössler, 2016, p. 29).

Women and men differ in **what they perceive as a life crisis**. For example, Kendler, Thornton and Prescott (2001) point out that women report more about interpersonal relationships (housing problems, loss of trust, crises and problems, conflicts with people in their network and illnesses of people in their own network), whereas men refer more to legal and work-related stressful life events (job loss, legal problems, involvement in a robbery and problems at work) when it comes to naming stressful life events. A large study by Pilar Matud (2004) with 2000 men and women participants confirmed strong gender differences in perceiving life crises. She found that although there was no difference in the number of life events identified over the previous 2 years, these life events were rated more negatively by women and were considered less controllable by them than by men. Women more frequently named family and health-related events, while men highlighted relationship, financial and work-related events. The author further emphasises that women achieved significantly better results than men in emotional coping styles and avoidance coping, but men scored better in rational and distanced coping. The results of this study also showed that women suffer more stress than men and that their coping style is more emotionally focused than that of men. In a meta-analysis of studies exploring the gender-specific risks of potentially traumatic events and post-traumatic stress disorder, Tolin and Foa (2006) were able to show that the real risks of certain crisis-triggering events also differ for men and women. These authors found that women were more likely than men to experience sexual assault and child sexual abuse but less likely to experience accidents, nonsexual assault, death or injury, disaster or fire and combat or war.

Men and women also differ in their **coping behaviour** (Filipp & Aymanns, 2018, p. 251 and 360). Women are more likely to turn to other people in particularly stressful situations—Taylor et al. (2000) refer to the tending and befriending patterns of women—while men appear to prefer fight or flight patterns. In crisis situations, women also rely less exclusively on their partner and more on their social networks. This also seems to be evident across several cultures (Filipp & Aymanns, 2018, p. 237). It appears that women are more heavily burdened by the illness of a partner than vice versa (Filipp & Aymanns, 2018, p. 250). In a study of parents whose child had died, Wijngaards-de Meij et al. (2008) found that the mourning behaviour of men was positively influenced when the women were more forward-looking again and that this had a positive effect on the men's depression. The coping behaviour of women, however, was not positively influenced in the opposite case.

Another very relevant difference seems to be that women are more inclined to **rumination**, to think about a crisis repeatedly or to lose themselves in endless loops of thought (Johnson & Whisman, 2013). Studies also identify rumination as a particular vulnerability factor, as it can lead to a spiral of negative thinking, depression and inability to act or problem-solve but can also trigger social isolation, as rumination may lead to a loss of social attention and support (Filipp & Aymanns, 2018, p. 178; Johnson & Whisman, 2013; Jose & Brown, 2007; Krause et al., 2017).

3 Life Crises and Shame

Life crises are often associated with shame. As traumatic events, they can be caused by shameful experiences (The Finnish Association for Mental Health 2018). However, shame can also be a concomitant or consequence of a life crisis (Hilgers, 2019; Mayer, Vanderheiden & Oosthuizen, 2019, pp. 8–13). It can be a reaction to the experienced loss of control or orientation or violation of boundaries (Lammers, 2016), an expression of embarrassment or loss of face (Hilgers, 2019) or frustration at not having lived up to one's own expectations and values or social norms.

Increasingly, shame is also perceived as a resource in research (Briegleb, 2014; Mayer & Vanderheiden, 2019; Vanderheiden & Mayer, 2017; Wong, 2011, 2019; Wurmser, 2010, 2015) and can therefore also provide new perspectives for discussion in connection with coping with life crises.

3.1 Shame and Gender

Shame can be regarded as a "gender-responsive" phenomenon (Hernandez & Mendoza, 2011). Tangney and Dearing found that, regardless of age, females "consistently report greater levels of shame than their male counterparts" (Tangney & Dearing, 2002, p. 154; see also Brown, 2008, 2012). Riecher-Rössler (2003) confirms that women were more often and more intensively ashamed, especially with regard to their bodies, their performance and their social competence. According to Benetti-McQuoid and Bursik (2005), although women report a greater propensity for guilt and shame, men report more characteristics of guilt. Both men and women with traditionally female gender roles are more prone to guilt and shame, while a traditionally male self-concept is associated with less shame among women.

Miller-Prieve (2016) was able to prove that shame occurs significantly more often in women than in men. She attributes this to social and cultural norms that are imposed on women and that cause negative self-assessments in women if these norms are not observed. Similar conclusions are also made by Velotti, Garofalo, Bottazzi and Caretti (2016), who found in a study ($n = 380$; 66.1% women) that women reported higher degrees of shame (especially physical and behavioural shame) than men. Men in the study had higher levels of self-esteem, emotional repression and physical aggression. They found shame was associated with low self-esteem, hostility and psychological stress in a consistent manner across all genders. Associations between character shame and emotional repression, and between physical shame and anger, were found only in women. In addition, character shame and physical shame contributed to the prediction of low self-esteem, hostility and psychological distress beyond the influence of character shame. Finally, emotional suppression in women mediated the influence of character shame on hostility and psychological distress.

In their study, Ludwig, Fellner-Röhling and Thoma (2017) investigated the analytical connection between self-assessment and observability depending on gender. They found that women downgraded their self-assessment based on observability, while men did not. Women avoid the shame they might feel when others observe that they have overestimated themselves. However, men do not seem to be similarly shameful. This gender difference may be the result of different societal expectations: The authors suspect that men are expected to be overconfident, whereas this is not the case for women. Ludwig et al. (2017) conclude that this contempt for shame leads, for example, to women shying away from competition, demanding jobs and wage negotiations, because entering these situations requires confidence in one's own abilities.

A recent study by Nyström, Kjellberg, Heimdahl and Jonsson (2018) comes to quite different conclusions. These authors investigated gender differences in interpersonal sensitivity and internalised public coping strategies in 252 students and found that women show a higher degree of interpersonal sensitivity than men and that they use internalised public coping strategies to a higher degree. The results also showed that interpersonal sensitivity is strongly correlated with shame management strategies. However, in contrast to previous studies, no gender difference was found, and gender did not significantly cause a correlation between interpersonal sensitivity and internalised public coping strategies.

3.2 Shame and Culture

Shame is universal (Harper, 2011, p. 1); it is a social emotion (Casimir & Schnegg, 2002) which is culture-specific in terms of its perception, experience and expression (Brown, 2008, 2012; Lindisfarne, 1998; Miller, 1996). It is strongly connected to the cultural space a person is socialised and living in and to the contextual influences of religion and the Zeitgeist (Greiner, 2014, p. 19). However, questions of power are also very important, as Archana Krishnamurthy confirmed in her studies with Indian women when she examined the functioning of shame in connection with gender norms in a post-colonial context. "The body vocabulary of shame ... is an expression of condensed experience of power relations" (Krishnamurthy, 2018, p. 181).

Among others, Bhawuk (2017) and Saraswati (2018) have pointed out that the cultural concept of shame differs widely. Some understandings of shame, such as lajja in Hindi/Sanskrit (Bhawuk, 2017, 2019) or malu in Indonesia (Cucuani, Sulastiana, Harding & Agustiani, 2021; Saraswati, 2018), are much more positive than in the Western context, which are often negatively connotated.

4 Life Crises and Digital Resources

With regard to the relevance of digital services for coping with life crises, research is only just beginning but has been gaining importance since the turn of the millennium and relates primarily to online and e-therapies, coaching or counselling (see Amichai-Hamburger, Klomek, Friedman, Zuckerman & Shani-Sherman, 2020; Cook & Doyle, 2002; Recupero & Rainey, 2006). Increasingly, social media are also establishing themselves as a field of research in terms of coping with crises (see Rasmussen & Ihlen, 2017). At the same time, digital resources based on artificial intelligence or on integration with the management of crises are gaining relevance (e.g. Crisis Text Line, 2020; Pestian, Nasrallah, Matykiewicz, Bennett & Leenaars,

2010) as well as digital wearables (e. g. smart watches, glasses, smart applications invisibly attached in clothing or implanted in the body) (Landesanstalt für Medien Nordrhein-Westfalen, 2020) especially in the diagnosis of emotional and mental states in connection with crises and well-being (Chan, Estève, Fourniols, Escriba & Campo, 2020; Marzano et al., 2015; Olff, 2015).

For the participants in the present study, it is communication and interaction offerings provided by social media that are of particular relevance to them. In line with the findings of other studies, for example, Naslund, Aschbrenner, Marsch and Bartels (2016) found that even people with severe mental illness increasingly turn to popular social media, including Facebook, Twitter or YouTube, to share their experiences of illness or seek advice from others with similar health problems. Naslund et al. (2016) found that people with mental illness benefit from this peer-to-peer support, for example, through greater social connection, a sense of belonging to a group and the sharing of personal stories and strategies for coping with the everyday challenges of living with mental illness. They also gain access to interventions for mental and physical well-being offered through social media and experienced mutual support. At the same time, these authors point out the unforeseen risks posed by misleading information, exposure to hostile or derogatory comments from others or the increase in uncertainty about one's own health status. Overall, however, the authors come to the conclusion that peer-to-peer benefits outweigh the potential risks that can undoubtedly be associated with social media.

The significance of social media in shaping social relationships has been sufficiently proven, even if the media are discussed ambivalently in this context. Some researchers such as Bevan, Gomez and Sparks (2014); Neumann-Braun and Autenrieth (2011); and Kadler-Neuhausen (2020) emphasise contradictory or negative effects of social media, while others such as Orben, Dienlin and Przybylski (2019); Tang (2010, 2012); Sinus Institut (2018); or Vanderheiden (2020b) emphasise the media's opportunities and chances. Digital media also play an increasingly important role in shaping intimate or romantic relationships (Ben-Ze'ev, 2020; Fahr & Graf, 2012; Kirchner, 2014; Linke, 2010; Utz & Beukeboom, 2011; Vanderheiden, 2020c, 2020d).

Increased global migration movements have brought the relevance of social media in the context of migration and flight increasingly into the focus of research interests. For example, in a study with a representative survey of 404 refugees in Germany—mainly from Syria, Iraq, Afghanistan, Pakistan and Iran—on media use behaviour of refugees before, during and after flight, Emmer, Richter and Kunst (2016) found that for respondents, communication was the most important function of the Internet. The study also confirmed the major importance of interpersonal communication for refugees. Information conveyed via interpersonal communication enjoyed the greatest trust among all those questioned in the study, whereas information from television and the Internet other than personal contact was relatively untrusted.

Several other studies—such as that of Komito (2011) in the context of 65 Polish and Filipino migrants in Ireland—show that the use of social media particularly supports the binding of capital and transnational communities in a hitherto unknown way. Wei and Gao (2017) demonstrated that the use of social media can contribute to the social integration of migrants, including the building of social identity, social networks and real social participation. Dekker and Engbersen (2014) were able to demonstrate that social media not only represent new communication channels in migration networks but also that they actively change the nature of these networks and thereby facilitate migration in a sustainable way. In this way, digital resources contribute to facilitating migration in four ways. First, they improve the opportunities to maintain strong ties with family and friends; second, they address weak ties that are relevant for the organisation of the migration and integration process. Third, they can help build a new infrastructure, and finally they provide a rich source of inside knowledge about migration that is discreet and unofficial.

5 Research Methodology

The present study, the results of which are presented in this chapter, focuses on qualitative research as defined by Yin (2009). The study is based on a retrospective autobiographical research approach, in which adults were interviewed about a past life crisis. By definition, a crisis is an episode, referring to a defined temporal period in someone's life with a beginning and an end. Episodes can only be described in retrospect as part of a life story (McAdams, 1993). This has the advantage of a retrospective approach, allowing a distinction to be made between life before and life after the crisis. The contributions of the participants are evaluated with regard to shame occupation and digital media and are analysed and interpreted according to common patterns of interpretation (Creswell, 2013; Hussy, Schreier & Echterhoff, 2010).

5.1 Data Collection, Analysis and Reporting

This chapter is based on the results of an ongoing study that the author is currently conducting on the subject of life crises. In an online questionnaire (English or German) which is available on the Internet (Vanderheiden, 2019a, 2020a), participants are asked to define what they understand by a life crisis, how they evaluate it and which coping strategies they have experienced as successful.

The first 15 questions of the questionnaire refer to biographical data. The remaining 23 questions ask what the person affected understands by the term "life crisis", what their life crisis consists of, what metaphor they have associated it with, what factors they experienced as conducive or obstructive to overcoming the crisis, what consequences this crisis had for them, what aspects were relevant to them in overcoming the crisis (e.g. faith, love, pride, humour, educational opportunities, digital resources) and what further comments they wish to add. This is based on a biographical approach, which starts with life crisis events, their evaluation and how they are dealt with in the lives of the interviewees. It is assumed that these events "have become engraved in the autobiographical memory of those affected" (Filipp & Aymanns, 2018, p. 36) and are still relevant for those affected decades later.

With 39 questionnaire replies received so far, only a relatively narrow database is currently available, so that generalisability or representativeness is not assured. According to Mayring (2010, p. 23; 2016), however, this survey could serve as a pilot study for further research.

Gräf (2010) emphasises the increasing relative importance of online survey forms (Gräf, 2010, p. 10), with regard to respondents, who have the advantage of controlling the time they spend answering and enjoying the process. The survey carried out is a self-recruited survey (Gräf, 2010, p. 16), which is characterised, above all, by the fact that anyone who becomes aware of this survey can take part. Participants were initially recruited by personal contact in personal and professional networks and according to the snowball sampling. In addition, a homepage was developed and made available (Vanderheiden, 2019a), and the survey was advertised via LinkedIn. In the meantime, the snowball sampling method has become an important resource, especially for online surveys in the context of existing network structures, as explained by Jackob, Schoen and Zerback (2009) and Gräf (2010, p. 81). This has proven to be a successful recruitment strategy with greater chances of success than anonymous contact attempts. This is because the trust built up from personal contact in social networks and the reciprocal relationships that exist there represent a reliable resource for empirical data collection (Jackob et al., 2009, p. 189). A particular advantage of the online survey is that it ensures no direct contact between the interviewer and interviewee. This can be advantageous for a topic such as shame, which is perceived by many people as very intimate, because people may find it easier to address or elaborate on certain potentially shameful topics, e.g. in the context of sexuality.

5.2 *Sample*

Participants were found based on a purposeful sampling (Naderifar, Goli & Ghaljaie, 2017). At the time of writing this chapter, 39 people have answered the questionnaire (30 persons in German, 9 in English). Because the study is ongoing, no final research findings are presented yet, but sample case studies are featured.

The to date age range of participants varied from 11 to 82 years, with 28 female and 11 male participants. The participants come from or live in Germany, South Africa, Iran, Vietnam, India, Mexico, Lebanon, Turkey, Afghanistan, Australia, the USA and Canada. Fifteen participants were married, three were in homosexual marriages and one person was living in a partnership but not married. Further six participants were single, two were married but separated, five were widowed, five divorced and one person gave no relationship status information. Twenty-five participants live in more urban areas, while 14 live in more rural areas. Twenty-four persons have a university degree, ten have completed vocational training, three persons have a school-leaving qualification but not yet completed vocational training or studies and two individuals have not yet completed school (Vanderheiden, 2019a).

In total, 4 persons described themselves as Christians, 20 as Roman Catholics, 1 as catholic and worshipping Maria, 8 as Lutherans, 2 as Muslims and 1 each as agnostic, spiritual and without religious affiliation.

As far as educational background is concerned, the participants had 17 high school certificates plus 1 ongoing, 1 was doing Grade 10 IGCSE, 4 had secondary school certificates, 2 doctoral degrees, 8 masters degrees and 2 diploma degrees, 1 habilitation (postdoctoral), 1 magister artium and 2 bachelor's degrees. The sample also included three managers in leading positions, two professors, two lawyers/judges, two project managers, four office managers/bank clerks, three students, two teachers, two therapist/psychiatrist, two entrepreneurs, two gardeners/construction workers, one engineer, one accountant, one social workers, one educator and one ministerial officer, one retired salesperson, one retired tailor, a volunteer, one retiree, one organisational consultant and one artist.

Table 12.1 provides an overview of the biographical details of the participants.

5.3 Limitations

This study also has limitations. It is not representative because it is a self-recruited survey of the respondents and anyone who had knowledge of the survey could participate. Very open questions were deliberately asked, and no definitions were given, for example, with regard to what is individually understood by life crisis, what definition of shame the study is based on and what is meant by digital sources. This decision was made deliberately in order to allow the greatest possible diversity and freedom of response, also with regard to individual, gender and cultural differences. On the other hand, it must be accepted that answers can sometimes be less clear and specific than in more formalised survey procedures. The interviewees were also unaware of the questions themselves and their consequences, i.e. they did not know that they would be asked about aspects such as shame or digital media in the course of the survey in view of their life crisis. They could therefore not select their reported crisis specifically against this background.

6 Findings of the Study

As explained in the methodology section, the study examined the role of shame in the context of a life crisis. The relevance of digital media in coping with this crisis was also investigated. A total of 39 people took part in the studies (ongoing). In the following sections, the focus will be on what was experienced by the interviewees as a life crisis, what reference was made to shame, what special significance digital

Table 12.1 Biographical data of participants (author's own construction)

Code	Sex	Age	Nationality	Religion	Family status	Educa Education	Profession
P 1	F	60	German	Catholic	Divorced	Master	Judge
P 2	F	55	German	Catholic	Married	Master	Therapist
P 3	F	43	German	Lutheran	Married	Master	Project manager
P 4	F	55	German	Catholic	Married	High school certificate	Office employee
P 5	F	20	German	Agnostic	Single	High school certificate	Volunteer in an adult education organisation
P 6	F	82	German	Catholic	Widowed		Retired tailor
P 7	F	50	German	Lutheran	Married	Diploma	Office employee
P 8	F	41	German	Catholic	Married in a gay marriage	Master	Teacher
P 9	F	57	German	Catholic—worships Maria	Married in a gay marriage	Bachelor	Accountant
P 10	F	70	German	Catholic	Married	Master	Retiree
P 11	M	45	German	Catholic	Single	Secondary school certificate	Gardener
P 12	M	57	Luxembourgers	Catholic	Married but separated	High school certificate	Engineer/entrepreneur
P 13	M	37	Italian	Lutheran	Single	High school certificate	Social worker
P 14	F	58	German	Lutheran	Widowed	Diploma	Freelance organisational consultant
P 15	F	45	German	Catholic	Married	High school certificate	Self-employed
P 16	M	41	German	Lutheran	Divorced	High school certificate	Executive manager
P 17	M	63	German	Lutheran	Widowed	Master	Retired organisational consultant
P 18	M	64	German	Catholic	Married	Magister artium	Project manager
P 19	F	52	Dutch	Catholic	Married	Secondary school certificate	Retired sales person
P 20	F	55	German	Catholic	Married	Doctorate	Professor
P 21	F	43	German	Lutheran	Married	Bachelor	Ministerial officer

(continued)

Table 12.1 (continued)

Code	Sex	Age	Nationality	Religion	Family status	Educa Education	Profession
P 22	F	50	German	Catholic	Divorced	High school certificate	Retired bank clerk
P 23	F	56	German	Catholic	Single	Doctorate	Leading manager
P 24	F	48	German	None	Married	Master	Manager
P 25	F	53	German	Catholic	Married	Master	Lawyer
P 26	F	71	German	Catholic	Married	High school certificate	Retired physiotherapist
P 27	F	55	German	Catholic	Single	High school certificate	Teacher
P 28	F	38	German	Lutheran	Single	High school certificate	Bank clerk
P 29	M	23	German	Catholic	In a relationship	Secondary school certificate	Construction worker
P 30	F	38	German	Catholic	Widowed	High school certificate	Educator
P 31	F	43	German	Catholic	Married but separated	Habilitation	Professor
P 32	F	18	German	Christian	Single	Grade 10 IGCSE	Student
P 33	M	11	South African	Christian	Single	High school (ongoing)	Student
P 34	F	47	Iranian	Muslim	Widowed	High school certificate	Professor
P 35	M	43	Mexican	Christian	Married but separated	High school certificate	Self-employed
P 36	F	60	Lebanese	Christian	Divorced	High school certificate	Psychiatrist
P 37	M	50	Turkish	Muslim	Married in a gay marriage	High school certificate	Engineer
P 38	F	70	German	Spiritual	Divorced	High school certificate	Artist
P 39	M	19	Afghan	Muslim	Single	Secondary school certificate	Student

resources had in this context and which of the resources were actually involved. These findings are presented in detail.

6.1 *Character of the Crisis Experienced*

The questions were deliberately formulated very openly so that participants had as much freedom as possible in answering the questions. First, they were asked which event they can remember in their biography that they perceived as a life crisis. The power to define what was perceived as a life crisis was left entirely to the participants. In a subsequent question, the participants were asked to describe the crisis in more detail. Another follow-up question raised their thoughts and feelings in this situation. Most participants named several life crises. Table 12.2 provides an overview of participants' responses.

As Filipp and Aymanns (2018, p. 81) emphasise, the naming shows that critical life events are either perceived as externally acting burdens or as results of the subjective evaluation of a particular event or chain of events. Life crises are temporary situations in which people become aware—usually unexpectedly and

Table 12.2 Character of the crisis experienced (author's own construction)

Life crisis	Number of total nominations	Nominations by female participants	Nominations by male participants
Death	12 (9♀, 4♂)	P1, P2, P4, P8, P33, P10, P14, P23, P24	P11, P17, P38
Disease (own or in social environment)	10 (7♀, 3♂)	P8, P10, P14, P19, P20, P22, P25	P16, P32, P34
Relationship topics (divorce or separation)	8 (4♀, 4♂)	P1, P14, P37, P28	P11, P17, P18, P36
Loneliness	8 (7♀, 3♂)	P1, P2, P4, P23, P24, P37, P28	P1
Family issues	7 (7♀, 3♂)	P3, P10	P12, P32, P34, P36, P38
Migration topics	6 (2♀, 4♂)	P21, P23	P34, P36, P38, P39
Educational topics	6 (4♀, 2♂)	P3, P7, P15, P26	P38, P29
Unfulfilled life dreams	6 (5♀, 1♂)	P15, P19, P33, P37, P21	P11
Questions of identity	5 (4♀, 31♂)	P15, P25, P27, P28	P13
Sexual topics	3 (2♀, 1♂)	P35, P27	P13
Mobbing, bullying	3 (3♀, 0♂)	P3, P5, P31	
Depression	3 (2♀, 1♂)	P5, P37	P32
Workplace-related problems	2 (2♀, 0♂)	P3, P30	
Addiction issues	2 (1♀, 1♂)	P6	P11
Financial topics	2 (1♀, 1♂)	P6	P11
Loss of meaning in life	2 (2♀, 0♂)	P1, P2	

abruptly—that the structure of the relationship between them and their environment is falling apart, but cannot be restored by a simple corrective intervention.

The majority of respondents describe loss crises such as death (12: 9♀, 4♂) and disease (10: 7♀, 3♂), connected to relationship topics (8: 4♀, 4♂), loneliness (8: 7♀, 3♂) or migration topics (6: 2♀, 4♂), workplace-related problems (2: 2♀, 0♂) and loss of meaning in life (2: 2♀, 0♂). Hofer-Moser et al. (2020) recommend drawing distinctions between archetypal loss crises such as death and the other loss crises in the context of separation, migration, job loss, health integrity and, as a third category of loss crises, the loss of values. This would apply to the study participants with regard to educational topics (6: 4♀, 2♂), unfulfilled life dreams (6: 5♀, 1♂) and loss of meaning in life (2: 2♀, 0♂).

6.1.1 Life Crises as Descriptions of Breaks in Development and Life Courses

Many participants describe the life crisis as a milestone, break or turning point in their lives. An example is P12, a 57-year-old male Belgian freelance engineer who talks about his life crisis, triggered by the 24-hour disappearance of his then 13-year-old son:

> My son happened to overhear a telephone conversation I had been having with my (current) partner, who was my lover at the time, while I was still maintaining the supposedly harmonious family life with my wife. I thought he was at school, but he was sick in bed and had heard the conversation and then ran away from home. There had been suicides and attempted suicides in his school and the criminal investigation department found a suicide note on his computer. He was picked up in the early hours of the morning several hundred kilometres away and brought home, but I thought all the time, I'll never see him again.

After his son was found again, he decided to talk to his wife and to separate from her and confess to his partner. For him, the life crisis thus becomes the decisive turning point in his life, which he actively uses to give his life a direction that is less orientated to social norms and more towards his own needs and desires.

Another example is P29, who is 23 years old, a German construction worker:

> I have had many crises, but when my daughter was born and I realised I have to change something. I have problems with reading and writing. my girlfriend helps me to write this and when my daughter was born I realised I have to change something. she should be proud of her daddy she is one and a half years old now and often she comes to me with her toys to play with her but with a book she always goes to her mother. as if she knew that I can't read. so I can already read the letters and our names and write other words too. but don't write texts. for my little one I'll do that now.

This is a common phenomenon in the description of life crises. In the retrospective description, the crises are perceived as events that have irrevocably changed the direction of one's life. Here, life crises become the object of (auto)biographical diagnosis (Jäger & Booth, 1984, p. 150), in the sense that they are perceived by those affected as a caesura or nodal point and biographical particularity.

6.1.2 Life Crises as Marker in the Reconstruction of One's Own Biography

On the other hand, life crises represent markers in the subjective reconstruction of one's own life. In this context, life and self-analysis are also significant, as are the activities that people proactively initiate to bring them about.

This is illustrated by P36, from Lebanon, now a US 60-year-old psychiatrist, when she explains:

> I have three daughters. Meanwhile they are grown up and I am grandmother. When my eldest daughter was 5 years old, I found out that my husband was sexually harassing her. My daughter told me what my husband did or tried to do to her. He touched her sexually when I wasn't in the house. At first I was totally shocked, I couldn't believe it. But then I became very fast active and brought the children to safety. I was in a panic, wondering how long it had been for, whether I had perhaps overlooked early signs that my child would have had to protect earlier. Then it quickly became unpleasant, because there were legal consequences, I moved out, my daughters no longer know him alone with him, the right of residence had to be arranged, maintenance issues clarified. I was still a student at the time, that was not easy. Nor was there such an open debate about sexualised violence, especially not and the family, which was still very taboo. At that time, children were warned not to go with strangers. I felt very guilty, too.

In terms of effective coping strategies, it seems helpful and useful for people not to feel at the mercy of coincidences, but to be able to understand, explain and handle what they experience (Antonovsky, 1979, 1987; Wilson & Gilbert, 2008). This may also explain why people in the context of life crisis narratives take responsibility for certain events, even though they are not directly responsible for a certain event in the narrower sense. However, this behaviour seems to contribute to regaining control over the situation (Filipp & Aymanns, 2018, pp. 197–198) and to experiencing oneself as self-effective again. Bandura (1997) has pointed out the importance of self-efficacy expectations in the sense of trust in one's own abilities and in one's own actions in order to achieve the desired goals. So this competence may possibly be considered a key competence in overcoming life crises.

6.1.3 Life Crises as an Explicative Concept

Life crises are often understood by those affected as an explicative concept in the sense that they are used as an explanation for changes in natural event variables that have almost fatefully steered the behaviour and feelings of those affected in one direction or another.

P6, 82 years old, a female German former tailor, now retired, describes it like this:

> Four years after I was married, a crisis began for me. I was 24 years old, had three children and realised that my husband was turning more and more to alcohol. I could no longer work outside the home because of the three children, sewing day and night for private individuals from home and making changes for clothing stores so that we had enough household income. That was in 1964, when the term single parent didn't exist, but actually I was. I stood alone with everything.

The life crisis is described here as a massive event of restriction and loss, both in terms of original life plans (for a harmonious partnership, shared responsibility for the children, life in material security) and in terms of very real loss of resources (the actual loss of the partner and loss of income from alcohol addiction). In this context, the question of blame of the other or self-blame as an explanatory pattern gains particular importance (Filipp & Aymanns, 2018, p. 197), because it is from this that the self-definition of those affected is derived and it opens or closes options for coping with and transforming the crisis. Equally crucial is the question of how to deal with loss—both at the value level and at the level of actual loss.

6.1.4 Relevance of Life Crises

The majority of participants (24 of 39 = 62%) rate the life crisis as very relevant to the question of meaning, with an extremely high proportion of women coming to this conclusion (16♀, 7♂). Another 18% of participants (7 of 39) conclude that the life crisis was not relevant to their understanding of the meaning of life, while 20% (8 of 39) state that it was somewhat relevant. The answers make it clear that some participants, although explicitly asked about the meaning, generally name the positive outcomes (benefits). Examples are that they have learnt something positive from the crisis, that unexpected new opportunities have arisen or that they have experienced love and solidarity coming from their social environment. This is also in line with the results of research. Filipp and Aymanns (2018) speak in this context of benefit-finding, i.e. the positive that was found in the events or the re-interpretation of the events in the sense of positive reappraisal or refining (Filipp & Aymanns, 2018, p. 201). In their view, this must be distinguished from the construction of meaning.

6.2 Relationship Between Life Crises and Shame

Life crises often trigger feelings of shame in those affected (Blawat & Ehrig, 2010; Hilgers, 2019; Marks, 2010, 2015; Worth, 2021). The close connection between life crises and feelings of shame is confirmed by the present study, as Table 12.3 and Fig. 12.1 convincingly show.

For the majority of participants, life crises are particularly shameful events: 21 participants perceive them as very shameful, 7 as somewhat shame-loaded and 6 participants see no connection between shame load and life crisis.

Of those who do not create a connection between their life crisis and shame, most are people who have lost their partner to cancer and death. Only one person indirectly mentions shame in this context—P14, who is a widow, 58 years old and an organisational consultant in Germany:

Table 12.3 Relevance of shame with regard to life crisis (author's own construction)

Relevance of shame re life crisis	Number of total nominations	Nominations by female participants	Nominations by male participants
Not relevant at all	6	P20, P22, P24	P17, P18, P33
Somewhat relevant	7	P7, P14, P25, P31, P34	P11, P12
Very relevant	21	P1, P3, P5, P6, P9, P10, P15, P19, P21, P23, P26, P27, P28, P30, P32; P36, P38	P13, P29, P35, P37
Totals	34	25	9

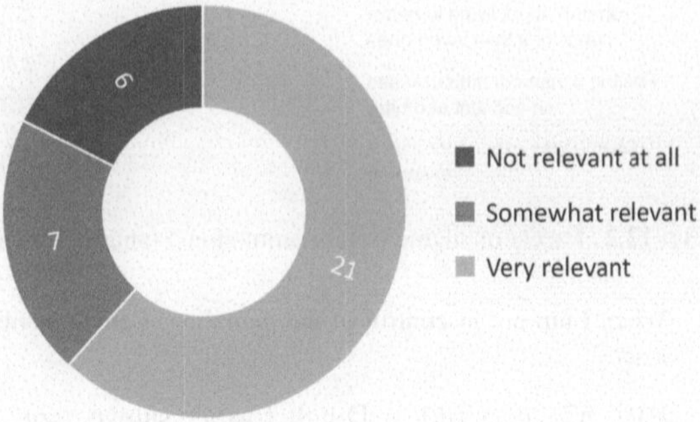

Fig. 12.1 Relevance of shame with regard to life crisis (author's own construction)

> I felt shame for my husband because it was about dependence and loss of control and privacy. On the other hand, the care was not filled with shame for me. Depending on the definition of shame, there were moments when I was impatient, sometimes because I was at the end of my tether or because his behaviour seemed temporarily very strange to me due to the [brain] tumours. Moments that I regret again and again until today, moments that I feel sorry for, even if everyone says that it is nonsense. But it's there and I can't change it anymore. I'm sorry for that. And I ask him to forgive me.

For most of the interviewees, however, shame—especially in its especially when unexamined—is a constant side effect of the life crisis.

P6, the 82-year-old German former tailor, now retired, states:

> I was often ashamed when he [my husband] came home and got drunk again. and everyone saw him, I wanted to hide there too. When he would stagger through the streets and whistle loudly at the front door so that I would press the door opener, that was really no pleasure.

P7, 50 years old, a female German business teacher, notes:

> I was ashamed to admit to myself that I had not found the right career path for me. I was also ashamed of not being very successful in my studies. I felt that studying economics did not suit me, so I did not enjoy it and I often felt that I had to struggle. Nevertheless I finished it.

P11, a 45-year-old German construction worker addicted to gambling, writes about a crisis that was triggered because he lost more in one night than he can earn in a month:

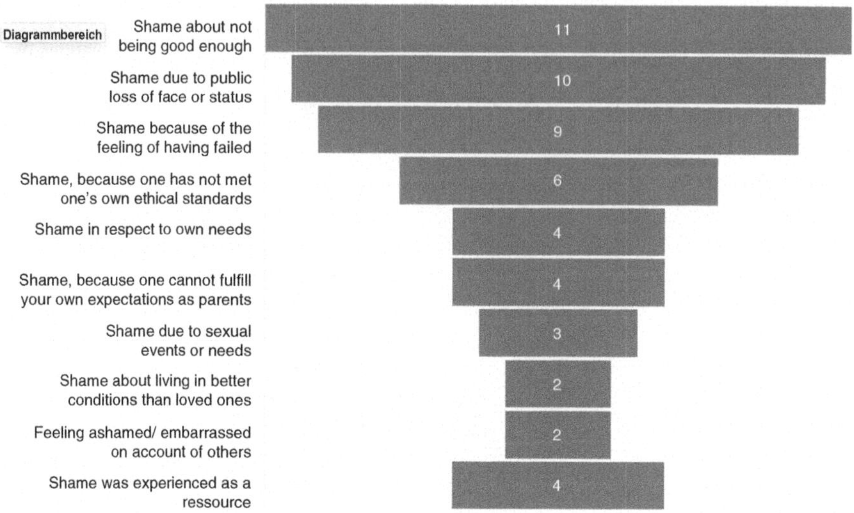

Fig. 12.2 Facets of shame (total nominations) (author's own construction)

> When I am not in control of the gambling, I am sometimes deeply ashamed. I feel like a loser.

P19, 52 years old, a Dutch former salesperson, now unable to work owing to illness, feels a deep shame about her appearance and describes it as follows:

> Shame plays a big part. I was ashamed to have an abortion. In my first relationship I was often beaten, but I never told anyone that and he always did it in such a way that you couldn't see it as long as I wore clothes and always turned it around so that it was my fault. I was ashamed of that too. And for my appearance, that I am so fat and can move so badly, although I am still relatively young. Especially when I'm with doctors who always tell you that if you just lost weight, everything would be fine. But of course it is not like that. I also suffer from incontinence, and sometimes I feel ashamed of it because I am still so young. Even if I go outside with my oxygen equipment and people stare at me and maybe they think she would just lose weight, she wouldn't need that thing. Then I feel ashamed.

As a point of interest, Fig. 12.2 also shows that some participants experience their shame as explicitly positive and as a resource.

Thus P9, a female 57-year-old German accountant, reports after a crisis caused by the death of her mother from cancer:

> Shame has shown me where there are real borders to watch out for. If I perceived them, it helped me to tackle necessary changes.

Some participants succeed in explicitly defining and using shame as an initial point for change and further development, for example, P29, the 23-year-old German gardener whose life crisis was caused by his lack of literacy skills. The birth of his daughter triggered a change. He writes:

> I am very ashamed. for a long time. for a long time I thought that only I am too stupid. but now I know that this is not so. and that I am not stupid I just can not read and write so well so far. I'm changing that now.

Also P13, 37 years old, a German-Italian social worker living in Germany, describes similar things. He reports the following event as the trigger for his life crisis:

> When I was 32, I met a woman at a training course in a hotel who took me to her hotel room. That's when I understood that I like to pass on the responsibility for my sexuality to someone else. This was tremendously pleasurable, but it also caused a great crisis to learn about myself.

Regarding his experience of shame, he adds:

> In the beginning shame played a very important role. In the beginning I was also very ashamed of my sexual needs. Also for my lust. Not anymore, even if I am insulted for it, e.g. when I address women on online platforms in a friendly and polite way. Today I stand by myself and my lust.

P28, a German female bank employee, writes about shame in relation to the life crisis:

> The beginning of the crisis was my 30th birthday. I had the feeling that I had only been busy with my job in my twenties and that I had achieved nothing in my private life, that I had not lived my life. . . . The feeling of shame prevented me at first to get out of the crisis. At some point I learned to look more closely behind the feeling or the trigger and learned to deal with it in a positive sense in order to reduce and counteract the feeling of shame and thus the area of attack.

These results reflect what the recent literature on shame is increasingly showing, namely, that shame has to be seen as a resource for personal development (Mayer & Vanderheiden, 2019; Vanderheiden & Mayer, 2017; Wurmser, 2010, 2015), as a resource for creativity and well-being (Briegleb, 2014; Mayer et al., 2019) and can actually contribute to individual happiness by transforming toxic experiences of shame (Vanderheiden, 2019a, 2019b).

The study reveals distinct and diverse gender differences, both in the overall view and when examining individual cases. It is clear that the more the life crisis is seen or experienced in connection with shame, the greater the gender difference becomes (Fig. 12.3).

These results are also in line with earlier research findings as shown in Fig. 12.4.

Women show a much stronger sense of shame about not meeting their own standards or failing in any way and about not being good enough or standing up for their own needs, including sexual needs. Men feel shame above all when they live in better living conditions than their families (these are without exception migrants who live abroad and care for their families from there) (see McKay, 2021).

P35, a 43-year-old Mexican living in the USA, who works as a cleaner in a restaurant and at the same time is self-employed with a small cleaning company, expresses it this way:

> At first I was paralysed, hoping and praying that Trump would not win and that this nightmare would not become truth. I had hoped to be able to bring my children here

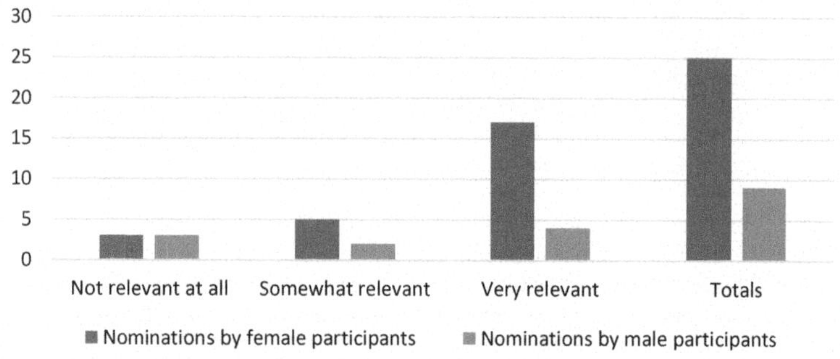

Fig. 12.3 Gender difference: relevance of shame with regard to life crises (author's own construction)

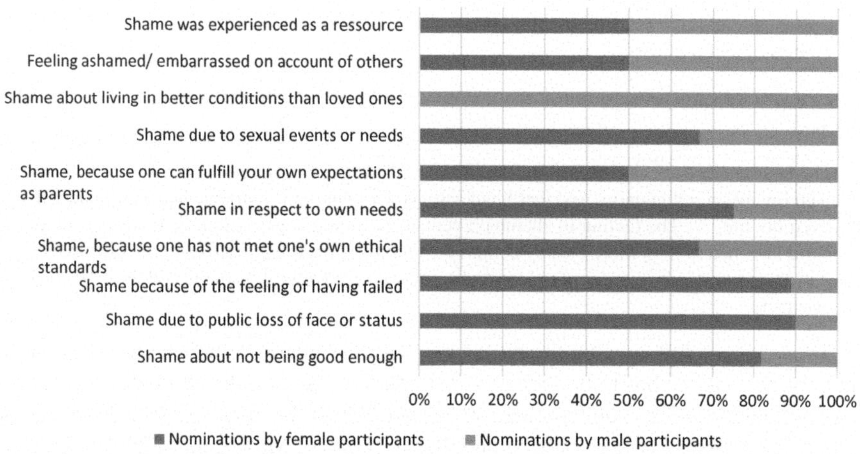

Fig. 12.4 Facets of shame according to gender (author's own construction)

> sometime, to meet my son once, but this has become very unlikely. That's very sad, but I'm not giving up hope. By having two jobs for a long time, I often have stress and severe headaches. Most of the time I couldn't afford a car either, which is very unusual in the USA, had to do everything by bike, that's sometimes difficult, after two job shifts a work so much and so hard, send what I can to my children, but still I am ashamed because I am better off here than they are. And when the restaurant closes late at night and it storms or rains heavily. I don't have health insurance either. I work so much and so hard, send what I can to my children, but still I am ashamed because I am better off here than they are in Mexico.

P39, who at 19 is a refugee from Afghanistan, living in Germany and lost his parents in their flight, says:

> I would have been ashamed if I hadn't managed to come here and create what my parents wanted for me. Sometimes I also feel ashamed towards other family members or friends who are still in Afghanistan that I can now live in security and freedom and no longer have to fear for my life every day, that I was allowed to go to school and do my vocational training.

Some recent studies, such as Bauwens (2017) and United Nation's Human Development Report (UNDP, 2020), also confirm the strong correlation between the burden of being a refugee or migrant and sensitivity for shame. Although their study did not directly refer to life crises, Orth, Robins and Soto (2010) showed that age, gender and cultural differences in shame, guilt and two forms of pride can be observed throughout the life span. They examined 2611 people aged from 13 to 89 years and found that shame decreased from adolescence into middle adulthood, reaching a low point around the age of 50, and then increased with age. On average, women reported more shame and guilt; black people reported less shame and Asians more pride than other ethnic groups. Throughout life, shame and arrogant pride tended to be negatively related to psychological well-being, and shameless guilt and authentic pride showed positive relationships with well-being. Overall, the results of the study by Orth et al. (2010) support the maturity principle of personality development and suggest that people become more susceptible to psychologically adaptive, self-confident emotions such as guilt and authentic pride as they grow older and less susceptible to psychologically maladaptive ones such as shame and hubristic pride.

6.3 Relevance of Digital Resources in Overcoming the Crisis

Progressive digitalisation—also known in certain contexts as the Fourth Industrial Revolution (see Mayer and Vanderheiden 2021)—will lead to far-reaching changes in all areas of life. There are signs of the effects of digitalisation (both toxic and otherwise) in profound upheavals in the context of shame and shaming, but researchers are only just beginning to understand its connection with the triggering of, perception of, and coping with life crises. Accordingly, two questions of the online questionnaire referred to the extent to which digital media or resources were considered relevant for coping with life crises and which of these were relevant. The responses to these questions so far appear to be quite contradictory as shown in Fig. 12.5.

It became apparent that most participants had little or no digital services available at the time of their life crisis. This is where the age distribution of the respondents comes into play, as the following figure (Fig. 12.6) shows.

On the other hand, it must be taken into account that the life crisis for most of the interviewees already dates back several years, sometimes even decades. Thus, it can be understood that 16 participants state that digital resources were not relevant for coping with the life crisis, while 3 others explicitly state that digital media did not exist at the time of the crisis. For 15 people they were very important and for 3 others, somewhat relevant.

The study shows that especially for the middle-aged respondents (15 participants aged 51 to 60 years) and for the 4 respondents older than 60 years, digital media were often less important in coping with their crisis. This is related to the fact that these media were not yet available to them at the time of the crisis, as most respondents

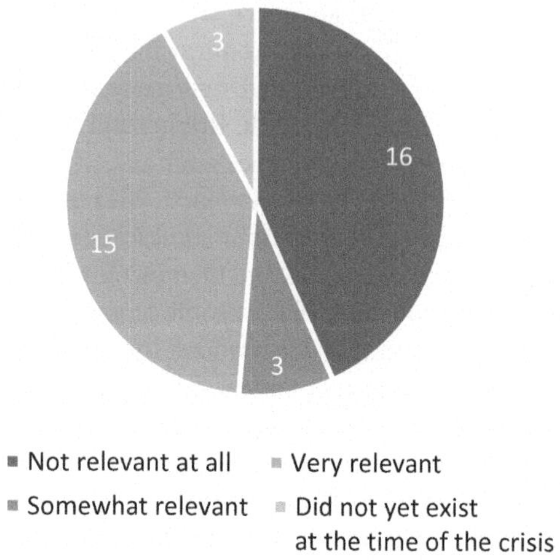

Fig. 12.5 Significance of digital resources with regard to life crisis (total) (author's own construction)

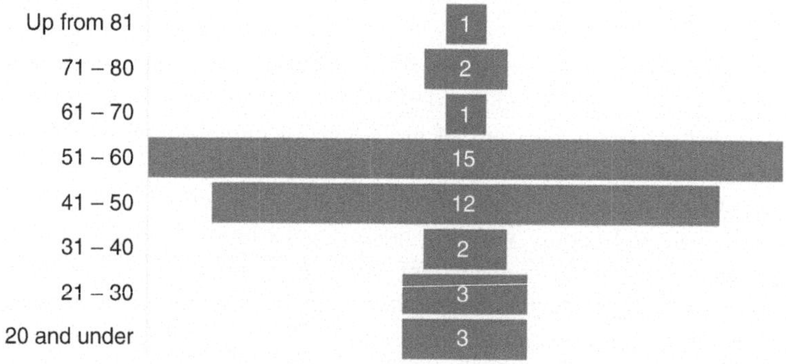

Fig. 12.6 Age distribution in the study (author's own construction)

report crises from their youth or young adult life. With the exception of one participant—P19, who refuses digital media for fundamental reasons because she feels she is too old at 52 years to learn new things—the majority of participants provide examples of how they use digital media today in comparable situations to overcome crises.

Here again, a clear gender difference is evident: the statement "did not exist at the time of the crisis" is only relevant for women, as is the statement that they did. In the category "very relevant", the ratio is balanced; in the category "not relevant", the proportion of women clearly predominates (Fig. 12.7).

At the same time, it became clear that digital media play an important role for the majority of those surveyed, even in the case of crisis-ridden events in current life

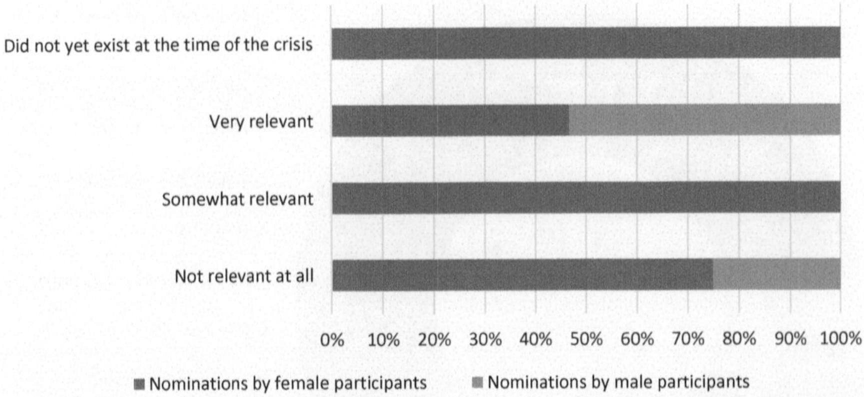

Fig. 12.7 Significance of digital resources with regard to life crisis by gender (author's own construction)

contexts. For most of them, digital services (messenger services, social media services, video calls) are an important way of staying in touch with friends and family (12 total, 9♀, 3♂), with their partner (3 total, 1♀, 2♂) or with their cultural group of origin (4 total, 2♀, 2♂). For others, it was or is a resource to come into exchange and contact with like-minded people or people in a similar situation (2 total, 1♀, 1♂) or to obtain information about the disease in question (3 total, 3♀) or the factors causing the crisis (3 total, 1♀, 2♂) or is a therapeutic resource (1 total, 1♀). Four participants use digital services for educational purposes (4 total, 1♀, 3♂), two for job search (2 total, 2♀) and one to compensate for limited reading and writing skills (1 total, 1♂). In addition, specific services such as online dating (1 total, 1♀) or online shopping during her husband's cancer illness (1 total, 1♀) were used in the context of life crisis management (Fig. 12.8).

P35, the 43-year-old Mexican in the USA, working as a cleaner and at the same time self-employed, states:

> Facebook and Whatsapp are very important for me. I can stay in contact with my family. I talk to them every day. I have never seen my son other than on video, my daughter not since she is 3 years old. Now she's a young lady. I also stay in contact with my parents, siblings and friends.

P39, the 19-year-old refugee from Afghanistan, living in Germany, who lost his parents, comments:

> This is very important. It allows me to stay in touch with family members and friends in my home country, but also internationally, through Messenger Services. It also helped a lot with learning. It is also an important part for my education as a media specialist, almost everything goes digital, the recordings, the planning, the movie and sound editing. I even have my own YouTube channel.

P38, a female artist, 70 years old in Australia, migrated from Germany. After her separation, which was completely unexpected because her husband fell in love with another woman and left her within a few days, she started looking for a new partner online:

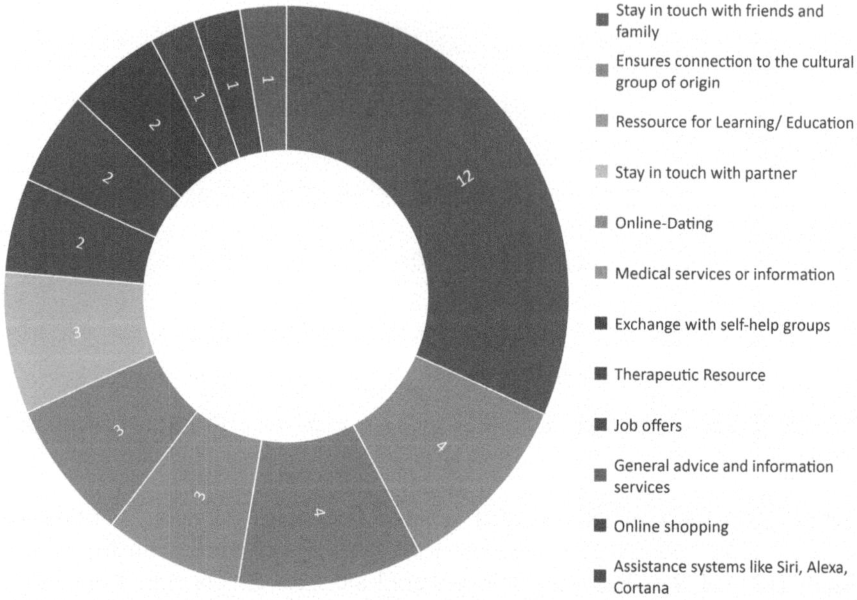

Fig. 12.8 Character of relevant digital resources (total) (author's own construction)

> I was married for over forty years, then my husband left me because he fell in love with another woman. This happened completely unexpected. I wanted a new relationship, started looking around on online dating platforms. I started a relationship with a man, he called me every day, there was even a video contact. He wanted to come visit me, then it turned out that he was a so-called love scammer. Never heard of that before. I felt so stupid and ashamed. At least I was clever enough not to transfer any money.... Anyway I did not give up. I have friends all over the world, with which I stay in touch. Through digital media. This is important for my emotional and my life and love balance. Seven years ago I found my cyberlover. We have a close connection, also energetically. We chat and we do video calls, sometimes for hours.

P4, who is 55, a female German office employee, writes with regard to digital support in her life crisis caused by two miscarriages:

> Digital offerings were very important to me in overcoming the crisis, because I used a computer program to calculate ovulation. Ultimately, this helped me to get pregnant.

P1, 60, a female Dutch judge, names several life crises: a divorce and other separations, an abortion, the death of her father. She writes in reference to digital media:

> When I was young, they did not exist, or they were not available to me. But today, in a crisis, they are important in terms of coping from many different angles: some of my friends live on other continents, with them I can easily stay in touch by video, message or mail. This is very important to me—especially in view of the loneliness I often feel. They are indispensable in terms of information gathering. But also on the compensatory level: as meditations or empowerment videos on YouTube have already been a great help to me in many a crisis.

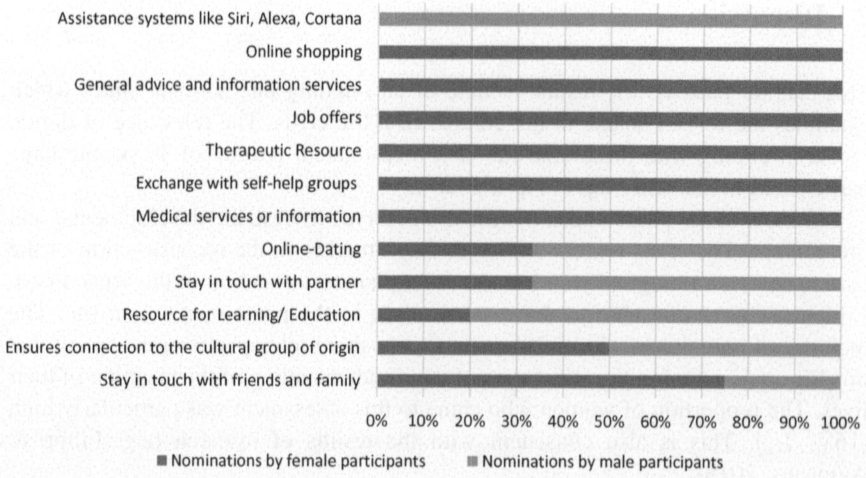

Fig. 12.9 Character of relevant digital resources by gender (author's own construction)

> In principle, online therapy would also be an option for me, even though I have no experience with it so far.

There are some clear gender-specific differences in usage behaviour of digital media. For participants of both sexes, digital media are important for being in contact with family and friends, but for women, the value is three times higher (12 total, 9♀, 3♂). In terms of the value of digital media for educational purposes, the proportion of men is significantly higher than for women (5 total, 1♀, 4♂). The motivations are quite different: P1 (female) and P18 (male), both Germans, and P30 ♀, South African, describe themselves as persons for whom continuous learning processes are a constitutive part of their self-image and thus also a logically obvious strategy for overcoming a life crisis and a natural part of their use of digital media. For P39 as a young refugee from Afghanistan, his vocational training in Germany is decisive for his future chances and also the legal basis for his stay in Germany. For P29, German, who has difficulties with the written language, the birth of his daughter is the motivation for him to start a new attempt to learn to read and write as an adult. Up to now, he has been using digital assistance systems for many issues, mainly to avoid reading and writing. Online dating (3 total, 2♀, 1♂) and staying in contact with the partner through digital media (3 total, 1♀, 2♂) are named somewhat more frequently by men than by women.

Services such as medical services or information, exchange with self-help groups, therapeutic resource, job offer, general advice and information services and online shopping are named exclusively by women.

This is also essentially true of some of the participants who belong to the group of refugees and migrants, such as P35 and P39 (Fig. 12.9).

7 Discussion

This chapter presents the results to date of an ongoing international study which examines the role of shame in the context of a life crisis. The relevance of digital media in coping with these crises is also investigated. A total of 39 people have participated in the study (up to April 2020).

For most of the participants, the life crisis serves to describe developmental and life courses. The crisis represents a significant marker in the reconstruction of the participant's own biography and serves an explanatory function in the sense that it explains why certain changes have taken place in the participant's own life. The majority of participants (24 of 39) came to a positive retrospective assessment that this life crisis was significant in terms of their understanding of the meaning of their lives. The proportion of women who came to this assessment was particularly high (16♀, 7♂). This is also consistent with the results of research (e.g. Filipp & Aymanns, 2018).

The results show that for the majority of the respondents, the experience of life crises was associated with shame; this was particularly true for the female participants. The majority of the participants experienced shame as rather painful and stressful. However, a very interesting result of the study is that a total of four participants (4 of 39) stated that they experienced shame as a resource. For them, the experience of shame was either an impulse for self-protection and mindfulness or for self-awareness and initiation of personal development processes. This complements findings in earlier publications (Briegleb, 2014; Mayer & Vanderheiden, 2019; Vanderheiden & Mayer, 2017; Wong, 2011, 2019; Wurmser, 2010, 2015).

The study could also show that for the majority of the respondents, digital media played an important role in coping with crisis events in current life contexts, even though many of the older respondents did not yet have access to them as coping resources for past crisis events. Messenger services, social media services and video calls were identified as particularly relevant digital offerings as an important way to stay in touch with friends and family, with a partner and cultural group of origin, or to exchange information with like-minded people or people in a similar situation.

The study contributes to new findings by supporting the previously cited literature.

8 Recommendations for Further Research

This chapter presents the results of an international study that examined the role of shame in the context of a life and the relevance of digital media in coping with this crisis (up to April 2020). It would be desirable to extend the number of respondents even further and thus to put them on an even broader footing.

It could be a worthwhile research project to examine the relationship between life crises, shame and the search for meaning more closely in further analyses. The relationship between life crises, shame and education is also a worthwhile field of research. A more detailed examination of the relationship between life crises and the experience of shame, especially from the perspective of Positive Psychology 2.0 (Wong, 2011, 2019), could also provide new insights and valuable impulses to move forwards with research.

Research into the relevance of digital means in coping with life crises could also be further expanded. Here, the use of artificial intelligence in particular could prove to be a worthwhile field of research, especially with regard to differences in various cultural contexts.

The current corona pandemic is leading to a variety of crisis situations worldwide. What will be reflected in this context in the form of life crises cannot be estimated at this point but will certainly become an important field of research in the future.

With regard to people with a history of flight, trauma research is now broadly based, but the focus on life crises is largely absent. This would be an exciting and worthwhile field of research.

Acknowledgement I would like to thank those who took the time to participate in my research: the people who shared their crisis experiences with me and completed my online surveys. For many individuals this meant exposing themselves again to very painful events. I am deeply grateful for this. I was and am very touched by the openness of their answers and the manifold resources that these people were able to activate, by their high level of creativity and their strength to transformatively overcome these life crises. I am very grateful to my friend and colleague, Claude-Héléne Mayer, for her inspiration in the realisation of this research project.

References

Amichai-Hamburger, Y., Klomek, A., Friedman, D., Zuckerman, O., & Shani-Sherman, T. (2020). The future of online therapy. Retrieved 15 March 2020, from https://www.researchgate.net/publication/267573372_The_future_of_online_therapy

Antonovsky, A. (1979). *Health, stress and coping*. San Francisco: Jossey-Bass.

Antonovsky, A. (1987). *Unraveling the mystery of health. How people manage stress and stay well*. San Francisco: Jossey-Bass.

Bandura, A. (1997). *Self efficacy: The exercise of control*. New York: Freeman.

Bauwens, D. (2017, December 12). Migrants in Italy: ‘Shame is keeping us here’. *IPS News*. Available at: http://www.ipsnews.net/2017/12/migrants-italy-shame-keeping-us/.

Benetti-McQuoid, J., & Bursik, K. (2005). Individual differences in experiences of and responses to guilt and shame: Examining the lenses of gender and gender role. *Sex Roles, 53*, 133–142. https://doi.org/10.1007/s11199-005-4287-4.

Ben-Ze’ev, A. (2020). Cyberspace: The alternative romantic culture. In C.-H. Mayer & E. Vanderheiden (Eds.), *International handbook of love*. Cham: Springer.

Bevan, J., Gomez, R., & Sparks, L. (2014). Disclosures about important life events on Facebook: Relationships with stress and quality of life. *Computers In Human Behavior, 39*, 246–253. https://doi.org/10.1016/j.chb.2014.07.021.

Bhawuk, D. (2017). lajjA in Indian psychology: Spiritual, social, and literary perspectives. In E. Vanderheiden & C.-H. Mayer (Eds.), *The value of shame. Exploring a health resource in cultural contexts* (pp. 109–134). Cham: Springer.

Bhawuk, D. (2019). lajjA: Learning, unlearning and relearning. In C.-H. Mayer & E. Vanderheiden (Eds.), *The bright side of shame. Transforming and growing through practical applications in cultural contexts* (pp. 35–50). Cham: Springer.

Blawat, K., & Ehrig, C. (2010). Rituale puffern den Schock ab. Retrieved May 2, 2020, from https://www.sueddeutsche.de/wissen/psychologie-rituale-puffern-den-schock-ab-1.1018114

Briegleb, T. (2014). *Die diskrete Scham.* Frankfurt: Insel.

Brown, B. (2008). *I thought it was just me (but it isn't).* New York: Gotham Books.

Brown, B. (2012). *Daring greatly.* New York: Gotham Books.

Casimir, M. J., & Schnegg, M. (2002). Shame across cultures: The evolution, ontogeny and function of a "moral emotion". In H. Keller & Y. H. Poortinga (Eds.), *Between culture and biology: Perspectives on ontogenetic development* (pp. 270–200). New York: Cambridge University Press.

Chan, M., Estève, D., Fourniols, J., Escriba, C., & Campo, E. (2020). Smart wearable systems: Current status and future challenges. *Artificial Intelligence in Medicine, 56* (2012) 137–156. https://doi.org/10.1016/j.artmed.2012.09.003

Cook, J., & Doyle, C. (2002). Working alliance in online therapy as compared to face-to-face therapy: Preliminary results. *Cyberpsychology & Behavior, 5*(2), 95–105. https://doi.org/10.1089/109493102753770480.

Creswell, J. W. (2013). *Qualitative inquiry and research design: Choosing among five approaches* (4th ed.). Thousand Oaks, CA: Sage.

Crisis Text Line. (2020). Crisis text line. Retrieved March 15, 2020, from https://www.crisistextline.org

Cucuani, H., Sulastiana, M., Harding, D., & Agustiani, H. (2021). The meaning of shame for malay people and the role for tackling counterproductive work behaviour. In: C.-H. Mayer, E. Vanderheiden, & P. T. P. Wong (Eds.), *Shame 4.0: Investigating an emotion in digital worlds and the fourth industrial revolution.* Cham: Springer.

Dekker, R., & Engbersen, G. (2014). How social media transform migrant networks and facilitate migration. *Global Networks, 14*(4), 401–418.

Emmer, M., Richter, C., & Kunst, M. (2016). *Flucht 2.0. Mediennutzung durch Flüchtlinge vor, während und nach der Flucht.* Retrieved April 16, 2020, from https://www.polsoz.fu-berlin.de/kommwiss/arbeitsstellen/internationale_kommunikation/Media/Flucht-2_0.pdf

Fahr, A., & Graf, A. (2012, May 17). Is Facebook for lovers? Beziehungsmanagement auf Facebook. Vortrag auf der Jahrestagung der DGPuK, Berlin.

Filipp, S., & Aymanns, P. (2018). *Kritische Lebensereignisse und Lebenskrisen* (2nd ed.). Stuttgart: Kohlhammer.

Gesundheitsförderung Schweiz. (2016). Psychische Gesundheit über die Lebensspanne. Grundlagenbericht. Retrieved March 8, 2020, from https://gesundheitsfoerderung.ch/assets/public/documents/de/5-grundlagen/publikationen/psychische-gesundheit/berichte/Bericht_006_GFCH_2016-04_-_Psychische_Gesundheit_ueber_die_Lebensspanne.pdf

Gräf, L. (2010). *Online-Befragung. Eine praktische Einführung für Anfänger.* Berlin: Lit.

Greiner, U. (2014). *Schamverlust.* Reinbek bei Hamburg: Rowohlt.

Harper, J. (2011). Regulating and coping with shame. Pvsps.cz. Accessed May 1, 2016, from http://www.pvsps.cz/data/document/20110715/12_Shame.pdf?id=690

Hernandez, V., & Mendoza, C. (2011). Shame resilience: A strategy for empowering women in treatment for substance abuse. *Journal of Social Work Practice In The Addictions, 11*(4), 375–393. https://doi.org/10.1080/1533256x.2011.622193.

Hilgers, M. (2019). Wenn wir uns vor der Welt verstecken wollen. *Geowissen. Lebenskrisen Überwinden, 62*, 74–77.

Hofer-Moser, O., Hintenberger, G., Schwarzmann, M., Dominicis, R., & Brunner, F. (2020). *Krisenintervention Kompakt. Theoretische Modelle, Praxisbezogene Konzepte Und Konkrete Interventionsstrategien*. Göttingen: Vandenhoeck & Ruprecht.

Hoffmann, N., & Hofmann, B. (2017). *Anpassungsstörung Und Lebenskrise. Material Für Therapie, Beratung Und Selbsthilfe* (2nd ed.). Weinheim: Beltz.

Hussy, W., Schreier, M., & Echterhoff, G. (2010). Qualitative Analyseverfahren. In: *Forschungsmethoden in Psychologie und Sozialwissenschaften für Bachelor*. Berlin: Springer.

Jackob, N., Schoen, H., & Zerback, T. (2009). *Sozialforschung im Internet. Methodologie und Praxis der Online-Befragung*. Wiesbaden: VS Verlag für Sozialwissenschaften | Springer Fachmedien Wiesbaden GmbH.

Jäger, R., & Booth, J. (1984). *Diagnostische Urteilsbildung In Der Psychologie*. Göttingen u.a.: Hogrefe.

Johnson, D., & Whisman, M. (2013). Gender differences in rumination: A meta-analysis. *Personality and Individual Differences, 55*(4), 367–374. https://doi.org/10.1016/j.paid.2013.03.019.

Jose, P., & Brown, I. (2007). When does the gender difference in rumination begin? Gender and age differences in the use of rumination by adolescents. *Journal of Youth and Adolescence, 37*(2), 180–192.

Kadler-Neuhausen, I. (2020). Beziehungen im Kontext von Online Social Networks. Retrieved March 21, 2020, from https://medienbildung.hypotheses.org/5793

Kendler, K., Thornton, L., & Prescott, C. (2001). Gender differences in the rates of exposure to stressful life events and sensitivity to their depressogenic effects. *American Journal of Psychiatry, 158*(4), 587–593.

Kirchner, J. (2014). Schatz, ich hab dich gegruschelt! Nutzung von Social Network Sites in Fernbeziehungen. *Medienkommunikation In Bewegung*, 155–169. https://doi.org/10.1007/978-3-531-19375-5_9

Komito, L. (2011). Social media and migration: Virtual community 2.0. *Journal of the American Society for Information Science and Technology, 62*(6), 1075–1086. https://doi.org/10.1002/asi.21517.

Krause, E., Vélez, C., Woo, R., Hoffmann, B., Freres, D., Abenavoli, R., et al. (2017). Rumination, depression, and gender in early adolescence: A longitudinal study of a bidirectional model. *The Journal of Early Adolescence, 38*(7), 923–946.

Krishnamurthy, A. (2018). *Scham Macht Geschlecht. Körperdialoge In Südindien*. Opladen: Verlag Barbara Budrich.

Lammers, M. (2016). *Emotionsbezogene Psychotherapie Von Scham Und Schuld*. Stuttgart: Schattauer.

Landesanstalt für Medien Nordrhein-Westfalen. (2020). Wearables. Retrieved May 1, 2020, from https://www.medienanstalt-nrw.de/fileadmin/user_upload/lfm-nrw/Foerderung/Digitalisierung/Digitaltrends/Digitaltrends_Wearables.pdf

Lindisfarne, N. (1998). Gender, shame and culture: An anthropological perspective. In P. Gilbert & B. Andrews (Eds.), *Shame. Interpersonal bahaviour, psychopathology, and culture* (pp. 246–261). Oxford: Oxford University Press.

Linke, C. (2010). *Medien im Alltag von Paaren*. Wiesbaden: VS, Verl. für Sozialwiss.

Ludwig, S., Fellner-Röhling, G., & Thoma, C. (2017). Do women have more shame than men? An experiment on self-assessment and the shame of overestimating oneself. *European Economic Review, 92*, 31–46.

Marks, S. (2010). *Die Würde des Menschen*. Gütersloh: Gütersloher Verlagshaus.

Marks, S. (2015). *Scham - die tabuisierte Emotion* (5th ed.). Mannheim: Patmos.

Marzano, L., Bardill, A., Fields, B., Herd, K., Veale, D., Grey, N., et al. (2015). The application of mHealth to mental health: Opportunities and challenges. *The Lancet Psychiatry, 2*(10), 942–948. https://doi.org/10.1016/s2215-0366(15)00268-0.

Matud, M. (2004). Gender differences in stress and coping styles. *Personality and Individual Differences, 37*(7), 1401–1415.

Mayer, C.-H., & Vanderheiden, E. (2019). *The bright side of shame. Transforming and growing through practical applications in cultural contexts*. Cham: Springer.

Mayer, C.-H., & Vanderheiden, E. (2021). Shame in the fourth industrial revolution, industry 4.0 and the age of digitalisation. In C.-H. Mayer, E. Vanderheiden, & P. T. P. Wong (Eds.), *Shame 4.0: Investigating an emotion in digital worlds and the fourth industrial revolution*. Cham: Springer.

Mayer, C.-H., Vanderheiden, E., & Oosthuizen, R. (2019). Transforming shame, guilt and anxiety through a salutogenic PP1.0 and PP2.0 counselling framework. *Counselling Psychology Quarterly,* 1–17. https://doi.org/10.1080/09515070.2019.1609421

Mayring, P. (2010). *Qualitative Inhaltsanalyse*. Beltz: Weinheim.

Mayring, P. (2016). *Einführung in die qualitative Sozialforschung*. Basel: Beltz.

McAdams, D. P. (1993). *The stories we live by: Personal myths and the making of the self.* New York: Guilford Press.

McKay, G. (2021). A place for 4IR in transforming shame in returning migrants. In C.-H. Mayer, E. Vanderheiden, & P. T. P. Wong (Eds.), *Shame 4.0: Investigating an emotion in digital worlds and the fourth industrial revolution*. Cham: Springer

Miller, S. B. (1996). *Shame in context*. Hillsdale, NJ: Analytic Press.

Miller-Prieve, Vienna. (2016). Women, shame, and mental health: A systematic review of approaches in psychotherapy. Retrieved from Sophia, the St. Catherine University repository website: https://sophia.stkate.edu/msw_papers/630

Naderifar, M., Goli, H., & Ghaljaie, F. (2017). Snowball sampling: A purposeful method of sampling in qualitative research. *Strides in Development of Medical Education, 14*(3), e67670.

Naslund, J., Aschbrenner, K., Marsch, L., & Bartels, S. (2016). The future of mental health care: Peer-to-peer support and social media. *Epidemiology and Psychiatric Sciences, 25*(2), 113–122. https://doi.org/10.1017/s2045796015001067.

Neumann-Braun, K., & Autenrieth, U. (2011). *Freundschaft und Gemeinschaft im Social Web*. Baden-Baden: Nomos, Edition Reinhard Fischer.

Nyström, M., Kjellberg, E., Heimdahl, U., & Jonsson, B. (2018). Shame and interpersonal sensitivity: Gender differences and the association between internalized shame coping strategies and interpersonal sensitivity. *Bulletin of the Menninger Clinic, 82*(2), 137–155.

Olff, M. (2015). Mobile mental health: A challenging research agenda. *European Journal of Psychotraumatology, 6*(1), 27882. https://doi.org/10.3402/ejpt.v6.27882.

Orben, A., Dienlin, T., & Przybylski, A. (2019). Social media's enduring effect on adolescent life satisfaction. *Proceedings of the National Academy of Sciences, 116*(21), 10226–10228. https://doi.org/10.1073/pnas.1902058116.

Orth, U., Robins, R., & Soto, C. (2010). Tracking the trajectory of shame, guilt, and pride across the life span. *Journal of Personality and Social Psychology, 99*(6), 1061–1071. https://doi.org/10.1037/a0021342.

Pestian, J., Nasrallah, H., Matykiewicz, P., Bennett, A., & Leenaars, A. (2010). Suicide note classification using natural language processing: A content analysis. *Biomedical Informatics Insights, 3*, BII.S4706. https://doi.org/10.4137/bii.s4706

Rasmussen, J., & Ihlen, Ø. (2017). Risk, crisis, and social media. *Nordicom Review, 38*(2), 1–17. https://doi.org/10.1515/nor-2017-0393.

Recupero, P., & Rainey, S. (2006). Characteristics of E-therapy web sites. *The Journal of Clinical Psychiatry, 67*(09), 1435–1440. https://doi.org/10.4088/jcp.v67n0915.

Riecher-Rössler, A. (2003). Psychotherapie von Frauen - Chancen dun grenzen der Geschlechtersensibilität. *Psychodynamische Psychotherapie, 2*, 91–101.

Riecher-Rössler, A. (2016). Weibliche Rollen und psychische Gesundheit. In B. Wimmer-Puchinger, K. Gutiérrez-Lobos & A. Riecher-Rössler (Eds.), *Irrsinnig weiblich-Psychische Krisen im Frauenleben* (pp. 19–37). Heidelberg: Springer.

Saraswati, L. (2018). "Malu": Coloring shame and shaming the color of beauty in transnational Indonesia. *Feminist Studies, 105*(1), 221–224. https://doi.org/10.1353/ind.2018.0012.

Sinus Institut. (2018). *Deutsche haben 3,7 enge Freunde – Offene Kommunikation und Fürsorge in einer Freundschaft am wichtigsten*. Retrieved from https://www.sinus-institut.de/sinus-loesungen/sinus-milieus-deutschland/

Tang, L. (2010). Development of online friendship in different social spaces: A case study. *Information Communication and Society, 13*(4), 615–633. https://doi.org/10.1080/13691180902998639.

Tang, L. (2012). Online friendship. *Encyclopedia of Cyber Behavior*, 412–421. https://doi.org/10.4018/978-1-4666-0315-8.ch035.

Tangney, J., & Dearing, R. (2002). *Shame and guilt*. New York: Guilford Press.

Tavrovetska, N. (2020). *Empirical study of an individual's basic beliefs in the context of overcoming life crises*. https://doi.org/10.32626/2227-6246.2019-45.358-380

Taylor, S., Klein, L., Lewis, B., Gruenewald, T., Gurung, R., & Updegraff, J. (2000). Biobehavioral responses to stress in females: Tend-and-befriend, not fight-or-flight. *Psychological Review, 107* (3), 411–429.

The Finnish Association for Mental Health. (2018). *Traumatic crises*. Retrieved from https://www.mielenterveysseura.fi/en/home/mental-health/crises/traumatic-crises

Tolin, D., & Foa, E. (2006). Sex differences in trauma and posttraumatic stress disorder: A quantitative review of 25 years of research. *Psychological Bulletin, 132*(6), 959–992.

UNDP. (2020). Scaling fences: Voices of irregular African migrants to Europe. Retrieved May 1, 2020, from https://www.undp.org/content/dam/rba/docs/Reports/UNDP-Scaling-Fences-EN-2019.pdf

Utz, S., & Beukeboom, C. J. (2011). The role of social network sites in romantic relationships: Effects on jealousy and relationship happiness. *Journal of Computer-Mediated Communication, 16*, 511–527.

Vanderheiden, E. (2019a). Study life crisis. Online questionnaire. Retrieved from https://crisis.jimdosite.com

Vanderheiden, E. (2019b). In C. -H. Mayer & E. Vanderheiden (Eds.), *"Nothing I accept about myself can be used against me to diminish me" - Transforming shame through mindfulness* (pp. 505–519). Cham: Springer.

Vanderheiden, E. (2020a). "Ever tried. Ever failed. No matter. Try again. Fail again. Fail better". Life crisis and failure as a resource. In E. Vanderheiden & C.-H. Mayer (Eds.), *Mistakes, errors and failures across cultures: Navigating potentials*. Cham: Springer. Available at: https://doi.org/10.1007/978-3-030-35574-6. Accessed 11 Jan 2020.

Vanderheiden, E. (2020b). "A friend? A single soul dwelling in two bodies." Friendship - A special kind of love . In C.-H. Mayer & E. Vanderheiden (Eds.), *International handbook of love*. Cham: Springer.

Vanderheiden, E. (2020c). "I have a friend with benefits, whom off and on I see." Friends with benefits relationships. In C. Mayer & E. Vanderheiden (Eds.), *International handbook of love*. Cham: Springer.

Vanderheiden, E. (2020d). "A matter of age?" Love relationships between older women and younger men – The so-called "cougar" phenomenon! In C. -H. Mayer & E. Vanderheiden (Eds.), *International handbook of love*. Cham: Springer.

Vanderheiden, E., & Mayer, C.-H. (2017). *The value of shame: Exploring a health resource in cultural contexts*. Cham: Springer.

Velotti, P., Garofalo, C., Bottazzi, F., & Caretti, V. (2016). Faces of shame: Implications for self-esteem, emotion regulation, aggression, and well-being. *The Journal of Psychology, 151*(2), 171–184. https://doi.org/10.1080/00223980.2016.1248809.

Wei, L., & Gao, F. (2017). Social media, social integration and subjective well-being among new urban migrants in China. *Telematics and Informatics, 34*(3), 786–796. https://doi.org/10.1016/j.tele.2016.05.017.

Wijngaards-de Meij, L., Stroebe, M., Stroebe, W., Schut, H., Bout, J., Van Der Heijden, P., et al. (2008). The impact of circumstances surrounding the death of a child on parents' grief. *Death Studies, 32*(3), 237–252.

Wilson, T. D., & Gilbert, D. T. (2008). Explaining away a model of affective adaptation. *Perspectives on Psychological Science, 3*(5), 370–386.
Wong, P. T. P. (2011). Positive psychology 2.0: Towards a balanced interactive model of the good life. *Canadian Psychology, 52*(2), 69–81. Retrieved from http://www.drpaulwong.com/positive-psychology-2-0-towards-a-balanced-interactive-model-of-the-good-life/
Wong, P. T. P. (2019). Foreword: From shame to wholeness: An existential positive psychology perspective. In C.-H. Mayer & E. Vanderheiden (Eds.), *The bright side of shame. Transforming and growing through practical applications in cultural contexts* (pp. v–xi). Cham: Springer.
Worth, P. (2021). A re-conceptualisation of Erikson's life cycle: A proposed process to address individual experiences of 'shame' . In: C.-H. Mayer, E. Vanderheiden, & P. T. P. Wong (Eds.), *Shame 4.0: Investigating an emotion in digital worlds and the fourth industrial revolution.* Cham: Springer.
Wurmser, L. (2010). Die Maske der Scham. Eschborn/Frankfurt, M.: Klotz.
Wurmser, L. (2015). Primary shame, mortal wound and tragic circularity: Some new reflections on shame and shame conflicts. *International Journal of Psychoanalysis, 96*, 1615–1634. Blackwell. https://www.highbeam.com/doc/1P3-3956053881.html
Yin, R. K. (2009). *Case study research: Design and methods*. London: Sage.

Elisabeth Vanderheiden is a pedagogue, theologian and intercultural mediator. She is the CEO of the Global Institute for Transcultural Research and the President of Catholic Adult Education in Germany. Her publishing activities focus on pedagogy, in particular on the further education of teachers and trainers in adult education, vocational and civic education, but also on the challenges of digitalisation. She has also edited books on intercultural and transnational issues. Her most recent publications deal with shame as a resource as well as with mistakes, errors and failures and their hidden potentials in the context of Culture and Positive Psychology 1.0 and 2.0. Current research projects deal with love in transcultural contexts, life crises as well as humour in the context of Positive Psychology 2.0. Another focus of her work is design thinking in transcultural contexts.

Part III
Shame 4.0 in Philosophy, Religion and Belief Systems

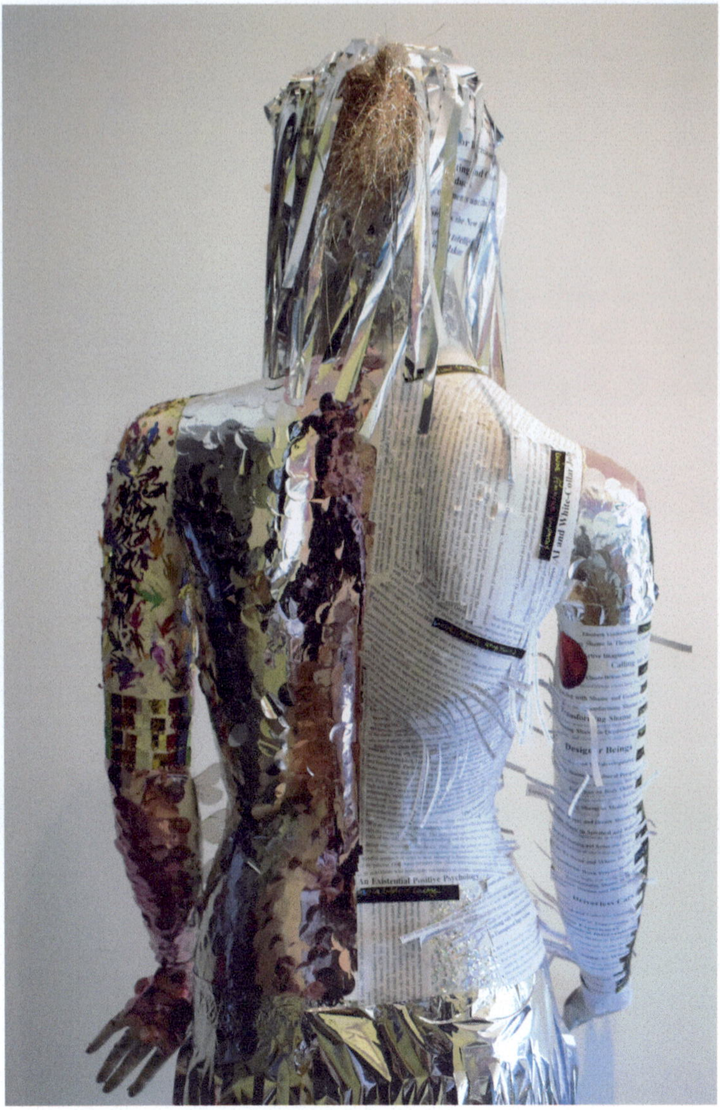

Chapter 13
Lessons Learnt from Baruch Spinoza: Shame and Faith Development in the Light of Challenges in Contemporary Society

Claude-Hélène Mayer and Paul J. P. Fouché

> *The more clearly you understand yourself and your emotions, the more you become a lover of what is.*
>
> *Baruch Spinoza*

1 Introduction

Psychobiography describes the study of extraordinary individuals through the application and analysis of their life by using psychological theories. It is therefore viewed as a psychological subdiscipline with a growing importance in the field (Fouché & Van Niekerk, 2010; Mayer & Kóváry, 2019; Schultz, 2005). Previous psychobiographies focused on analysing the life of outstanding writers, actors, entrepreneurs and (political) leaders (Holm-Hadulla, 2012; Runyan, 2005). This psychobiographical investigation explores the life of a philosopher, Baruch Spinoza, who contributed to philosophy through new religious interpretations and the invention of inspirational and philosophical approaches to self and society, as well as ethics (Spinoza, 1677/2001).

This study focuses on two topics in the life of Spinoza, namely, shame (SH) and faith development (FD). Previously, **shame** has been defined as a negative emotion; however, during recent years, research has pointed out that SH can be viewed and experienced as a resource with its own value (Mayer & Vanderheiden, 2019; Vanderheiden & Mayer, 2017). If treated as a dualistic emotion, which contains

C.-H. Mayer (✉)
Department of Industrial Psychology and People Management, University of Johannesburg, Auckland Park, Johannesburg, South Africa

Kulturwissenschaftliche Fakultät, Europa Universität Viadrina, Frankfurt (Oder), Germany

P. J. P. Fouché
Department of Psychology, University of the Free State, Bloemfontein, Republic of South Africa
e-mail: fouchejp@ufs.ac.za

C.-H. Mayer et al. (eds.), *Shame 4.0*, https://doi.org/10.1007/978-3-030-59527-2_13

negative and positive aspects, shame can greatly impact a person's development and growth (Scheff, 2013; Wong, 2016).

James Fowler's **faith development theory** (FDT) defines faith as "... our way of discerning and committing ourselves to centres of value and power that exerts ordering forces in our lives" (Fowler, 1981, pp. 24–25). Fowler provides a stage framework for comprehending the individual's struggle for greater awareness of the self and the Divine (i.e. God). FD correlates with development in other areas, such as Piaget's cognitive development theory, Erikson's psychosocial development theory, Kohlberg's moral development theory, Selman's social development theory and Levinson's work in FDT (Burnell, 2013; Fowler, 1981, 2004; Wing, 1997). For Fowler, faith refers to "... the human activity of composing meaningful worlds in which to live out the fabric of day-to-day experience with other human beings, institutions, values and visions" (Dykstra, 1982, p. 59).

This **study aims** to explore SH and FD and how Spinoza dealt with these issues throughout all his life's challenges, albeit from a positive psychology perspective (PP). This psychobiographical investigation not only adds to research on psychobiography from a PP perspective but also contributes to transferring the gained knowledge into lessons learnt from Spinoza, which will be applied in contemporary society and ultimately in Industry 4.0.

1.1 Lessons to Learn in Industry 4.0

Industry 4.0 is characterised by rapid lifestyle changes, technologisation, digitalisation, changing relationship patterns, human-machine and globalised interaction and new ascriptions to the meaning of life and work as a global phenomenon (Mayer, Van Niekerk & Fouché, 2020). In Industry 4.0, individuals have to cope with increases in diversification, as well as multi- and pluralistic worldviews (Johannessen, 2019; Palti, 2017), increasing cross-cultural interaction, the implementation of mart systems, digital workspaces as well as artificial intelligence (Coetzee, 2019). Workplace competition will expand, with specific knowledge and skills being on demand and different types of mental health and well-being issues that will manifest; thus it is assumed that a strong faith and the ability to deal with negative emotions, such as shame, will aid in coping (Mayer, 2017; Mayer et al., 2019, 2020).

In contemporary societies and Industry 4.0, meaning and meaning systems change and individuals will have to search for new meaning in life, anchored in the individual and the environment. It will be important to address top issues such as climate change, environmental protection and nature (Mayer et al., 2020). Spinoza's radical development and break with traditions and ideas of his time were directed by a radical new way of democratic freedoms and the spirit of solidarity, redefining notions of the society on a global scale. Negri (2020) has pointed out that Spinoza's idea enables present time individuals to reconstruct a revolutionary perspective, keeping a critical view on power and power struggles, multitude, liberty and necessity. It is argued in this chapter that this critical thought is needed when it comes to agreeing to or opposing the radical changes of the Fourth Industrial Revolution.

It is further argued that consciousness about FD contributes to transforming negative emotions such as shame and increases mental health and well-being (Ryan, 2019) in diverse, pluralistic, hyper-rapid and technologised realities. These might have resulted in the loss of societal abilities to guide individuals in terms of fixed sets of faith, values and strategies to deal with self-embodied emotions (Campbell & Garner, 2016). Therefore, the authors focus on the life of Spinoza, who has transformed shame and developed his faith throughout his life, ultimately leading to highly innovative and creative ideas, complex understandings and a pioneering framework—all that is needed to drive Industry 4.0 processes in a healthy way.

2 Psychobiography in Research and Practice and Its Potential Impact on Contemporary Issues and Industry 4.0

Psychobiography, originally grounded in the psychoanalytic tradition of psychology (Mayer & Kóváry, 2019; Runyan, 2005), has increased importance during the past decades and gained significant, theoretical rigour and methodological diversification (Mayer & Kóváry, 2019). Often criticised in the past as elitist, subjective in nature, reductionist and nonsystematic (Elms, 1994, 2007), scientists have expanded its impact remarkably, transdisciplinary and in terms of PP perspectives (Mayer & Kóváry, 2019).

Since the start of the Industry 4.0 movement, individuals find themselves interwoven in rapid changes and challenges to cope (Morley, 2013; Stubbings, 2018). Within these changes, emotions and meaning alter and call for recreation, since concepts of work, lifestyle and meaning change and request new definition and concepts which relate to changes in workplaces, technologisation and digitalisation (Coates & Morrison, 2016; Johannessen, 2019; Mayer, 2019). New topics, such as remote workplace management, cyber-marginalisation (e.g. being marginalised due to cyberbullying; being marginalised due to limited access, for example, to cyber spaces; etc.), cyberbullying and exclusion, occur on different levels (Mayer & Vanderheiden, 2021). It is argued here that the exploration of extraordinary individuals' lives can provide insights on how to deal with negative emotions within the newly created context of Industry 4.0. The authors focus on Baruch Spinoza to deal with SH and FD to see which lessons can be learnt from him.

Previous studies in psychobiography have focused on extraordinary individuals with backgrounds in writing, politics, philosophy and acting, for example (Schultz, 2005; Mayer & Kóváry, 2019). This chapter focuses on exploring the life of Baruch Spinoza, a Dutch philosopher, writer and scholar who, despite his life challenges, became a world-known scholar and influencer. The research questions posed and responded to in this chapter are as follows: (1) How did Spinoza deal with and transform the experienced shame in his life? (2) How did the development of faith happen in his life? (3) How are shame and faith development connected? (4) Which lessons can be learnt from Spinoza's life for dealing with the new challenges in Industry 4.0?

3 Baruch Spinoza: A Synoptic Biography of His Life and Work

Baruch Spinoza—his family called him Bento, Baruch and Benedictus, translated as "blessed person" (Nadler, 2019)—was a Dutch philosopher and one of the original thinkers related to the Enlightenment age and modern biblical criticism. This included radical conceptions of the self and the universe (The New Republic, 2012; Yovel, 1992). His naturalistic views of the Divine, or God, and the human being lay the foundations for a strongly democratic political thought and a deep critique of Scripture and sectarian religion (Nadler, 2019). Among the great philosophers of the early modern period, Spinoza is the most mysterious and fascinating of them all (Nadler, 2009); he died at the age of 45 due to a lung disease which was most probably caused by his profession of being a lens grinder, inhaling glass dust (Ratner, 2011).

4 Shame Experiences and Their Transformation

SH is a self-conscious emotion which is described as strongly negative since it is connected to the action and reaction of other individuals or groups towards the self (Lewis, 2011). It is based on an external impact and occurs when people feel that they have failed to stand up to their ego ideal (Freud, 1930). For Tangney and Dearing (2002), SH is related to the ascription of a negative personality trait rather than a negative behaviour as perceived when feeling guilty. Shame regulates moral behaviour and refers to the experience of social failure, mistakes or transgressions, often experienced as impacting the entire self and his/her identity (Deonna, Rodogno & Teroni, 2012). According to Lewis (2011), the impact of shame on a person can be so strong that she/he would like to disappear, hide or even die. It is painful and associated with exclusion and marginalisation from the social context or the group of origin or belonging (Bahrs & Henze, 2019). The shamed person might be—after certain rituals—be reintegrated into the social context and group.

During the past years, the perspective has been applied in shame research and practice (Mayer & Vanderheiden, 2019; Vanderheiden & Mayer, 2017; Wong, 2019), with shame being seen as a source of personal growth, development and well-being. This can happen when the individual develops a positive and healthy self-consciousness and self-worth to transform for a greater good or the betterment of the person (Marks, 2011). Wong (2019, p. v) highlighted that shame is an existential emotion which provides a great potential for growth, since "the greatest potential for growth only comes from the most intense pain". It is human in nature. As previously highlighted by Wong (2019), shame needs to be treated as dualistic. It should be explored from its negative and unhealthy as well as positive and healthy side for the individual to reach optimal health and functioning. In Mayer and Vanderheiden (2019), various therapies and ways of dealing with shame have been presented by different authors; however, in this article, it is emphasised that shame does not necessarily have to be treated through counselling and therapy, but can also be transformed by the individual through self-reflection and self-work. Wong (2016, 2019, p. ix) (see Chap. 7 in this book) emphasised the following points for transforming shame positively through therapeutic practice or self-work:

- Self-awareness, acceptance and acknowledgement of one's failures and limitations
- Self-forgiveness and self-compassion
- Self-affirmation through reauthoring and reframing
- Self-affirming the intrinsic value and sacredness of life
- Taking personal responsibility for positive change
- Seeking a support group
- Focusing on the meaning people attach to events
- Seeking deeper meaning and self-transcendence
- Seeking deeper understanding through verbalising one's emotions and dreams

Within the context of self-exploration, self-transcendence, new meaning-seeking and the transformation of shame, it is assumed that faith plays a certain role in self-development and healing (Fowler, 1981; Freund & Gill, 2018). Researchers have highlighted that faith can support an individual to transform negative emotions, such as shame, and create new perspectives, as well as transformational forces to support individuals to deal with shame constructively and positively (Mayer, 2017; Ryan, 2019).

5 Fowler's Faith Development Theory (FDT)

FDT is a stage model of spiritual or religious expression and offers a non-sectarian model of spiritual growth that allows for the comprehension of spiritual development apart from the specifics of various faith traditions (Parker, 2011). Fowler (1987, 2001) identified four convictions which underpin FDT, namely, that (a) humans are genetically potentiated for partnership with the Divine; (b) potentiation does not necessarily translate into the realisation of the partnership with the Divine; (c) the realisation of the partnership with the Divine takes place within a specific context of interaction and interrelatedness with the Divine, as well as fellow humans; and

(d) the interaction with, and dependence upon, the Divine and our environment starts in a non-conscious manner. Based on these convictions, Fowler developed his theory with the identification of the following different stages of faith development: (a) pre-stage: primal faith and the incorporate self, (b) intuitive-projective faith and the impulsive self, (c) mythical-literal faith and the imperial self, (d) synthetic-conventional faith and the interpersonal self, (e) individuative-reflective faith and the institutional self, (f) paradoxical-conjunctive faith and the interindividual self and (g) universalising faith and the Divine-grounded self (Burnell, 2013; Mayer, 2017).

In 1987, when Fowler extended his faith development stages, he also added dimensions of selfhood, with a particular focus on the work of Robert Kegan (1982). Kegan made an important contribution to the constructivist developmental theory by extending the theories of Kohlberg and Piaget to include ego development and personality theory. Kegan's (1982) theory provided a developmental account or explanation of the self in motion and its process of meaning-making. This extended the developmental dynamics of faith (Fowler, 1987, 2001):

> To be a self means at the outset, to be a human being with structuring patterns that shape a distinctive style of being as a person ... A major concern of the stage theories ... is with understanding the development of those capacities by which we construct self-other, self-self and self-ultimate or God relationships. (Fowler, 1987, pp. 55–56)

As social perspective-taking evolves through the stages of faith development and selfhood, each new level allows for extended self-knowledge and the potential to greater intimacy with others and God (Burnell, 2013). As humans evolve through the levels, various forms of self-deception also emerge, making it possible to trace the development of cunning and capacity for evil within an individual's developmental history (Fowler, 1981, 1987). With the development of self, humans become capable of shaping and expressing; Fowler refers to this as "disposition of faith" (1987, p. 56), indicating that both emotive and cognitive aspects are involved (Burnell, 2013). According to Fowler, "faith is a construing of the conditions of existence" (1987, p. 56), and it also attempts to make sense of our daily existence "... in light of some accounting for the ultimate conditions of our existence" (Fowler, 1987, p. 56). Next, the faith development stages are discussed sequentially.

5.1 Pre-stage (Stage 0): Primal Faith and the Incorporate Self

The pre-stage commences at birth, before the development of language and conceptual thought (Fowler, 1981, 1987). Babies are affected in utero by the environment surrounding pregnancy, which is communicated by the emotional state of the mother biochemically, as well as through mediation (Fowler, 1987). When babies experience their caregivers as dependable realities, the caregivers constitute the baby's initial experience of a super-ordinate power (Fowler, 1981, 1984). On the foundation of trust or mistrust rests all that emerges in subsequent stages in terms of faith (Fouché, Burnell, Van Niekerk & Nortjé, 2016; Straughn, 2010). During the first 2 years of life, a baby develops cognitive and relational separation, while differentiation also occurs (Fowler, 1987; Mayer, 2017). During this time, the predictable presence of the mother or caregiver substitute is essential "... for mediating experiences of separation and return and for the important mirroring that conveys a deep regard and a clear focusing of self as other to the mother" (Fowler, 1987, p. 59).

5.2 *Stage 1: Intuitive Projective Faith and the Impulsive Self*

This stage coincides with language development from the age of two and continues to the preschool years (Dykstra, 1982; Fowler, 1981). Language enables a reflexive awareness concerning the self and the environment, as well as wider access to stories and symbols. From stories, children form images that bind their reality with meaning and awe, including their understanding of God (Burnell, 2013; Croucher, 2010; Fowler, 1981, 1984). However, the child does not possess the logic that necessitates the questioning of perspectives or fantasy, but this stage does involve a growing and dynamic faith (Straughn, 2010). An awareness of a larger reality occurs, as well as a sense of the taboos instilled by the child's family and culture (Fowler, 1984, 1987). The child can pair feelings of profound guilt or terror, as well as love and ecstasy, with the religious symbols and images of "good and evil". Children at this stage can also form long-standing emotional and image orientations and connotations to faith (Burnell, 2013; Fouché et al., 2016; Fowler, 1981, 1987; Straughn, 2010).

5.3 *Stage 2: Mythical-Literal Faith and the Imperial Self*

Mythical-literal faith develops between the ages of 6 and 8, at school-going age, until the ages of 10–12 (Croucher, 2010; Fowler, 1981). The child's experiences are now less dependent on feeling and fantasy (Fowler, 1981). This stage may be referred to as the *stage of concrete functioning* (Croucher, 2010). The child's world becomes more orderly and predictable (Fouché et al., 2016). Stories embody how experiences are valued (Fowler, 1984). Stories are recounted with more accuracy, but the child is not yet ready to reflect upon their full meaning (Straughn, 2010).

Furthermore, children start to recognise the perspectives of others as different from their own (Fowler, 1981, 1987) and possess the ability to include God's perspective (Fowler, 1981). In terms of faith, the child does not interpret or reproduce symbols or myths since the child does not yet neurocognitively function at an abstract level. Therefore, faith becomes a matter of reliance on the stories, rules and values of the family and immediate community (Dykstra, 1982; Fowler, 1984). The latter provides the mythical-literal stage with a striking feature: "... the orientation to narrative and story as the principal means of constructing conserving and sharing meanings" (Fowler, 1987, p. 61). This stage lacks the feature of *interiority*, which refers to an individual's internal world composed of motives and personality (Fowler, 1987). Children at this stage do not possess a sense of themselves as separate personalities, but rather a sense of who they are in context to their experiences and the stories related to their family and community (Fowler, 1987).

5.4 Stage 3: Synthetic-Conventional Faith and the Interpersonal Self

Synthetic-conventional faith evolves in late childhood or early adolescence, between the ages of 11 and 13. During this stage, faith development coincides with the child's ability to think abstractly (Burnell, 2013; Fowler, 1981; Straughn, 2010). This stage is also marked by an awareness of the interiority of oneself and others in terms of personality traits, ideas and experiences (Croucher, 2003; Fowler, 1984, 1987). Furthermore, it coincides with a broader social perspective of life (Fowler, 1984, 1987). As young individuals develop their interpersonal perspective, they also attune themselves to the expectations of significant others around them, such as teachers, parents and peers. Due to a greater connection to others and more advanced self-knowledge, the individual experiences feelings of being linked to what Fowler refers to as *ultimacy* (Dykstra, 1982; Fowler, 1981, p. 153). This stage is referred to as the *faith community stage* (Croucher, 2010). Individuals primarily conform to majority views and are attuned to the judgement and external authority of significant others. Beliefs are often stereotyped, and individuals feel that the rules have to be followed (Croucher, 2003; Fowler, 1981).

5.5 Stage 4: Individuative-Reflective Faith and the Institutional Self

Individuative-reflective faith most often develops in young adulthood but could also emerge during the 30s or 40s. The transition depends on changes in the individual that coincide with the development of an executive ego, which means that individual authority is relocated within the self (Fowler, 1981, 1984). Traditional answers no longer "make sense", and the individual questions previously unquestioned beliefs. The rational ability develops to evaluate tradition critically, and as such, this stage may also be referred to as the *rational constructs stage* (Burnell, 2013; Croucher, 2010; Fowler, 1981). During this stage, two significant changes take place. Firstly, changes regarding the orientation towards the self take place. A new sense of self-authorisation develops instead of the individual being defined by mere social roles. Social relationships are assessed (Fowler, 1984, 1987; Straughn, 2010), reliance on external authority is interrupted and authority is relocated within the self (Fowler,

1981). The second change entails the clarification of one's beliefs, characterised by greater accountability to one's beliefs and values. This process may be disruptive to the social system and confusing for the individual (Fowler, 1981, 1984; Straughn, 2010). A third-person perspective is established, and the individual develops an enhanced recognition of his or her own ideology, as well as an improved understanding of others' ideologies (Fowler, 1981, 1987). This new perspective facilitates the careful appraisal of others' and one's own views and expectations (Dykstra, 1982; Fowler, 1981, 1987). More clarity regarding social boundaries and identity also develops (Straughn, 2010). Fowler (1981) identified certain tensions during this stage, namely, (a) individuality vs. group membership, (b) subjectivity and the power of emotions vs. objectivity and critical reflection, (c) self-fulfilment or self-actualisation vs. service to and for others as primary concern and (d) the question of commitment to the relative vs. struggle with the possibility of an absolute. Transition to this stage is difficult due to the individual's resistance to let go of the authority of others and the fear that relationships may end when the reliance dynamic changes (Fowler, 1981). Anxiety also exists about expressing one's own beliefs, and individuals may feel as if they are abandoning their community (Croucher, 2003; Fowler, 1981, 1987, 2001, 2004). This may result in a traumatising transition for the person (Straughn, 2010). Since this stage involves emotional upheaval, the process may be protracted for 5–7 years (Fowler, 1981). Sometimes only one of the two changes mentioned above occurs, and the individual then stabilises in a transitional position and finds himself/herself caught between the previous stage (i.e. *synthetic-conventional faith*) and this stage (*individuative-reflective faith*) (Dykstra, 1982; Fouché et al., 2016 ; Fowler, 1984).

5.6 Stage 5: Conjunctive Faith and the Interindividual Self

This stage emerges in the mid-stage of life (i.e. 35–40 years) or beyond. It involves a more dialogical and dialectical way of thinking (Fowler, 1981, 1987, 2004) and is based on the work of Nicholas of Cusa (1401–1464) who developed the idea of God as *coincidence of opposites*, the being wherein all opposites and contradictions meet and are reconciled (Fowler, 1984, 1987). This stage is a mature stage of faith development and is rarely reached by individuals (Dykstra, 1982; Mayer, 2017). It is referred to as a *Numinous Supernatural* or *Mysterious Universe* (Croucher, 2010). The individual is no longer reflecting the views of the group or taking an individual stance (Fowler, 1984), but rather grasps the interconnectedness of things (Fouché, Burnell & Van Niekerk, 2015; Fowler, 1981). *Conjunctive faith* allows the individual to come to terms with the dialectical dimensions and paradoxes in faith and allows the individual to manage opposite tensions without collapsing in one direction or another (Burnell, 2013; Fowler, 1981, 1984, 1987). The name of the stage implies that the clarity of boundaries and ideas of the self achieved in the previous stage of faith must be relinquished in order to move towards the re-joining of what may have been separated previously (Fowler, 1981, 1987). Thus, the person strives to unify opposites in beliefs and experience and is open to paradox and the truth in apparent contradiction (Fouché et al., 2016; Fowler, 1984). A more confident ego develops an awareness of the importance of interpersonal respect and the impact of the archetypal unconscious on behaviour. This implies the acceptance of behaviour we may never be able to change, as well as coming to terms with death and our own mortality (Dykstra, 1982; Fowler, 1981; Straughn, 2010). Individuals recognise that the symbols and doctrines of their traditions are partial and incomplete, enabling them to look beyond their own traditions (Fowler, 1981). In *conjunctive faith*, the individual recognises the error of the "old way" and can celebrate the possibility of transformation. However, the person may still have some attachments to the "old way" that may make transformation anxiety-provoking and costly. The danger of *conjunctive faith* is that the individual may become immobilised or stuck between these two opposites. As these individuals long for transformation, their loyalties or commitments to persons or institutions may keep them stuck (Fouché et al., 2016). Individuals stuck in *conjunctive faith* may experience a sense of homelessness or loneliness (Fowler, 1981, 1984). This stage remains divided, living and acting between a vision of a renewed world and the reality of an untransformed world (Fowler, 1981). At this stage, individuals are prepared for interpersonal connections with different persons and can make allegiances beyond their own cultural constraints and taboos (Burnell, 2013; Straughn, 2010).

5.7 Stage 6: Universalising Faith and the God-Grounded Self

Universalising faith is the most mature stage in faith development but is seldom reached (Croucher, 2010; Fowler, 1984). Individuals move beyond the paradoxical awareness and embrace polar tensions (Fowler, 1981, 1984, 1987), also called the *stage of selfless service* (Croucher, 2010). According to Fowler (1984), this stage is best recognised by a radical *decentration* from the self and relinquishment of the self (i.e. an objective way of perceiving the world). As individuals move through the different faith development stages, their circle of "those who count" expands, from the family relations to peers and friends, to those who share their political and religious beliefs and then beyond to humankind (Croucher, 2010; Fowler, 1981, 1984). It implies, "... knowing the world through eyes and experiences of persons, classes, nationalities and faiths quite different from one's own" (Fowler, 1984, p. 69). Individuals display a kind of detachment from self and finite centres of value and are drawn into a new quality of participation and grounding in God or "Principle of Being" (Fowler, 1987; Straughn, 2010). The individual "... participates in a kind of identification with God's way of knowing and valuing other creatures" (Fowler, 1987, p. 75). Universalising faith enables individuals to engage in fellowships with any other person at another stage of faith development and other faith traditions. This stage gives rise to activist efforts to transform unjust social conditions (Dykstra, 1982; Fowler, 1984, 1987). Therefore, people at this stage are often viewed as subversive of political and religious structures and can invest in a greater cause without a concern with personal cost (Croucher, 2010; Fouché et al., 2016).

6 Findings and Discussion: Shame and Faith in Baruch Spinoza's Life

In the following psychobiography, accounts will be presented in the context of Baruch Spinoza's life and work, which respond to the research questions under each life development section:

1. How did Spinoza deal with and transform the experienced shame in his life?
2. How did the development of faith happen in his life?
3. How are shame and faith development connected?
4. Which lessons can be learnt from Spinoza's life for dealing with the new challenges in Industry 4.0?

6.1 Baruch Spinoza's Family Background

Baruch (Benedictus) Spinoza was born on 24 November 1632 in Amsterdam as a son of Jewish Sephardim Marrano immigrants from Portugal; Spinoza died at the age of 45. According to Garrett (1996), Spanish was the cultural language among the Sephardim Marranos, Jews, whose forefathers had been expelled from Spain to Portugal. Spinoza's parents were among those Marranos who forcibly converted to Christianity but, in fact, continued to practice Judaism in secret. After being arrested, tortured and condemned by the inquisition in Portugal, many Sephardim Marranos escaped to Amsterdam (Popkin, 2019), including Spinoza's family.

Baruch's father, Michael Spinoza (born in 1587 in Vidiger, Portugal), was a respected member of the Jewish community in Amsterdam. He earned his living as a merchant who traded in dried citrus fruits (Klever, 1996). They lived in a Jewish community in Amsterdam (Feld, 1989), known as Vlooienburg, where today the Music House and Townhall are erected (Garrett, 1996). Michael was married three times. According to Klever (1996), his first wife, Rachel de Spinoza, died in 1627; his second wife, Hanna Debora Espinosa, died in 1638 (just before Baruch Spinoza's sixth birthday); and, lastly, he was married to Ester d'Espinosa who died in 1653. Two children, Isaac and Rebecca, were born to Michael and Rachel. Baruch, Mirjam and Gabriel were born to Michael and Hanna Debora.

6.2 *Childhood and Adolescence of Baruch Spinoza (1632–1650)*

Sparse information exists on the infancy and early childhood of Baruch, except that his mother died when he was 6 and that he hardly felt at home in the Netherlands since his family always held a migrant status as Jews who fled to escape prosecution (Carlisle, 2011).

In the early years of his childhood, **shame** was most probably experienced by Baruch unconsciously and collectively in terms of belonging to a population group that was prosecuted in earlier decades in different cultures and who had to flee the country of their origins. The experienced marginalisation and exclusion from previous generations of his religious group might have brought a feeling of collective shame to Baruch that might not have occurred consciously. Furthermore, he might have unconsciously experienced collective shame, belonging to a group who was seen as migrants, but also in terms of having to convert officially to a new religion and practice their religion in secrecy. Shame might most probably have been experienced as a collective group shame, co-consciously manifested.

Baruch was the middle son in a prominent family of moderate means and was seen as intellectually gifted (Nadler, 2019). Baruch's mother-tongue was Portuguese, although he also knew Spanish, Dutch, Hebrew and later Latin (Garrett, 1996). He grew up under the watchful eyes of the rabbis of Amsterdam's Portuguese Kehilla. As a child, he attended the elementary school of the United Talmud Torah congregation (Nadler, 2009). At this Jewish school, founded in 1638 (Popkin, 2019), Baruch was particularly educated in theology and commerce (Deleuze, 1988). As Judaism was included in the curriculum, Baruch probably was also taught Hebrew and Jewish philosophy (Popkin, 2019). According to Nadler (2019), Baruch was groomed for a career as a Rabbi and, at the age of 15, was seen as one of the most brilliant pupils of Rabbi Saul Levi Morteira (Ratner, 2011). However, he never achieved to pass the upper levels of the curriculum, which required the advanced study of the Talmud, because he was too critical and claimed that the Bible was rather insufficient and unsatisfactory (Ratner, 2011). At the age of 17, after the death of his elder brother Isaac, he was forced to cut short his formal studies to assist with the running of the family's import business, also grinding glass lenses (Nadler, 2019).

He might have experienced shame by dropping out of the Jewish educational system, not coming to pass the upper levels of the curriculum (Nadler, 2019); however, no evidence could be found about this in the literature.

About the primal **FD** stage, nothing is known about Baruch, the pregnancy and his mother's experiences during pregnancy, including his first unconscious experiences of trust and mistrust and the experiences of the mother as a super-ordinate power (Fowler, 1981, 1984). It is assumed that Baruch grew up close to his mother until her death.

Concerning his faith, Baruch was educated and brought up in the context of Judaism which can be viewed as his base for language learning, his base to stories and symbols and the formation of reality and meaning (as in Burnell, 2013; Fowler, 1981, 1984) and which is connected with stage 1 (Fowler, 1981). Since he grew up in the Jewish community who was in a state of exile, it might be assumed that Baruch was able to form a long-standing emotional bond with Judaism and its image orientations, as well as connotations to faith (Burnell, 2013; Fouché et al., 2016; Fowler, 1981, 1987; Straughn, 2010). Although he could learn complex issues and develop his cognitive skills well, being supported by the United Talmud Torah congregation (Nadler, 2009), Baruch must have experienced a break regarding his faith when, at the age of 6, he experienced that his father did not give him the inheritance of his late mother that was rightfully his, nor "did he receive any capital" returns (Cohen, 2002, p. 146). Baruch must have experienced this as a shame for himself as the son of his mother and also as a break with the religious beliefs and traditions. The decision of the father and the Jewish community to keep the inheritance with the father and not to share it with Baruch was probably based on the fact that the father belonged to the Jewish elite, viewed as a responsible businessman who, at the same time, held various important positions in the Jewish community (Cohen, 2002).

Due to life circumstances, Baruch did not advance his studies in Talmud. Still, he was groomed as a future Rabbi (Nadler, 2019) due to his brilliant intelligence and his leadership potential for the Jewish community, holding a deeper understanding of the religious meanings, as explained in Fowler's stage 2 of FDT, which usually occurs between 10 and 12 years of age (Fowler, 1981). Furthermore, Baruch probably strongly relied on stories, values and rules (Dykstra, 1982; Fowler, 1984) of the immediate Jewish community since this community was relatively closed and a strong frame of reference for his life experiences (Fowler, 1987). Since children at this stage do not possess a sense of themselves as separate personalities, but rather a sense of who they are in context to their experiences and the stories related to their family and community (Fowler, 1987), the religious belonging might have given Baruch strengths to grow and develop within his strict religious context.

Stage 3 in FDT usually evolves between 11 and 13 years of age, and as Baruch, individuals in this stage usually conform to majority views and are attuned to the judgement and external authority of significant others (Croucher, 2003; Fowler, 1981). Since Baruch went to a Jewish primary school with strict traditions and focused on the Jewish curriculum, it can be assumed that at this age, he conformed to the majority religious assumptions.

The first signs of stage 4 of FD are visibly acknowledged in Baruch from the age of 17 years when he had to take over the family business. This shift in his life brought about the relocation of authority within himself (Fowler, 1981, 1984), and he used his time at the business to think about theology, philosophy and religion (Deleuze, 2001). This stage, however, turned into full swing in early adulthood.

6.3 Early Adulthood (1650–1660)

After the death of Baruch's father in 1654, he and his brother Gabriel managed the family business (Garrett, 1996). During his early adulthood, Baruch started critically evaluating tradition (Ratner, 2011), as presented in Fowler's **stage 4** as *rational constructs stage* (Burnell, 2013; Croucher, 2010; Fowler, 1981). In early adulthood, he developed a new orientation towards himself, a self-authorisation which allowed him to cross the boundaries of the previously defined social roles he had to adapt to. With the death of his father, a shift in the family relationships occurred due to running the business with his brother Gabriel and his renunciation of the father's inheritance (Cohen, 2002). The shift towards full responsibility of the business and the experience of the death of his father might have supported a new assessment of the social relationship (as in Fowler, 1984, 1987; Straughn, 2010), as well as the experience of disruption of external authority in his life. By this strong relocation of authority within himself, he analysed, criticised and questioned not only the social community but also the religion and the assumption of religious authority within the community (Ratner, 2011). During this time, he also clarified his own belief system (as described in Fowler, 1981, 1987), which is typical in this FD stage. Spinoza was soon seen as a threat and dangerous influence by the leaders of the Jewish community since he had different perspectives on the Jewish religion and believed that God did not create the world, but that the world was part of God (Carlisle, 2011). This movement is often described as Pantheism, which includes the idea that God and the world are one—however, Spinoza distinguished his thoughts and maintained that God and the world are two (Carlisle, 2011). He argues that God and the world are not two different entities, but merely two different aspects of a single reality, which countered Christian and Jewish worldviews (Carlisle, 2011).

Despite mainly being educated in Hebrew in his childhood, he was also taught Latin by an anonymous German in early adulthood, who opened the world of thinkers and philosophers to him, such as Descartes. Ratner (2011) states that Franciscus van den Enden (1602–1674)—a Dutch Jesuit, Neo-Latin poet, physician, philosopher and art dealer—became a great influencer of Spinoza who taught a few selected students Latin and ethical-political realism. Until today, there is a huge controversy around the question of who influenced whom—Spinoza Van den Enden or vice versa (Gullan-Whur, 2000; Klever, 1990; Meinsma, 1983).

Through these new influences, Baruch gained an improved understanding of others' ideologies (Fowler, 1981, 1987) and facilitated his own views and expectations (Dykstra, 1982; Fowler, 1981, 1987). Within this context, Baruch redefined his identity and shifted the social boundaries, described as an important step during this stage (as in Straughn, 2010). This led to strong tensions between himself, his family and the (religious) community and, according to Fowler (1981), the tensions manifested. According to Gullan-Whur (2000), Spinoza was a very arrogant and ascetic person who was divided by the need for love and solitude, sexual feeling and self-discipline, as well as reasoned and mystical approaches to God. Due to his specific perspective on the Bible and God, he was caught up in tensions about individuality and group membership (a) (Fowler, 1981). However, he also felt torn about the subjectivity and the power of emotions, objectivity and critical reflection and experienced tensions about how to deal with emotions and reason simultaneously (b) (Fowler, 1981). Spinoza suffered from emotional outbursts, as well as the ideal of ascesis and reason (Gullan-Whur, 2000).

Furthermore, Spinoza was highly occupied with self-fulfilment and self-actualisation, always seeking for the truth and new knowledge (Gullan-Whur, 2000), rather than developing a primary concern of service to and for others, which created tensions within himself and interpersonally between himself, other family members and the community (c) (Fowler, 1981). Parts of Spinoza's struggle and inner divides were also concerned with the question of commitment to the relative vs. the struggle with the possibility of an absolute (d) (Fowler, 1981). He, however, came to the decision that man should strive for the eternal totality, thereby referring to God as an endless, limitless and boundless energy (The Book of Life, 2020) and thereby leaned rather towards the absolute than towards relativity.

Fowler (1981) emphasises that the transition of stage 4 is often difficult due to the individual's resistance to letting go of the authority of others and the fear that relationships may end when the reliance dynamics change (Fowler, 1981). However, concerning Spinoza, this is not necessarily true since he clearly took for a stance towards his own argument and accepted the excommunication—the *cherem*[1] was launched by the leaders of the Jewish community in 1656 when Spinoza was aged 23 (Ratner, 2011)—from his religious group, consciously knowing that he had thereby lost his career as a member and also as a potential religious leader within the community (Deleuze, 1988; Garret, 1996; Gullan-Whur, 2000; Klever, 1996). He had to cope with feelings of abandonment of the community (Croucher, 2003; Fowler, 1981, 1987, 2001, 2004). He was thus personally abandoned from a group that had previously experienced collective exclusion from different countries too. He was therefore abandoned twice: as a group member on collective and as an individual on individual levels. It can be assumed that Spinoza's **experiences of shame** might have erupted fully with the confrontational discourses with the Jewish leaders about religion, worldviews and the concept of God, as well as the interpretation of the Hebrew Bible (Ratner, 2011). The event of excommunication must have been experienced as very shameful for him and his family since he was marginalised and excluded by his social and religious group of belonging (Bahrs & Henze, 2019), as well as from his family; which must have been a very painful experience (Lewis, 2011). It impacted strongly on his entire self, his life and his identity (Deonna et al., 2012). However, when the excommunication was spelt out, he was not in Amsterdam but, later on, wrote a letter responding with "grace and humour of a cultured mind", taking the action of changing his name from Hebrew "Baruch" to Latin "Benedict" (Ratner, 2011, p. 2), indicating his shift in identity, his new orientations.

[1]Cherem is defined as one of the three forms of ecclesiastical excommunication and seen as its most severe form, used by rabbis or other officials of a synagogue or community, in sentencing wrongdoers, usually for an indefinite period of time (Merriam-Webster Dictionary, 2020).

From thereon, he referred to the Jews as "the race (to) which he did not belong" (Ratner, 2011, p. 2), taking the excommunication as a conscious act of boundary-spanning. It can also be assumed that Baruch took the excommunication as a self-developmental step, developing a rather positive, active and healthy attitude towards the abandonment, using it to self-develop, opening up new worlds and social relationships and transforming the shame towards the establishment of his own philosophy and religious concepts and for the betterment of himself and the people (as described in Marks, 2011). Through his pain of abandonment from the community and the family, he aimed at being true to himself, seeking deeper understanding, knowledge and truth, thus working on himself, increasing his self-awareness, the reaffirmation and reframing of authority and truth, self-responsibility, meaning creation, self-transcendence and deeper understanding of himself and his emotions (as suggested by Wong, 2019). Baruch took on a PP2.0 perspective, working through the pain and vulnerability (Wong, 2016) to develop his own faith and theory of God and nature, which contributed to the healing of shame and a deeper development of faith and self-worth (as in Fowler, 1981; Mayer, 2017; Ryan, 2019).

6.4 *Middle Adulthood (1660–1677) to His Death Aged 45*

In continuation of van den Ende's tradition, Spinoza enjoyed the ideas of the Italian political insurgent Masaniello (1622–1647)—who fought against the rule of Habsburg Spain in Naples, Italy—as well as Machiavelli's (1469–1527) influence, who saw religion only as a political tool to establish social order (Machiavelli, 1513/2013). Spinoza's political mindset was influenced by Machiavelli's political philosophy, which referred to morals, religion, the establishment of power and real-life political scenario rather than philosophical principles (Machiavelli, 1513/2013). Spinoza's approach to gender, gender inequality and misogyny (Gullan-Whur, 2000) has often been discussed, since he described women as unequal to men and excluded them from participation in politics (Gullan-Whur, 2002), arguing that women were disempowered by nature, excluding them from democratic participation in society (Lord, 2011).[2]

During the last years of his life, Spinoza wrote his book *Ethics* (Spinoza, 1677/2001), which is said to be the most remarkable and important book in the history of philosophy because it is multidisciplinary, drawing on metaphysics, knowledge, philosophical psychology, moral philosophy and political philosophy, referring to God, nature, human being and happiness. Nadler (2009) highlighted that Spinoza's

[2]This discourse is not deepened here due to its relative irrelevance to faith development and shame issues. However, it might be important that the degradation of women in Spinoza's mindset might be related to the early death of the mother, the patriarchic upbringing in the Jewish community and the frustrations with love relationships of Spinoza which might have caused him to feel shamed and unfaithful with regard to his involvement with women on a personal note. Please see Gullan-Whur (2000, 2002) for a detailed insight.

approach is still relevant today since he highlighted that salvation can only be reached when humans expand their minds towards an intuitive understanding of God in interaction with nature and its laws (Carlisle, 2011). Spinoza challenged the main tenets of Judaism by highlighting that God is not a person who stands outside nature and by rejecting the assumption that there is anyone to hear the prayers, to create miracles and to punish humans for misdeeds (Spinoza, 1677/2001). Spinoza also emphasised that there is no afterlife, that man is not God's chosen creature and that the Bible was written by ordinary individuals (Spinoza, 1677/2001). Carlisle (2011) further points out that Spinoza, within his writings, argued for a life based on spiritual practice aiming to reach happiness and liberation. He also emphasised that the representation of God as a person is a projected imagination. He did not see himself as an atheist, but rather created his own idea of God which contains the perspective that God is found in a deep interdisciplinary understanding which should not only be viewed under the aspect of time (*sub specie durationis*), but rather under the aspect of eternity (*sub specie aeternitatis*), thus participating in eternal totality (The Book of Life, 2020).

This worldview and interpretation of God and life in the context of nature can be seen as an important aspect of Spinoza's conjunctive **faith (stage 5)** and the development of the interindividual self, as described in stage 5 of Fowler's stage theory. Although this stage is rarely reached by individuals (Dykstra, 1982; Mayer, 2017), it can be assumed that Spinoza expressed this stage through no longer reflecting the views of the group or taking an individual stance (Fowler, 1984), but rather grasps the interconnectedness of things (as described in Fouché et al., 2015; Fowler, 1981). Through his belief and writings on ethics, Spinoza showed his ability to re-join different sciences and gain an interdisciplinary understanding of ethics and faith (Spinoza, 1677/2001), typical to stage 5, trying to find the truth in apparent contradictions (Fouché et al., 2016; Fowler, 1984). He envisioned a life based on freedom, being free from guilt, sorrow, pity and shame (The Book of Life, 2020). His major work laid the groundwork for the eighteenth-century Enlightening movement as well as for modern biblical criticism, having been indexed by the Catholic Church after its publication (Ratner, 2011).

As indicated for stage 5, Spinoza also created an awareness of the importance of interpersonal respect towards his community, his family and the elders and saw the impact of the archetypal unconscious on behaviour. He referred to shame as a feeling, not as a virtue, and considered it as good because it shows that the person who feels shame inherits a desire to live honourably (Rotenstreich, 1965). However, shame shows that the concern for the opinion of others is too big (Deigh, 1983). Furthermore, he viewed shame as a very painful emotion that is related to a person's action which others might blame (Isenberg, 1949). Spinoza, therefore, clusters shame as a passion that is "sad", thus lowering the energy and decreasing the power of a person to act and to think, since the focus is on the pain which does not only diminish the power of the person but also strives to decrease the power of the people surrounding the person (Sullivan, 2011). Accordingly, Spinoza defines shame as a "weakness of the spirit" (*animi impotentia*) (Green, 2016, p. 80). It is viewed as an opposite to honour but can, according to Spinoza, motivate a person to act morally (Green, 2016) and therefore might be seen as an experience with a positive aspect or even a resource for transformation.

Spinoza further views shame in the context of regret as well as sympathy and evaluates it as a partly positive emotion. It is also seen as a universal emotion without interpersonal dimensions. This is based on the perspective that since the person is a part of God, as well as part of the universal system, shame is not only part of interpersonal relationships, but rather a universal emotion (Hartmann, 1984). Spinoza accepted shame as a "sad passion" and agreed with several authors (Dykstra, 1982; Fowler, 1981; Straughn, 2010) highlighting (as typical for stage 5 in FDT) that the individual implies the acceptance of behaviour, which they may never be able to change, as well as come to terms with death and their own mortality. Cohen (2002), for example, emphasises that Spinoza has highlighted that there is no behaviour in humans he has not seen and that he is prepared to accept humans' behaviour (no matter how it plays out). However, it might be assumed that Spinoza struggled his entire life with the rigidness and narrow-minded view of the Jewish community on his extraordinary religious viewpoints and with his (philosophical) enemies who worked against the publishing of his last book during his lifetime (Nadler, 2019).

Spinoza recognised that the symbols and doctrines of his traditions are partial and incomplete and was able to look beyond his own traditions, even defining himself in a very new view with a different perspective (Fowler, 1981). He recognised the errors in his community of faith and celebrated his own transition, as stated in Fowler (1981). At the same time, he also felt loyalties and commitments to certain individuals from the Jewish community, such as his family who had banned him—however, he did not feel stuck in *conjunctive faith* (Fowler, 1981), but felt a sense of homelessness and loneliness at times (Fowler, 1981, 1984). He envisioned a renewed worldview, but saw—not at least due to his excommunication—that the broader community is still bound to an untransformed world (Fowler, 1981), which led to negative emotional responses and frustrated him (Feuer, 2017). He built relationships within a new community of thinkers (Feuer, 2017), as described by Fowler (1981, 1987), and made allegiances beyond their own cultural constraints and taboos (Burnell, 2013; Straughn, 2010). According to Damasio (2003), he belonged nowhere and everywhere at the same time.

Concerning the experience of **SH** and based on his exclusion from the community, he most likely transformed this shame in middle adulthood further towards a source of personal growth and energy. He did not get caught up in feelings of anxiety, frustration, irritation, anxiety and fear or depression, but used the exclusion to rebuild himself; to develop his thinking, new relationships and friendships; and to learn and transform the negative feeling of shame towards a source of personal growth (Feuer, 2017). Through his philosophy, he attempted to create a new mindset and spirituality which freed individuals from shame as a community-based negative feeling (Ratner, 2011). However, it is assumed that, based on the changing environmental and political aspects in the Netherlands, he died lonely and frustrated due to an illness caused by working with glass fibre. It might further be assumed that had he not died that early; he might have even transformed further in FD towards stage 6.

7 Conclusions and Recommendations

This study aimed to contribute to psychobiographical research on Baruch Spinoza with special regard to shame and faith development in his life. Also, the study aimed to explore what the lessons learnt from Spinoza's life (also referring to Negri, 2020) could be for the times of Industry 4.0—in which diversity and counteracting worldviews increase and in which people can also see a radicalisation in movements towards one's own group and belief system. This point will be addressed within the conclusions. The following can be concluded regarding the research questions:

7.1 How did Spinoza Deal with and Transform the Experienced Shame in His Life?

The experience of shame can be described as follows in Baruch Spinoza's life:

During childhood and teenage years, Spinoza mainly experienced shame about his own group, albeit an unconscious, collective shame that impacted him, being a member of a prosecuted group living in exile. On an intrapersonal level, it might have also been shameful for him that he did not inherit his share from his late mother since the father kept his inheritance for himself. It might also have been shameful for him that he could not finalise his studies of the Talmud due to personal circumstances. Baruch most probably experienced shame on collective and individual levels in more or less conscious ways. Since there is hardly any reference to Baruch's personal feelings during this time of his life, these assumptions are interpretative.

In early adulthood, Baruch might have experienced shame because he criticised his Jewish religious leaders and later due to his excommunication from the group. Although not shown to the outside world, this exclusion from his group of origin must have caused deeply experienced shame in himself. However, he managed to transform this shame by opening new doors for himself, deepening his knowledge, getting into new social relationships, self-developing and working for his own betterment and the development of his theory of faith, understanding of the world, meaning and God. He managed successfully to work through the experienced pain (as described by Wong in PP2.0) to grow in new areas and further develop.

Finally, in middle adulthood, Baruch worked towards a world free of shame and the transformation through shame towards a greater self-development, inner freedom, betterment of self, self-worth and new perspectives and learnings. He finally saw shame as an opportunity to develop honour and morals and to free the spirit from the weaknesses that are expressed by the experience of shame (Table 13.1).

Table 13.1 Spinoza's SH

Baruch Spinoza's life development	Shame experience
The childhood, adolescence and teenage years (1632–1650, until aged 17)	• (Unconscious) collective shame experience based on marginalisation and exclusion from the Jewish community in Spain and Portugal • Shame when his father did not give him the inheritance from his late mother nor his capital returns later on in his life • Shame of stopping his advanced studies due to family circumstances
Adolescence and early adulthood (1650–1660, aged 18–28 years)	• Individual shame experience due to critical view on own religion and excommunication from the Jewish community • He renounced the inheritance of the father aged 22 when the father died, not believing in possessions and not wanting further involvement in inheritance court cases (Cohen, 2002) • Shame of being excommunicated by the Jewish community and leaving the family business behind, becoming a craftsman • Transforming shame towards self-development, inner freedom, betterment of self, self-worth and new perspectives and learnings
Middle adulthood (1660–1677, aged 28–45), death at the age of 45 years	• Transforming shame towards self-development, inner freedom, betterment of self, self-worth and new perspectives and learnings • Striving to a life free of shame, defining it as a chance to live honourably • Transforming shame as a "weakness of the spirit" towards a proactive attitude, a desire for honour and moral behaviour

7.2 How Did the Development of Faith Happen in His Life?

In his childhood and teenage years, Baruch grew up strongly involved in the Jewish community, being supported and promoted by the Rabbis due to his intellectual abilities. However, he quickly developed through Fowler's stages of FDT to reach stage 4 already early in adolescence. Having firstly developed strongly framed within the Jewish community's belief and their conventional interpretations of symbols, meaning and life, Baruch already reached stage 4 of FDT during teenage years, criticising the interpretations, relocating the authority within himself, criticising traditional religious interpretations and ways to understand God and becoming a threat to the Jewish community.

In early adulthood, Spinoza gained new knowledge by learning Latin, which opened up new philosophies and new thinking to him. The death of his father led to a final break with the Jewish community and his excommunication from religion and also from the family business. By taking up a new profession, namely, becoming a lens maker and craftsman, the teachings of Van den Enden on philosophy and

Table 13.2 Spinoza's FD

Baruch Spinoza's life development	Faith development stages in Baruch Spinoza						
	Stage 0	Stage 1	Stage 2	Stage 3	Stage 4	Stage 5	Stage 6
The childhood, adolescence and teenage years (1632–1650, until aged 17)	x	x	x	x	x		
Adolescence and early adulthood (1650–1660, aged 18–28 years)					x	x	
Middle adulthood (1660–1677, aged 28–45), death at the age of 45 years						x	

political realism and the joining of a club of gifted scholars, Baruch fully advanced into stage 4 of the FDT, shifted social boundaries and redefined his identity and meaning in life. Fowler (1981) highlighted four aspects, which usually lead to tensions during this state of mind, with the literature analysis also showing that Baruch experienced all four tensions during early adulthood, as shown in the analysis. The working through the pain must have led Baruch to a stronger faith and the urge to develop his own theory.

During middle adulthood, Spinoza established the idea that conventional religion existed only to establish social order—from a political philosophy viewpoint—and aimed at developing a theory which contributed to the meaningfulness of God and nature as integrated parts which is a central part of stage 5 in Fowler's FDT, grasping the interconnectedness of the systems in the world, showing an interdisciplinary knowledge and understanding, exploring contradictions and truths and envisioning a life based on freedom, free from guilt, sorrow, pity and shame. He saw the incompleteness of the doctrines of the Jewish religion and celebrated his own transition towards a new understanding and knowledge, sometimes getting frustrated with his enemies and the rigidness of the Jewish community.

It might be assumed that, had he lived longer, he would have had the potential to reach stage 6 of the FDT (Table 13.2).

7.3 How Are Shame and Faith Development Connected?

SH and FD appear to be connected topics in the life of Spinoza. In childhood and adolescence, shame is strongly connected to the experiences of his primary religious group of belonging, and collective and individual shame is experienced based on collective religious shame experiences in connection with faith. Individual shame is experienced by the breaking of the traditions and religious laws, not inherited from his mother and through breaking through the principles of faith believed by his religious reference groups. Thus, shame is intertwined on collective and individual levels (intra- and interpersonal experiences). During early adulthood, Spinoza experienced shame based on his public break with his religious group of belonging, by renouncing his inheritance from his father, as traditional in Judaism, and by leaving behind the family business. Again, all of these aspects are bound to his childhood faith system and the foundations of faith by his primary group of belonging. At the same time, the excommunication freed him from his entire sociocultural and economic system and provided him with the freedom to transform shame through self-development and through the development of his own theoretical framework, which provided him with the strengths and worldview to transform his shameful experiences into a fruitful new worldview. The development of his own reference to faith simultaneously allowed him to transform his emotions. Lastly, his new social environment strengthened him too in transforming both faith and shame and coming up with new frames of references for the integration of new cognitive and emotional concepts: transformation based on pain towards joy, happiness and new meaningfulness in life (Table 13.3).

7.4 *Which Lessons Can Be Learnt from Spinoza's Life for Dealing with the New Challenges in Industry 4.0?*

The following learnings can be taken from Spinoza's life developments in terms of SH, SH transformation and FD for the changing societies in the twenty-first century within the context of Industry 4.0.

7.4.1 The Person and Personal Development of Spinoza

Spinoza, as an extraordinary person of great giftedness, can be seen as a role model for contemporary gifted learners who are congenial thinkers, and creative and innovative contributors to contemporary society with an approach of liberal thinking (Ratner, 2011), which is particularly needed in times of technological and digital revolutions and new settings of human-machine interaction. Spinoza can be a role model in terms of ethics, moral and honourable behaviour and the transformation of negative experiences, thoughts and emotions towards positive impact and self-development.

7.4.2 Topics of Spinoza for Contemporary Society

Spinoza's lessons to be learnt deal with the defining and redefining of concepts such as meaning, meaningfulness, religion and faith; the rational function and utility of the human mind and humankind; the importance of critical thought within societal development, hesitation and change; and the emotional and cognitive strengths needed to transform challenges and pain towards positive concepts, based on

Table 13.3 Spinoza's FD, SH and SH transformation

Baruch Spinoza's life development	Learnings for dealing with faith development and shame in the Fourth Industrial Revolution	
	Faith	Shame
The childhood, adolescence and teenage years (1632–1650, until aged 17)	*Stage 0 to stage 4* Faith development within the strict communities of Jewish rabbis Break in faith regarding Jewish traditions and rituals when he did not inherit the mother's inheritance Religious Jewish community as a strong frame of reference At 17 years, a shift of authority to relocate within himself (taking over the business from the late brother)	• (Unconscious) collective shame experience based on marginalisation and exclusion for the Jewish community in Spain and Portugal • Shame when his father did not give him the inheritance from his mother nor his capital returns later on in his life • Shame of stopping his advanced studies due to family circumstances
Adolescence and early adulthood (1650–1660, aged 18–28 years)	*Stage 4 and partly stage 5* Judaism as a base to interpret meaning, stories and symbols strongly established through the Jewish community in exile, educational system and promotion of his strong abilities Conscious break with faith and religious traditions by renouncing the inheritance of his father Break with Judaism through strong critical views on the interpretation of the Talmud	• Individual shame experience due to critical view on own religion and excommunication from the Jewish community • He renounced the inheritance from the father aged 22 when the father died, not believing in possessions and not wanting further involvement in inheritance court cases (Cohen, 2002) • Shame of being excommunicated by the Jewish community and leaving the family business behind, becoming a craftsman • Transforming shame towards self-development, inner freedom, betterment of self, self-worth and new perspectives and learnings
Middle adulthood (1660–1677, aged 28–45), death at the age of 45 years	*Stage 5* Developing his own theory and philosophy of ethics Integrating conventional learnings and newly learnt philosophies Creating interdisciplinary knowledge and views on faith with a systemic approach of interconnectedness of the world, humans, nature and God	• Transforming shame towards self-development, inner freedom, betterment of self, self-worth and new perspectives and learnings • Striving to a life free of shame, defining it as a chance to live honourably • Transforming shame as a "weakness of the spirit" towards a proactive attitude, a desire for honour and moral behaviour

courage which is to the extent of excommunication relatively seldom seen in individuals, acting against the collective group's faith and threats to life, thus implementing innovative thoughts "in a religious spirit and calm manner", as Spinoza did (Ratner, 2011, p. 8).

Furthermore, his philosophy is important for the contemporary world, since its central idea is that all things are determined in nature, seeing God as identical with the universe, nature and humans. According to Spinoza, "if man is to be free, he must be guided by the laws of his own being" (Ratner, 2011, p. 11). Thus, for a world that becomes more and more driven by robots, artificial intelligence and technology, humankind needs to re-think and overthink processes occurring in contemporary society. Spinoza can remind us of our origin, our connectedness and our universal being and guide us in an environmental, spiritual, respectful and honourable way to treat the environment, which includes humans, as elements of the entire system.

Faith, in Spinoza's as well as in Fowler's mind, refers to the human activity of composing a meaningful world, with fruitful visions and values, based on faith. This seems to be often missing in Industry 4.0-driven societies that strive for speed, technological innovation and action, no time to think through new concepts of meaning and visions which are sustainable and human in nature.

As Nadler (2019) highlighted, Spinoza's approach is still relevant today; salvation can only be reached when humans expand their minds towards an intuitive understanding of God in interaction with nature and its laws (Carlisle, 2011). New concepts of contemporary societies and Industry 4.0 require extraordinary thinkers who remind us of faith, God, nature and intuitive understanding, particularly when robots and machines (still) seem to miss this. They remind us of the importance of thinkers who think "out of the box", who dare to counteract rising trends and fast-speeding actions, extraordinary individuals who have the courage to be innovative rather than productive.

Spinoza challenged the main tenets of Judaism by highlighting that God is not a person who stands outside nature and by rejecting the assumption that there is anyone to hear the prayers, to create miracles and to punish humans for misdeeds. Radical self-responsibility regarding faith and regarding concepts of God to sustain life on earth is needed, which Spinoza calls for. Spinoza, in these days of contemporary society, could even guide nonbelievers to return to God and guide churches and other religious institutions to become attractive again to nonbelievers by displaying the integration of science and religion, God and nature, humans and God, subsequently presenting valuable concepts which support morals and ethics within a digitalised, technology-driven world which seems to be far removed from nature, self and any belief that goes beyond the ego and the self. Spinoza can guide humans more than ever, the ever-stressed and burnt-out individuals, based on his idea of spiritual practice aiming to reach happiness and liberation (Carlisle, 2011).

God, according to Spinoza, is found in a deep interdisciplinary understanding which should not only be viewed under the aspect of time (*sub specie durationis*) but rather under the aspect of eternity (*sub specie aeternitatis*), evidently participating in eternal totality (The Book of Life, 2020). Therefore, Spinoza represents what is needed in today's complex world for its own good. It needs complex understanding, a knowledge that is human-based and founded in values which think beyond the present day and which think eternally and thereby support sustainability and the love for upcoming generations, which should experience joy and happiness as the most important meaning in life.

Spinoza finally stands in for individuals who work across boundaries and who are transdisciplinary, but also transcultural, trans-lingual, transformed and (self-) developed and spiritual in nature, building their relationship to the world through combining faith and science and through innovation, independent thinking and creativity overcoming negative emotions, such as shame, transforming them while self-developing towards a higher consciousness that strives for the interweaving of all things. With this approach, the driving of technologised environments can work well when based on that complex understanding with a loving attitude and "joyful passions" on the one hand (Spinoza, 1677/2001) and the revolutionary, critical view of Spinoza (Negri, 2020) on the other hand. This requires more in-depth research, which will support these ideas through further empirical investigations.

References

Bahrs, O. & Henze, K.-H. (2019). From shame to pride – Initiation of de-stigmatisation processes in review dialogues. In C. -H. Mayer & E. Vanderheiden (Eds.), *The bright side of shame. Transforming and growing through practical applications in cultural contexts* (pp. 363–380). Cham: Springer.

Burnell, B. (2013). *The Life of Beyers Naudé: A Psychobiographical study*. Unpublished Doctoral dissertation. Submitted in fulfilment of the requirements for the degree of Philosophiae Doctor in Psychology. Faculty of the Humanities, at the University of the Free State, Bloemfontein, RSA.

Campbell, H. A., & Garner, S. (2016). *Networked theology (engaging culture): Negotiating faith in digital culture*. Grand Rapids, MI: Baker Academic.

Carlisle, C. (2011, February 7). Spinoza, part 1: Philosophy as a way of life. *The Guardian*. Retrieved from https://www.theguardian.com/commentisfree/belief/2011/feb/07/spinoza-philosophy-god-world

Coates, K. S., & Morrison, B. (2016). *Dream factories. Why universities won't solve the youth job crisis*. Toronto, ON: Dundurn.

Coetzee, M. (2019). *Thriving for digital workspaces. Emerging issues for research and practice*. Cham: Springer.

Cohen, A. (2002). The excommunication of Baruch Spinoza: A struggle between Jewish and Civil Law. In J. Israel & R. Salverda (Eds.), *Dutch Jewry. Its history and secular culture (1500-2000)*. Leiden: Brill.

Croucher, R. (2003). *Fowler's stages of faith in profile*. Retrieved from: http://www.jmm.aaa.net.au/articles/2219.htm [5 Aug 2011].

Croucher, R. (2010). *Fowler's stages of faith*. Retrieved from http://jmma.aaa.net.au/Articles/23318.htm [24 Dec 2019].

Damasio, A. (2003). *Looking for Spinoza: Joy, sorrow, and the feeling brain*. Orlando, FL: Harcourt.

Deigh, J. (1983). Shame and self-esteem: A critique. Ethics. *An International Journal of Social, Political, and Legal Philosophy, 93*(2), 225–245.

Deleuze, G. (1988). *Spinoza: Practical philosophy* (pp. 3–14). San Francisco: City Lights Publications.

Deleuze, G. (2001). Life of Spinoza. In: G. Lloyd (Ed.), *Spinoza: Critical Assessments of Leading Philosophers* (pp. 100–110). London: Routledge.

Deonna, J., Rodogno, R., & Teroni, F. (2012). *In defense of shame.* Oxford: Oxford University Press.

Dykstra, C. R. (1982). Transformation in faith and morals. *Theology Today, 39*(1), 56–64.

Elms, A. C. (1994). *Uncovering lives: The uneasy alliance of biography and psychology.* New York: Oxford University Press.

Elms, A. C. (2007). Psychobiography and case study methods. In R. W. Robbins, R. Fraley, & R. F. Krueger (Eds.), *Handbook of research methods in personality psychology* (pp. 97–113). New York: Guilford Press.

Feld, E. (1989). Spinoza the Jew. *Modern Judaism, 9*(1), 101–119.

Feuer, L. S. (2017). *Spinoza and the rise of liberalism.* New York: Routledge.

Fouché, J.P., Burnell, B. & Van Niekerk, R. (2015). The spiritual wellness of Beyers Naudé: A psychobiographical study of a South African anti-apartheid theologian. *Journal of Psychology in Africa, 25* (5), x–xx. https://doi.org/10.1080/14330237.2015.110126

Fouché, J. P., Burnell, B., Van Niekerk, R., & Nortjé, N. (2016). The faith development of the anti-apartheid theologian Beyers Naudé: A psychobiography. *Spirituality in Clinical Practice, 3*(4), 276–288. https://doi.org/10.1037/scp0000105.

Fouché, J. P., & Van Niekerk, R. (2010). Academic psychobiography in South Africa: Past, present and future. *South African Journal of Psychology, 40*(4), 495–507.

Fowler, J. W. (1981). *Stages of faith: The psychology of human development and the quest for meaning.* San Francisco: Harper & Row.

Fowler, J. W. (1984). *Becoming adult, becoming Christian. Adult development and Christian faith.* New York: Harper-Collins.

Fowler, J. W. (1987). *Faith development and pastoral care.* Philadelphia, PA: Fortress Press.

Fowler, J. W. (2001). Faith development theory and postmodern changes. *International Journal for the Psychology of Religion, 11*(3), 159–172.

Fowler, J. W. (2004). Faith development at 30: Naming the challenges of faith in a new millennium. *Religious Education, 99*(4), 405–421.

Freud, S. (1930). Das Unbehagen in der Kultur. In A. Freud & E. Bibring (Eds.), *Gesammelte Werke. Chronologisch geordnet (XIV: Werke aus den Jahren 1925–1931), hg. von Anna Freud u.a.* (pp. 1948–1968). London.

Freund, R.R. & Gill, C.S. (2018). Understanding the development of spirituality, religion, and faith in the client's life. In C. S. Gill & R. R. Freund (Eds.), *Spirituality and religion in counselling. Competency-based strategies for ethical practice.* New York: Routledge.

Garrett, D. (1996). *The Cambridge companion to Spinoza.* Cambridge, UK: Cambridge University Press.

Green, K. (2016). Spinoza on self-hatred. *The Jerusalem Philosophical Quarterly, 65*, 73–95.

Gullan-Whur, M. (2000). *Within reason: A life of Spinoza.* New York: St Martins Press.

Gullan-Whur, M. (2002). Spinoza and the equality of women. *Theoria, 68*(2), 91–111.

Hartmann, F. (1984). The corporeality of shame Px and Hx at the bedside. *The Journal of Medicine & Philosophy, 9*(1), 63–74.

Holm-Hadulla, R. M. (2012). Goethe's anxieties, depressive episodes and (self-) therapeutic strategies: A contribution to method integration in psychotherapy. *Psychopathology, 46*, 266–274.

Isenberg, A. (1949). Natural pride and natural shame. *Philosophy and Phenomenological Research, 10*(1), 1–24.

Johannessen, J.-A. (2019). *The workplace of the future: The Fourth revolution, the Precariat and the death of hierarchies.* New York: Routledge.

Kegan, R. (1982). *The evolving self: Problem and process in human development.* Cambridge, MA: Harvard University Press.

Klever, W.N.A. (1996). Chapter 1: Spinoza's life and works. In D. Garrett (Ed.), *The Cambridge companion to Spinoza* (p. 13). Cambridge, UK: Cambridge University Press.

Klever, W. (1990). Hume Contra Spinoza?. *Hume Studies, 16*(2), 89–105.
Lewis, M. (2011). The self-conscious emotions. In M. Lewis (Ed.), *Encyclopaedia on early childhood development.* Institute for the Study of Child Development, UMDNJ-Robert Wood Johnson Medical School, Child Health Institute. http://www.child-encyclopedia.com/sites/default/files/dossiers-complets/en/emotions.pdf
Lord, B. (2011). Disempowered by Nature#: Spinoza on the political capabilities of women. *British Journal for the History of Philosophy, 19*(6), 1085–1106.
Machiavelli, N. (1513/2013). *The Prince* (Original: De Principatibus). Vancouver, BC: CreateSpace Independent Publishing Platform.
Marks, S. (2011). *Scham—die tabuisierte Emotion.* Düsseldorf: Patmos.
Mayer, C.-H. (2017). *The life and creative works of Paulo Coelho: A psychobiography from a positive psychology perspective*. Gewerbetrasse: Springer.
Mayer, C.-H. (2019). Key factors of creativity and the art of collaboration in twenty-first-century workplaces. In M. Coetzee (Ed.), *Thriving in digital workplaces: Innovations in theory, research and practice* (pp. 147–166). Cham: Springer Nature.
Mayer, C.-H., & Kóváry, Z. (2019). *New Trends in psychobiography*. Cham: Springer.
Mayer, C.-H., & Vanderheiden, E. (2019). *The bright side of shame. Transforming and growing through practical applications in cultural contexts*. Cham: Springer.
Mayer, C.-H., & Vanderheiden, E. (2021). Naming and shaming in cyber space: Effects and counter-strategies. In C.-H. Mayer, E. Vanderheiden, & P. T. P. Wong (Eds.), *Shame 4.0: Investigating an emotion in digital worlds and the fourth industrial revolution*. Cham: Springer.
Mayer, C.-H., Vanderheiden, E., & Oosthuizen, R. (2019). Transforming shame, guilt and anxiety through a salutogenic pp1.0 and pp2.0 counselling framework. *Counselling Psychology Quarterly, 32*(3-4), 436–452.
Mayer, C.-H., Van Niekerk, R. & Fouché, P.J. (2020). Holistic wellness in the life of Angela Merkel: A call to revise Wheel of Wellness in the light of new Positive Psychology movements and socio-cultural changes. *International Review of Psychiatry,* 625–637. https://doi.org/10.1080/09540261.2020.1735317.
Meinsma, K. O. (1983). *Spinoza et son cercle*. Paris: Vrin.
Merriam-Webster Dictionary. (2020). Cherem. https://www.theschooloflife.com/thebookoflife/baruch-spinoza/
Morley, L. (2013). The rules of the game: Women and the leaderist turn in higher education. *Gender and Education, 25*(1), 116–131.
Nadler, S. (2009). The Jewish Spinoza. *Journal of the History of Ideas, 70*, (3), 491–510. https://www.jstor.org/stable/20621904
Nadler, S. (2019). *Baruch Spinoza* (E. Zalta, Ed.). Stanford, CA: The Stanford Encyclopedia of Philosophy. https://plato.stanford.edu/archives/spr2019/entries/spinoza/
Negri, A. (2020). *Spinoza then and now*. Cambridge, UK: Polity Press.
Palti, I. (2017). Creativity will be the source of our next industrial revolution, not machines. Quartz, 11.
Parker, S. (2011). Spirituality in counselling: A faith development perspective. *Journal of Counselling and Development, 89*(1), 112–119.
Popkin, J. (2019). *A study of Spinoza by James Martineau* (3rd ed.). Macmillan. https://www.britannica.co/contributor/Richard-H-Popkin/2352
Ratner, J. (2011). *Baruch Spinoza. The philosophy of Spinoza: Life, work and the philosophy of Spinoza*. Vancouver, BC: CreateSpace Independent Publishing Platform.
Rotenstreich, N. (1965). On shame. *The Review of Metaphysics, 19*(1), 55–85.
Runyan, W. M. (2005). Evolving conceptions of psychobiography and the study of lives: Encounters with psychoanalysis, personality psychology and historical science. In W. T. Schultz (Ed.), *The handbook of psychobiography* (pp. 19–42). New York: Oxford University Press.
Ryan, T. (2019). Transforming shame: Strategies in spirituality and prayer. In C. -H. Mayer, & E. Vanderheiden (Eds.), *The bright side of shame. Transforming and growing through practical applications in cultural contexts* (pp. 187–198). Cham: Springer.

Scheff, T. (2013). *The S-word: Shame as a key to modern societies. Global summit on diagnostic alternatives.* http://dxsummit.org/archives/1286. Accessed 1 May 2016.

Schultz, W. T. (2005). *Handbook of psychobiography*. New York: Oxford University Press.

Spinoza, B. (1677/2001). *Ethics*. Hertfordshire, UK: Wordsworth.

Straughn, H. F. (2010). *Stages of faith: Interview with James Fowler.* Retrieved from http://jmm.aaa.net.au/articles/23318.htm [5 Aug 2011].

Stubbings, C. (2018). *Workforce of the future: The competing forces shaping 2030.* PwC. https://www.pwc.com/gx/en/services/people-organisation/publications/workforce-of-the-future.html

Sullivan, S. (2011). Sad versus joyful passions. Spinoza, Nietzsche, and the transformation of whiteness. *Philosophy Today, 55*(suppl), 231–239.

Tangney, J., & Dearing, R. (2002). *Shame and guilt*. New York: Guilford Press.

The Book of Life (2020). Chapter: Western philosophy. Baruch Spinoza. https://www.theschooloflife.com/thebookoflife/baruch-spinoza/

The New Republic (2012). Destroyer and builder. https://newrepublic.com/book/review/book-forged-hell-spinoza-treatise-Steven-Nadler

Vanderheiden, E., & Mayer, C.-H. (2017). *The value of shame. Exploring a health resource in cultural contexts*. Cham: Springer.

Wing, K. A. (1997). *Adult faith development: Current thinking*. Retrieved from http://www.hope.edu/academic/psychology/335/webrep/fiathdev.html

Wong, P. T. P. (2016). Self-transcendence: A paradoxical way to become your best. *International Journal of Existential Psychology and Psychotherapy, 6* (1). Retrieved from http://journal.existentialpsychology.org/index.php/ExPsy/article/view/178/141

Wong, P.T.P. (2019). Foreword: From shame to wholeness: An existential positive psychology perspective. In C.-H. Mayer & Vanderheiden, E. (Eds.). *The bright side of shame. Transforming and growing through practical applications in cultural contexts* (pp. v–xi). Cham: Springer.

Yovel, Y. (1992). *Spinoza and other heretics: The adventures of immanence*. Princeton, NJ: Princeton University Press.

Claude-Hélène Mayer (Dr. habil., PhD, PhD) is a Professor in Industrial and Organisational Psychology at the Department of Industrial Psychology and People Management at the University of Johannesburg, an Adjunct Professor at the European University Viadrina in Frankfurt (Oder), Germany and a Senior Research Associate at Rhodes University, Grahamstown, South Africa. She holds a Ph.D. in Psychology (University of Pretoria, South Africa), a Ph.D. in Management (Rhodes University, South Africa), a Doctorate (Georg-August University, Germany) in Political Sciences (sociocultural anthropology and intercultural didactics), and a Habilitation (European University Viadrina, Germany) in Psychology with focus on work, organisational, and cultural psychology. She has published several monographs, text collections, accredited journal articles, and special issues on transcultural mental health and well-being, sense of coherence, shame, transcultural conflict management and mediation, women in leadership in culturally diverse work contexts, constellation work, coaching, and psychobiography.

Paul J. P. Fouché (D Phil) is a full-professor in Counselling Psychology in the Department of Psychology at the University of the Free State, Bloemfontein in South-Africa. Paul has published psychobiographical and psychohistorical articles in various journals. His interest is in the field of psychobiography and psychohistory and he acts as research supervisor to post-graduate scholars undertaking life history research.

Chapter 14
lajjA and the Fourth Industrial Revolution (4IR): The Need for Pause

Dharm P. S. Bhawuk

1 Introduction

Researchers are still grappling with the idea of the Fourth Industrial Revolution (4IR), and the agreed-upon definition is yet to emerge. Some think we are in the midst of the Third Industrial Revolution (Greenwood, 1997; Liu & Grusky, 2013; Rifkin, 2011), whereas others propose that we are in 4IR (Bloem et al., 2014; Maynard, 2015; Petrillo, Felice, Cioffi, & Zomparelli, 2018; Prisecaru, 2016; Rabeh, Husam, & Saeed, 2017). Schwab (2016) has been preparing to deal with issues emerging from the Fourth Industrial Revolution by organizing a community under the auspices of the World Economic Forum, and he posits that 4IR is characterized by the speed of technological breakthroughs, the geographical and industrial scope of changes taking place, and the impact these changes have on production, management, and governance systems (see Chap. 1 in this book).

A historical reflection shows that the First Industrial Revolution started with the invention of steam engine powered by coal, which led to mechanization of production systems in textile and steel industries. The Second Industrial Revolution was characterized by the transition from coal to oil, use of electricity, establishment of scientific management (Taylor, 1911), and Fordist mass production (Womack, Jones, & Roos, 1991) that was perfected in the assembly line for automobiles. The Third Industrial Revolution refers to the introduction of electronics in the automation of production and service industries. This phase also refers to the shift of the economy from manufacturing to service, use of nuclear energy, computers, robotics, and globalization of markets (Levitt, 1983). Finally, the Fourth Industrial Revolution (4IR) is characterized by, to name a few of its defining attributes, the emergence of

D. P. S. Bhawuk (✉)
Honolulu, HI, USA

University of Hawai'i at Manoa, Honolulu, HI, USA
e-mail: Bhawuk@hawaii.edu

C.-H. Mayer et al. (eds.), *Shame 4.0*, https://doi.org/10.1007/978-3-030-59527-2_14

the information age fired by the Internet, development of bio- and nano-technologies, artificial intelligence, availabilities of gadgets like the cell phone that control communication and a host of home and office gadgets, Internet of Things, and blockchain. Prisecaru (2016) proposed a timeline for the four industrial revolutions as 1760–1900, 1900–1960, 1960–2000, and 2000 onward and that the transition periods for the four phases were 1860–1900, 1940–1960, 1980–2000, and 2000–2010. Even if we are still in the Third Industrial Revolution, there is no doubt that rapid changes are taking place and we may be on the cusp of the next industrial revolution. For the purpose of the discussion here, we will proceed with the assumption that we are in 4IR.

It should be noted at the outset that these phases are presented from the Western perspective and generally presented as positive development for humankind. Clearly, this is not the case. Colonization was bolstered by these industrial revolutions, and what used to be the economic First World until 1760 (Kennedy, 1989), China and India, became impoverished and a part of the Third World. Western scholars untiringly credit the technological innovation of steam engine and the First Industrial Revolution for the British and European economic success, whereas the draconian policies and unethical practices that systematically destroyed the industrial production systems of the colonies are only becoming apparent now (Broadberry & Gupta, 2015; Maddison, 2007, see Chapter 3, pp.111–179; Robins, 2006). Arrighi, Silver, and Brewer (2003) empirically demonstrated that the rapid industrialization of the colonized nations under the changing banners of development, globalization, and Washington Consensus did not help reduce the North-South income divide during the last 40 years of the nineteenth century. Therefore, we should be open to the possibility that the hyped 4IR may also cause the North-South economic divide to grow. It is best to be cautious about imagining how 4IR will make human experience positive and exciting (see Seke, 2019, for a discussion of 4IR as a buzz word for the Emerging Markets of Africa).

In this chapter a critical review of 4IR is presented to show both the positive and negative aspects of the changes and those that are impending. The behavioral consequences of 4IR and how *lajjA* will be shaped and shape human behavior in the new context of 4IR are discussed. There is evidence that *lajjA* is an important virtue that guides human behavior in Asia (e.g., Fung, 1999; Lebra, 1983) in general and India in particular (Bhawuk, 2017, 2019a; Menon & Shweder, 1994, 2003; Sinha & Chauhan, 2013). This chapter extends how *lajjA* will work in the virtual space in the context of 4IR. It is clear that one of the defining characteristics of 4IR is speed and *lajjA* proposes a *pause* for keeping a check on behaving appropriately. Implications for our global village are discussed.

2 Two Faces of 4IR

To illustrate the positive and negative faces of 4IR, two aspects of each are presented. The first positive aspects of 4IR pertains to the ever optimistic business managers euphoria about change, and all change is good captured in the edict by the Greek philosopher Heraclitus—change is the only constant in life—and the possibility of the emergence of a new model of business. An example can be found in how businesses are touting the dawn of a great change, a paradigm shift, for 4IR as they did for the previous industrial revolutions. Oracle has a website ("Plan your path", n. d.) where it provides information that 56% of manufacturers are ready to invest in IR4 initiatives (Oracle uses both 4IR and IR4 in its message).

Oracle provides an approach to the new world and has created an interactive guide for orientation to survey the landscape of 4IR for the purpose of planning. It presents five steps, the last being how Oracle can help, which is an effort to sell their technology to other organizations. The first step is understanding that everything starts with the customer. This has been the slogan of businesses for the longest time as preached in all marketing textbooks starting with Kotler's classic (1967). In the second step, organizations are required to decide if the change they are seeking will be operational or at the business model level, which is a fundamental question of strategy that has been applicable to organizations in the previous industrial revolutions as well (Roth, Schweiger, & Morrison, 1991). For 4IR the importance of connected enterprise is touted, which was also championed by management people under the label of boundaryless organization previously (Ashkenas, Ulrich, Jick, & Kerr, 1995).

Finally, organizations need to align people, process, and technology, which is the fundamental of management, and has always been present in the previous industrial revolutions going back to Fayol's (1916/1949) principles of general management. Whether 4IR is here or not, people are preparing for it, and there are organizations like Oracle that are helping prepare to ride the wave of this new industrial revolution. This has always been true of business organizations with the dawn of new technologies, and they always paint a positive face, for in business everything is an opportunity!

The second positive face of 4IR pertains to the emergence of public-private partnership and social entrepreneurship in meeting various global human needs like poverty alleviation. Even before the dawn of 4IR, or even 3IR, many models of excellent business existed, and Amul, Grameen Bank, and Mondragon are illustrious organizations that have stood the test of time employing principles of community psychology (Bhawuk, Mrazek, & Munusamy, 2009). Aravind Eye Hospital (Naidoo, 2012) is another example of healthcare initiative that has been successful. Mohammad Yunus, the founder of the Grameen Bank, is one of the champions of the new model of business through private-public partnering, what he calls building social businesses (Yunus, 2011) to serve the needs of people that fall outside the world of multinationals. For example, Grameen Health Care Services, a sister organization of the Grameen Bank, partnered with Aravind Eye Hospital and with half a million dollar funding from Green Children Foundation, USA, opened its first eye hospital in Bangladesh in 2007, and with its success, the second one in 2009. A third one was opened in 2013 with the support of SEVA Foundation, USA.

Social entrepreneurship offers a positive business model with four characteristics, namely, addressing issues that are often neglected by the market mechanism, presenting sustainable solutions, having positive externalities, and empowering local communities (Santos, 2012; see also Bhawuk et al., 2009, for the discussion of community psychology principles found to be present in Amul, Grameen Bank, and Mondragon), and has emerged on a big scale, which 4IR could claim some credit for. Many colleagues and I were involved with the Istanbul International Center for Private Sector in Development of the United Nations Development Program and produced a document for enhancing public-private partnership to serve the need of the people in the base of the pyramid (Ali et al., 2014). It is fair to say that though social entrepreneurship and private-public partnership are not new ideas, it is plausible that they will grow and get institutionalized in 4IR.

The negative face of 4IR is captured by democratic deficit and the speed of information flow that has an adverse impact on the well-being of workers and the efficient functioning of organizations. The idea of democratic deficit sprang from Jeunes Européens Fédéralistes (JEF or Young European Federalists), who presented it in their manifesto in the Berlin Congress in 1977 (Richard, 1977). Democratic deficit is referred to decisions made by governments without regard to the need of people and without their participation in the decision-making process. It applies to both the struggle against power of capital as well as the state and its agencies. Democratic deficit is caused by centralization by the state at the cost of participation at the local levels, missing out on cultural insights embedded in the community (Bhawuk et al., 2009). With the growth of large multinationals, workers have become fungible and unimportant, and conflict between management and worker has continued from the First to the Fourth Industrial Revolution. With globalization, a similar democratic deficit can be seen in how the affluent North dictates unreasonable terms to the developing South through institutions like IMF and the World Bank (Stiglitz, 2007).

Historically, Fordist production system is known to have dehumanized work by taking away the five characteristics of work—skill variety, task identity, task significance, autonomy, and feedback from the task itself (Hackman & Oldham, 1975)—that make tasks inherently motivating. Nevertheless, Fordism has expanded the world over. Toyota and other Japanese auto manufacturers have succeeded in creating learning organizations in which, through job rotation, workers learn to do a host of tasks first under supervision and then independently and finally are able to train other new employees to learn those tasks, which continues over a career span of 40 years (Morishima, 1995). This has helped with job enrichment. However, that is only true for less than 30% of the workers of large organizations in Japan, who have what is called lifetime employment, i.e., they are not laid off for economic reasons. The plight of daily wage earners and even the ones working on assembly line barely makes up for workplace democracy in Japan, according to some researchers (Mehri, 2006) (see Chap. 3 in this book).

Even worse is the treatment of workers in the Japanese and German organizations with factories in the southern states of the USA (Waldman, 2017), though organizations in these countries are known for quality circles and work councils, respectively, in their home countries. The decline of union movement should also be a reminder that there is democratic deficit in the workplace even in the Western world, and there is some evidence that computerization leads to decline in unionization (Kristal, 2019), and so 4IR is likely to cause a bigger democratic deficit in the workplace.

Norris (2011) examined democratic deficit resulting from the gap between public expectations and democratic performance of a government in 50 societies worldwide. He found that democratic deficit was shaped by three factors, namely, people's desire for democracy, the performance of the government institutions and their structure, and news, often negative, about the government. Social media has a significant impact on all three of them, and so in 4IR there will be a gap between real democratic deficit and a perception of it, and perceptions will sway people with the power of social media. This brings us to the second dark side of 4IR, its speed. Though champions of 4IR (Schwab, 2016) see much scope in public-private partnership, and there are some success stories as noted above, it is likely that 4IR will create a bigger gap between the haves and the have-nots and affect the well-being of people due to the global informational connectivity.

The Internet has led to global *informational connectivity*, and news is no more dependent on news agency; a common person can post online what is happening in some place with the help of a cell phone, and it is available to everybody who has access to the Internet. It guarantees neither sensitivity nor understanding, and acting compassionately and responsibly is a far cry to expect, which had already started to emerge in the analogue world of 3IR interactions. This informational connectivity is also creating *information load*, and it is becoming difficult, if not impossible, to be able to process all the available information to make a rational or wise decision. The information load is converting people into *pleasure seekers* as the inability to process the available information creates the desire to enter one's cave of comfort, a safety zone, away from the issues facing the global community and indulge into pleasurable activities like streaming movies, playing video games, or simply surfing on the net; none of which serves anybody, anywhere. It simply makes one an escapist and hungry for endless pleasures. We have all become a bundle of insatiable desires and seek immediate solutions on the net, and not finding what we want, we become frustrated, angry, violent, or chronically depressed. The wisdom tradition of India has warned us about how desires lead to greed and anger (see Bhawuk, 2011, Chapter 7), and the speed of the Internet has amplified the level of our desires for all kinds of services, further raising the level of greed and frustration.

Let us examine the implications of mobile phone and social media on individuals, which should provide an understanding of the scale of changes we face. First, people do not have to dwell on an event for long, and they can respond by texting and using emoji. For example, if one is at a funeral, one has to dress for the occasion, act somber, and commit to be physically there for the ceremony. In the virtual space, one could simply send an emoji capturing sadness and be done with it in less than a minute. It takes less time than even ordering flowers, if one did not want to go to a funeral. Second, people are able to choose what event they want to focus their time and energy on in the virtual space, whereas in the physical social context, one may find oneself simply stuck in the specific behavioral setting, which determines one's behavior. For example, one could send emojis to many people in less than a minute and share happy emoji, excited emoji, shy emoji, sad emoji, proud emoji, gratefulness emoji, and love emoji. It is not possible to feel so many emotions in the social context so quickly.

Third, we are able to avoid people and situations in the virtual space, which is not possible in the social context, barring work contexts like video conferencing. A general outcome of interactions in the virtual space is that people become extremely individualistic and self-centered—they only engage in what they want to. Friendship in virtual space is all about me, rather than the other. Communication in the virtual space is all about what I want to say, rather than listening to what others have to say. In fact, one is able to terminate communication at will without any consequence, with many easy copout solutions (my phone died, call dropped, I had to address another person who was in my face, and so forth), which are not available in face-to-face interactions since the other can see us.

Fourth, powered by high-speed gadgets and the relentless pursuit of objects, goals, and ideas, people inevitably lead to speedup, which is "an employer's demand for accelerated output without increased pay" (Bauerlein & Jeffery, 2011). Focus on productivity has not only led to the dumbing down of America (Bluestone & Bluestone, 1992) in the mindless simplification of work found in fast food restaurants but also increased demand on multitasking and the use of telephone and e-mail at home to perform work-related task. McEwen (2011) noted that at least a third of the people in the USA report that they have no time to reflect on what they are doing and always feel rushed. Speeding up leads people to have no patience for slow-moving social interactions or events.

Fifth, there is confusion about the ownership of downloaded information without processing it. Students think they know the material because they have downloaded it on their computer or phone. The gap between the ability to download texts and processing them can paralyze even the best minds.

Other possibilities include new forms of citizen participation in governance like liquid democracy (Blum & Zuber, 2016) (see Chap. 24), which is a model of collective decision-making that could allow people to vote directly on policies or representative who champion those policies, binding the representatives to a priori pre-election policy positions. This is a possibility because of the technological innovation of 4IR. We may also find new forms of work and learning. But they are all likely to be related to artificial intelligence or speed of decision-making through technology. Indeed, we need to be open about the possibilities, yet being cautious about the managerial euphoria, especially in light of democratic deficit in the workplace, may be wise.

Speedup is not conducive to creativity and often causes stress, and spiritual practices help avoid the demands of speedup. Only focusing on the outward journey often leads to such consequences (Bhawuk, 2019b). McEwen (2011) noted that being silent and purposefully not doing anything, e.g., simply having a cup of coffee, doing yard work, listening to music, and so forth, lead to creativity. Csikszentmihalyi (1996) noted how many European physicists discovered their most influential ideas while climbing mountains or gazing at stars. Purposefully not doing anything work-related is a process of simply being or cultivating an internal journey (Bhawuk, 2019b). Leisure has been viewed as a spiritual need by some (Doohan, 1990) and as a source of spiritual well-being and mental health by others (Heintzman, 2002). Slowing down, interjecting pauses in life, and leisure need to be cultivated, since they are much needed not only to pursue an internal journey but also to have some balance in life and to be creative (Bhawuk, 2019b). In what follows we will examine how *lajjA* worked in the social context and how it may work in the virtual space with the ever-growing technological speed of phone, computers, and other gadgets. Clearly, to manage the speed of communication requires enhanced sense of responsibility.

3 What We Know About *lajjA*

Bhawuk (2017) examined dictionary meanings, synonyms, and antonyms of *lajjA* in *saMskRtam* and *hindI* and analyzed the usage of the word in two popular scriptural texts, namely, the *bhagavadgItA* and *durgA saptazatI*. He further examined the uses of *lajjA* in the literature in *kAmAyanI*, a modern *hindi mahAkAvya* or epic as well as in daily communications and proverbs. This multi-method approach resulted in a web of meaning, a sort of thick description (Geertz, 1973; Ryle, 1949, 1971) of the construct, showing that *lajjA* is a positive construct, one of the 26 *daivik sampadA* or virtues enumerated in the *bhagavadgItA* that guides human behavior. Scholars consistently define *lajjA* as a prohibitive feeling that arises when one considers doing something inappropriate (*akAryakaraNe lajjA*), which prevents one from doing such a task. Subjective norms, or what others would say, also play a role. For example, the moment one thinks about doing an inappropriate task, the negative evaluation that others would make of the act is made salient in the *manas*[1] or mind, thus restricting the performance of such an activity (*akAryapravRttyArambhe tatpratibandhikA lokalajjA*). This internal prohibitive mechanism is *lajjA* (or its synonyms, viz., *hrIH* and *vrIDA*).

There is general agreement among scholars about the meaning of *lajjA* as a reflective evaluation process that is automatically called into the cognitive process

[1]*manas* in *saMskRtam* or *mana* in *hindi* is the center for cognition, affect, and behavior (Bhawuk, 2011), and, therefore, it is difficult to translate it in English. Mind is a widely used translation, which only captures the cognitive function of *manas*, but not the affective and behavioral functions. See Bhawuk (2011, Chapter 4) for a definition and discussion of *manas*, *buddhi*, *ahaGkAra*, and *antaHkaraNa*. The closest translation of *ahaGkAra* would be ego, which comes at the cost of much loss of meaning. And *antaHkaraNa* is the composite internal organ or agent combining *manas*, *buddhi*, and *ahaGkAra*.

restricting the performance of certain tasks that ought not to be done or are considered inappropriate by the *zAstras* or scriptures. The same process prohibits the non-performance of tasks that ought to be done (e.g., showing respect to one's parents or teachers, being charitable to the needy, and so forth). Thus, *lajjA* has both internal and external aspects or guilt and shame elements. Other researchers (Menon & Shweder, 1994, 2003; Sinha & Chauhan, 2013) have similarly concluded that *lajjA* is associated with being shy, having modesty, and showing deference to elders. Having *lajjA is* akin to being a civilized person who knows his or her place in the society and acts properly as demanded by one's duties and responsibilities. Thus, *lajjA* prevents people from any transgressions.[2] Sinha and Chauhan (2013) also showed that *lajjA* is used by Indian women in defining their identity, and it seems to be the core of womanhood. Such a structure is at odds with the Western literature that views guilt and shame as distinct and independent constructs (Creighton, 1990; Lewis, 1971; Tracy & Robins, 2006).

Socially unacceptable behaviors like showing disrespect to elders, smoking, drinking alcohol, gambling, going to a prostitute, adultery, and so forth have trickled down from the scriptures as behaviors that one ought not to do, and doing them causes *lajjA*. In the Indian worldview, there are six enemies of spiritual practice—*kAma* (desire), *krodha* (anger), *lobha* (greed), *moha* (attachment), *ahaGkAra* (ego), and *mAtsarya* (jealousy) (see Bhawuk, 2011, Chapter 7; Figure 7.1)—that are associated with a host of behaviors that would also fall in the "ought not to do" category and cause *lajjA*. Those who cannot detach themselves from these evils would be involved in so many behaviors that would lead to the experience of *lajjA* for themselves as well as their families.

lajjA is a social psychological construct that we learn through the socialization process (see Fung, 1999, for how shame is used to socialize children in China so that they can develop a sense of right or wrong). Bhawuk (2019a) showed that *lajjA* is learned and unlearned under certain behavioral settings through interaction between socialization, conformity, and personal choice (see also Chaps. 15 and 20 in this book). Researchers have given more importance to conformity and neglected the importance Asch (1955, 1956) ascribed to independence, which alludes to using personal choice in the face of pressure from the group. Twenty-five percent of the participants in the studies by Asch were found not to conform, which tends to be neglected in the conformity literature (see Friend, Rafferty, & Bramel, 1990). Beyond the individual, institutions play a significant role as they provide the social space that is necessary for the enactment of the behaviors in the learning and unlearning process. Because of personal choice, we can find much individual

---

[2]Bible also calls knowing what one ought to do and not doing it as inappropriate or even a sin in more than one place. James 4.17: Therefore to him that knoweth to do good, and doeth it not, to him it is sin. Luke 12.47: That servant who knows his master's will but does not get ready or follow his instructions will be beaten with many blows. John 9.41: "If you were blind," Jesus replied, "you would not be guilty of sin. But since you claim you can see, your guilt remains." 2 Peter 2.21: It would have been better for them not to have known the way of righteousness than to have known it and then to turn away from the holy commandment passed on to them.

difference in how *lajjA* is learned, unlearned, or relearned (Bhawuk, 2019a). Gender differences also suggests that there may be other group-level differences in the process of acquisition or shedding of *lajjA*. Therefore, the *zeitgeist* of 4IR is likely to influence how *lajjA* will be learned, unlearned, or relearned (see Bhawuk, 2011, Chapter 3 for a discussion of how the *zeitgeist* shapes human behavior).

We should also note that socialization and personal choice operate in a social space, and institutions provide the social space for enactment of thought, speech, and action. Abusive workplaces have existed for decades since institutions provided the supportive environment for the abusers to act inappropriately. The "#MeToo" movement has brought down many abusers that had gotten away in the past (Bennett, 2017). Organizations can also take positive steps to create policies to address racism and sexism under the umbrella of diversity management (Bhawuk, Podsiadlowski, Graf, & Triandis, 2002) (see Chaps. 18 and 24). Therefore, the power of institutions in helping us cultivate undesirable behaviors that would naturally cause us *lajjA* should not be underplayed, as can be seen in the growth of democratic deficit both in public life and organizations mentioned above. At the same time, we can be hopeful that institutions can create a supportive environment for people to acquire appropriate behaviors and relearn *lajjA* in the process as can be seen in the private-public partnerships noted above.

In making decisions we employ *viveka* (or discretion), which is housed in *buddhi*[3] or intellectual faculty. *viveka* becomes salient when we make a *saGkalpa* or form an intention about doing an action (see Fig. 14.1). If we decide that it is not prudent to perform that intention because it is not proper, for whatever reason, then the *saGkalpa* ends in *akarma* or inaction right there. However, if we decide that we want to pursue that *saGkalpa* or intention, then we may realize that it is leading us to either *karaNIya* (what ought to be done) or *akarNIya* (what ought not to be done). If it is *karaNIya*, and we decide to perform it, then we perform a *karma* or *sakarma* (proper action). If we decide not to perform the *karaNIya*, then we experience *lajjA*, and if we are guided by *lajjA*, then we would perform the action, but if we neglect *lajjA*, then we will end up not doing something that ought to be done, which is *vikarma* or *niSiddha karma* (or prohibited action like not showing respect to an elder, not following a company policy, and so forth).

There is a parallel path for *akaraNIya* or what ought not to be done (see Fig. 14.1), and if we decide not do it, we end with inaction. However, if decide to go forward with the *akaraNIya*, then we will experience *lajjA*. If we heed *lajjA*, then we will not do the action. However, if we are not guided by *lajjA*, then we will perform the action that is *akaraNIya*, which results in performing a *vikarma* or *niSiddha karma* (prohibited action). Thus, not heeding *lajjA* always leads to *vikarma* or improper behavior, whereas being guided by *lajjA* may help us either do what we

---

[3] *buddhi* is often translated as the intellectual faculty that is involved in reasoning and judging. It is closest to the super-ego in Freudian parlance, but without ego, which makes the similarity rather superficial. See Bhawuk (2011, Chapter 4) for a definition and discussion of *manas*, *buddhi*, *ahaGkAra*, and *antaHkaraNa*.

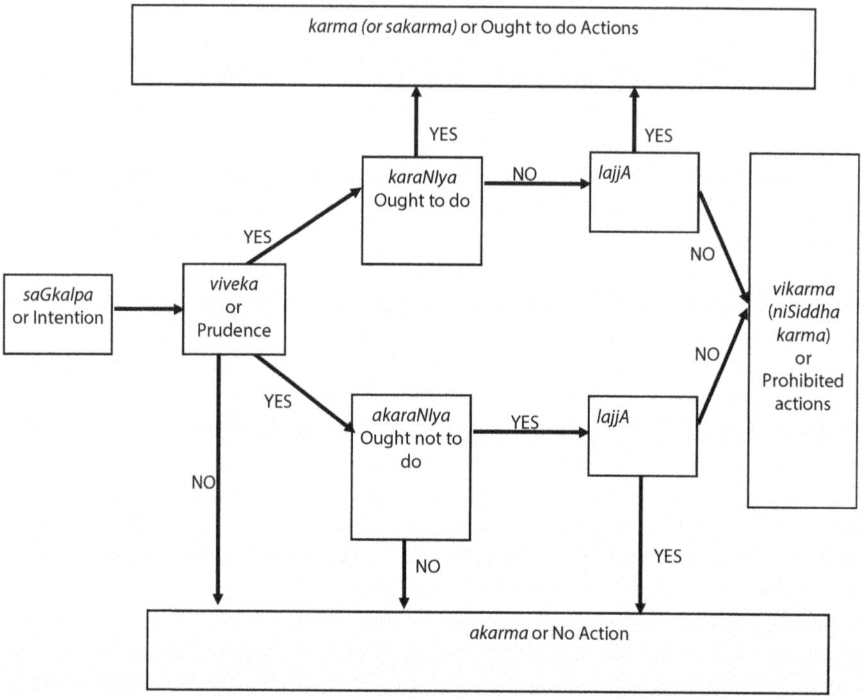

Fig. 14.1 How *lajjA* and *viveka* shape *karma*, *akarma*, and *vikarma* (ought to do, ought not to do, and inaction)

ought to do or simply not take any action. What is *karaNIya* and *akaraNIya* should be guided by professional code of behavior at work and social mores in other settings. The process of using *viveka* and *lajjA* in making decisions about *akarma* (inaction), *karma* (action), and *vikarma* or *niSiddha karma* (improper action) is presented schematically in Fig. 14.1. The definitions of these terms are presented in verses 15–18[4] of Canto 4 of the *bhagavadgItA*.

[4]Verse 4.15: *evaM jJAtvA kRtaM karma pUrvairapi mumukSubhiH, kuru karmaiva tasmattvaM pUrvaiH pUrvataraM kRtam.* You should perform *karma* (actions that are ought to be done, or your duties) the way those desirous of *mokSA* (or freedom from birth and death cycles) performed their duties in the past.

Verse 4.16: *kiM karma kimakarmeti kavayo'pyatra mohitAH, tatte karma pravakSyAmi yajjJAtvA mokSyase'zubhAt.* Even the wise get confused about what is *karma* (action) and what is *akarma* (inaction); therefore, I will instruct you about *karma* (action) so that you can achieve *mokSa* (or freedom from birth and death cycles) from the inauspicious consequences of *karma.*

Verse 4.17: *karmaNo hyapi boddhavyaM boddhavyaM ca vikarmaNaH, akarmaNazca boddhavyaM gahanA karmaNo gatiH.* One should know about *karma* (action that ought to be done), *akarma* (inaction or not performing actions), and *vikarma* (prohibited karma or actions), for it *karma* is a complex subject.

Verse 4.18: *karmaNyakarma yaH pazydakarmanI ca karma yaH, sa buddhimAnmanuSyeSu sa yuktaH kRtsnakarmakRt.* One who seems *akarma* in *karma* and *karma* in *akarma* is a wise person, *viveka* is similar to *lajjA* in that both serve us in doing what we ought to do (*karaNIya*) and not doing what we ought not to do (*akaraNIya*). Ideally, when *viveka* guides us properly, we act properly. However, our *viveka* may be clouded by strong desires for certain products or social outcomes or for favoring people we love. These are the situations where we are likely to experience *lajjA* both while making the decision and later when we face the outcome. But if we consider such situations as having the absence of *viveka* (or we are being *vivekahIna*), then we could say that absence of *viveka (or vivekahInatA)* leads to *lajjA*.

In the virtual space, it is easier to slip into not doing what ought to be done and doing what one ought not to do. The speed with which actions will be taken using gadgets in 4IR, the likelihood of slipping is more pronounced. For example, it is natural to respond to an unpleasant e-mail negatively in the heat of the moment since the person is not present in front of us. A practice that has stood this author in good stead is to type the response e-mail but sending it to oneself, allowing a pause to the speedy action and only send it in a day or two allowing *viveka* or discretion to prevail.

lajjA is an instrument of *buddhi*, and it is associated with *buddhi* in mediating thought and action (Bhawuk (2017). It is a fleeting emotion (or a *saJcarI bhAva*). *viveka* also is an instrument of *buddhi*, but whereas *lajjA* is associated with emotion, *viveka* does not seem to be associated with emotion and is rather associated with *tejas* (fiery energy, vital power, or efficacy). The highest level of *viveka* is associated with discriminating the spiritual from the material, and, in so doing, one does not get confounded with desires and passions. Thus, there are many levels of *viveka*, and there will be differences in the *viveka* of a worldly and that of an enlightened person (Bhawuk, 2019a). Also, *viveka* is often related to the quality rather than appropriateness of decisions.

Conscience refers to an inner feeling or voice that guides a person to appropriate behavior. It is a sense of being right and wrong and leads to right or moral rather than wrong or unethical behavior. When one does not follow the conscience, he or she often has a guilty conscience about the behavior. Sometimes one's conscience does not allow the person to keep silent or inactive, as is the case of whistleblowers. Therefore, conscience is akin to *vivek* and *lajjA*.

4 *lajjA*, Responsibility and 4IR: Need for Pause

With the increasing speed of the Internet, we are able to use video communication using the Internet (FaceTime, Skype, etc.), telephone communication, voice messages, texting, e-mails, document-sharing, and so forth, which make the boundary of virtual and face-to-face interactions become blurred. Since a good proportion of

and though he or she may be engaged in all kinds of actions, he or she remains unaffected by the bondage of *karma* or actions.

communication is through e-mails and text messages, in using this medium, there is a loss of degrees of freedom. When one says something, one still has the opportunity to withdraw or not to do what one says. When one writes a message, the message can often become the action (for a discussion of how to do things with words; see Austin, 1962).

In Indian philosophy, spiritual aspirants (or *sAdhakas*) monitor themselves at the levels of *vicAra* (i.e., thoughts, the *manas* referred to as *manasA*), *vacana* (words or vAcA), and *karma* or actions (*karma* done by the *kAyA* or actions done by the body). As in the Western psychology, *karma* is an overt response, but *vicAra* is a covert response. *vacana* falls in between and supposedly translates *vicAra* into *karma. lajjA* guides people at all the three levels. Awareness of one's motives and intentions is purely internal; crafting one's words and deeds is seen by observers and are external. Smoking, drinking alcohol, disrespecting elders, and neglecting one's duties to the needy are examples of socially undesirable behaviors. When one displays such acts, he or she is effectively snubbing *lajjA* as if *buddhi* (see footnote 3) is unable to guide *manas*.

At the level of speech, the use of foul language is the obvious *akaraNiya* (or something we ought not to do) and evokes *lajjA*, but not to a bully. Other areas of improper speech would include the use of inappropriate language with one's elders, which includes one's parents, uncles and aunts, older siblings, teachers, older people in the community, and so forth. There is also a decorum for communication between men and women. For example, men may discuss sex among themselves, but not with women (except with their wives), or in the presence of women. There is also an appropriate way to communicate with children, younger people, or our subordinates in the workplace. Therefore, there are many ways one can experience *lajjA* in communication, and if not careful, one can become insensitive in one's speech and lose *lajjA*. In 4IR where speed of communication is high, such lapses are likely to happen more, and we need to cultivate a stronger sense of *lajjA* that would catch us in time before we hit the enter button.

One's *buddhi* (see footnote 3) is the citadel of *lajjA*. *buddhi* uses *lajjA* to guide behaviors, such as choosing right over wrong or healthy over unhealthy. As *lajjA* is a *sancarI bhAva* or a fleeting emotion (Bhawuk, 2017), it stops appearing in our *manas* when it is ignored or flouted a few times by indulging in behaviors that are improper. Therefore, if our speech and acts are polluted, our thoughts will be polluted. And if our speech and acts are polluted in a wide range of domains, our thoughts are likely to be equally polluted. Purifying the thoughts would require the purification of actions and speech. In the context of 4IR, purifying the thought would require shaping one's texting (used as a general term for all written communication like e-mailing) behavior. And pausing will need to be cultivated.

5 Discussion

The tragedy of September 11, 2001, led Triandis (2009) to emerge out of his retirement to write an insightful book about how to avoid self-deception that is prevalent in all domains of human endeavor by synthesizing half a century of his understanding of culture and human psychology. He prophetically recommended that we should remember that we are creatures of chance of evolution, we should be modest for it is good for our mental health, we should minimize our desires following the recommendation of Buddha, and we should pursue the noble goal of life—to make life on this planet as good as it can be for as many people as possible while preserving the environment (p. 204). I think the four *karaNIya* or ought to do—being modest, minimizing desires, making life of as many people as possible good, and preserving the environment—presented by Triandis could be a starting point for us to cultivate *lajjA* and thus shape 4IR different from the other three revolutions.

These four criteria could help amend the historical lapses (what ought to have been done or what ought not to have been done) of the three previous industrial revolutions. The moral basis for helping people in places one may never see is derived from the work of Singer (1972), who argued that being passive is morally wrong when people can act to help in some way despite being far away from those affected. Singer used the example of a child drowning in a shallow pond and argued that a bystander had the moral duty of saving the child at the cost of muddying his or her clothes. He argued that with global connectivity, those with resources have become bystanders and ought to help those who need help because of a natural calamity or political discord in places far away from one's own residence. There is a lot of help going from one part of the world to another, and this needs to become one of the ought-to-do values for the global connectivity and speed to serve as many people as possible.

Bhawuk et al. (2009) noted the limitations of the problem-solving paradigm of engineering, which is likely to be championed by people in the technologically dominated 4IR, and presented a prototype for social change by drawing from the community psychology literature. A social change agent should pay attention to the following five principles of community transformation: being a facilitator who is embedded in the community, working with the community to define problems (it resolves democratic deficit), employing multiple methods and perspectives to measure the problem (it avoids the positivist bias derived from the sciences), implementing solutions in collaboration with the community (again, resolves democratic deficit), and always being flexible. These five principles could be another set of *karaNIya* or ought to do, and not following them should arouse *lajjA*. Such a framework would allow nurturing and building the capacity of people so that they can transform their communities from within, which will go a long way to generate positive stories on the world connected with the Internet. The case studies of Amul, Grameen Bank, and Mondragon showed that they have followed these principles all through the Second and Third Industrial Revolutions and should be exemplars for 4IR also.

The green revolution seems to be a part of 4IR and presents a significant positive step toward a new world. We do not need to force the naysayers to convert to green technology. We should continue to dialogue, for imposition would lead to democratic deficit, which is an ought not to. Creating businesses and other community-based organizations that provide a good life to many people as possible is also emerging from the ventures of social entrepreneurs that are growing significantly. It is the taming of the multinationals, not through legislation, but from within, developing a sense of *karaNIya* and *akaraNIya* that arouses *lajjA*, which is a daunting task. The private-public partnerships that are growing do show a promise, and it is likely that MNCs will slowly become more responsible outgrowing the value of profit as their raison d'être employs multiple criteria including people and environment (Elkington, 1994).

Partnerships built by the US Environmental Defense Fund (EDF) are exemplary since it has been a pioneer in working with companies like McDonalds and General Motors (Elkington, 1998). In the last 30 years, EDF has cultivated partnership with hundreds of organizations that has led to positive environment results (EDF, n.d.). For example, Walmart successfully met its goal of reducing greenhouse gas by 30% (about 36 million metric tons of emission) by managing its supply chain. Similarly, a partnership with McDonald's led to discontinuing the use of Styrofoam clamshell packaging and 300 pounds of waste. Working with FedEX led to the use of hybrid delivery trucks (65% reduction in emission), and partnership with KKR led to Green Portfolio Program that generated $1.2 billion in financial capital (reducing 2.3 million metric tons of greenhouse gas emission). The good work of Walmart with EDF should neither be used to cover the loss of life for more than 100 people in the garment factory fire in Bangladesh on November 24, 2012, which was a part of its supply chain (Anbarasan, 2012), nor to justify its negligence on many fronts that is reported in the documentary, *Walmart: The High Cost of Low Price* (Gilliam, 2005, 1:33).

Another notable example of private and public partnership can be found in the work done by Bill & Melinda Gates Foundation (BMGF). It has worked with pharmaceutical companies like Merck, Eisai, and GlaxoSmithKline, governments (USA, UK, UAE), and international organizations (the World Bank and others) to serve health needs related to neglected tropical diseases (NTD), which led to the London Declaration on NTD to eradicate ten NTDs by the end of 2020. BMGF has also worked on the eradication of malaria, better sanitation to the developing world, and numerous other projects that are exemplars of private-public partnerships and well captured in a three-part documentary series on Bill Gates (Guggenheim, Osisek, & Leckart, 2019, 2:37).

To summarize, what we ought to do has been neglected from the beginning of the industrial revolutions, all four of them, and we have lost the sense of *lajjA*, which could have guided us to be responsible for the all-round (physical, mental, and spiritual) health of people and the care of the environment. We have seen the dark side of slavery, but we are still enamored by capitalism. We have seen the dark side of autocratic rulers but are still enamored by the power of elected presidents and prime ministers. We have seen the dark side of destructive technology but are still enamored by science. We have accumulated much wisdom over thousands of years, yet we are enamored by information and speed. Unless we learn from history, and the repulsive consequences of the industrial revolutions, one after another, we are likely to continue to make the same mistakes. With the connectivity we have, and the speed with which we can express our anger, it is plausible that we will bring upon ourselves tragedies of such proportions that what we have seen historically will pale in comparison. It is time to pause. It is time to reflect and identify what is important for humanity as a collective on this only planet that we have. It is time to cultivate *paJcazIla*, the commitment to nonviolence, non-stealing, non-lying, non-intoxication, and faithfulness in relationship, as a part of our personal code of behavior so that *lajjA* can guide us constantly in our interactions. These values are time tested and have stood such leaders as Buddha and Gandhi in good stead. Cultivating these values will allow us to translate the notion of *vasudhaiva kuTumbakam*, or the whole world is my family, which is not merely poets' imagination but seers' vision that is knocking on our door with the global connectivity that 4IR has sprung upon us. We need to learn from history and set a course individually and collectively to cultivate what we ought to do for the planet and other fellow human beings, rather than create silos of gated community and nations that can live at the cost of others, which is not sustainable in the long run for anyone.

References

Ali, A., Bhawuk, D., Blustein, D. L., Bullock, H. E. Carr, S. C., Gloss, A., et al. (2014). *Barriers and opportunities at the base of the pyramid.* UNDP: Istanbul International Center for Private Sector in Development.

Anbarasan, E. (2012, November 25). Dhaka Bangladesh clothes factory fire kills more than 100. *BBC News*. Retrieved from https://www.bbc.com/news/world-asia-20482273.

Arrighi, G., Silver, B. J., & Brewer, B. D. (2003). Industrial convergence, globalization, and the persistence of the North-South divide. *Studies in Comparative International Development, 38* (1), 3–31.

Asch, S. E. (1955). Opinions and social pressure. *Scientific American, 193*(5), 33–35.

Asch, S. E. (1956). Studies of independence and conformity: I. A minority of one against a unanimous majority. *Psychological Monographs: General and Applied, 70*(9, Whole No. 416), 1.

Ashkenas, R., Ulrich, D., Jick, T., & Kerr, S. (1995). *The boundaryless organization: Breaking the chains of organizational structure.* San Francisco: Jossey-Bass.

Austin, J. L. (1962). *How to do things with words*. London: Oxford University Press.

Bauerlein, M., & Jeffery, C. (2011, August 14). The speedup. *Los Angeles Times*, A 14.

Bennett, J. (2017, December 1). The #MeToo moment: When the blinders come off. *The New York Times*, Section A, p. 2.

Bhawuk, D. P. S. (2011). *Spirituality and Indian psychology: Lessons from the Bhagavad-Gita*. New York: Springer.

Bhawuk, D. P. S. (2017). *lajjA* in Indian psychology: Spiritual, social, and literary perspectives. In E. Vanderheiden & C.-H. Mayer (Eds.), *The value of shame—Exploring a health resource across cultures* (pp. 109–134). New York: Springer.

Bhawuk, D. P. S. (2019a). *lajjA*: Learning, unlearning, and relearning. In E. Vanderheiden & C.-H. Mayer (Eds.), *The bright side of shame: Transforming and growing through practical applications in cultural contexts* (pp. 35–49). New York: Springer.

Bhawuk, D. P. S. (2019b). Toward a spirituality-based theory of creativity: Indigenous perspectives from India. In K. -H. Yeh (Ed.), *Asian indigenous psychologies in the global context* (pp. 139–168). London: Palgrave MacMillan. https://doi.org/10.1007/978-3-319-96232-0_7.

Bhawuk, D. P. S., Podsiadlowski, A., Graf, J., & Triandis, H. C. (2002). Corporate strategies for managing diversity in the global workplace. In G. R. Ferris, M. R. Buckley, & D. B. Fedor (Eds.), *Human resource management: Perspectives, context, functions, and outcomes* (pp. 112–145). Englewood Cliffs, NJ: Prentice-Hall.

Bhawuk, D. P. S., Mrazek, S., & Munusamy, V. P. (2009). From social engineering to community transformation: Amul, Grameen Bank, and Mondragon as exemplar organizations. *Peace & Policy: Ethical Transformations for a Sustainable Future, 14*, 36–63.

Bloem, J., Van Doorn, M., Duivestein, S., Excoffier, D., Maas, R., & Van Ommeren, E. (2014). *The fourth industrial revolution: Things to tighten the link between IT and OT.* https://www.sogeti.com/globalassets/global/special/sogeti-things3en.pdf. Downloaded on 29 Mar 2020.

Bluestone, B., & Bluestone, I. (1992). *Negotiating the future*. New York: Basic Books.

Blum, C., & Zuber, C. I. (2016). Liquid democracy: Potentials, problems, and perspectives. *Journal of Political Philosophy, 24*(2), 162–182.

Broadberry, S., & Gupta, B. (2015). India and the great divergence: An Anglo-Indian comparison of GDP per capita, 1600–1871. *Explorations in Economic History, 55*, 58–75. https://doi.org/10.1016/j.eeh.2014.04.003.

Creighton, M. R. (1990). Revisiting shame and guilt cultures: A forty-year pilgrimage. *Ethos, 18*(3), 279–307.

Csikszentmihalyi, M. (1996). *Creativity, flow and the psychology of discovery and invention.* New York: HarperCollins.

Doohan, L. (1990). *Leisure: A spiritual need.* Notre Dame, IN: Ave Maria Press.

EDF. (n.d.). Our work with business and industry. Retrieved from https://www.edf.org/partnerships/business-and-industry.

Elkington, J. (1994). Towards the sustainable corporation: Win-win-win business strategies for sustainable development. *California Management Review, 36*(2), 90–100.

Elkington, J. (1998). Accounting for the triple bottom line. *Measuring Business Excellence, 2*(3), 18–22. https://doi.org/10.1108/eb025539.

Fayol, H. (1916/1949). *General and industrial management* (C. Storrs, Trans.). London: Sir Isaac Pitman & Sons. First published in 1916 as *Administration Industrielle et Generale,* Dunod, Paris. Originally published in the *Bulletin de la Societe de l'Industrie Minerale*, 5th series Vol. 19, 1916).

Friend, R., Rafferty, Y., & Bramel, D. (1990). A puzzling misinterpretation of the Asch 'conformity' study. *European Journal of Social Psychology, 20*(1), 29–44.

Fung, H. (1999). Becoming a moral child: The socialization of shame among young Chinese children. *Ethos, 27*(2), 180–209.

Geertz, C. (1973). *The interpretation of culture*. New York: Basic Books.

Gilliam, J. (Producer), & Greenwald, R. (Director). (2005). *Wal-Mart: The high cost of low price* [Documentary]. United States: Brave New Films.

Greenwood, J. (1997). *The third industrial revolution: Technology, productivity, and income inequality (No. 435).* Washington, DC: American Enterprise Institute.

Guggenheim, D., Osisek, B., Leckart, S. (Producers), Guggenheim, D. (Director). (2019). *Inside Bill's brain: Decoding Bill Gates*. United States: Netflix.

Hackman, J. R., & Oldham, G. R. (1975). Development of the job diagnostic survey. *Journal of Applied psychology, 60*(2), 159–170.

Heintzman, P. (2002). A conceptual model of leisure and spiritual well-being. *Journal of Park and Recreation Administration, 20*(4), 147–169.
Kennedy, P. (1989). *The rise and fall of the great powers: Economic change and Military conflict from 1500 to 2000*. London: Fontana Press.
Kotler, P. (1967). *Marketing management: Analysis, planning and control*. Englewood Cliffs, NJ: Prentice-Hall.
Kristal, T. (2019). Computerization and the decline of American Unions: Is computerization class-biased? *Work and Occupations, 46*(4), 371–410.
Lebra, T. S. (1983). Shame and guilt: A psychocultural view of the Japanese self. *Ethos, 11*(3), 192–209.
Levitt, T. (1983). The globalization of markets. *Harvard Business Review*, May-June, pp. 2–11.
Lewis, H. B. (1971). Shame and guilt in neurosis. *Psychoanalytic Review, 58*(3), 419.
Liu, Y., & Grusky, D. B. (2013). The payoff to skill in the third industrial revolution. *American Journal of Sociology, 118*(5), 1330–1374.
Maddison, A. (2007). *Contours of the world economy, 1–2030 AD: Essays in macro-economic history*. Oxford University Press. ISBN 978-0-19-922720-4.
Maynard, A. D. (2015). Navigating the fourth industrial revolution. *Nature Nanotechnology, 10* (12), 1005–1006.
McEwen, C. (2011, August 14). Don't just do something: Stand there. *Los Angeles Times*, A14.
Mehri, D. (2006). The darker side of lean: An insider's perspective on the realities of the Toyota production system. *The Academy of Management Perspectives, 20*(2), 21–42.
Menon, U., & Shweder, R. (1994). Kali's tongue: Cultural psychology and the power of "Shame" in Orissa, India. In S. Kitayama & H. Markus (Eds.), *Emotion and culture: Empirical studies of mutual influence*. Washington, D.C.: American Psychological Association.
Menon, U., & Shweder, R. (2003). Dominating Kali: Hindu family values and tantric power. In R. McDermott & J. Kripal (Eds.), *Encountering Kali: In the margins, at the center, in the west*. Los Angeles, CA: University of California Press.
Morishima, M. (1995). The Japanese human resource management system: A learning bureaucracy. In L. F. Moore & P. D. Jennings (Eds.) *Human resource management on the Pacific Rim: Institutions, practices, and attitudes* (pp. 119–150). New York: Walter de Gruyter.
Naidoo, J. (2012, May 15). An infinite vision: The story of Aravind Eye Hospital. *Huffington Post*, p. 15.
Norris, P. (2011). *Democratic deficit: Critical citizens revisited*. Cambridge University Press.
Petrillo, A., Felice, F. D., Cioffi, R., & Zomparelli, F. (2018). Fourth industrial revolution: Current practices, challenges, and opportunities. *Digital Transformation in Smart Manufacturing*, 1–20.
"Plan your path". (n.d.) *The fourth industrial revolution: Plan your path to success*. https://www.oracle.com/webfolder/assets/digibook/plan-your-path-to-IR40/index.html
Prisecaru, P. (2016). Challenges of the fourth industrial revolution. *Knowledge Horizons Economics, 8*(1), 57–62.
Rabeh, M., Husam, A., & Saeed, M. (2017). The fourth industrial revolution (industry 4.0): A social innovation perspective. *Technology Innovation Management Review, 7*(11), 12–20.
Richard. (1977). The first use of the term "democratic deficit." https://federalunion.org.uk/the-first-use-of-the-term-democratic-deficit/. Downloaded on 29 Mar 2020.
Rifkin, J. (2011). *The third industrial revolution: How lateral power is transforming energy, the economy, and the world*. New York: Macmillan.
Robins, N. (2006). *The corporation that changed the world: How the East India Company shaped the modern multinational*. London: Pluto Press.
Roth, K., Schweiger, D. M., & Morrison, A. J. (1991). Global strategy implementation at the business unit level: Operational capabilities and administrative mechanisms. *Journal of International Business Studies, 22*(3), 369–402.
Ryle, G. (1949). *Concept of the mind*. London: Hutchinson.
Ryle, G. (1971). *Collected papers. Volume II collected essays, 1929-1968*. London: Hutchinson.

Santos, F. M. (2012). A positive theory of social entrepreneurship. *Journal of Business Ethics, 111*(3), 335–351.
Schwab, K. (2016). *The fourth industrial revolution.* London: Penguin Random House.
Seke, M. M. (2019). The fourth industrial revolution-4IR: A New buzz concept for the emerging markets of Africa. *i-Manager's Journal on Cloud Computing, 6*(2), 1–12.
Singer, P. (1972). Famine, affluence, and morality. *Philosophy & Public Affairs*, 229–243.
Sinh, A. M., & Chauhan, V. (2013). Deconstructing LajjA as a marker of Indian womanhood. *Psychology and Developing Societies, 25*(1), 133–163.
Stiglitz, J. E. (2007). Democratizing the World Bank. *Brown Journal of World Affairs, 8*(2), 79–86.
Taylor, F. W. (1911). *The principles of scientific management.* New York: Harper.
Tracy, J. L., & Robins, R. W. (2006). Appraisal antecedents of shame and guilt: Support for a theoretical model. *Personality and Social Psychology Bulletin, 32*(10), 1339–1351.
Triandis, H. C. (2009). *Fooling ourselves: Self-deception in politics, religion, and terrorism.* Westport, CT: Praeger.
Waldman, P. (2017, March 22). Inside Alabama's auto jobs boom: Cheap wages, little training, crushed limbs. The South's manufacturing renaissance comes with a heavy price. *Bloomberg Business*, 46–51.
Womack, J. P., Jones, D. T., & Roos, D. (1991). *The machine that change the world: How Japans secret weapon in the global auto wars will revolutionize western Industry.* New York: Harper.
Yunus, M. (2011). *Building social business: The new kind of capitalism that serves humanity's most pressing needs.* London: Public Affairs.

Dharm P. S. Bhawuk is a Professor of Management and Culture and Community Psychology at the University of Hawai'i at Manoa, USA. His research interests include indigenous psychology and management (focused on India and Nepal), cross-cultural training, individualism and collectivism, intercultural sensitivity, diversity in the workplace, culture and quality, culture and entrepreneurship, and political behavior in the workplace. Bhawuk is a citizen of the USA and was born and raised in Nepal. He received his early education at the Laboratory School, Kathmandu. He has BTech (Hons) in Mechanical Engineering from IIT Kharagpur (1979), MBA from the University of Hawai'i at Manoa (1989), and PhD from the University of Illinois at Urbana-Champaign (1995). He is the author of the book Indian Psychology: Lessons from the Bhagavad-Gita (2011) and coeditor of the book Asian Contributions to Cross-Cultural Psychology (1996). He has published more than 90 papers and book chapters and made over 250 presentations internationally. He is a Founding Fellow of the International Academy of Intercultural Research (IAIR). He was a H Smith Richardson Jr. Visiting Fellow, Center for Creative Leadership, Greensboro, North Carolina (2009–2010). He has received many awards and honors including Distinguished Scholar Award, Management Department, College of Business Administration (2000); the Best Paper Award from the Academy of Management (1996 and 2009); the Distinguished Service Award from the East West Center (1989); and the Lum Yip Kee Outstanding MBA Student Award from the College of Business Administration, University of Hawaii (1990).

Chapter 15
Relooking at Shame as a Cultural Phenomenon Through a Generational Perspective

Sowmya Puttaraju and Tony Brian D'souza

1 Introduction

The dilemma of shame begins with its numerous definitions; some refer to it as devaluing of self (either global or specific) based on a behaviour or lack of it implying an inadequacy. This line of thought has most endorsements as it distinguishes it from guilt, which is task-specific devaluation of the behaviour and the doer. The next most popular aspect of shame is its maladaptive nature (Fedewa, Burns & Gomez, 2005), research ties mental ill health and the experience of shame into resulting in emotional disorders, personality disorders, eating disorders and sometimes fatal acts like self-harm and even suicide (Vizin & Unoka, 2015). When we next place the variable of culture in the study of shame, an intriguing aspect of shame appears, there are shame-oriented cultures and guilt-oriented cultures (Wong & Tsai, 2007), and while shame is looked at as a bitter pill, in a socio-cultural aspect, lack of shame is more disastrous than shame (Baron, 2017). With inclusion of culture, the self-conscious emotion,[1] shame is now seen in the light of

[1]Refer: Jessica L. Tracy, Richard W. Robins, and June Price Tangney (2007). *The Self-Conscious Emotions Theory and Research.* ISBN 9781593854867

S. Puttaraju (✉)
Bangalore, Karnataka, India

Jain University, Bangalore, Karnataka, India

Department of Psychology, Mount Carmel College, Bangalore, Karnataka, India

T. B. D'souza
Bangalore, Karnataka, India

Department of Psychology, St. Joseph's College (Autonomous), Bangalore, Karnataka, India

C.-H. Mayer et al. (eds.), *Shame 4.0*, https://doi.org/10.1007/978-3-030-59527-2_15

moral emotions[2], with presence of shame being read as an acknowledgment of the moral fracture and shamelessness as devoid of accountability (Mason, 2010). While in research we have the luxury and it is even prescribed to look at a phenomenon of interest in fragments and then arrive at it as a whole, actual human experience does not enjoy this privilege. The current study again focuses on fragments and based on some assumptions proposes to understand and view shame by connecting fragments already present. The study does not look at adding pieces to a jigsaw puzzle, but placing the existing pieces next to each other to see how they fit and what picture of shame emerges.

The study attempts to comprehend culture as a medium of transmission of information that allows for adaptation of progressive generations. It specifically focuses on stories that are passed down across generations, as vehicles that carry the required template to allow for adaptation within a group. The researchers attempt to examine the influence of culture through the medium of stories on the emotional topography of an individual. Emotions are culturally, evolutionarily and psychologically looked at as adaptive tools that allow any individual to navigate social spaces well within socially accepted and prescribed boundaries (Mesquita & Leu, 2007; Gendron & Barrett 2009) (see Chap. 1). Especially the secondary or self-conscious emotions like shame, pride, embarrassment, jealousy, etc., are regarded as crucial for maintaining the integrity of social fabric by developing a stable, familiar and accountable atmosphere of functioning.

The study also attempts to understand if Millennials express shame similar to the older generation. To explore this, the study unfolds in two parts, where the first part attempts to understand the cultural cause for adaptive and maladaptive forms of shaming and part two attempts to understand the generational perspective. This will also help us understand if the rising context of 4IR has played any influence in modifying or retaining shame and its processes in individuals.

Looking at the contemporary 4IR multicultural and multigenerational melting pot of Indian culture, if culture is an adaptive tool and so are emotions, then would shame have an adaptive value in a specific culture[3]? Could culture become a vehicle for transmission of shame-educative information and how does it go about accomplishing it? And just as a tool can be adaptive and maladaptive with simple changes in either the tool or the environment or both, could shame too encompass both adaptiveness and maladaptiveness? Lastly, could the presence of other cultural values be the antidote or the precursor to adaptive value or maladaptiveness of shame (see Chaps. 3, 4, 5, 7, 8, 14 and 20 in this book)? Again the above questions are too large in their scope; the study only focuses on a more specific component in each question. Does shame serve an adaptive role in an intermediate culture comprising

---

[2]Refer: Tangney, June & Stuewig, Jeffrey & Mashek, Debra. (2007). Moral Emotions and Moral Behavior. Annual review of psychology. 58. 345–72. DOI: 10.1146/annurev.psych.56.091103.070145.

[3]Refer: Rodogno, R. (2008). Shame and Guilt in Restorative Justice. Psychology, public policy and law. 14 (2). 142–176. DOI: 10.1037/a0013474

elements of individualistic and collectivistic culture like India, if it does why and how? If shame does have a maladaptive role, can that be understood in the cultural context? If culture does influence shame and its adaptive and maladaptiveness, could stories passed on in one's culture be a way of transmitting shame-related education? If shame is a tool, then what is the goal that this tool tries to achieve in the specified culture? Could it be other cultural values like forgiveness, worthiness and fairness?

2 Methodology

The study design involves a mixed approach, with a quantitative measure and a qualitative component that are used as complementary processes, to better understand the emotion of shame as experienced (objectively) and as conceptualized by an individual (subjectively). The study recorded responses from 115 participants from India. The study incorporated the snowball sampling method. The compass of shame scale developed by Jeff Ellison, Randy Lennon and Steven Pulos[4] on Nathanson's compass of shame theory was used to assess objectively the shaming style of a participant. Followed by a narration of a story (cultural) as remembered by the participant that involves the theme of transgression. The cultural stories or folktales or mythologies are mostly religious in origin, which in turn is treated as a cultural product. In the context of a participant's inability to recall, a priorly designed list of titles of stories that tackles the theme of transgression was read out to the participant. The list was prepared after consulting psychologists, academicians and religious head who were briefed about the intent of the study [5] The narration of the story is followed by a series of questions to identify the emotions of the protagonist, the affected party, investigate the sense of worthiness (of the transgressor) and identify whether the focus was on forgiveness or fairness in the aftermath of the transgression.[6]

---

[4]Refer: Elison, Jeff; Lennon, Randy and Pulos, Steven. Investigating the Compass of Shame: The development of the Compass of Shame Scale.Social Behavioural Personality, 2006, 34(3), 221–238

[5]Dr. Leemamol Mathew, Psychologist, Guest Faculty at Bangalore University, Dr. Lakshmi Kuchibhotla, Faculty and Academic Mentor at Banjara Academy, an Islamic religious head and Mrs. Zakia Siraj, former Dean and Department Head of Psychology, Mount Carmel College

[6]The method of using a story by treating it as a cultural product has been used earlier, in the study titled Kali's Tongue. The authors used a picture of Goddess Kali biting her tongue and asked their participants to narrate the story that led to the point of the incident illustrated in the picture. The authors aimed to study the experience of shame as the associated emotion with the Goddess in the picture and used a Guttman scale to measure a progressive narration that started with a factual narration to articulating the larger objective of comprehending shame. - Menon, U., & Shweder, R. A. (1994). Kali's tongue: Cultural psychology and the power of shame in Orissa, India. In S. Kitayama & H. R. Markus (Eds.), Emotion and culture: Empirical studies of mutual influence (p. 241–282). American Psychological Association. https://doi.org/10.1037/10152-007

3 Results and Discussion

Part I: Does shame serve an adaptive role in an intermediate culture comprising elements of individualistic and collectivistic culture like India, if it does why and how? And if shame does have a maladaptive role, can that be understood in the cultural context?

Nathanson's compass of shame scale describes the scripts that underlie the coping mechanism in the experience of shame. While Nathanson's definition of shame[7] is vague, the response styles are definitive. The original theory of Nathanson (1992) and thereafter the construction of the compass of shame scale by Elison et al. (2006) only described four maladaptive styles. Among the four styles, withdrawal and attack self define the individual as acknowledging the experience as negative, valid and withdrawing or getting angry with self. While in the avoidance style, the individual does not acknowledge the experience as either negative or valid and merely behaves as though in denial, whereas in attack other, the experience could be evaluated as negative, but the individual holds others responsible for it and targets the others (Elison et al. 2006).[8] Uptill the COSS 3, the scale only measured the maladaptive styles, but with COSS version 5,[9] additional ten items were added, to assess adaptive strategies that could be utilized to restore or initiate reparative actions towards the transgression.

The study recorded responses from 115 participants. For the purpose of this study, the data collected was grouped based on age (millennials, middle-aged and old-aged) and gender (female and male). Based on their responses on the compass of shame scale, over 91% of the 115 participants recorded higher on adaptive shaming responses as compared to the maladaptive shaming styles. But this does not mean that the other (maladaptive) shaming styles are not used. The questionnaire (original component) provides four choices of responses for each item outlining a "shame-related scenario", with every choice representing a specific style of maladaptive shaming and no provision for adaptive response or no response with a later addition of items that provide an adaptive shaming response. Another interesting feature that such a differentiated construction of questionnaire would give is to provide a way to circumvent social desirability as every individual will receive a score on adaptive shaming and other maladaptive shaming styles separately. The scale takes for granted that individuals would demonstrate both.[10] Allowing for a comparison of

[7]"Shame is the negative effect felt in response to any impediment to the ongoing experience of interest or joy" (Tomkins, 1963) ; Tomkins, S. S. (1962–1991). Affect/imagery/consciousness. Vols. 1–3. New York: *Springer*. Nathanson, fleshed out Tomkins definition of shame

[8]Refer: Elison, Jeff; Lennon, Randy and Pulos, Steven. Investigating the Compass of Shame: The development of the Compass of Shame Scale.*Social Behavioural Personality*, 2006, 34(3), 221-238.

[9]The guilt proneness items in COSS 5 are not considered in the study.

[10]Research trends indicate that there is plurality in shame evoked reaction behaviours, with most opting a polarized view, of shame reaction behaviours constituting either adaptive (Rodogno, 2008)

Table 15.1 Represents age-wise mean of scores on COSS-5 for styles of shaming

Age	Percentage score for avoidance dimension	Percentage score for attack self dimension	Percentage score for withdrawal dimension	Percentage score for attack other dimension	Percentage score for adaptive dimension
Millennials (18–30)	58	52.3	52.51	37.25	72.59
Middle age (31–50)	51.36	45.64	49.24	35.36	70.45
Old age (51–92)	55.54	44.46	52.83	29.02	69.24

frequency of adaptive shaming responses to maladaptive styles both between and within individuals. Also the predominant maladaptive styles are highlighted for comparison across individuals. The proximity between the adaptive score and maladaptive scores can be used to compare the frequency of the behaviours in the individuals.

The finding demonstrates the significance of shame in a collectivistic culture. Around 83% of respondents identified that the protagonist in their story would experience "shame and guilt".[11] Of the 115 participants, 107 recorded a higher adaptive score than maladaptive with only 8 scoring higher on the maladaptive dimension. The difference between the adaptive score and maladaptive ranged between a percentage of 6 and 59. Of the four maladaptive shaming responses, the avoidance response was largely the most frequently chosen response, followed by withdrawal, and attack other is the least chosen response, even when the population was segregated according to age (Table 15.1) and gender (Table 15.2). There is a significant difference between avoidance and withdrawal dimension ($p < 0.05$) and also significant difference between cluster of avoidance and withdrawal versus attack self and attack other scores ($p < 0.01$), indicating that avoidance and

---

or maladaptive behaviours (Fedewa et al., 2005). With few researchers signifying a blend of both (Miceli & Castelfranchi, 2011)

Refer: Rodogno, R. (2008). Shame and Guilt in Restorative Justice. *Psychology, public policy and law*. 14 (2). 142–176. DOI: 10.1037/a0013474.

Refer: Fedewa, B.A., Burns, L.R. & Gomez, A.A. 2005. Positive and negative perfectionism and the

shame/guilt distinction: adaptive and maladaptive characteristics. *Personality and Individual Differences*, 38: 1609–1619.

Refer: Miceli, M., & Castelfranchi, C. (2011). Forgiveness: A cognitive-motivational anatomy. *Journal for the Theory of Social Behaviour*, 41, 260–290. DOI: 10.1111/j.1468-5914.2011.00465.x

[11] After shame and guilt, the next most common response was as low as 10%, with participants identifying "regret" as the emotion in the protagonist post transgression, and only 6% identified the protagonist as being "angry": this anger was mostly directed at self (with the exception of one, where the anger was directed at the affected party) in the protagonist for having committed the transgression. Around 2% identified only guilt and (only) shame as the emotional response or were unable to identify no emotional response in the protagonist.

Table 15.2 Represents gender-wise mean of scores on COSS-5 for styles of shaming

Gender	Avoidance dimension	Attack self dimension	Withdrawal dimension	Attack other dimension	Adaptive dimension
Female	30.49	26.74	28.30	19.57	36.03
Male	31.14	28.08	28.61	19.68	35.27

Table 15.3 Represents mean of scores on COSS-5 for styles of shaming

Styles of shaming	Avoidance dimension	Attack self dimension	Withdrawal dimension	Attack other dimension	Adaptive dimension
Population	55.82	49.42	51.64	35.65	71.55

withdrawal are the two most frequently used responses, while attack self and others are the least frequently used ones (Table 15.3).

According to Hofstede ratings, India scores a 48 (an intermediate score) on the individualism dimension.[12] Thus demonstrating both collectivistic and individualistic tendencies. In accordance with the Hofstede model, a collectivistic culture prioritizes the interests of the collective over the individual and vice versa in an individualistic culture. An intermediate score might indicate both an individual accountability towards the collective and a collective accountability towards the individual welfare thereby creating an exquisite web of expectations that influences the slightest of decisions an individual would make. Perhaps in such a scenario, an individual often weighs the societal implications of his/her behaviour, like "what will people say/think ?" becomes a very pertinent question. In reciprocation such an individual could also feel "entitled" to "returns" from the society, often wondering "what did I get for all that I did?" If the give and take (between the collective and the individual) is perceived as fair, there is gratitude and if the deal is short (disfavouring the individual) it is either attributed to intangible powers like "destiny" or the philosophy of "karma"[13] leading to disgruntlement and distrust. Perhaps culture's prescriptive role gains more prominence, as these expectations need to be effectively communicated to maintain the intricacy of social fabric. The intermediate score in individualism and collective dimension is often interpreted in the academic discipline of management as in-group loyalty, conformity and individual accountability towards how one's life turns out to be. The later largely attributed to the philosophy promoted in the dominant religion of the country. The current study does not focus

[12]Refer: Hofstede, G., Hofstede G. J., & Minkov, M. (2010). *Cultures and organizations: Software of the mind*. Revised and Expanded 3rd Edition. New York: McGraw-Hill. and/or

Refer: Hofstede, G. (2001). Culture's consequences: Comparing values, behaviors, institutions, and organizations across nations. Thousand Oaks, CA: *Sage Publications*.

[13]Karma is defined as the sum of a person's actions in this and previous states of existence, viewed as deciding their fate in future existences (in Hinduism and Buddhism – religious idea and contemporary also viewed with a philosophical lense)- Devdutt, Pattnaik. (2014).Karma is the new swastika. https://devdutt.com/articles/karma-is-the-new-swastika/

on the source or the philosophy, but it's inevitable influence on the individual-social interaction.

The report of both guilt and shame in the respondents is supported by the Hofstede findings. Research findings mostly associate, guilt with individualistic cultures (Fessler, 2010)[14] and shame with collectivistic cultures (Fessler, 2010).[15] In the context of a transgression, for the maintenance of social fabric, accountability on behalf of the transgressor is essential to restore trust. Thus the presence of shame in the transgressor could be interpreted as a sign of acknowledgement and accountability in the transgressor and even culturally treated as the beginning of reparative action. And lack of shame could lead to social isolation, as interdependency (prevalent in collectivistic cultures) is unmet, challenged and compromised.

Researchers have also successfully discerned between the two emotions, though in layman's parlance and comprehension, the two emotions could be used as synonyms. Researchers (Wong & Tsai, 2007) have distinguished guilt and shame based on "what" is evaluated and "who" is evaluated. While guilt is considered internally oriented, self-evaluation (negative) for not meeting one's own expectation and is task specific. Shame is externally oriented, meaning a negative self-evaluation for not meeting the expectations of others and unlike guilt is not task specific but a devaluation of one's global self. And there is a general consensus that both emotions qualify to be labelled as moral emotions, experienced in the context of transgression or violation of a socially accepted norm. While shame can be considered a moral emotion, it is not restricted to moral transgressions alone but also to nonmoral acts, as in a discrepancy as discussed by Miceli and Castelfranchi (2011) between "one's actual self and one's ideal self..." entails shame, while guilt is a result of violating one's moral self.

Also the popular trend in research is to consider guilt more than shame leading to reparative actions. This has been relooked at by de Hooge, Zeelenberg and Breugelmans (2010), stating that guilt entails reparative action when there is conscious admission and accountability of the wrongdoing in the transgressor. The authors highlight the play between "self-defence manoeuvers" with contextual accountability, intentionality and intensity of the transgression and the credibility or the status of the affected party, to influence the path to "making amends".[16] Thus steering clear from a linear relationship between a specific emotional domain and an action tendency.

The authors discuss the function of shame as significant for social cohesion. They delineate two categories of motives and the entailed behaviours that could emanate

[14]"Shame is overshadowed by guilt in individualistic cultures." Fessler, Daniel, 2010. Shame in Two Cultures: Implications for Evolutionary Approaches. *Journal of Cognition and Culture* 4.2

[15]"Shame is more prominent in Bengkulu, a collectivistic culture, than in California, an individualistic culture" Fessler, Daniel, 2010. Shame in Two Cultures: Implications for Evolutionary Approaches. *Journal of Cognition and Culture* 4.2

[16]Refer: Miceli, M., & Castelfranchi, C. (2018). Reconsidering the Differences Between Shame and Guilt. Eur J Psychol. 2018 Aug; 14(3): 710–733. Published online 2018 Aug 31. doi: 10.5964/ejop.v14i3.1564

Table 15.4 Represents number of individuals whose scores indicate adaptive and maladaptive shame

Total	115	Difference	
Adaptive	107	Min = 6%	Max = 59%
Maladaptive	8		

in the aftermath of shame experienced by transgression: the motive to "restore one's threatened self-image" and the motive "to protect one's self image from further damage". When the threat to self is perceived as manageable, it leads to acquisition of skills and re-attempting a flawed performance. Perhaps this explains the feelings of shame associated with performance that fails to meet expectations[17] both socially (e.g. when the parent considers himself/herself a failure at the misbehaviour of a child) and professionally (e.g. a student who has received a low score or has failed). The protect motive of shame kicks in when the restorative efforts are perceived as overwhelming leading to withdrawal behaviours.

Gausel, Vignoles and Leach (2016) endorsed the dual motive theoretical conception of shame. They term the self-defensive and pro-social motives as paradoxical effects of shame. Depending on the individual's appraisal of either improving one's self-image or salvaging one's social image. The authors position shame as the result of self-critical (negative) appraisal of a self-defect (specific and not global) perceived as a moral failure. Therefore the individual experiencing shame is highly motivated to improve the perceived defect and alleviate the failure. Contingent to the plausibility of the specific flaw's correction entailing improvement in one's self-image. The second path that Gausel et al. (2016) propose as moral failure is the result of condemnation by others awareness of one's self-defect (specific and not global). Thus, any failures of the self can adversely affect one's social image. Authors explain it as people having a "need to belong" and disapproval due to one's defect, could lead to defensive behaviours like avoidance and covering up in the individual.

The conceptualization of shame by de Hooge et al. (2010) and Gausel et al. (2016) is better suited to explain shame in a collectivistic cultural context than the predominant view. Over 90% of the respondents recorded higher on adaptive shaming style, demonstrating a willingness to make amends in the aftermath of shame, with less than 10% scoring higher on maladaptive style[18] (Table 15.4). The current study findings are in line with the above insights. This allows for shame to be looked at as essaying a functional adaptive role, motivating the transgressor for making amends and indicating to the larger collective to consider reinstating them as dependable, trustworthy members of the social fabric. For instance, in stories (as narrated by participants) such as "The Prodigal Son", shame identified in the

[17]For these expectations to be potent in the creation of shame, they cannot be only looked at externally imposed criteria but also internalized or accepted by the individual experiencing shame. This is done to delineate between shame and fear of disapproval and not shame at not meeting expectations. For more information refer to Miceli and Castelfranchi (2018).

[18]The range of difference between the adaptive and the nearest maladaptive style being – 6–59%.

transgressor is met with forgiveness in the affected party, thereby allowing for transgressor to be reaccepted in the social fabric.

The identification of shame in the transgressor having an adaptive quality in the context of the collective can further draw support from cultural framework as delineated by Hofstede and Schwartz. According to the latest report published on Hofstede ratings[19,20] and as mentioned earlier in the study, it may not just account for the presence of guilt as associated with individualistic dimension but also account for the "adaptiveness" of shame. The report also gives a high score of 77 on the dimension of power distance that measures the expectation and acceptance of unequal distribution of power. The presence of an indomitable hierarchy and the inevitable expectation of compliance is also reflected in Schwartz's cultural analysis of nations.[21] Hofstede ratings provide an individual nation rating. Schwartz's framework is a group-based inference where nations similar in cultural heritage are grouped together. India features in the category of South Asian nations. Schwartz evaluates the South Asian nations as being highly embedded and lower in egalitarianism and autonomy. The presence of hierarchy in the social structure and the emphasis on obedience and obligations to maintain social order further underlines the "adaptiveness" value of shame in the current population as a cultural prescriptive and expected behaviour in the view of transgression from an (in group) individual. Therefore the nature of transgressions that fall under the purview of a social context and concerns the "social image", in anticipation of "rejection" or "condemnation"

---

[19]Refer: Hofstede, G., Hofstede G. J., & Minkov, M. (2010). *Cultures and organizations: Software of the mind*. Revised and Expanded 3rd Edition. New York: McGraw-Hill. and/or

Refer: Hofstede, G. (2001). Culture's consequences: Comparing values, behaviors, institutions, and organizations across nations. Thousand Oaks, CA: *Sage Publications*

[20]If culture does play an adaptive role, how stable are the ratings?

To answer the first question, whether Hofstede ratings or the cultural dimensions are in fact stable over time, authors refer to the work of Beugelsdijk, Maseland, and van Hoorn (2015), who addressed both sides of the debate and used the survey scores from two birth cohorts (mean birth year 1941 & 1971), to address the changes brought about by globalization, economic, scientific advances on the practice of culture in contemporary times. As the predominant view is to look at the economic, government and other institutions as the result of the country's cultural mindset and not the other way around. The study based its approach on Inglehart (1990) socialization theory that an individual's socialization is determined largely by their early years (childhood and adolescence) and centres their efforts in procuring what they perceived as lacking in the growing, impressionable years. The results of the study affirm Hofstede's earlier claim that cultural differences across countries remain stable. The results for national cultural dimensions have changed, more so for some dimensions than others. Also the change in the national cultural dimensions is discussed as a global trend, and global averages are presented and do not provide country specific changes. Indicating that while changes at the level of country could follow the global trend, the actual change could deviate from the global averages. The research findings demonstrate that individualism is the dimension that has recorded the most change followed by power distance and indulgence. Countries have on the whole moved towards individualism, scoring lower on power distance than adopting an increasingly egalitarian view and exercising less restraint.

[21]Refer: Schwartz, S.H. (2004) *Mapping and interpreting cultural differences around the world*. In Vinken, H., Soeters, J. and Ester, P. (Eds.): Comparing Cultures, Dimensions of Culture in a Comparative Perspective, Brill, Leiden, The Netherlands, 43–73.

(Gausel & Leach, 2011) with the motive of restoring one's image (Miceli & Castelfranchi, 2011), shame could entail adaptive behaviours.

Along the same lines of hierarchical dominance, in the course that the transgressor is unable to restore one's self-image, in accordance to de Hooge et al. (2010), they would demonstrate defensive behaviours especially withdrawal. Here the authors challenge the view that withdrawal is a defensive behaviour. They present evidence that re-conceptualizes withdrawal in a pro-social light, as a sign of surrender and appeasement that evokes empathy and forgiveness in others. For example from the qualitative data, subjects who have discussed The Prodigal Son[22] story have narrated the instance when the younger son, after losing all his money and while staying in a pigsty, decides to return to his father. He does so after realizing his mistake and feeling ashamed of it. He decides to ask for forgiveness and requests his father to allow him to live in the house even as a servant. As it would still fare better than boarding with the swine family. On his return the prodigal son is forgiven and restored his prior place in the family and the household. The prodigal son's surrender to his father's mercy could be viewed as withdrawal and acknowledgement of hierarchy, evoking empathy in the father and is awarded with forgiveness and reinstatement into his original social position. The current study supports the prior mentioned research insights and records the next most widely used style (after adaptive) as avoidance followed by withdrawal (the least used styles are self-attack and other attack). Again the hierarchical arrangement and the social value placed on obligations towards the hierarchy could explain the "adaptive" value of the maladaptive styles of avoidance and withdrawal (over self and other attack). The generality of the style of maladaptive patterns across age groups and gender found in the study also affirms the overarching cultural significance of the ubiquitous hierarchical structure.

In line with Gausel & Leach (2011) view, the items in the compass of shame scale that checked for adaptive and maladaptive responses were further divided into self-image-oriented (items that focused on skills or lack of it in self) and social image-oriented (items that focused on unfavourable evaluation by others) (Table 15.5). If the Gausel et al.'s view were to be true, then the population studied would show higher adaptive responses in self-image when compared to social image. The population will also demonstrate significant difference between maladaptive responses, with social image-related responses recording a higher maladaptive

[22]The Prodigal Son: "So it starts off with a wealthy family, the father has two sons, where the younger one is pampered and first born is hard working. When the time comes to split the wealth, the younger one takes the money and goes to distant exotic land and spends it. And when he is done spending it, he also has friends who take advantage of his gullibility, they all spend his money, and he ends up working in a pig farm, where he is mistreated so badly that he has to eat the pigs' food. And then one day while eating food he realizes that the servants at his fathers' home are treated better and they have better food and so he decides to go back to his father's house and ask forgiveness and at least be a servant if not a son I suppose, and then while he is coming back to his father's home, I think somebody notices him, and the father says 'Ohh my son is returning' and then a fast is ordered. This upsets the older son, but the younger son is taken back with open and loving arms."

Table 15.5 Represents *t*-test values for Maladaptive and Adaptive responses from the Shame Scale and its comparison with self-image and social-image

Sl. no	Mean Item name	Mean	Item name	Mean	Significance	*t*-test value	Results
1	Maladaptive	48.137	Adaptive	71.559	$p < 0.01$	1.39E-33 (0.000)	Significant
2	Adaptive self image	3.8112	Adaptive social image	3.717	$p > 0.01$	0.354	Not significant
3	Maladaptive self image	8.790	Maladaptive social image	10.267	$p < 0.01$	0.0000441	Significant
4	Adaptive self image	3.8112	Maladaptive self image	8.790	$p < 0.01$	1.60E-42 (0.000)	Significant
5	Adaptive social image	3.717	Maladaptive social image	10.267	$p < 0.01$	1.60E-42 (0.000)	Significant
6	Avoidance	55.830	Withdrawal	51.644	$p < 0.05$	0.01711	Significant
7	Avoidance/ withdrawal	53.737	Attack self/ attack other	42.538	$p < 0.01$	2.31E-13 (0.000)	Significant

mean. Also avoidance would emerge as the most frequently used maladaptive style (Table 15.5), with the exception of one of the study findings corroborating the other assumptions. While the *t*-tests between adaptive shaming responses to self-image and social image were not significant, the *t*-tests between maladaptive responses to self-image and social image were highly significant, with social image-related responses recording a higher mean (Table 15.5). Also among the styles of maladaptive shaming, avoidance was the most frequently used style and showed a significant difference from other styles. Gausel et al. have neither consulted nor laid a reference to Nathanson's compass of shame or that of shame essaying a social cohesive role in a collectivistic culture. This highlights the need to integrate the diverse perspectives used to study shame to arrive at a comprehensive understanding.

In accordance with de Hooge et al.'s (2010) view, to understand shame as function from a restorative motive and if overwhelmed, transition to a self-defensive protective motive. Authors define shame as a self-conscious emotion that indicates a threatened self, which could elicit restorative and protective behaviours based on the plausibility of neutralizing the threat. The questionnaire items were clustered into adaptive scores and maladaptive scores, with the understanding that adaptive scores demonstrate reparative and amendment making behaviours, thus demonstrating the restorative motive. Whereas the protective motive is demonstrated in maladaptive behaviours, when the restorative behaviours are considered overwhelming. *t*-test was done to see if the responses for each category were significantly different.[23] Restorative (adaptive) and protective (maladaptive) were found to be different at a significance level of 0.01, with restorative (adaptive) behaviours scoring a higher mean than the protective (maladaptive) behaviours (Table 15.5). Also the higher

[23]Please refer to the tables for the *t*-test values.

scored maladaptive styles emerged as avoidance and withdrawal followed by attack self and attack other (Table 15.3).[24]

The maladaptive styles of avoidance and withdrawal emerging as the more frequently used maladaptive styles are in line with Gausel et al. (2016) and de Hooge et al. (2010), who mentioned avoidance and withdrawal as frequently used behaviours to defend and protect a threatened social image and/or self-image (Table 15.3). The maladaptive behaviours also can be understood in the light of Hofstede's cultural dimensions of power distance and masculinity. The stress on obedience (power distance) and competition/achievement (masculinity) constantly brings to fore the comparisons to others and the importance of external validation. With disobedience, failures and inadequacies inviting negative appraisals, threatening self- and social image.

So does shame serve an adaptive role in an intermediate culture comprising elements of individualistic and collectivistic culture like India? The answer from the research findings seems to be yes. To answer, why and how—it does so to acknowledge and conform to the inherent hierarchical structure embedded in the culture of the social fabric. The findings show that even the maladaptive styles of shame especially avoidance and withdrawal too maintain social cohesion and can be viewed as pro-social behaviours than as defensive behaviours. But this would require a more elegant alignment of theoretical understanding of shame and the development of a corresponding instrument to assess shame in a culturally adaptive context.

PART II—Difference in generational perspective: Did millennials learn from their elders the consequences of social transgression and yet are independent of it?

If culture does influence shame and its adaptive and maladaptiveness, could stories passed on in one's culture be a way of transmitting shame-related education? And if shame is a tool then what is the goal that this tool tries to achieve in the specified culture, could it be other cultural values like forgiveness, worthiness and fairness?

The study focused on two interconnected sources of qualitative data. The narration of the cultural story and the answers to questions framed to understand the aftermath of transgression. The narrative and the answers for the questions were analysed separately and interrelated.

The questions asked following the narration are as follows:

- What emotion is the protagonist in the story feeling? Participants were encouraged to name an emotion, if they used an evaluative adjective like bad or good.
- Because the protagonist felt and expressed ______ what was the reaction of the opposite/affected/other/aggrieved party? In the context of your story.
- What if the protagonist didn't feel __________ then what would be the reaction of the affected/other/opposite/aggrieved party? In the context of your story.
- Does the protagonist become unworthy for having committed the mistake?

---

[24]Please refer to the tables above.

- If the worth is lost then how is it regained?
- If not forgiven, what do you think the protagonist should do next?

The analysis of the answers for the above questions revealed two predominant themes—forgiving and unforgiving. The two themes were selected on the basis of forgiveness being mentioned as the consequential emotion in the aggrieved or affected party, as the reciprocal response to the shame experienced in the protagonist (transgressor). The responses that did not align themselves to forgiving mentioned higher-intensity emotions like anger, insult, hurt and shocked which were followed up by action tendencies like revenge, curse and punishment. Emotions that did not mention forgiveness but others like regret, disappointment, patience, etc., were grouped under forgiving as they led to repentance and forgiveness-oriented action tendencies like making amends, reconciliation efforts and persistently asking for forgiveness. The question of worth of the protagonist, in the aftermath of transgression, if unaffected or regained through repentance or reconciliatory efforts were grouped under forgiving. If the worth of the protagonist was remarked as lost or contingent to repetition of mistakes, then they were grouped in the unforgiving theme as they were followed by punitive action tendencies. For the last question if unforgiven what would become of the protagonist, the replies that spoke of non-adverse circumstances awaiting the protagonist like moving on, making newer efforts to repent and continuing seeking forgiveness were grouped under forgiving. The responses that entailed adverse circumstances befalling the protagonist for not being forgiven, like doomed, continues making mistakes, continues feeling shame, is helpless etc., were grouped under unforgiving. As the study focused on the aftermath of transgression and the expectation of probable emotions and action tendencies of the aggrieved/affected party, the emotion of the protagonist was not considered in the current analysis.

The answers of the participants were given a score of 1, for every forgiving and unforgiving response. The total score of unforgiving and forgiving are subtracted from each other to arrive at a final score. The difference is coded as predominantly forgiving (Pf) if forgiving is a higher score, predominantly non-forgiving (Pnf) if unforgiving is a higher score and dualistic tendency (Dt) if the difference is 0, i.-e. equal number of forgiving and unforgiving responses are recorded. The nature of forgiveness that emerged in the analysis was mostly a blend of conditional forgiveness, the kind given under certain conditions like "apology, acceptance and change in unacceptable behaviour" and authentic process forgiveness, "unconditional, self-regarding, prosocial, altruistic motive, to avoid revenge for the good of both" transgressor and the affected party. The above two definitions are from the topology of seven types of forgiveness as outlined by Walrond-Skinner (1998).[25] The authors would like to highlight that they identify the other group as non-forgiving and not unforgiving as all groups demonstrated forgiving and unforgiving behaviours, even the non-forgiving group recorded forgiving behaviours but lesser as compared to the

[25]Refer: Walrond, Skinner S (1998) The function and role of forgiveness in working with couples and families: Clearing the ground. *J Fam Ther* 20: 3–19.

Table 15.6 The table categorizes the answers to the questions into the two dominant themes of forgiving and unforgiving

Forgiving	Questions	Unforgiving
• Forgiveness • Regret • Disappointment • Patience • Grief • Sad • Unconditional love • Depressed • Disheartened • Glad • Proud • Unaffected[a] • Afraid • Happy • Acceptance • Sympathy • Peaceful • Composed • Self-awareness • Redemption • Obedience[b] • Love • Surprised • Embarrassed	Because the protagonist felt and expressed ______ what was the reaction of the opposite/affected/other/aggrieved party? In the context of your story What if the protagonist didn't feel __________ then what would be the reaction of the affected/other/opposite/aggrieved party?	• Anger • Indifference • Insult humiliated • Hurt • Shocked • Guilty • Hopeless • Betrayed • Wrath • Authoritative (righteous anger) • Furious • Upset • Frustrated • Helpless • Unforgiving • Vengeful • Arrogance[c] • Destroyed • Disgusted • Turmoil • Stubborn
• Worth unaffected/intact • Regained after receiving forgiveness • No • Not really[d]	In the context of your story. Does the protagonist become unworthy for having committed the mistake?	• Yes • Yes, with regard to the affected party[e]
• Work to regain it • Making amends • Doing one's duty • Ask forgiveness • Considering the other's perspective (empathy) • Obedience • Accepting faults • Teach their children not to make the same mistakes[f] • Letting go • Apologizing	If the worth is lost then how is it regained?	• Avoid repeating mistakes • It is difficult to get it back • What is lost is lost • Cannot regain
• Marry (reconciliatory action) • Look for shelter elsewhere • Move on/leave[g] • Make amends (work for women's rights) • Rectify mistakes • Seeking forgiveness • Convince/persuade to receive	If not forgiven, what do you think the protagonist should do next?	• Never return, leave • Exile • Nothing • Defiance—refuse fire test • Continues to live in shame • Death

(continued)

Table 15.6 (continued)

Forgiving	Questions	Unforgiving
forgiveness • Engage the affected party in a discussion • Evoke empathetic response in the affected party by urging to take the protagonist perspective • Take rectifying steps to not repeat mistakes • Ask for mercy		• Continue to live in deplorable conditions (live with the pigs)[h] • Sulking • Walk away from the protagonist[i] • Suicide[j] • Revenge

[a]Unaffected is followed by non-adversarial action tendency

[b]In the context of Rama and Sita, the participant has interpreted the story as Rama as the transgressor and Sita the affected who obeys Rama's command to go through the fire test

[c]The story the participant referred to was the Lakshmana and Surpanaka story and the affected party is Surpanaka whose provocative responses lead to Lakshmana committing the transgression

[d]As the response was followed by non-adversarial action tendency

[e]This response as categorized as unforgiving as the response was followed up by adversarial action tendency

[f]Participant responded so in reference to Adam and Eve story

[g]The participant was referring to the story of Rama and Sita, with Sita choosing to leave Rama after all ordeals are over

[h]Participant was referring to the story of the—The Prodigal Son

[i]Participant refers to the story of Karna and Kunti. Karna the protagonist choosing to walk away when refusing to comply by his mother's (Kunti) anguished plea

[j]Participant refers to the story of Adam and Eve, in the eventuality of not receiving divine forgiveness

Table 15.7 Represents scores classified under predominantly forgiving, predominantly non-forgiving and dualistic

	Predominantly forgiving (Pf) (Total number: 70)	Predominantly non-forgiving (Pnf) (Total number: 26)	Dualistic tendency (Dt) (Total number: 19)
Population identified as adaptive (Total number: 107)	91.5%	100%	89.5%
Population identified as maladaptive (Total number: 8)	8.5%	0	10.5%

predominantly forgiving group. The dualistic group on the other hand demonstrated not a predominance but a unique blend of both forgiving and unforgiving behaviours, discussed in a later section.

The participants were thus grouped into predominantly forgiving (Pf), predominantly non-forgiving (Pnf) and dualistic tendency (Dt). Table 15.7 provides the distribution of population identified as adaptive or maladaptive using the compass of shame scale assessment across the three groups (Pf), (Pnf) and (Dt).

Table 15.8 Representing t-tests scores for of Predominantly forgiving—maladaptive (Pf(M)), Predominantly forgiving—adaptive (Pf(A)), Dualistic—maladaptive (Dt(M)), Dualistic—adaptive (Dt(A)), Predominantly non-forgiving—maladaptive (Pnf(M)), Predominantly non-forgiving—adaptive (Pnf(A))

Item	Significance	*t*-test value	Results
Pf (A) & Dt (A)	$p > 0.01$	0.2190381058	Not significant
Pf (A) & Pnf (A)	$p > 0.01$	0.4888203951	Not significant
Dt (A) & Pnf (A)	$p > 0.01$	0.5340315971	Not significant
Pf (M) & Dt M)	$p < 0.01$	0.0034109206	Significant
Pf (M) & Pnf (M)	$p > 0.01$	0.1589043179	Not significant
Dt (M) & Pnf (M)	$p > 0.01$	0.2799851898	Not significant
Pf (A) & Pf(M)	$p < 0.01$	3.15E-26 (0.000)	Significant
Dt (A) & Dt(M)	$p < 0.01$	0.0000003339	Significant
Pnf (A) & Pnf(M)	$p < 0.01$	0.0000000008	Significant
Pf (A) & Dt&Pnf (A)	$p > 0.01$	0.2238718808	Not significant
Pf (M) & Dt&Pnf (M)	$p < 0.05$	0.0103846748	Significant
Pf (A) & Dt&Pnf (A)	$p > 0.01$	0.2238718808	Not significant
Pf (M) & Dt&Pnf (M)	$p < 0.05$	0.0103846748	Significant
Pf&Pnf (A) & Dt(A)	$p > 0.01$	0.2178561412	Not significant
Pf&Pnf (M) & Dt(M)	$p < 0.01$	0.0033276947	Significant

Interestingly of the eight people identified as maladaptive in the study, none fall into predominantly non-forgiveness inclined category. The groups were then compared on their adaptive and maladaptive scores. While the adaptive scores did not differ across each group. The maladaptive scores differed between the forgiving (Pf) and dualistic tendency (Dt), with Dt recording a higher mean score (please refer to Table 15.8 for scores). The mean for the predominantly non-forgiving group (Pnf) fell in between the mean of Pf and Dt, with Pf recording the lowest mean. To check whether the group Pnf behaved more like Pf or like Dt, the scores of Pnf were combined with Pf and Dt, and a *t*-test was done. The combined group of Dt and Pnf differed at the 0.05 level with Pf, whereas the combination of Pf and Pnf differed at the 0.01 level. Indicating that the group Dt behaved very distinctly and worse compared to Pf and Pnf in maladaptive dimensions. The Dt group is the smallest of the three groups 16.5%, the highest is the forgiving group that comprises a little over 60%, and the Pnf group accounts for the rest of 22.6% of the population in the study (Table 15.11).

In accordance with de Hooge et al. (2010), all the groups demonstrated no difference in restorative motive but behaved significantly differently in their maladaptive or protective motive. Both Dt and Pnf group score higher than the adaptive mean for the whole population, with Pf group scoring the least, though marginally. (Refer to Table 15.6.) Both Dt and Pnf groups also score higher than the population's maladaptive mean and Pf group scored the lowest. The *t*-test between each group's adaptive and maladaptive dimensions was the same as that for the whole population.

Table 15.9 Representing mean of predominantly forgiving (Pf), dualistic (Dt) and predominantly non-forgiving (Pnf) in adaptive shaming style (A) and maladaptive shaming style (M)

Item	Mean Scores
Pf (M)	46.23
Pf(A)	70.45
Dt(M)	52.58
Dt(A)	74.49
Pnf(M)	49.61
Pnf(A)	72.24
Dt and Pnf (M)	50.87
Dt and Pnf (A)	73.19

The Dt group scored highest, the Pf group the lowest and the (Pnf) in between the two, in the adaptive and maladaptive dimensions, as compared to the total population's mean. The three groups differed at a significance level of 0.01, between their adaptive and maladaptive dimensions, scoring higher on the adaptive dimension. This meant that most participants demonstrated both forgiving and unforgiving behaviours, with some demonstrating a higher predominance or inclination for forgiving (Pf) or unforgiving (Pnf), and some others did not show any such clear inclination (Dt). The Dt group that demonstrates the propensity for either behaviours records a significantly higher mean 52.6 from the forgiving (Pf) group (least mean of 46.23) but not significantly from the unforgiving (Pnf) with the second highest mean 49.6. To understand whether unforgiving (Pnf) behaved more like the both (forgiving and unforgiving) (Dt) or the forgiving (Pf). The group Pnf was clubbed with Dt, the significance level of difference from the Pf group fell to 0.05 level, but when clubbed with (Pf), the significance of difference remained at 0.01 level. Thus it would be safer to say that Pf and Dt are closer to each other in terms of their maladaptive scores, but Pnf inching towards the similar level of maladaptiveness as the Dt.

To better understand the "why" Dt group behaved more maladaptively, the next level of qualitative analysis focused more on the narrated story of each participant. The stories differed in their complexities in connecting the protagonist, the transgression and the aftermath of the transgression. The aftermath of the transgression included the impact on the affected or the aggrieved party and the probable action tendencies of the affected. Sometimes the stories presented a very linear relationship between the cause (protagonist and transgression) and the effect (impact on the affected/aggrieved party). It was also observed that the complexities of the narration had little to do with the actual story lines but more unique to the participant narrating the story and their alignment to the three groups of Pf, Pnf and Dt.

The below boxes presents a selection of the same story title told by participants of the three groups.

Story I : Expulsion of Adam and Eve from the Garden of Eden

Story by an individual who belongs to Dt group

"...God created two perfect human beings because that was one of the- one of his finest creation, and he made a garden of Eden for them to live. So he made all those amenities there like fruits, flowers, beautification; everything he did, so that they won't feel lonely there; they would enjoy their life there, so, it was like that, but; there was Satan (Satan was Lucifer) who was God's one of the angels but he did some treason that's why he was discriminated from heaven... and he lost his position as Angel.......

..........Adam was very, like, loyal to God; he always knew, like, the God is the almighty and he'll be the follower of him. He's one of his creations so he won't do any trouble or any wrong.......

.......Eve had a dream like: if you get that fruit then you will get knowledge; with that knowledge, you can do more, more, more better things, so, she somehow tried to convince Adam,

Adam was sleeping. So, Eve went there and plucked that fruit and ate it. And suddenly, everything like thunder and lightning happened,......

...... Eve made the bigger mistake, so, women have to give birth to babies. So that is the more...like, like... higher...like (what I'll tell?) ... is the bigger... It's very painful for a woman to give birth. The biggest pain the woman got because she made the, like, crucial mistake and Adam, as he supported her, so he also got- went through some, like... he has to suffer all these pains: hunger, trust, everything came; so, like that it happened. The end of the story – the moral of the story is that: (according to what I have understood, Milton's Paradise Lost) it's like that, like: if you do a mistake, it's a crime, and if you support a mistake, it's also an equal crime... so maybe because of that, both got punishment... like.. whatever be the reason.........."

The underlined lines present a detailed background, an empathetic view of the characters and a stern conclusion of who and what is wrong justified elaborately.

Story by an individual who belongs to predominantly forgiving (Pf) group

"So God was alone and he decided to create a friend,Adam. God is happy but then he saw that Adam was alone and that Adam couldn't relate with God. So God makes another human form from Adam, another human called Eve. Adam was happy and loved Eve. Eve was a very curious person so she walks around the garden and see a beautiful red apple and she is attracted to it."

The underlined lines mention more positive words (emotions, positive adjectives) and an empathetic view of the characters but not as in detail as the (dt) group's. The conclusion is stern, but it does not justify the conclusion. Merely states it as an end.

Story by an individual who belongs to predominantly non-forgiving (Pnf) group

"God created heaven and Earth and he named the garden Eden and then he made man. Since Adam was alone, he made Eve. God told them to enjoy the garden but to stay away from the tree of knowledge. One day, the serpent came and convinced Eve to eat the fruit and she gave it to Adam. After eating it, they realized they were naked and hid from God and then God got angry and banished them from the garden."

The underlined lines highlight the factual, cause, effect and a sequential narration of the story and mentions the end tersely as the other groups and like the Pf group does not explain it.

Story II: Kunti and Karna

Story by an individual who belongs to Dt group

"Kunti was the daughter of Kuntibhoja. She got a boon from sage Dhurwasa such that she could invoke any God and could produce a child from him.……... As she was unmarried and her marriage was about to take place soon, she decided to abandon the child since it would bring disgrace to her virginity.….... Even though it was a painful incident it ended that way.……, Kunti informs Karna that she is his mother and Pandavas are his younger brothers. The epic clearly doesn't state that Karna was angry with this revelation but certainly it was painful for him as he was abandoned soon after he was born. He did express his grouse for her when he revealed his identity. Precisely he said to her that this act cause harm to his fame and achievements.………, Kunti never sought good for him and at last before the war starts, Karna stressed on the point that what Kunti did to him was never done by any enemy to him. So precisely he never cursed his mother.

I basically appreciate Karna for not crossing the limit in blaming his mother even though he certainly felt bad and got offended by the act. According to me, Kunti did a wrong thing in abandoning Karna and also came to him before the war for the greater good of Pandavas."

A similar pattern elaborates background, empathetic consideration of the characters and a clear conclusion of why and who is wrong.

Story by an individual who belongs to Pf group

"Yeah... Kunti, one of the days, when she is a young girl, she'll be wandering in the balcony, looking at the Sun God. And when she looks at the Sun she thinks, "Oh, it will be so nice if I had a son who is as powerful as the Sun, and as beautiful as the Sun."

Then, suddenly, she gets scared, 'what happened?' So, she's got a baby, baby child... um, she didn't know what to... do with the... baby. So, she thinks 'Oh, what will people say now? That I have a baby without, um, getting married. What will I do with this baby?' So becomes panicky and then, somehow, in a process to get rid of the baby, she sends the baby away with somebody, and the baby boy goes away from her.

She thinks, 'Okay, I have gotten rid of the baby'. She abandons the kid. Then, that boy, when he grows up understands – somebody for some- somehow, he comes to know about this part that Kunti is his mother and she had abandoned him. Um, when he understands this, he becomes very angry and then, um, uh, he joins with the enemy (kauravas) and then fights with Kunti's sons; his own brothers."

The narration again features an empathetic view of the characters, also highlighted is the disdain for factual information. The conclusion is not justified, merely stated.

Story by an individual who belongs to Pnf group

"Karna was the eldest son of Kunti. She didn't disclose the secret to the other sons and the rest of the family. He was good at many things, better than the rest of the sons. But she gave him away after birth. She recognized him when he grew up, but still didn't accept him or disclose the secret. Kunti did suffer because she in a difficult position."

The narration presents crucial pieces of information, lines it in cause and effect sequence, succinctly mentions the end and does not elaborate to justify it.

Story III: Rama and Sita

Story by an individual who belongs to Dt group

"Uh... so, as far as I remember, listening to these stories from my Grandmother, I believe that there was a ... there was a person from the lower community of whatsoever they used to call who came to Rama and who just- who told – or who developed, who made Rama develop some doubts about Sita when she was away; when she was taken away by Ravana. And...

(continued)

Rama kind of got succumbed to what he heard at that point of time and that made him actually go... I mean, put Sita through that Agni Pravesha or whatever she had to claim for her purity;

And... Sita had had children by then; she had Luv and Kush, so there was a lot of... I mean, people were passing a lot of judgements about her character and... of course,

Of course, being... because Rama has been considered as the epitome of a good husband and somebody who possesses all the qualities of niceness... but this... I don't know, it brings all the other traits down, is what I feel...

And... .Sita, well, she accepted to be a part of this, to go through the fire test, the Agni Pravesh, and she... as expected, nothing happened to her. She remained pure, she remained that...She... The fire couldn't destroy her, so that meant that she was as pure as the fire itself... So, that probably proved everyone around her wrong."

The narration again follows the previous pattern of larger setting, empathetic view of the characters and a well-explained justification of a stern judgement.

Story by an individual who belongs to Pf group

"In Ramayana, as we know Rama along with Laxman and Sita followed him in his exile to Ayodhya. Sita proved her faithfulness towards her husband because it was not necessary for her to follow him although she chose that path. When she was abducted by Ravana, we see how Rama fought to bring Sita back. I don't think that was anything compared to the faithfulness shown by Sita. But in the end Rama questions her faithfulness and purity. He claims that it's not because he doubts her but because he is the prince and people have expectations from him. So, he needs to do that for the sake of the mass. Sita passes the fire test. She stands on the fire, and it turns into ash without affecting her. Rama takes her back so happily but then Rama's faith on Sita is so less because he made her do the fire test when a simple washer man had doubt on her whether she was pregnant. That was the turning point of Ram's character where he sends Sita away without any further knowledge of what actually happened.

This is what Rama does with her. But in the end Sita forgives him since Ram was everything to her. He was the perfect husband she could have ever asked for."

A similar pattern of empathetic view of the characters but this time an explicit orientation towards forgiveness is made as the conclusion.

Story by an individual who belongs to Pnf group

"We consider Ram as a God, but there's something that bothers me. Why did he have to abandon Sita? She was struggling along with him for 14 years in the jungle. She did a lot for him. But still he made her undergo the fire test. If it was fair for rajas to have many wives, then why didn't Ram accept her? Women should be mentally prepared to be okay with other wives of their husbands, but if something goes wrong with the wife, he'll abandon her? Just for showing people, he sent her back to the jungle. He couldn't move on from her past. Later, she was so upset that she asked Mother Earth to take her in."

The factual narration is inundated with questions, and a very strong clear judgement of who and what is wrong is explained.

To summarize, forgiveness stories show more positive words and tend to present an empathetic view of the characters involved, while the unforgiving group looked at the story as a sequence of cause and effect connections. The Dt group did a bit of both and some more; they provided a larger background to understand the motivations of the characters involved. The predominantly forgiving and predominantly non-forgiving groups represent the forgiving and unforgiving sides of the same story, and the Dt group runs deeply into the two sides. The elaborateness of the story is reflected in the average word count of stories in the Dt group being the highest at 200; they also record the highest minimum number of words among the three groups. Table 15.7 mentions the average, minimum and maximum word counts for each group. The Dt group presents a confluence of forgiving and unforgiving thoughts but does not represent a lack of decision-making ability or confusion but more an ability to in detail discuss the different perspectives and contextual layers in the story.

Also interestingly the age group and the source of the story of the participants present another interpretation. Both Dt and the Pf have a predominant 18–30 age group (millennials). While the Dt has family as their source of the story, Pf indicates religious texts and institutions as their source. The Pnf group has predominant 30 and above age group and also refers to religious texts and institutes as their source (refer to the tables above). Probably the place of Dt can be understood as the lack of forgiveness objective, emphasized by a family member, when narrating the story or simply the option to debate the story is improved. As most religious sources emphasize obedience and conformity, the narration by a family member could be followed by discussions of the different perspectives involved in the story. Also a family member would probably be more accessible and less formidable than religious sources. A religious source could build an idealistic understanding of the working of the world which is seasoned into a more realistic world view as seen by the older group predominance in the Pnf group. The group has almost equal representation of the 18–30 (millennials) and the 30–50 age group; the latter gains dominance after the addition of the 50 and above group. Research trends indicate that with age individuals tend to get more forgiving (Cheng & Ying-Kit, 2008).

Table 15.10 Represents the response to the fairness question to both transgressor and aggrieved party by the groups - predominantly forgiving, dualistic and predominantly non-forgiving

	Fair to both transgressor and aggrieved party	Fair to transgressor but not to the aggrieved party	Unfair to the transgressor but fair to the aggrieved party	Unfair to both transgressor and the aggrieved party	Not answered/ omitted to answer
Predominantly forgiving	62%	11%	7%	14%	6%
Dualistic	36%	36%	5%	15%	8%
Predominantly non-forgiving	54%	19%	0	19%	8%

Table 15.11 Shows the percentage scores of the three groups responding to the question of the transgressor's worthiness

Items	Total population	Transgressor is worthy	Transgressor loses worth
Predominantly forgiving (Pf)	70 (60.9%)	85.7%	14.3%
Dualistic (Dt)	19 (16.5%)	84.2%	15.8%
Predominantly non-forgiving (Pnf)	26 (22.6%)	38.4%	61.5%
All the participants	115 (100%)	74.7%	25.3%

All groups recorded both forgiving and unforgiving behaviours; perhaps the Pnf group demonstrates motivations other than forgiveness. Another question that was posed to participants was, if forgiven (by the aggrieved party), was the conclusion of the story fair for both the transgressor and the aggrieved party (Table 15.10)? They were also questioned about the transgressor's worthiness. The Pnf group's answer as seen in Table 15.11 demonstrates a more judgemental attitude when compared to the other groups. More than half of the Pnf group considers the transgressor unworthy and the group records the highest percentage for evaluating the conclusion of the story as unfair for both the transgressor and the aggrieved parties (Table 15.11). The Dt group is more accepting of the transgressor and seems more stringent about fairness than the other two groups, as they recorded the lowest percentage in evaluating the conclusion as fair to both parties. The Pf group emerged as the most accepting of the worthiness of the transgressor and the fairness of the conclusion. Interestingly they have a predominance of the 18–30 age group (millennials), and their source of the story is identified as religious institutes and texts (Table 15.12). Perhaps their cultural education had an explicit emphasis on forgiveness and acceptance of human beings as fallible and still worthy. And their fairness orientation is less individualistically evaluated, and the collective harmony is prioritized above subjective fairness. But all the above insights would require more in-depth and specific analysis than what the current study attempted.

Table 15.12 Represents source of story, age and word count of dualistic (Dt), predominantly forgiving (Pf) and predominantly non-forgiving (Pnf) groups

The predominant source for the story attributed to in each group	Dt	Family
	Pf	Religious institutes or religious texts
	Pnf	Religious Institutes or religious texts
Age group distribution in each group	Dt	18–30 = 68% 30–50 = 26% 50 and above = 6%
	Pf	18–30 = 61% 30–50 = 22% 50 and above = 17%
	Pnf	18–30 = 46% 30–50 = 42% 50 and above = 12%
Minimum, maximum and average word count for stories narrated by each of the three groups	Dt	Min. word count—54 Max.—799 Avg word count—200
	Pf	Mi. word count—32 Max. word count—756 Avg. word count—157
	Pnf	Min. word count—43 Max. word count—440 Avg. word count—121

The millennials come across as eager learners, absorbing the lessons of life from the older generations, as demonstrated in the study. They seem to inherit both adaptive and maladaptive processing styles of shame. The presence of more humane cultural values like forgiveness and acceptance seems to determine whether their complex thinking could lead them away from maladaptive and towards adaptive ways of reintegrating back into society. Otherwise retain harsh judgemental views like the older generation in the predominantly non-forgiving group leading towards maladaptive shaming.

4 Implication for Future Studies

So does culture influence shame and its adaptive and maladaptiveness and could stories pass be culture's way of transmitting shame-related education? The research findings seem to point in the direction of yes. Only with a robust theory weaving culture as an integral part of shame, a more in-depth analysis of the thus collected stories and repetition of this method in different cultures could lead to more confident conclusions. The study also highlights the need to identify the end goal of shame and the play of other cultural values like forgiveness, worthiness, fairness and the role of aggrieved or the affected party. Especially when shame is experienced in a transgression context. As seen in the generational perspectives, while the millennials could debate both sides of the transgression, the emphasis on forgiveness could reduce the maladaptive impact of shaming. Along with the aforementioned, the complexity of transgression perceived as a lack of behaviour or the result of a behaviour, as well as the intentionality behind the behaviour, also needs to be accounted for in the conceptualization of shame in future studies.

Using cultural stories as narrated by participants would address the debate on lexical differences highlighted in cross-cultural psychology (Breugelmans & Poortinga, 2006). Considering the universal or relativistic utilization of emotion words and emotion processes to accurately capture emotional experiences, instead of imposing a non-native framework of emotion conceptualization (as indicated by the vocabulary). Scholars would need to contemplate an innovative solution to address disparity in emotional conceptualizations (as indicated in the vocabulary) and emotional experiences across cultures. This would enable us to cross-reference emotional experiences while maintaining their uniqueness than compromising it to achieve (a forced) universality that might facilitate academic discussions but undermine the very objective of such a discussion.

5 Conclusion

Part 1 of the study demonstrates that individuals in an intermediate culture in India which is a blend of individualistic and collectivistic culture express both adaptive and maladaptive styles of shaming. Even maladaptive behaviours like avoidance and withdrawal play a pro-social role in the given cultural context. Part 2 of the study's findings indicate that millennials like the older generations demonstrate both adaptive and maladaptive styles of shaming and are very receptive to cultural lessons. Unlike the older generation, they engage in more complex thinking in order to exercise shaming. Millennials are keenly observing and introspecting the ways of the world. Through cultural embodiment of forgiveness attitude towards transgression, an individual and a collective culture could temper shame into its adaptive healthier ways leading to amendments and reparative behaviour. Thus maintaining the sanctity of the whole in self and the collective.

6 Implications of the Study

The paper's primary finding highlights that in specific cultural contexts, even maladaptive styles of shaming like avoidance and withdrawal play a pro-social/positive role. Examining the aforementioned possibility in the context of Fourth Industrial Revolution, a probable future, with automated machines replacing human workforce, could result in shame, due to loss of social stature, unemployment leading to low self-efficacy and increase in "unoccupied" or "leisure" time making individuals vulnerable to negative thinking, behaviour and habits. The findings of the paper suggest that a culture with collectivistic dimensions would allow for better adaptation as individuals would experience adaptive shame as compared to cultures with more individualistic dimensions.

The current research findings could help understand the plausibility and mechanics of the application of restorative justice. The framework of restorative justice utilizes the adaptive value of reintegrative shaming and significance of forgiveness, when facilitating formal justice procedures (Gavrielides, 2007). The process especially addresses the "impersonal" treatment received by the affected party and provides possibilities of "psychological closure" achieved through personal interaction between the perpetrator and the victim. The "ashamed" behavioural expressions and the proposed psychological amends facilitate a personal accountability towards the transgression and its unique impact on the affected party. The "shaming" in this framework is said to fulfil a reintegrative function, enabling the rehabilitative process of the perpetrator and thereby reducing recidivism, thus accomplishing a fundamental function of justice in and for a civil society. The current study reiterates the adaptive value of shaming as serving a reintegrative purpose in enabling a path for the perpetrator to reform and rejoin the society. And also the pivotal role of forgiveness in tempering the shaming process to remain adaptive for the perpetrator, affected party and the society. Restorative justice could be instrumental in the context of 4IR as advances with technology could also bring cyber bullying and cyber security-related challenges among other activities deviating from the law and order. Restorative justice could play an influential role in the justice system with this regard. The research findings also highlight the role of forgiveness as crucial to the aftermath of transgression in facilitating the adaptiveness of shame experienced by the transgressor. Forgiveness when culturally emphasized allows the acceptance of fallibility of human beings, the importance of dissociating deed from the doer—thus treating the transgressor as worthy and making justice restorative rather than punitive. Thus, the shame experience in the transgressor gains adaptive value, when demonstrated in culture imbibing the value of forgiveness.

In the near future, advanced technology, artificial intelligence and digitization would significantly alter the way we live, work and even build relationships. Scholars and researchers have hypothesized that while it could be towards betterment of civilization, it depends on the individual to make a positive or negative transformation implying strongly that there could be "shame" involved in terms of finding (or failure in finding) meaning and value in "living". The paper's secondary findings highlight that millennial's unique processing of "shame" as compared to the older/previous generations, is more nuanced and complex enabling deep analysis before arriving at "shame". The ability to analyse in depth could play a significant positive role in empowering millennials to address uncertainty and adversity of the unseen future. Millennials would be able to unpack the context in which change in their environment has occurred and be in a position to view it objectively and subsequently work, handle and manage their "shame"-related perceptions of inadequacies. It would be within reason to hypothesize that millennials are more capable to adapt to the 4th revolution compared to the previous generation (baby boomer generation and Generation X).

Appendix 1: Structured Interview Questions

(A) Do you remember a story from your culture on the theme of mistake/transgression? Could you please narrate it?

Or

(B) Here is a list of stories on the theme of mistake/transgression, can you narrate one that best captures the theme?

1. How do you think the protagonist is feeling? (If participant says bad/horrible/terrible, gently guide them to emotion words like joy, happy, sad; record any words or word they say).
2. Because the protagonist felt and expressed ______ (guilt/shame or any other word they used to answer question 1) what was the reaction of the opposite/affected/other/aggrieved party? In the context of your story. (If participant says forgetting/letting go or some other synonyms, ask if they mean forgiveness, if they agree then record it as forgiveness)
3. What if the protagonist didn't feel __________ (answer from question 1), then what would be the reaction of the affected/other/opposite/aggrieved party? In the context of your story.
4. Does the protagonist become unworthy for having committed the mistake?

   Ask the below question only if the answer to the above is "yes".

5. If the worth is lost then how is it regained?
6. In the conclusion of the story what was given more importance—justice or forgiveness and why? (If the participant gives another answer, then do not correct them or repeat the question—only record their answer.)

   Ask question 7/8 only if forgiveness is mentioned in the above answers:

7. If forgiven, do you think the ending was fair to the protagonist? Do you think the ending was fair to the aggrieved party?
8. If not forgiven, what do you think the protagonist should do next?
9. How did you come about hearing this story? (trying to find out the source)
10. When did you first hear about the story? (developmental stage—childhood adolescence/young adulthood, etc.)
11. In what context did you hear this story? (why were you told this story?)

Appendix 2: Story Titles

Christianity:

1. The Expulsion of Adam and Eve from the Garden of Eden
2. The Curse of Cain or The Mark of Cain
3. King David, Bathsheba and Uriah (The Transgression of King David)
4. The Prodigal Son
5. Zacchaeus the Tax Collector

Hinduism:

1. Bhishma with regard to Amba
2. Yudhishthira with regard to the dice game and the "lie" on the battlefield
3. Draupadi with regard to Ashwatthama
4. Kunti for abandoning Karna
5. Rama with regard to the fire test and for sending Sita away
6. Bharata on his mother's act of sending Rama away

Islam:

1. Messenger/Prophet Yusuf and Zakia
2. Messenger/Prophet Dawood and his 99 wives
3. Messenger or Prophet Mohammed and Aisha

Appendix 3: Story Narration

Story I : Expulsion of Adam and Eve from the Garden of Eden

Story by an individual who belongs to dualistic (Dt) group "So, there is a story of Adam and Eve, maybe this I read when I was in my college...maybe first year, second year... Paradise Lost! The story is like: Adam and Eve – God created two perfect human beings because that was one of the- one of his finest creation, and he made a garden of Eden for them to live. So he made all those amenities there like fruits, flowers, beautification; everything he did, so that they won't feel lonely there; they would enjoy their life there, so, it was like that, but; there was Satan (Satan was Lucifer) who was God's one of the angels but he did some treason that's why he was discriminated from heaven... and he lost his position as Angel. So, he was termed as Satan; he blamed himself and punishment got through him and he was angry with God because without him- without his power. He didn't know about this human being creation of Adam and Eve... and...yes...and...so, he was very anxious to know about why Adam and

(continued)

Eve was created and to destroy what God's motive was, so... that was his main intention.

Adam was very, like, loyal to God; he always knew, like, the God is the almighty and he'll be the follower of him. He's one of his creations so he won't do any trouble or any wrong. So, they were living peacefully on Garden of Eden and Eve had one dream: like, Satan came and spoke to, like, in his ears, like... that... fruit of... some fruit was there... so apple tree was there and (forbidden fruit!) ... So, God told that you don't eat that fruit only; that is the tree of knowledge. Except that, whatever you are eating, or taking things, or making things – leaves, you do whatever you want; you just go- don't go to that area.

So, Adam was very obedient and he used to, like, maintain that distance with that thing; but Eve had a dream like: if you get that fruit then you will get knowledge; with that knowledge, you can do more, more, more better things, so, she somehow tried to convince Adam, but Adam was very obedient to God; he never wanted to go and eat that fruit.

So, once, Adam was sleeping. So, Eve went there and plucked that fruit and ate it. And suddenly, everything like thunder and lightning happened, and God realized the Eve had like... done a treason sort of thing which he has told her, she has not obeyed him, so... God came down... And Adam loved Eve very much. He never- he loved because Eve was created from Adam's rib, eleventh rib, so... Adam loved Eve more than himself. So, he thought that only Eve would get punishment..so.. I'll do one thing: I'll eat one – like – I'll take one bite.

So, Adam took one bite, but he wasn't able to swallow it down so, the boy's have their Adam's apple around here (makes gesture with hand) and the problem is that God found both guilty. When he came down, he found that both were guilty.

So... he told like.. you both have disobeyed my rules and things, so you both will leave some... you had to stay in the garden of Eden, I made it for you only, you guys. But you will have to go through all the pains, sufferings, which I thought I won't give you all; I'll only give you a good life to live in.

But, because of Eve's like, too much of knowing things, or maybe because of Satan's like stimulating her (like: go and eat that fruit), maybe, Eve got into that; Adam never got into that. Because of Eve's like... fault, Adam also got punishment.

But... it's also true; as Eve made the bigger mistake, so, women have to give birth to babies. So that is the more...like, like... higher...like (what I'll tell?) ... is the bigger... It's very painful for a woman to give birth. The biggest pain the woman got because she made the, like, crucial mistake and Adam, as he supported her, so he also got- went through some, like... he has to suffer all these pains: hunger, trust, everything came; so, like that it

(continued)

happened. The end of the story – the moral of the story is that: (according to what I have understood, Milton's Paradise Lost) it's like that, like: if you do a mistake, it's a crime, and if you support a mistake, it's also an equal crime... so maybe because of that, both got punishment... like.. whatever be the reason.. like.. whoever does the crucial crime, is not the matter – like – other people supporting that crime is also – like – equally criminal...

So, that's my story."

Story by an individual who belongs to predominantly forgiving (Pf) group

"So God was alone and he decided to create a friend,Adam. God is happy but then he saw that Adam was alone and that Adam couldn't relate with God. So God makes another human form from Adam, another human called Eve. Adam was happy and loved Eve. Eve was a very curious person so she walks around the garden and see a beautiful red apple and she is attracted to it. She finds the snake who convinces her to eat the apple. She eats it and realized that she knows more things. She then shares it with Adam and then they knew that they did something wrong. So then they feel shame because of their nakedness. They feel shame and guilty. God then comes and he is angry, he then banishes them."

Story by an individual who belongs to predominantly non-forgiving (Pnf) group

"God created heaven and Earth and he named the garden Eden and then he made man. Since Adam was alone, he made Eve. God told them to enjoy the garden but to stay away from the tree of knowledge. One day, the serpent came and convinced Eve to eat the fruit and she gave it to Adam. After eating it, they realized they were naked and hid from God and then God got angry and banished them from the garden."

Story II: Kunti and Karna

Story by an individual who belongs to Dt group

"Kunti was the daughter of Kuntibhoja. She got a boon from sage Dhurwasa such that she could invoke any God and could produce a child from him. While she was unmarried, she invoked Surya deva and gave birth to her child Karna. As she was unmarried and her marriage was about to take place soon, she decided to abandon the child since it would bring disgrace to her virginity. That's how she decided to abandon Karna. She kept him in a basket and immersed that in the river and it flows away. Even though it was a painful incident it ended that way. Years after, Karna, the first born of Kunti comes face to face with rest of Pandavas. Before the great war of Mahabharata,

(continued)

Kunti informs Karna that she is his mother and Pandavas are his younger brothers. The epic clearly doesn't state that Karna was angry with this revelation but certainly it was painful for him as he was abandoned soon after he was born. He did express his grouse for her when he revealed his identity. Precisely he said to her that this act cause harm to his fame and achievements. Further, he was deprived of his Kshatriya identity and he lost the right to follow all the kstariya traits. He felt that as a mother, Kunti never sought good for him and at last before the war starts, Karna stressed on the point that what Kunti did to him was never done by any enemy to him. So precisely he never cursed his mother. I basically appreciate Karna for not crossing the limit in blaming his mother even though he certainly felt bad and got offended by the act. According to me, Kunti did a wrong thing in abandoning Karna and also came to him before the war for the greater good of Pandavas."

Story by an individual who belongs to forgiving (Pf) group

"Yeah... Kunti, one of the days, when she is a young girl, she'll be wandering in the balcony, looking at the Sun God. And when she looks at the Sun she thinks, "Oh, it will be so nice if I had a son who is as powerful as the Sun, and as beautiful as the Sun."

So, she just makes a wish like that, and it just so happens that her wish comes true and, immediately, she will get a baby...um, in front of her who is very beautiful.

Then, suddenly, she gets scared, 'what happened?' So, she's got a baby, baby child ... um, she didn't know what to... do with the... baby. So, she thinks 'Oh, what will people say now? That I have a baby without, um, getting married. What will I do with this baby?' So becomes panicky and then, somehow, in a process to get rid of the baby, she sends the baby away with somebody, and the baby boy goes away from her.

She thinks, 'Okay, I have gotten rid of the baby'. She abandons the kid. Then, that boy, when he grows up understands – somebody for some- somehow, he comes to know about this part that Kunti is his mother and she had abandoned him. Um, when he understands this, he becomes very angry and then, um, uh, he joins with the enemy (kauravas) and then fights with Kunti's sons; his own brothers."

Story by an individual who belongs to Pnf group

(continued)

"Karna was the eldest son of Kunti. She didn't disclose the secret to the other sons and the rest of the family. He was good at many things, better than the rest of the sons. But she gave him away after birth. She recognized him when he grew up, but still didn't accept him or disclose the secret. Kunti did suffer because she in a difficult position."

Story III: Rama and Sita

Story by an individual who belongs to Dt group

"Uh... so, as far as I remember, listening to these stories from my Grandmother, I believe that there was a ... there was a person from the lower community of whatsoever they used to call who came to Rama and who just- who told – or who developed, who made Rama develop some doubts about Sita when she was away; when she was taken away by Ravana. And...

Rama kind of got succumbed to what he heard at that point of time and that made him actually go... I mean, put Sita through that Agni Pravesha or whatever she had to claim for her purity; That's what Rama wanted to test, because it was told to him that, "Sita was away for so many years and... she was with Ravana. How sure are you that there was no physical relationship between Ravana and Sita?"

And... Sita had had children by then; she had Luv and Kush, so there was a lot of... I mean, people were passing a lot of judgements about her character and... of course, there's another version that says Rama was confident that nothing would happen to Sita and she would come out as pure as how she... she would come out in the same form even after the Agni Pravesh.

I somehow feel it wasn't for him to prove to anybody in the kingdom, he could have just... He could have had the trust in her and just shut the other people's mouth. So, that is my opinion. Of course, being... because Rama has been considered as the epitome of a good husband and somebody who possesses all the qualities of niceness... but this... I don't know, it brings all the other traits down, is what I feel...

And... Sita, well, she accepted to be a part of this, to go through the fire test, the Agni Pravesh, and she... as expected, nothing happened to her. She remained pure, she remained that... She... The fire couldn't destroy her, so that meant that she was as pure as the fire itself... So, that probably proved everyone around her wrong."

Story by an individual who belongs to forgiving (Pf) group

"In Ramayana, as we know Rama along with Laxman and Sita followed him in his exile to Ayodhya. Sita proved her faithfulness towards her husband because it was not necessary for her to follow him although she chose that

(continued)

path. When she was abducted by Ravana, we see how Rama fought to bring Sita back. I don't think that was anything compared to the faithfulness shown by Sita. But in the end Rama questions her faithfulness and purity. He claims that it's not because he doubts her but because he is the prince and people have expectations from him. So, he needs to do that for the sake of the mass. Sita passes the fire test. She stands on the fire, and it turns into ash without affecting her. Rama takes her back so happily but then Rama's faith on Sita is so less because he made her do the fire test when a simple washer man had doubt on her whether she was pregnant. That was the turning point of Ram's character where he sends Sita away without any further knowledge of what actually happened. He questions Sita's chastity and that made her go away. Sita was way beyond the perfect wife. She even followed Ram to exile, left everything behind and moved from the comfort zone and came to the forest. This is what Rama does with her. But in the end Sita forgives him since Ram was everything to her. He was the perfect husband she could have ever asked for."

Story by an individual who belongs to unforgiving (Pnf) group

"We consider Ram as a God, but there's something that bothers me. Why did he have to abandon Sita? She was struggling along with him for 14 years in the jungle. She did a lot for him. But still he made her undergo the fire test. If it was fair for rajas to have many wives, then why didn't Ram accept her? Women should be mentally prepared to be okay with other wives of their husbands, but if something goes wrong with the wife, he'll abandon her? Just for showing people, he sent her back to the jungle. He couldn't move on from her past. Later, she was so upset that she asked Mother Earth to take her in."

Appendix 4

Table 15.13 Represents scoring of predominantly forgiving (Pf), dualistic (Dt) and predominantly non-forgiving (Pnf)

Sl. no	1. How do you think the protagonist is feeling?	2. Because the protagonist felt and expressed ______ what was the reaction of the opposite/affected/other/aggrieved party? In the context of your story	3. What if the protagonist didn't feel ______ then what would be the reaction of the affected/other/opposite/aggrieved party? In the context of your story	4. Does the protagonist become unworthy for having committed the mistake?	5. If the worth is lost, then how is it regained?	8. If not forgiven, what do you think the protagonist should do next?	Forgiving inclined	Non forgiving inclined	Scoring Pf, Pnf and Dt
1	Sad	Sad and guilty	He'll still feel sad and guilty	No		Never return, leave	4	1	Pf
2	Iblees (the protagonist) felt that he did the right thing. He did not feel guilty. He felt vengeful, bitter and angry.	God (the affected party) did not forgive Iblees; He was sad; God had faith in himself to forgive humanity and swore to keep on fighting till the end; even if humans would be led astray, he would forgive them	If Iblees did not feel vengeful, then God would have likely forgiven him. However, since Iblees did not feel guilty, and felt vengeful and bitter instead, God did not forgive him	Yes	Iblees can regain his worth in God's eyes by asking for forgiveness and remaining obedient to Him	The protagonist should go and ask for forgiveness	4	2	Pf

3	Sita: sad	Ram: sad and guilty	He'll still feel sad and guilty	No		Never return. Leave	4	1	Pf
4	Bad-guilty	Krishna did not feel angry. Yudhishthira lied for a good cause to allow Pandavas to win	Krishna, as a manipulator, would not have cared	No		Confront the party affected the most but feel guilty as Bhishma was gone before he could confess	3	2	Pf
5	Bhishma: no emotion	Amba: anger	If he would be guilty, Amba would be less angry. She wouldn't take revenge	No		Marry her	3	1	Pf
6	Guilty and confused	Angry	She'll hate him and be very angry	Yes	He can't	Exile	0	5	Pnf
7	Happy	Opponents felt insulted and called Krishna for help	Aggrieved party would have felt happy	Yes	By asking for forgiveness	Not move on	1	3	Pnf
8	Guilty/filled with shame	Happy, glad, forgiving	Would have initially forgiven but wouldn't have forgiven if the mistake was repeated	No, I don't think so, everyone commits a mistake (but if repeated yes!)	NA	Work hard, amend mistakes, live decently	4	2	Pf
9	Guilt	Angry and disappointed	Disappointment	No		Ask for forgiveness	4	1	Pf

(continued)

Table 15.13 (continued)

Sl. no	1. How do you think the protagonist is feeling?	2. Because the protagonist felt and expressed ______ what was the reaction of the opposite/affected/other/aggrieved party? In the context of your story	3. What if the protagonist didn't feel ______ then what would be the reaction of the affected/other/opposite/aggrieved party? In the context of your story	4. Does the protagonist become unworthy for having committed the mistake?	5. If the worth is lost, then how is it regained?	8. If not forgiven, what do you think the protagonist should do next?	Forgiving inclined	Non forgiving inclined	Scoring Pf, Pnf and Dt
10	(Eve) scared and frustrated	Angry and authoritative	Shocked	No		Nothing	1	3	Pnf
11	Guilty and ashamed.	Forgiving and happy.	Polite and welcoming.	No.		Looked for shelter elsewhere	4	0	Pf
12	Guilt, regret	Disheartened	Angry	Yes	He shouldn't repeat the mistake and stop others as well	He should work on women's rights	2	3	Pnf
13	Regret but joyful when his father accepts him back	Overjoyed and forgiving	Father would still have forgiven him	No		He would have tried to stay and then move on	4	0	Pf
14	Sad, angry, hurt	Sad and hurt	Shocked	No		Don't give fire test	2	3	Pnf
15	Guilty	Humiliated	Furious	No		Not forgiving	1	3	Pnf
16	Angry	Afraid	Unaffected	No		Ask for apology	2	2	Dt

17	Guilty and regret.	Forgiveness	He was only guilty after the prophet Nathan came and spoke to him	Yes	He would have prayed to God	Live in deep shame and regret	2	3	Pnf
18	Regrets his mistakes	Happy that his son has come back	The father would have been depressed and shocked	No		Chased him out of the house and the son would run away	3	2	Pf
19	Regret	Forgiveness	Still forgive the protagonist	No		Give explanation and apologize for the same	4	0	Pf
20	Guilt, devastated	The father was happy, did not judge his son, forgave him	Would have been angry yet given the son another chance	No		Begged and asked for forgiveness, tried to prove his repentance	4	1	Pf
21	Shame and regret	Anger and betrayed	Punish her more severely	No		Repent for her actions. Make up for the act	2	2	Dt
22	Guilty	Wrath	Disappointed	Yes	Asking for forgiveness	Repent	3	2	Pf
23	Guilty but helpless	Patient	Still patient	Not really		Should reflect upon her actions	4	0	Pf
24	Confusion	Sadness	Happiness	No		Keep their trust on their partners and not believe rumours	4	0	Pf

(continued)

Table 15.13 (continued)

Sl. no	1. How do you think the protagonist is feeling?	2. Because the protagonist felt and expressed ______ what was the reaction of the opposite/affected/other/aggrieved party? In the context of your story	3. What if the protagonist didn't feel ______ then what would be the reaction of the affected/other/opposite/aggrieved party? In the context of your story	4. Does the protagonist become unworthy for having committed the mistake?	5. If the worth is lost, then how is it regained?	8. If not forgiven, what do you think the protagonist should do next?	Forgiving inclined	Non forgiving inclined	Scoring Pf, Pnf and Dt
25	The protagonist is feeling happy that his father took him back	The father was happy too; he forgave his son, while the older brother questioned his father's judgement	The father would still forgive the protagonist. He would make his son understand his mistake and also make him realize the mistake	No		The protagonist would have gone back to his old ways and continue his mistakes	3	2	Pf
26	The farmer's wife (protagonist) is feeling very guilty. She regrets acting hastily. She is sad, upset and	The mongoose (affected party) would have felt anger, but it would have accepted her apology and forgiven her	It would have been angry and haunted her. It would have tried convincing her of her wrongness	Yes, she does become more unworthy after having committed the mistake. She should have been more patient. She was	She can regain the lost worth by not committing the same mistake again. She was taught a lesson	As she can't ask for forgiveness, she should have taken it as a lesson and not repeated the mistake	3	3	Pnf

	angry with herself			the one who wanted the pet, yet she killed it					
27	Guilty	Forgiveness	Anger	No		Ask for forgiveness	3	1	Pf
28	Scared and nervous	Anger	Wrath	No	Make up for their mistakes	Work towards being better and not repeating any mistakes	3	2	Pf
29	Sita: angry and sad	Ram: guilty	Angry	No		Make Rama understand and stand up for herself	2	2	Dt
30	Regret	Forgiveness	Opposite party would forgive	No		Ask for forgiveness	4	0	Pf
31	Joyful	Proud and happy	Would feel let down	No	By making up for the wrong actions with the right ones	He should live a life worth getting forgiveness	4	1	Pf
32	Hurt, shameful and regret	Forgiveness	Grieved over the loss of his son	No		Leave since he was not forgiven	4	0	Pf
33	Kans: no emotion	Confused and sad	He would for-give him	Yes	Accepting his mistakes and submitting himself	Don't repeat such mistakes	3	2	Pf
34	Guilt	Punishment But gave another chance through redemption	Ignore	Yes	Ask for forgive-ness with deep repentance	Seek for forgiveness	4	2	Pf

(continued)

Table 15.13 (continued)

Sl. no	1. How do you think the protagonist is feeling?	2. Because the protagonist felt and expressed ______ what was the reaction of the opposite/affected/other/aggrieved party? In the context of your story	3. What if the protagonist didn't feel ______ then what would be the reaction of the affected/other/opposite/aggrieved party? In the context of your story	4. Does the protagonist become unworthy for having committed the mistake?	5. If the worth is lost, then how is it regained?	8. If not forgiven, what do you think the protagonist should do next?	Forgiving inclined	Non forgiving inclined	Scoring Pf, Pnf and Dt
35	Regret	Forgiveness after punishment, forgave but didn't forget	The punishment would've been more severe	Yes	Repentance and seeking his parents' forgiveness	Not answered	2	3	Pnf
36	Regret and guilt	Upset, not ready to forgive	Would continue to act the same	No		Ask for forgiveness	2	2	Dt
37	Guilty, shameful	God was angry and hurt	No change in God's punishment or anger towards them	No, they were just curious about the knowledge of good and evil	NA	NA	1	2	Pf
38	Shameful	Disappointment	God would've been patient with them	No	Not answered	Should've have asked for forgiveness and amended their mistake	4	0	Pf

39	Guilty	Acceptance and forgiveness	Still would have forgiven	No	N/A	Should've stayed as a servant for his father	3	1	Pf
40	Furious, sad	Stubborn	Will continue to understand	No		Just leave the opposite party	3	1	Pnf
41	Kaikeya (the protagonist) has been punished by the loss of her husband. Her son is unhappy. She has realized her mistake of listening to poisonous advice. She feels regret and a sense of guilt. She has lost her face with the other wives. She is feeling wretched, shocked, lost and sad	Rama (the affected party) is such that he values his duties as a priority. When you perform your duty, you are responsible for you action and have to bear the consequences. He sympathizes with Kaikeya. He could have returned to Ayodhya to assuage her guilt, but he doesn't do that. At a personal level, he feels no bitterness against her	Rama's character is such that he would be indifferent	No, she is not unworthy; it is a human frailty. Her action were governed by four things 1. She put motherly affection above her role as a queen. 2. She misjudged Bharata's ambitions and thought she would be serving the cause of Bharata. 3. She was weak-minded for listening to Mantara 4. She misused her boon		She has to rectify her mistake by serving people and doing the right thing. She should that Bharata is doing his job well; she could derive some solace by that. She could also go and join Rama in the forest	4	0	Pf

(continued)

Table 15.13 (continued)

Sl. no	1. How do you think the protagonist is feeling?	2. Because the protagonist felt and expressed ______ what was the reaction of the opposite/affected/other/aggrieved party? In the context of your story	3. What if the protagonist didn't feel ______ then what would be the reaction of the affected/other/opposite/aggrieved party? In the context of your story	4. Does the protagonist become unworthy for having committed the mistake?	5. If the worth is lost, then how is it regained?	8. If not forgiven, what do you think the protagonist should do next?	Forgiving inclined	Non forgiving inclined	Scoring Pf, Pnf and Dt
42	Confused, fear, they hide, shame	God wasn't really angry, he punished them for their actions, and he forgave them	He would have still done the same thing	No		They should have apologized because I heard they never apologized	4	0	Pf
43	Ashamed	Sadness; he expected them to follow the rules	Extremely disappointed due to no sense of repentance	No	Not answered	Convince God that they are repentant	4	0	Pf
44	Guilty, shameful	She didn't care. She was still angry and upset. Wanted justice	Even more angry	No		He should have taken care of her	2	2	Dt
45	Kunti (the protagonist) is feeling stupid about her action. She	He is angry and sad. He wants to take revenge	If Kunti had not felt fear, then Karna would have been	No, because it is not entirely her fault; it is the fault of the		She should ask for his forgiveness	2	1	Pf

	has a fear of what others will think. She is indifferent towards Karna. She feels no regret		happily raised by his own mother	unaccepting social system which caused her to commit the mistake					
46	Dharmaraya/ Yuddishthira (the protago-nist) is feeling sad. He was party to a lie. He was instrumen-tal in killing his own teacher by wrong means. He knew the consequences of his actions	Ashwatthama (the affected party) would feel betrayed. At that moment, he would have felt no empathy. In a battle field, no one believes in ethics and morals; sides are more impor-tant (Yudda-Dharma). Dharmaraya was justified in his actions. It is hard to forgive such mistakes. Ashwatthama would have spared Dharmaraya, but not forgiven him	Wars do not have individual significance. Dharmaraya has immense respect for his teacher, so, Ashwatthama would not hold a grudge against him. It would not affect Ashwatthama personally	No, because he was following a war strategy, and it was team decision		Dharmaraya will try to convince Ashwatthama. If he does not get convinced, the Dharmaraya would just ignore Ashwatthama; he is the king, after all	4	1	Pf

(continued)

Table 15.13 (continued)

Sl. no	1. How do you think the protagonist is feeling?	2. Because the protagonist felt and expressed ______ what was the reaction of the opposite/affected/other/aggrieved party? In the context of your story	3. What if the protagonist didn't feel ______ then what would be the reaction of the affected/other/opposite/aggrieved party? In the context of your story	4. Does the protagonist become unworthy for having committed the mistake?	5. If the worth is lost, then how is it regained?	8. If not forgiven, what do you think the protagonist should do next?	Forgiving inclined	Non forgiving inclined	Scoring Pf, Pnf and Dt
47	Disappointed, shameful	Upset	God would've punished them	Yes	After making the mistake, they then obeyed God's instructions	They would've died in the garden	1	4	Pnf
48	Guilty	They were punished but later on forgiven	A much harsher punishment	No		Beg for forgiveness and lived his whole life repenting	3	3	Dt
49	Remorse, ashamed	Forgiveness and acceptance	It would be the same, unconditional love	Yes but the father makes him worthy	By others making us feel worthy	Should've stayed with the pigs	4	1	Pf
50	Sita feels helpless. She understands her husband's conflict of interest, but wants him	Rama didn't pay much heed to Sita's feelings	If Sita would have been frustrated, Ram would have been too. He would have	No		She should have tried to talk to Rama once	2	2	Dt

	to take her side and not abandon her. She was sad, frustrated. She wasn't guilty		shown anger by isolating her. Rama believes she's wrong						
51	Not guilty	Never felt bad	Disappointment	No		Try to make the opposite party understand the circumstances under which the mistake was committed. Later, ask for forgiveness	4	0	Pf
52	Regret	Forgiveness	Still forgive him	No		Ask for forgiveness. Repent on mistakes	4	0	Pf
53	Sad	Forgiveness	Angry	Yes	He should apologize	Ask for forgiveness	3	2	Pf
54	Guilty	God probably felt let down but he clothes them before they left the garden of Eden	Even more disappointed and not admitting one's guilt would've been a greater sin	No	N/A	They should seek to mend the relationship between themselves and God	4	1	Pf
55	Bad-sad	Bad—letting go. . .does not mention forgiveness	Neutral reaction	No		Move on	4	0	Pf

(continued)

Table 15.13 (continued)

Sl. no	1. How do you think the protagonist is feeling?	2. Because the protagonist felt and expressed ______ what was the reaction of the opposite/ affected/other/ aggrieved party? In the context of your story	3. What if the protagonist didn't feel ______ then what would be the reaction of the affected/other/ opposite/ aggrieved party? In the context of your story	4. Does the protagonist become unworthy for having committed the mistake?	5. If the worth is lost, then how is it regained?	8. If not forgiven, what do you think the protagonist should do next?	Forgiving inclined	Non forgiving inclined	Scoring Pf, Pnf and Dt
56	Sita: sad	Ram: guilty	Shame	No		Whatever she did was correct. She maintained her dignity	1	3	Pnf
57	Regret, lost , repented, bad, guilty	God was angry, punished them and forgave them	Still forgiven	No		Come back and asked for forgiveness, did whatever God wants them to do	4	1	Pf
58	Guilty, ashamed	Forgiveness, the brother felt angry	Would be sad but still forgiving	No	Not answered	He would've gone back to being a slave	3	2	Pf
59	Eve felt tremendous guilt, betrayal, disappointment	God felt betrayed and disappointed. But still forgave them	God would have probably felt angry	Yes, because she disobeyed God	She might have to let go of a few things in order to escape the greater punishment of death	She would have faced death	2	4	Pnf

60	Guilty and regretful	Joy and happiness	The opposite party would have been accepting	Yes	By asking for another chance	Try again	4	1	Pf
61	The protagonist is feeling repentance and regrets the way he used to live. He feels ashamed	The opposition party forgives the son. He loves his son and the father realizes is mistake	He would still forgive only if he came back home; it was the son's choice to come back.	No		He would have stayed and sulked about it, and he would feel ashamed	3	1	Pf
62	He didn't care and he humiliated her. So isn't feeling anything	She was sad and angry. She felt helpless. She gets frustrated	If he felt bad for her, then she would have forgiven him	Yes	What is lost is lost .	He couldn't do much	1	4	Pnf
63	Shame, sad and regret	Cursed and punished the protagonist	Would have punished severely	No		Ask for forgiveness	2	2	Dt
64	He did not want to be associated with Jesus; he wants to protect himself and at the end feels regret. Scared, and shamed	Jesus was peaceful; he forgave Peter	Jesus would not have done anything, he still would have forgiven Peter	No		He would have pleaded for Jesus to forgive him	4	0	Pf

(continued)

Table 15.13 (continued)

Sl. no	1. How do you think the protagonist is feeling?	2. Because the protagonist felt and expressed ______ what was the reaction of the opposite/affected/other/aggrieved party? In the context of your story	3. What if the protagonist didn't feel ______ then what would be the reaction of the affected/other/opposite/aggrieved party? In the context of your story	4. Does the protagonist become unworthy for having committed the mistake?	5. If the worth is lost, then how is it regained?	8. If not forgiven, what do you think the protagonist should do next?	Forgiving inclined	Non forgiving inclined	Scoring Pf, Pnf and Dt
65	They feel ashamed and they felt sorry and asked for forgiveness	God punished, he was upset that they were not obedient; he felt betrayed	God regrets creating Adam and Eve	No, they are human, and humans make mistakes		They would try to ask for forgiveness	3	1	Pf
66	Sita (the protagonist) is feeling sad and scared. She regrets disobeying Lakshmana	Ram is sad and worried	He would be sad if she did not feel regret	No, people have fickle minds. She just wanted to give alms; she meant no harm to anyone. She did not mean to disregard Lakshmana		Sita should ask for his forgiveness	4	0	Pf
67	Ok	Curious and clueless	Explanatory	No		Seek forgiveness Yes	3	0	Pf

68	Guilty	Forgiveness	Would forgive the protagonist	No		Ask for forgiveness	4	0	Pf
69	Sad, regret, guilt	Forgiveness	Will wait for his son	No		Ask for forgiveness	4	0	Pf
70	Horrible by doing it right	He was angry	Would have been frustrated	Yes	By giving him what he deserves	Give him what he deserved	2	3	Pnf
71	Guilty, need to rectify	Ready to for-give, happy, realization	Make under-stand, learn the lesson	No		Wait, don't leave	4	0	Pf
72	Karna: sad, frustrated	Kunti: sad	Sad	Yes	It's difficult to get it back	Karna should walk away	2	3	Pnf
73	Regret	Forgiveness	Will curse the protagonist	No		Ask for forgiveness	3	1	Pf
74	Guilty and unhappy	God felt bad and hurt, but in the end he for-gave them	God would have still forgiven them, but they should not feel this way	No	NA	Commit suicide	3	1	Pf
75	Part1: He felt bad Part2: He felt guilty and ashamed	Part 1: He felt happy Part 2: He felt angry	Wouldn't matter	No		Part 1: He had to consult his stakeholders before making decisions Part 2: He had to verify the facts before making announcements, statements and decisions	2	3	Pnf

(continued)

Table 15.13 (continued)

Sl. no	1. How do you think the protagonist is feeling?	2. Because the protagonist felt and expressed ______ what was the reaction of the opposite/affected/other/aggrieved party? In the context of your story	3. What if the protagonist didn't feel ______ then what would be the reaction of the affected/other/opposite/aggrieved party? In the context of your story	4. Does the protagonist become unworthy for having committed the mistake?	5. If the worth is lost, then how is it regained?	8. If not forgiven, what do you think the protagonist should do next?	Forgiving inclined	Non forgiving inclined	Scoring Pf, Pnf and Dt
76	Ashamed, humiliated, guilty, humbled, happy	Father—forgiving, helping Brother—did not forgive	Father—the same , still forgave Brother—turmoil, tried to put the one at fault down	No, everyone is human		Begged for forgiveness	4	2	Pf
77	Sita: angry and sad	Ram: guilty and helpless	More guilty	No		Should've questioned him and other people	1	3	Pnf
78	Guilty	Composed	Sad and disgusting	No		Seek forgiveness and explain	4	1	Pf
79	Eve, the protagonist, is feeling horrible. She and Adam only had each other, and they both	Adam loved Eve very much. He came to rescue her when she ate the apple. He	If she didn't feel remorse for what she had done, Adam would be very angry with her	No, she does not become unworthy. People do commit mistakes and then learn from		If not forgiven, she would feel neglected and sad. She should try to convince Adam by her	2	2	Dt

	suffered. Eve is feeling sad and pathetic	shared her punishment as he felt sympathy for Eve. Yet, he is feeling sad as he has disobeyed God and is no longer in the Garden of Eden		them. However, we may become unworthy if we make the same mistake again and again		actions or her words. If he still doesn't forgive her, she would be very sad			
80	Guilt, shame, realization, fear, anger	Disappointed but no hatred	Disappointed and wrath	Yes	Obedience to commandment	Can do nothing	3	3	Dt
81	Jealous	Forgiveness	Happy	No, but what she did was wrong		She should've done something to make up for her mistake	4	0	Pf
82	Sad, angry	He felt bad but due not forgive them completely	Made it worse for them	Yes	Teach their children not to make the same mistakes	NA	2	3	Pnf
83	Pain doubt shame	Not happy	Betrayed	Yes	Begging sorry, respecting	Leave	3	2	Pf
84	Rama (the protagonist) is feeling guilty. He could consider his hasty actions and behave rationally. He feels sad	Sita (the affected party) would feel little good about Rama if he expressed guilt	Sita would have walked away. She would have felt resentment and thought that the whole affair of proving her virginity was very childish	No, people make mistakes. If there is regret, then, there is a chance for redemption		Rama should try to convince her. He should accept her judgement and believe that whatever she does is Karma coming back to him	2	2	Dt

(continued)

Table 15.13 (continued)

Sl. no	1. How do you think the protagonist is feeling?	2. Because the protagonist felt and expressed ______ what was the reaction of the opposite/affected/other/aggrieved party? In the context of your story	3. What if the protagonist didn't feel ______ then what would be the reaction of the affected/other/opposite/aggrieved party? In the context of your story	4. Does the protagonist become unworthy for having committed the mistake?	5. If the worth is lost, then how is it regained?	8. If not forgiven, what do you think the protagonist should do next?	Forgiving inclined	Non forgiving inclined	Scoring Pf, Pnf and Dt
85	Repentance, ashamed and regret	Forgiveness. he loves his son	He would still forgive his son	No—he still loves his son unconditionally		He would have stayed and sulked about it	3	1	Pf
86	Ashamed, guilty	He felt bad but wanted them to learn a lesson	He might have destroyed them	Yes	Accepting fault, repentance, making amends, avoiding repetition	Repent and try to make amends	3	3	Dt
87	Ashamed, disgusted	He was angry, unforgiving, felt cheated	His reaction would have been even worse	No, "unworthy" is too heavy. All she did was deal with the mistake she committed poorly		The protagonist could've tried harder to make amends, accept him for who he is or give him space	2	2	Dt
88	Angry, betrayed, sad	Supposed to be sad	Reacts the same way. Angry if not sad	Not unworthy.		Should have left Rama	4	1	Pf

89	Guilty, ashamed, humiliated	Self-awareness, happiness, forgive	No joy	No		Make father understand	4	0	Pf
90	Angry	Embarrassed	Arrogance. Nothing would have changed	No, he does not		Ask for forgiveness, be mature adults, and talk about it instead of cutting off body parts	3	2	Pf
91	Sad, guilty	Guilt, but patient and forgiving	Angry	Yes	By asking forgiveness	Should be punished	2	4	Pnf
92	Bhishma (the protagonist) thinks that he is justified in his actions. Even Parashurama comes to tell Bhishma that he is wrong, but to no avail; Bhishma ends up fighting with his own teacher There are these famous lines that Bhishma says: “Whether it is your Guru or your elders, you cannot let	Amba (the affected party) is feeling helpless, angry and upset. She feels that injustice has been done to her. She does not care about the vow; she knows the entire world thinks that the vow is wrong	If Bhishma showed a little guilt or remorse, Amba would have felt a little better/happier; she would at least feel understood and would have kept trying to marry him	No, Bhishma does not become unworthy. A person is not evaluated by only one act/mistake. Everybody makes mistakes. A person’s worthiness or unworthiness is the sum-total of everything But... he is definitely unworthy in Amba’s eyes		Bhishma should have been practical and married her We should modify our opinions and judgements with the changing time	2	3	Pnf

(continued)

Table 15.13 (continued)

Sl. no	1. How do you think the protagonist is feeling?	2. Because the protagonist felt and expressed ______ what was the reaction of the opposite/affected/other/aggrieved party? In the context of your story	3. What if the protagonist didn't feel ______ then what would be the reaction of the affected/other/opposite/aggrieved party? In the context of your story	4. Does the protagonist become unworthy for having committed the mistake?	5. If the worth is lost, then how is it regained?	8. If not forgiven, what do you think the protagonist should do next?	Forgiving inclined	Non forgiving inclined	Scoring Pf, Pnf and Dt
	anyone pressure you into doing wrong things" Bhishma is very stubborn and self-righteous. He is feeling happy and satisfied								
93	Guilty yet powerful	Dominant and authority, angry	Angrier and vengeful	No		Try to put forward his opinion on his action	1	3	Pnf
94	Sad, angry	Sad, regret	Happiness	Yes	Take back her wish and ask forgiveness	Admit her mistake	4	1	Pf

95	Happy his father took him back	Father was happy as well	Father would still be happy and would still forgive his son	No		He would have gone back to his old ways	3	1	Pf
96	Guilty and sad	Upset, hurt	Anger	No		He should try bringing her back	3	2	Pf
97	Guilty	Disappointed	Hopeless	Not really		Move on	2	2	Dt
98	Guilty and sad because she is a mother too	Anger	More angry, he might have even fought with her	Yes, in the eyes of Dasharatha and Bharata	She realized her mistake in the end and apologized to Rama, Dasharatha, Kausalya and Bharata	Good deeds so people can notice, change herself, think good about people, not do the same mistake	2	4	Pnf
99	Shock, shame, humiliation	Compassion, redemption, forgiveness	The affected party would have still forgiven the woman	No		She should have pleaded for mercy	4	0	Pf
100	Scared and ashamed.	Jesus was peaceful and forgave him	Jesus would still have forgiven him	No		Tried to get Jesus to forgive him	4	0	Pf
101	Fear, shame	Sad	Anger	Yes	Ask forgiveness, obey commands	There is nothing to do cause there's death	2	3	Pnf
102	Rama (the protagonist) is feeling sad as his wife can no longer be with	Sita (the affected party) is angry. She wonders why Rama can't	She would be even more angry	Yes, Rama does become unworthy for having committed this mistake. Sita is	He can regain the lost worth by thinking logically from Sita's	Rama should apologize and understand her. Instead of banishing her, he	2	2	Dt

(continued)

Table 15.13 (continued)

Sl. no	1. How do you think the protagonist is feeling?	2. Because the protagonist felt and expressed ______ what was the reaction of the opposite/ affected/other/ aggrieved party? In the context of your story	3. What if the protagonist didn't feel ______ then what would be the reaction of the affected/other/ opposite/ aggrieved party? In the context of your story	4. Does the protagonist become unworthy for having committed the mistake?	5. If the worth is lost, then how is it regained?	8. If not forgiven, what do you think the protagonist should do next?	Forgiving inclined	Non forgiving inclined	Scoring Pf, Pnf and Dt
	him. There is also the added fact that she was pregnant when he sent her away. Rama is conflicted	accept her if he loves her. She doesn't feel that there is ant use of Rama being sad unless some action is taken.		his wife, not the wife of the city. He should make her feel secure and value her love over others' opinion	perspective and asking her to come back	should try to convince the townsfolk			
103	Ashamed and regret	God punished them	God would have still punished them	No		They would have begged for forgiveness	2	2	Dt
104	Regret and shame	Anger	An even more severe punishment	Yes	Asking for forgiveness	Ask for another chance at forgiveness	2	3	Pnf
105	Kunti (the protagonist) is feeling immense guilt. She made	Karna (the affected party) is initially shocked. He	He would still forgive her and accept his fate	No, Kunti is not unworthy; a mother has to choose between		There is nothing she can do if he doesn't forgive her. She should	4	1	Pf

	him suffer twice. She felt sad	may empathize with her, but he is not fully convinced. He is feeling sad. He doesn't know how she could make him suffer so much. He feels lonely and lost		children sometimes. She is not an unworthy person; but she is not worthy of Karna		ask for his forgiveness and publicly announce that she is his mother			
106	Mohammed Bin Tughlaq (the protagonist) initially thought that the consequences to his action would be fruitful. He now feels guilty; due to him, the economy crashed and people went broke. He is angry at himself and his ancestors (from whom he claims to have gotten his ideas). He is feeling ashamed and is at unrest	His subjects (the affected party) are angry with him and disappointed in him. They cannot understand why he did what he did. They are worried about their livelihood. They feel betrayed and have lost their trust in him	If Mohammed did not feel guilt and regret, his subjects would have definitely revolted. They would have felt even more angry and would have disobeyed him. They would also have tried to put some sense in him	No, Mohammed does not become unworthy for having committed the mistake. However, he just needed good counsel and should have been more aware of his actions. He had good intentions		He should build their trust and make sure that he brings about changes for the good. He should show his subjects that he is looking out for them. He should try and understand their perspective	4	2	Pf

(continued)

Table 15.13 (continued)

Sl. no	1. How do you think the protagonist is feeling?	2. Because the protagonist felt and expressed ______ what was the reaction of the opposite/affected/other/aggrieved party? In the context of your story	3. What if the protagonist didn't feel ______ then what would be the reaction of the affected/other/opposite/aggrieved party? In the context of your story	4. Does the protagonist become unworthy for having committed the mistake?	5. If the worth is lost, then how is it regained?	8. If not forgiven, what do you think the protagonist should do next?	Forgiving inclined	Non forgiving inclined	Scoring Pf, Pnf and Dt
107	Guilty	Obedience; she was faithful to him	She probably would not have obeyed him	No		He should ask for forgiveness, and try not to believe what other people say	3	1	Pf
108	Shame, guilt, hopelessness	Happy	Anger	Yes	By being brave on the battlefield	Become a just king and no more wars	3	2	Pf
109	Regret	Anger and punishment	More severe punishment	No		Make sure not to repeat the mistake	2	2	Dt
110	Coveting, desire, shame, remorse, power, good, sorrow, repentance	He forgave David when he saw that David repented	Repentance would not have given	In the eyes of others yes, yet Bathsheba accepted him	If one loses self-worth, one must work to regain it. But if it is worth that has bestowed you, ask for it back	David should have given his kingship	2	3	Pnf

111	Bad, ashamed, felt sorry	God punished them; he felt betrayed	Regret making Adam and Eve	No. they are human, we all make mistakes		They would try to ask God for forgiveness	2	2	Dt
112	Let down, insulted	Disappointed	Surprised	No		Keep asking for forgiveness	4	0	Pf
113	Ashamed	Love and forgiveness	He would still feel love and forgiveness	No		The son would have stayed	3	0	Pf
114	Scared (Eve)	Anger	More anger	No		Try explaining	2	2	Dt
115	Sad	Forgiveness	Angry	Yes	By apologising	Ask for forgiveness	3	2	Pf

References

Baron, M. (2017). *Shame and shamelessness*. Philosophia: Springer. https://doi.org/10.1007/s11406-017-9933-x.

Beugelsdijk, S., Maseland, R., & Hoorn, A. (2015). Are scores on Hofstede's dimensions of national culture stable over time?. A cohort analysis. *Global Strategy Journal, 5*. https://doi.org/10.1002/gsj.1098.

Breugelmans, S., & Poortinga, Y. (2006). Emotion without a word: Shame and guilt among Rarámuri Indians and rural Javanese. *Journal of Personality and Social Psychology, 91*(6), 1111–1122. https://doi.org/10.1037/0022-3514.91.6.1111.

de Hooge, I., Zeelenberg, M., & Breugelmans, S. (2010). Restore and protect motivations following shame. *Cognition & Emotion, 24*(1), 111–127. https://doi.org/10.1080/02699930802584466.

Cheng, S.-T., & Yim, Y.-K. (2008). Age differences in forgiveness: The role of future time perspective. *Psychology and Aging, 23*(3), 676–680. https://doi.org/10.1037/0882-7974.23.3.676.

Devdutt, P. (2014). Karma is the new swastika. https://devdutt.com/articles/karma-is-the-new-swastika/

Elison, J., Lennon, R., & Pulos, S. (2006). Investigating the compass of shame: The development of the compass of shame scale. *Social Behavioural Personality, 34*(3), 221–238.

Fedewa, B. A., Burns, L. R., & Gomez, A. A. (2005). Positive and negative perfectionism and the shame/guilt distinction: adaptive and maladaptive characteristics. *Personality and Individual Differences, 38*, 1609–1619.

Fessler, D. (2010). Shame in two cultures: Implications for evolutionary approaches. *Journal of Cognition and Culture, 4*, 2.

Gausel, N., & Leach, C. W. (2011). Concern for self-image and social image in the management of moral failure: Rethinking shame. *European Journal of Social Psychology, 41*, 468–478.

Gausel, N., Vignoles, V. L., & Leach, C. W. (2016). Resolving the paradox of shame: Differentiating among specific appraisal-feeling combinations explains prosocial and self-defensive motivation. *Motivation and Emotion, 40*, 118–139.

Gavrielides, T. (2007). *Restorative justice theory and practice: Addressing the discrepancy*. Helsinki: Hakapaino Oy.

Gendron, M., & Feldman Barrett, L. (2009). Reconstructing the past: A century of ideas about emotion in psychology. *Emotion Review, 1*(4), 316–339. https://doi.org/10.1177/1754073909338877.

Hofstede, G. (2001). *Culture's consequences: Comparing values, behaviors, institutions, and organizations across nations*. Thousand Oaks, CA: Sage.

Hofstede, G., Hofstede, G. J., & Minkov, M. (2010). *Cultures and organizations: Software of the mind. Revised and Expanded* (3rd ed.). New York: McGraw-Hill.

Inglehart, R. (1990). *Culture shift in advanced industrial society*. Princeton, NJ: Princeton University Press.

Mason, M. (2010). On shamelessness. *Philosophical Papers, 39*(3), 401–425. https://doi.org/10.1080/05568641.2010.538916.

Mesquita, B., & Leu, J. (2007). The cultural psychology of emotions. In S. Kitayama & D. Cohen (Eds.), *Handbook for cultural psychology* (pp. 734–759). New York, NY: Guilford Press.

Miceli, M., & Castelfranchi, C. (2011). Forgiveness: A cognitive-motivational anatomy. *Journal for the Theory of Social Behaviour, 41*, 260–290. https://doi.org/10.1111/j.1468-5914.2011.00465.x.

Miceli, M., & Castelfranchi, C. (2018). Reconsidering the differences between shame and guilt. *Europe's Journal of Psychology, 14*(3), 710–733.

Nathanson, D. L. (1992). *Shame and pride*. New York: Norton.

Rodogno, R. (2008). Shame and guilt in restorative justice. *Psychology, Public Policy and Law, 14* (2), 142–176. https://doi.org/10.1037/a0013474.

Schwartz, S. H. (2004). Mapping and interpreting cultural differences around the world. In H. Vinken, J. Soeters, & P. Ester (Eds.), *Comparing cultures, dimensions of culture in a comparative perspective* (pp. 43–73). Leiden: Brill.

Tangney, J., Stuewig, J., & Mashek, D. (2007). Moral emotions and moral behavior. *Annual Review of Psychology, 58*, 345–372. https://doi.org/10.1146/annurev.psych.56.091103.070145.

Tomkins, S. S. (1962–1991). *Affect/imagery/consciousness* (Vols. 1–3). New York: Springer.

Tracy, J. L., Robins, R. W., & Tangney, J. P. (2007). *The self-conscious emotions theory and research*. New York: Guilford Press.

Vizin, G., & Unoka, Z. (2015). The role of shame in development of the mental disorders II. Measurement of shame and relationship. *Psychiatria Hungarica, 30*(3), 278–296.

Walrond-Skinner, S. (1998). The function and role of forgiveness in working with couples and families: Clearing the ground. *Journal of Family Therapy, 20*, 3–19.

Wong, Y., & Tsai, J. (2007). Cultural models of shame and guilt. http://www.gruberpeplab.com/teaching/psych3131_summer2015/documents/3.2_WongTsai_2007_CultureShameGuilt.pdf

Sowmya Puttaraju believes that her foremost skill is to be a learner and to be inquisitive about human behaviour. This has guided her in equipping herself with formal academic qualifications and guided her research pursuits as well. She presents her learning in specified group formats and in individual psychotherapy sessions. She has a PhD and MPhil in Psychology, where she tried to understand the important factors other than scholastic abilities that could effect academic performance. Her (PhD) research initiative was supported by free access to an online research program at Stanford. She was also provided grant facility to present her research initiative at Oxford by Indian Council of Social Science Research (ICSSR). Her publications have appeared in both international and national journals. She is also a certified psychotherapist from Albert Ellis Institute, USA. Endorsing the wisdom of the age old saying that "prevention is better than cure", she now plans to combine both her research and psychotherapy training to facilitate educational programs for children and adolescents to help build robust mental health in childhood that could run as an inherent part of mainstream education. Currently freelancing as consultant psychologist, counsellor, mind-coach, visiting-faculty at different spaces (from corporate to educational institutions) to diversify interests, especially in the social sector, having worked previously at a shelter for girl children as a consultant psychologist in an effort to improve their quality of life.

Tony Brian D'souza , while being an undergrad, does little to sum up his skill set and experience; his associated work as an intern in different spaces better represents his ambitions, of which the most significant ones are being part of a focused curriculum development team and later for 3 months as a part of pilot research and intervention design team member on WSHG (Women Self Help Groups) while at Udhyam Learning Foundation (NGO), Research assistant for a yearlong project at TRI (Training and Research Initiatives) and a research consultant at an ed-tech company, Walnut Knowledge Solutions, where he has led the development and design of Monitoring and Evaluation framework for two program verticals.

He has an undergraduate degree (Bachelor's degree in English, Journalism and Psychology) from St. Joseph's College (Autonomous), Bangalore and he aspires to contribute in the field of psychology and hope to earn a PhD in this field someday.

Chapter 16
"This Will Go Down on Your Permanent Record": Redeeming Shame in a World That Doesn't Forget

Simon Cozens

1 Introduction

One of the most consequential changes of the Fourth Industrial Revolution has been the creation of a permanent digital record of the lives of billions of citizens. Facebook, Twitter and Instagram record our daily activity, moods and reactions, while the search engine allows us to target an individual and instantly pull together "vast number of aspects of his private life and which, without the search engine, could not have been interconnected or could have been only with great difficulty" (Google Spain v AEPD, 2014, p. 80).

This has profound consequences for the handling of shame experiences. One coping strategy for shame which has persisted since antiquity has been the idea of self-reinvention: erasing the shameful self through self-imposed exile and reconstructing a new social identity in another place. We see this strategy in a wide variety of cultural contexts from ancient Athens (Ricoeur, 1967, p. 40), through nineteenth-century Australia (Clark, 2009), to contemporary Japan (Kraus, 1990, p. 212; Lewis, 2013, p. 203). Only 35 years ago, Heller could write that "[h]iding has become *easier* than before; we can change our social status, our domicile, even our names and start afresh. So the pressure of shame can be more easily alleviated" (Heller, 1985, 15, emphasis mine). The Fourth Industrial Revolution has made this self-reinvention impossible and has closed off such an avenue for evading shame, as our social identities are no longer atomic and localised; "when you're accused on the Internet... it's worldwide forever" (Ronson, 2015).

In this chapter, I will present insights on approaches to shame within Christian pastoral communities in the light of the permanent public record. My argument is

S. Cozens (✉)
Gloucester, UK

Worldview Center for Intercultural Studies, St. Leonards, TAS, Australia
e-mail: simon@simon-cozens.org

C.-H. Mayer et al. (eds.), *Shame 4.0*, https://doi.org/10.1007/978-3-030-59527-2_16

that the reservoir of ancient Christian theological experience contains valuable perspectives which can help transform an individual's relationship with their shame in this context and that these perspectives can, with some adaptation, be helpful beyond the faith community. In particular, I will demonstrate that the metanarrative of the Christian community poses critical questions about the link between shame and identity and highlights the need for a reconfiguration in worldview away from conditional models of self-acceptance based on perceived social value, in favour of an unconditional self-acceptance based on the concept of the intrinsic worth of the created person.

I will begin by examining the cultural changes brought about by the permanent public memory. Next, I will briefly outline a theological model of shame, before looking at two dimensions of how the early Christian community used worldview reconfiguration to process shame experiences. Finally, I will give a contemporary case study of actualising such a worldview reconfiguration in the context of an Australian church men's group.

While I acknowledge that not all readers will subscribe to some aspects of the proposed worldview, it is my belief that the elements of the approach—specifically, explicitly surfacing the social expectations surrounding shame and value, forming communities around new value structures and the deliberate construction of an unconditional self-regard based on external intrinsic worth—will serve as resources which can be adapted by practitioners to suit their context.

2 Shame and the Permanent Public Memory

In 1998, the Spanish government forced the sale of Mario Costeja González's property in order to recover social security debts, and this sale was advertised in the newspaper *La Vanguardia* (Google Spain v AEPD, 2014). The online version of these advertisements was indexed by Google, with the result that anyone searching for Costeja's name would soon discover that he was a defaulted debtor.

Before the advent of the 4IR, it was commonly held that "yesterday's newspapers are tomorrow's fish and chip papers"—that is, news was regarded as impermanent. Incriminating information about an individual's past would be difficult to determine without extensive archival research. Today, however, these archives are digitised and available online and easily retrievable through Internet search engines (Google Spain v AEPD, 2014, p. 80).

Costeja brought a case against Google, claiming that the information indexed about his debt was "inaccurate, irrelevant or no longer relevant" (David, 2014) and should therefore be removed from the search index, in essence removing it from the public memory. The court agreed and established a renewed form of the doctrine of "the right to be forgotten", based on "the fundamental need of an individual to determine the development of his life in an autonomous way, without being perpetually or periodically stigmatized as a consequence of a specific action performed in the past" (Mantelero, 2013). In essence, the court held that the stigmatisation potential inherent in the permanent digital record must be balanced by an opportunity for a "public forgetting" of information harmful to an individual's reputation. This is based on the principle that "a decent society needs to [find] ways to protect the dignity of its members against shame and stigma" (Nussbaum, 2004, p. 282).

From this we can see that permanent public memory of the Internet, and in particular its role in the stigmatisation of individuals, is sufficiently transformational as to require social and legal responses. The cultural changes brought by the pervasive nature of the Internet do not end there. Social media is providing both new sources of shame and self-image insecurity and also new mechanisms for shaming (Cozens, 2019, p. 142; Ronson, 2015).

To see this positively, the fact that shame in the Internet age can no longer easily be addressed by *evasion* is a welcome development: it highlights the opportunity for positive self-rediscovery and growth provided when shame experiences are not bypassed but rather faced, acknowledged, redeemed and integrated (Mayer, 2017). But this changed relationship with shame in turn requires new pastoral and therapeutic approaches which do not require the reputational damage to an individual to be expunged, spent or forgotten—because, given the permanent public memory, it cannot ever be—but which dig deeper into far more fundamental questions of wholeness, relationships and identity.

As we shall see, these very questions are explored in the Christian shame narrative of the Fall.

2.1 Shame in Christian Theology: A Problem of Perspective

The Bible's prototypical account of shame (Lewis, 1995, pp. 84–86), the Fall account of Adam and Eve in Genesis 3, is one of the first places where shame is discussed in world literature (see Chap. 15 in this book). This story is a foundational part of the Christian metanarrative and hence makes up a core part of the worldview of both historic and contemporary Christian communities. In order to understand how these communities have transformed shame and how this can help us in the context of the permanent public memory, we must first explore the narrative's depiction of shame and its relationship to identity.

It must be acknowledged that there is considerable diversity of opinion within theological circles as to how to interpret the Genesis 3 narrative and hence how to view shame from a Christian perspective. This diversity of opinion generally follows from differences in theological approach. Biblical theologians—those who begin their theological reflection from the text of the Bible—have generally dialogued with linguistics, literary criticism and, more recently, social anthropology and have generally seen shame as positive in its discretionary function.

While many Biblical commentators entirely omit the topic of shame—something which is explicitly mentioned in the text—and instead focus their discussion on Adam and Eve's *guilt*, something which does not explicitly appear in the narrative at all, those who do tackle the issue, such as Gunkel and Westermann, generally follow

Wellhausen in viewing the shame of Genesis 3 as the origin of the nudity taboo and thus interpret it positively as the development of sexual awareness and adult sensitivity (Westermann, 1994, pp. 250–51). It must be noted, however, that this was an *eisegesis*—that is, a bringing of contemporary (psychological) presuppositions to the text instead of reading it on its own terms. An accurate theological treatment of a psychological subject such as shame should not merely subject theological interpretation to psychological categories, but rather enter into a true dialogue between the disciplines (Charry, 2017; Watts, 2012).

Pastoral theologians—who begin by considering pastoral situations and applying theological doctrines to those situations—have on the other hand made use of the insights of psychology in their reflections (see Watts, 2001, 2012) and have been more interested in disgrace shame. The treatment of shame in pastoral theology has been almost wholly negative, seeing it as something which needs to be expunged from the individual through processes of atonement, confession and so on. (See Binau, 2002; Forrester, 2010, amongst others.)

We will take a biblical studies approach in this paper for two reasons: first, because as Gilligan (1997, pp. 70–73) argues, "the symbolism of shame" present in the biblical text, as a mythical and ritual description of shame, serves as "objective correlatives" for the emotions and thereby provides a rich source of psychological investigation, and second, because in the New Testament passages we will later consider, we see narrative and documentary evidence of a community taking an integrative approach to the situation of shame. The biblical record therefore operates as a "thick description" (Geertz, 2008) from which we can garner the community's understanding of shame and its reconfiguration. My own hypothesis, based on a close textual exegesis of the Genesis account (detailed in full in Cozens & Ochs, 2019), is that the prototypical biblical form of shame is neither portrayed negatively nor positively per se, but rather is used as *the symptom of a mis-derived identity*. Shame itself is not the problem to be solved; but the presence of shame is a signpost which draws our attention instead to the origins of our identity and self-worth.

Put briefly, before the Bible's Fall narrative, Adam and Eve received and reflected positive God-given affirmations about their identity as bearers of the image of God and about their fundamental goodness (Gen 1:27,31). God's affirmations about the goodness of creation reflect His continued exultation of humanity: "If God truly wants creation's flourishing he must exult when we love well, when we enjoy success at challenging tasks, and when we create adroitly. We, in turn, are encouraged by God's celebration of us as we succeed in living beneficiently" (Charry, 2017). Conversely, isolation and independence are flagged as negative factors (Gen 2:18); authentic existence is prefigured as only being possible through relationship.

As the narrative unfolds, Adam and Eve accepted these affirmations and appropriated them to themselves, and we find them in complete relational harmony with God, with self, and with one another, without the incursion of shame into their intrapersonal relationships (Gen 2:25). Instead, however, humanity chose to "be like God, knowing good and evil"—in other words, acting as an independent source of value judgements (3:5); but paradoxically this freedom caused their "eyes to be opened" (3:7), that is, gave them awareness of the possibility of *negative* judgements by others and the self (see Chaps. 7 and 15).

Because of this awareness, their interpersonal peace is shattered (symbolised by a realisation of their naked state), leading in turn to a psychic insecurity about their identity before one another. This insecurity is evidenced by shame behaviours: covering (3:7), hiding (3:8) and scapegoating (3:12–13). Hence shame was first experienced as the shift from purely receiving external, positive, definitive affirmation from the divine Other to a sensitivity to potential negative judgements from one's peers; as one would expect from its collectivist cultural context, shame in the Bible is predominantly social and relational, rather than internal and individual.

Hence the book of Genesis, anticipating Sartre by some 3000 years, first connects shame with what we would now call *le regard*, the opening of the eyes to the awareness of the "gaze of the other" and its consequent inducement of shame (see Wilson, 1987); it then portrays shame as the result of the *loss of faith in one's own goodness* and the individual's disconnection from, and disbelief in, identity-giving reference points based on positive affirmation—something which both psychological and popular writing on shame have since acknowledged.

But whereas secular authors have suggested the development of positive self-regard as a way to overcome the (negative) effects of shame (see, e.g. Brown, 2007; Gilbert, 2010), "a gap in Brown's research is the definition of humans as made in God's image, a concept termed *imago dei*" (Davis Nelson, 2016, p. 161). Within the Christian worldview, the origin of positive self-regard is the recognition of the image of God in oneself and in the other.

The function of shame in theological terms, then, is to highlight humanity's changed perspective: from the security of the identity-giving divine regard to the fallible and impermanent regard of the human other. Positive *self*-regard may ameliorate sensitivity to the negative judgements of the other, but it requires the shamed person (who is struggling with the very issue of self-regard) to effectively pull themselves up by their bootstraps; nor, from a Christian understanding of self, does positive self-affirmation restore people to the ultimate knowledge and experience of divine affirmation. In articulating "what Positive Psychology would look like if given theological [...] foundation..., we come to view *the basis* of human wellbeing as deriving from the divine wellbeing... and *the goal* of wellbeing as communion with the divine itself" (Anstey, 2017).

Having established that theological examination of shame serves to highlight the relationship between self and others and also between self and the image of the divine within the self, let us now examine how ancient Christian communities problematised these relationships in order to process their shame experiences. We will then see how these same principles can be applied today to situations of shame in the context of the permanent public memory.

3 Deconstructing the Shame System

Those coming to Christian faith in the first century CE were choosing to pledge their allegiance to a condemned and shamefully executed criminal, something which made them an object of scorn from surrounding society. The Alexamenos graffito, found near the Palatine Hill in Rome, satirises a Roman soldier worshipping a crucified donkey-headed figure, captioned "Alexamenos worships his God" (Lanciani, 1898, p. 122). How did they deal with this shame, and what can it tell us about shame situations today?

According to Neyrey (1994), one of the tasks of the Gospel writers was to equip the early churches with a coherent alternative metanarrative to the world's perception of them, displacing their shamed identity and reclaiming a shared positive self-understanding as the righteous and honourable people of God; this is not dissimilar to the task of those counselling the shamed today.

It is instructive to examine how the Gospel writers did this, as the early Christians were in a similar position to those shamed by the permanent public memory: their faith was a socially known fact about their public identity that they were not able to disown (Macmullen, 1981, p. 40; Neyrey, 1995). We can distinguish two components to the process of how these communities re-interpreted shame: first, through the deconstruction of the world's identity system, and second, through the re-construction of a new frame of reference for identity based on the gaze of the Other.

In terms of deconstructing the world's identity system, Neyrey (1998) highlights how Jesus' teaching was intended to expose and problematise assumptions about the origins of self-worth. Jesus pronounces God's blessing and affirmation upon the poor, mourning, meek and lowly and specifically upon "you when people insult you, persecute you and falsely say all kinds of evil against you because of me" (Matthew 5:3–11). These *makarioi* ("blessed") sayings form a programmatic introduction to his worldview-defining Sermon on the Mount. This teaching involves an ethical reconfiguration where reputation is not created, maintained or defended in worldly terms. Believers are not to defend their social worth by seeking satisfaction for public slights (5:22–25), nor should they find security in their property (5:40–42). In a society where good is often done "merely to be seen by people" (6:1) and hence to gain social reputation, believers are not to rely on peer affirmation of their behaviour but on the unseen regard of the God "who sees in secret" (6:4, 6:6, 6:18).

In other words, through his teaching:

> Jesus invites disciples to join his honourable world, where the opinions of neighbours do not count for much and where their expectations do not control one's behavior... Jesus' subversive commands would not be imaginable to disciples unless an alternative structure for worth, reputation, and respect were put in place, namely, honour from Jesus and rewards from one's heavenly Father. (Neyrey, 1998, p. 221)

deSilva (2010) similarly applies the same schema to the depictions of Jesus' crucifixion and death, particularly in the book of 1 Peter, arguing that "[t]he story at the center of the church's faith is one that forces a decision about the reliability of the world's estimation of honor and shame". For early Christians such as Alexamenos, choosing to be publicly identified with a crucified criminal *necessitates* a rejection of the world's value systems, and thus "the author calls the hearers to counter feelings of shame by *developing a healthy self-respect* based on the embodiment of ideals and virtues they know to be held in esteem both within the Christian subculture and the dominant culture" (Neyrey, 1994, emphasis mine).

For example, "because of his patient endurance of hardships, pain, and even death, Jesus should be seen as courageous. He voluntarily accepts his fate, and so he does not die a slave or a victim. His obedience to God's will indicates that he dies freely and nobly" (Neyrey, 1998). Pointing out that he was *not* seen as honourable in spite of these commonly held social virtues is intended to demonstrate to the new Christian communities that the world's perception and judgement is faulty and unreliable and so to wean them away from deriving their identity and self-image from the perceptions of others. In essence, Christians should not trust the world which tries to shame them, because it does not even play by its *own* rules correctly. Hence:

> [t]he negative evaluation outsiders form of and enforce on Christians is offset not only by considering the ignorance of these unbelievers, such that they are unable to form a reliable evaluation of worth, but also their dishonourable conduct, indeed, their utter shamelessness in the light of God's revelation of God's standards. To be shamed by the shameless is ultimately no shame at all. (deSilva, 2000, p. 63)

The New Testament narratives thus function counter-culturally, *conscientising* (Friere, 2005) the early Christians to the existence of the "shame system" and challenging them to an alternative source of standards and self-worth. As we shall see, this process of conscientising, deliberately surfacing the vacuity and fickleness of secular value systems of judgement as a basis for shaming, is a tool that can be used to build resilience against shame today.

4 "Consider Yourselves": Positive Image-Building in Community

But surfacing, naming and countering the social expectations which bring about shame is only the first part of the approach used by the early Christian communities; the second factor in this approach is a reconstructed social identity. In particular, returning to our understanding of shame in Genesis, the individual caught up in the evaluative gaze of the other must be *reconfigured* to once again receive the positive affirmation of the Divine. Early Christian communities did this by appropriating to themselves the inverted value systems we saw in the previous section and thereby considering themselves, and not their shaming oppressors, to be the true yardstick of human existence. This also gives us further hints about how to build shame-resilient communities today.

As an example, in Saint Paul's letters to the church in Corinth, he encourages them to see themselves as "saints" (*hagioi*; Paul's customary address at the beginning of each of his letters), "called to be his holy people" (1 Corinthians 1:2). Similar statements are made in Paul's letters to other churches, in which he calls them "heirs of God" (Romans 8:17), "sons of God" (Galatians 3:26), "members of God's household" (Ephesians 2:19) and so on. Paul is addressing them not just as *redeemed* people, but as utterly *exemplary* people—transformed to become the pinnacle of true humanity; and he does this in full knowledge of the fact that many of his correspondents had backgrounds and life experiences which were considered shameful by the moral standards of the time (1 Corinthians 6:9–11) and that they were on the whole considered socially inferior (1:26). By describing them in terms that are radically contrary from the world's understanding of them, he is directly challenging them to reconsider their own self-perception and self-regard; he is commanding them to "consider yourselves" (λογίζεσθε ἑαυτοὺς, Romans 6:11) in a different way. This is another example of how when "there is no reason or justification for being stigmatised by shame, ... shame is transmuted into pride as part of a strategy by individuals and groups to reverse the discourse" (Munt, 2008, p. 4).

In other words, Paul is encouraging the early Christian communities to rediscover a self-understanding based on the *imago dei* within themselves and pointing them back towards the identity-giving affirmation of the Divine. Even though their Christian identity might be a source of social stigmatisation by their peers outside of the church, Corinthian believers were to develop a worldview in which they were able to reject the received understanding of their social status and instead see themselves *first* in terms of God's acceptance and affirmation of them. Based on that affirmation, he then challenges them to align their own self-perception with this divine reality. For Paul, a *positive self-regard* develops out of a *positive God-regard*.

Finally, Paul's praxis demonstrates a communitarian approach to the transformation of shame. The process of transforming shame into authentic essence must take place through the community, because while "shame is shame of oneself before the Other... at the same time I need the Other in order to realize fully all the structures of my being" (Sartre, 1992, pp. 302–3). Paul's recurrent image of the church was as a unity, a body; the individual members as a collective made up the body of Christ (Romans 12:5; 1 Corinthians 12:27). We can understand the "body of Christ" in Paul's thinking to be synonymous with the "image of God" (as he states in Colossians 1:15). Therefore it was through the church that the image of God, the true humanity as expressed prior to the Fall, was fully present in the life of the individual.

The Christian community as imagined by Paul therefore serves to transform situations of shame in two ways. First, it is the locus in which true humanity is recovered and constituted. By identifying the image of God with the church, Paul simultaneously reminds the church members both of their external source of dignity and worth and also their need for one another in completing this dignity. Second, it acts as the primary bearer and guardian of the alternative metanarrative and value structure. That is to say, it is an idealised community in which the members operationalised an alternative social identity, valuing one another not in terms of social worth but based on the affirmations they had received from God.

For Paul, then, it was paramount that as a community which had rejected the world's shaming judgements, the churches did not reintroduce their own shaming behaviour. (See 1 Corinthians 6; Malina & Pilch, 2006, p. 82. For a contrary view, see Lau, 2020.) Indeed, through his "body of Christ" language, Paul portrays the whole body of the church as working *together* against shame. In particular, the more "presentable" members are to submit themselves to and to "treat with special honour" those who are considered shameful (1 Corinthians 12:22–24), not just as a means to transform their shame, but also as an acknowledgement that the worldly perspective is to be utterly rejected and instead replaced by the divine perspective: the church does not *bestow* honour upon the shamed, but rather *recognises* their intrinsic honour and worth that the world cannot see (Martin, 1999, p. 96).

5 Redeeming Shame Today

Unfortunately, we must admit that Paul's rejection of the shame system and reconstruction of a community based on alternative value lines has largely been forgotten by present-day churches. Indeed, churches can often themselves be tremendously shaming communities, because of such aspects as unhealthy social and religious expectations, judgementalism, pressure to conform and spiritual abuse (Nash, 2016). But a recent awareness of the role of shame within Christian ministry, and a burgeoning theological investigation of it—perhaps itself driven by the heightened interest in shame more generally in Western culture (Brown, 2007)—is causing some communities to rediscover these original concepts.

As part of a planned experiment in applying the worldview transformation, we have detailed above in the context of an Australian church, a group of men are having breakfast in the basement of a church. One of the men has been telling the others his life story, which has included his struggles with poverty, abuse, anger and alcohol misuse—not all of which are in the past. During the retelling, he breaks down, and another man puts an arm around him. "Mate, it's OK. That's not how God sees you. And that's not how we see you". Others begin to speak about their own experiences along similar lines.

Over the months that followed, it became apparent that this was the genesis of a new kind of community. In subsequent breakfast meetings, different men were able to discuss, unprompted, feelings of sexual inadequacy, addiction, financial shame and many other situations that they would ordinarily hide from one another. What was happening? It was not so much that shame was being acknowledged, claimed and mined for its transformative potential, as suggested by Ryan (2019), but rather that shame was *relativised* in favour of fundamental worth and identity. The men were able to accept their lives, including accepting their shame feelings, because they had established a communitarian self-regard wherein they no longer evaluated themselves according to the narrative of shame. Shame was still present, but it was dethroned.

That situation had not arisen spontaneously, but was the result of careful preparation. The initial men's meeting had been preceded by a teaching series on the book of 1 Corinthians which was designed to deconstruct systems of self-worth and identity based on reputation and achievement and instead build a united community around the *imago dei*. We had considered together the topic of reputation and why it was important to us and the desires for social recognition and merit that lay inside us. The initial self-disclosure in the men's group was deliberately timed to both demonstrate the strength of the community's changed value system and further develop it. It was an exercise designed to give these men the opportunity to prove—to themselves as well as to others—that they were living up to the values about the Other-based origins of identity and worth that they professed to belief. If the first man was a creature of God and that was all that mattered, then they would not enter into his shame—nor their own.

Within this context, the permanent public memory ceases to be a threat. Without the relativisation of shame and the development of a positive identity image rooted outside of one's social self-perception, there is a constant threat that shame feelings will be re-triggered by the rediscovery of shameful information. The next person we meet might find out that thing about us, and we are required to face our feelings about it once again and address the reputational damage. But when one has developed a self-image which is both externally anchored and unconditionally positive, while shame is not erased, it is no longer an existential, ontological threat. It becomes relativised by the gaze of the Other.

To put it another way, the guilt-based self-image will cause relationships to be dependent on what I have done; the shame-based self-image will cause relationships to be dependent on who I am; but the Other-based self-image will cause relationships to be dependent on *whose* I am. In our case study, the church had taken steps to internalise the idea that "[f]aith in oneself as a person is predicated on creation anthropology… As a created self or person we are of intrinsic value and worth" (Albers, 1995, pp. 118–19). By deconstructing the shame system and reclaiming as a community the importance of the *imago dei* within them, these men renewed their connection to the Divine source of affirmation which Adam had lost and restored their relational harmony with God, self and others.

6 Conclusion

In a culture transformed by social media and pervasive Internet access, where shame is "worldwide forever", shame can no longer be evaded nor erased. Addressing shame in this context requires instead consideration of the root causes of shame and reconfiguration of self-worth and identity. When I speak of reconfiguration, I am not merely referring to establishing a positive self-worth for the individual; reconfiguration instead seeks to deconstruct and reconstruct the concept and the origin of worth itself, including its social and reputational dimensions. Reconfiguration speaks of a change of worldview, and, in the Christian context, a reorientation of worth from conditioned human affirmation (or self-affirmation) to unconditional Divine affirmation.

In this chapter I have argued that ancient Christian practices point us towards methods of actualising such a reconfiguration today within a community dealing with shame. First, the Christian community subscribes to a common metanarrative, including the Fall narrative and its exploration of shame, which provides its members with a conceptual connection between shame and the source of identity and worth and highlights the loss of unconditional self-worth and the danger of finding worth in the eyes of others. Next, deliberate conscientisation serves to deconstruct shaming narratives of the world's systems for value, reputation and judgement, which is then reconstructed into an alternative worldview based on unconditionality and the divine regard. Finally, this alternative value system is entrusted to the community as a whole, which is given the opportunity and the challenge to act out its new values in practice, creating new social identities for its members.

In pastoral praxis, this reconfiguration is done through the concept of the *imago dei*, the creation of the individual in the image of God and the positive affirmation and acceptance of God towards His creation. With this reconfiguration complete and a reconfigured community established which reflects and reaffirms Original Goodness, the "painful ontological aspects of shame" (Wong, 2019, p. viii) become relativised and overcome. Shame still speaks, but the acceptance of the Other speaks louder.

References

Albers, R. H. (1995). *Shame: A faith perspective*. Psychology Press.

Anstey, M. P. (2017). 'And god saw it was good': The creation of wellbeing and the wellbeing of creation. In G. Ambler, M. P. Anstey, T. D. McCall, & M. A. White (Eds.), *Flourishing in faith: Theology encountering positive psychology* (pp. 55–64). Eugene, OR: Cascade.

Binau, B. A. (2002). When shame is the question, how does the atonement answer? *Journal of Pastoral Theology, 12*(1), 89–119.

Brown, B. C. (2007). *I thought it was just me (but it isn't): Making the journey from "what will people think?" to "I am enough"*. New York: Gotham.

Charry, E. (2017). Positive psychology and christian theology: an exchange of gifts. In G. Ambler, M. P. Anstey, T. D. McCall, & M. A. White (Eds.), *Flourishing in faith: Theology encountering positive psychology* (pp. 3–18). Eugene, OR: Cascade.

Clark, M. (2009). *For the term of his natural life*. London: Penguin.

Cozens, S. (2019). *Looking shame in the eye: A path to understanding, grace and freedom*. London: InterVarsity Press.

Cozens, S., & Ochs, C. (2019). 'Have you no shame?': An overlooked theological category as interpretive key in genesis 3. *Journal of Theological Interpretation, 13*(2).

David, E. G. (2014). Old and new domains of privacy: Towards the right to be forgotten (Comments on "Case Google, c 131/12, of 13 May 2014)". *ECJ Leading Cases*, 1–11.

Davis Nelson, H. (2016). *Unashamed*. Weaton, IL: Crossway Books.

deSilva, D. A. (2000). *Honor, patronage, kinship & purity: Unlocking new testament culture*. Downers Grove, IL: InterVarsity Press.

deSilva, D. A. (2010). Turning shame into honor: The pastoral strategy of 1 Peter. In R. Jewett, W. L. Alloway Jr, & J. G. Lacey (Eds.), *The shame factor: How shame shapes society*. Eugene, OR: Wipf & Stock.

Forrester, J. A. (2010). *Grace for shame: The forgotten gospel*. Toronto, ON: Pastor's Attic Press.

Friere, P. (2005). *Pedagogy of the oppressed*. New York: Continuum.

Geertz, C. (2008). Thick description: Toward an interpretive theory of culture. In *The cultural geography reader* (pp. 41–51). Routledge.

Gilbert, P. (2010). *The compassionate mind*. Oakland, CA: New Harbinger.

Gilligan, J. (1997). *Violence: Reflections on a national epidemic*. New York: Vintage Books.

Google Spain SL, Google Inc. v Agencia Española de Protección de Datos, Mario Costeja González. (2014). "European Court of Justice."

Heller, A. (1985). *The power of shame*. London: Routledge & Kegan Paul.

Kraus, C. N. (1990). The cross of reconciliation: Dealing with shame and guilt. In *Jesus Christ our lord: Christology from a disciple's perspective* (2nd edn., pp. 205–217). Scottdale, PA: Herald Press.

Lanciani, R. (1898). *Ancient Rome in the light of recent discoveries*. Boston, MA: Houghton Mifflin.

Lau, T.-L. (2020). *Defending shame: Its formative power in Paul's letters*. Ada, MI: Baker.

Lewis, M. (1995). *Shame: The exposed self*. New York: Free Press.

Lewis, D. C. (2013). *The unseen face of Japan, Revised*. Gloucester: Wide Margin Books.

Macmullen, R. (1981). *Paganism in the Roman Empire*. New Haven, CT: Yale University Press.

Malina, B., & Pilch, J. (2006). *Social-science commentary on the letters of Paul*. Minneapolis, MI: Augsburg Fortress.

Mantelero, A. (2013). The EU proposal for a general data protection regulation and the roots of the 'right to be forgotten'. *Computer Law & Security Review, 29*(3), 229–235. https://doi.org/10.1016/j.clsr.2013.03.010.

Martin, D. B. (1999). *The corinthian body* (new edn.). Yale University Press.

Mayer, C. -H. (2017). Shame—'a soul feeding emotion': Archetypal work and the transformation of the shadow of shame in a group development process. In *The value of shame: Exploring a health resource in cultural contexts*. Cham: Springer.

Munt, S. (2008). *Queer attachments: The cultural politics of shame. Queer interventions*. Surrey: Ashgate.

Nash, S. (2016). *Landscapes of shame in the church: A typology to inform ministerial praxis*. PhD thesis, University of Birmingham.

Neyrey, J. H. (1994). Despising the shame of the cross: Honor and shame in the Johannine passion narrative. *Semeia, 68*, 113–137.

Neyrey, J. H. (1995). Loss of wealth, loss of family and loss of honour: The cultural context of the original makarisms in Q. In P. F. Esler (Ed.), *Modelling early Christianity: Social-scientific studies of the new testament in its context*. London: Routledge.

Neyrey, J. H. (1998). *Honor and shame in the gospel of Matthew*. Louisville, KY: Westminster John Knox.

Nussbaum, M. C. (2004). *Hiding from humanity: Disgust, shame and the law*. Princeton, NJ: Princeton University Press.

Ricoeur, P. (1967). *The symbolism of evil*. New York: Harper & Row.

Ronson, J. (2015). *So you've been publicly shamed*. New York: Riverhead Books.

Ryan, T. (2019). Transforming shame: Strategies in spirituality and prayer. In C.-H. Mayer & E. Vanderheiden (Eds.), *The bright side of shame* (pp. 187–198). Cham: Springer.

Sartre, J.-P. (1992). *Being and nothingness*. New York: Washington Square Press.

Watts, F. (2001). Shame, sin and guilt. In *Forgiveness and truth* (pp. 53–70). Edinburgh: T & T Clark.

Watts, F. (2012). Doing theology in dialogue with psychology. *Journal of Psychology and Theology, 40*(1), 45–50. https://doi.org/10.1177/009164711204000109.

Westermann, C. (1994). *Genesis 1–11: A continental commentary* (J. J. Scullion, Trans.). Minneapolis, MN: Fortress Press.

Wilson, E. (1987). Shame and the other: Reflections on the theme of shame in French psychoanalysis. In D. L. Nathanson (Ed.), *The many faces of shame*. New York: Guilford Press.

Wong, P. T. P. (2019). Foreword: From shame to wholeness: An existential positive psychology perspective. In C.-H. Mayer & E. Vanderheiden (Eds.), *The bright side of shame*. Cham: Springer.

Simon Cozens is an adjunct lecturer in cultural anthropology at Worldview Center for Intercultural Studies, Tasmania, and the author of Looking Shame in the Eye. He worked for 7 years as a missionary in Japan and currently leads the ReThinking Mission think tank.

Part IV
Shame 4.0 in the Media

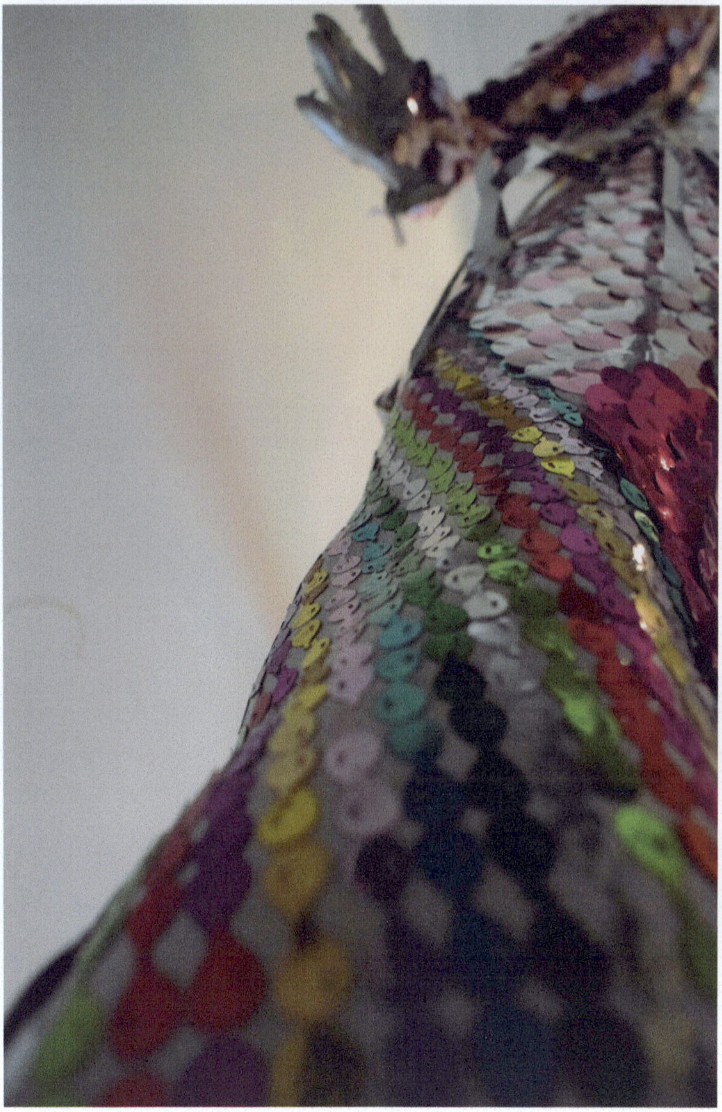

Chapter 17
Shame Dwells in the Eyes: Analysing Social Media Culture Using Aristotle's Perspectives

Anita Kasabova

1 Introduction

Traditionally, shame requires a witness, for "the way shame operates is how the subject feels under the eyes of another person" (Balick, 2019). With new technologies facilitating our use of social media and broadcasting our judgements, shame has gone through an industrial revolution (Scibona, 2019). We use social media to showcase ourselves how we would like to be seen, and 4IR technologies have made it easy to be seen by countless virtual witnesses. However, these same technologies also support the anonymous gaze of numerous users witnessing and judging behaviour that potentially breaks social norms. Social media shame ensues when our mistakes are retweeted and broadcast a million times and we are made aware that we have violated a social standard, as our failings elicit contempt and derision en masse. Aristotle says that shame dwells in the eyes. Owing to shame's industrial revolution, the witnessing gaze has been augmented to a multitudinous glare. 4IR's social media culture has become a feeding ground for online shame and shaming.

The author examines how Aristotle emphasizes the eyes in his conceptualization of shame and analyses his use of the words *aiskhyne* and *aidos*, exploring how they relate to a now familiar phenomenon in 4IR: social media shame. Aristotle's account of shame is reconstructed from the *Rhetoric* and the *Nicomachean Ethics*, and the semiotic square is used to map out the complex meanings of *aiskhyne* and *aidos*. The author argues that the Greek words provide a paradigm which can be used for analysing shame situations in social media culture. This chapter has two aims: first, to familiarize readers with Aristotle's theory of shame and show the relevance of past meanings of shame to a current phenomenon, social media shame, and second, to show how Aristotle's notions can help clarify the attitudes and behaviour

A. Kasabova (✉)
Department of Humanities, City Literary Institute, London, UK
e-mail: anita.kasabova@citylit.ac.uk

C.-H. Mayer et al. (eds.), *Shame 4.0*, https://doi.org/10.1007/978-3-030-59527-2_17

of groups on social media in regard to shame and shaming. The author argues that social disgrace, fear of social disgrace and taking social responsibility are features of shame shared by Aristotle and social media groups: both belong to cultures that value a social and visible self, defined by social relationships—and the public eye—rather than as a separate individual. Hence the paper aims to show how exploring *aiskhyne* and *aidos* could contribute to a better understanding of shame in social media culture, and it does so by examining an emotion that binds the values and behaviour of groups on social media. Besides discussing the negative aspects of shame, the paper also presents a positive perspective on shame, showing how *aiskhyne* and *aidos* can have a positive impact on our interaction with social network platforms and 4IR technologies. At a time when 4IR is reshaping social identity, cultural values and moral emotions, Aristotle's account is relevant for researching shame in social media culture. Therein lies the paper's contribution to the present volume.

2 Research Methodology

A mixed methodological approach is used in this paper, combining philosophical and semiotic analyses. A close reading of relevant passages in Aristotle's texts is offered for gaining a detailed understanding of his use of two Greek words, *aidos* and *aiskhyne*, translated as *shame*. The diverse meanings of these words are then analysed by using a tool from structural semiotics, called the semiotic square (Chandler, 2017). The paper highlights the relevance of Aristotle's account for examining shame in social media culture, by examining examples of recent shame situations on social networks.

3 Aristotle on Shame: *Aidos* and *Aiskhyne*

Aidos and *aiskhyne* are two Greek words usually translated as shame.[1] Yet they draw a slightly different picture from the English word, since the two languages express different social patrimonies. I argue that this picture can provide insights into the current English usage of shame. The Greek words partly overlap with *shame*, but, unlike the English word, *aidos* and *aiskhyne* relate shame to fear.[2] Besides feeling ashamed, *aidos* denotes modesty and a prospective, inhibitory affect akin to

[1] *Pace* Cairns (1993:14) who says that *aidos* is not shame. By contrast, Liddell and Scott (2007) list shame as a referent for *aidos* and *aideomai* (sense of shame).

[2] Plato (*Laws*, 1.646e4–647b7) relates shame to two kinds of fear: (1) respect or awe (*aidos*) and (2) fear of disgrace or contempt (*aiskhyne*). Euripides (*Hyppolitus*, 383–7) distinguishes between two kinds of *aidos*: modesty or an inner sense of shame and a respect for social approval. Aristotle defines *aidos* as "a kind of fear of disrepute" (*Nic. Eth.* 4.9.1128b12).

embarrassment. While detecting social threats, it also connotes awe and respect.[3] *Aiskhyne* oscillates between painful self-focused feelings, public humiliation, failure and loss. It also signals the choice to feel ashamed. Hence both words have a negative and positive import.

How does Aristotle use these two words translated as *shame*? Roughly, he considers shame a feeling related to a person's loss of reputation and social esteem. In feeling ashamed, I am painfully aware that others do not see me as I would like to be seen. This feeling kicks in when aspects I would like to conceal are exposed. Someone who feels ashamed [*aideomai*] does not want to be seen and is shamed [*aiskhynesthai*] by being exposed. Aristotle uses *aidos* and *aiskhyne* to address issues such as the fear of being seen with contempt, how feeling ashamed is a way for discerning or seeing what we have done wrong and how we can avoid being shamed. While *aidos* is inhibitory, a fear of disrepute and a respect for social conventions, *aiskhyne* is a painful feeling in response to disrepute which can also act as a deterrent. Aristotle argues that we feel *aiskhyne* when we "shrink from disrepute itself" (*Rhet* 1384a23-24). This conceptualization of shame as a response to a loss of social esteem indicates an emotion nested in social bonds, involving a painful perception of things that cause our public disgrace. Our witnesses may be real or imaginary, since *aiskhyne* has a timeline that spans past, present and future.

4 The Social Self: Common Ground Between Aristotle's Account and Social Media Culture

What is the link between an Ancient Greek philosopher's account of shame and social media shame manifesting through 4IR? Both Aristotle and social media belong to societies that value public opinion, reputation and the importance of being seen. Shame is a social emotion—it arises through painful exposure to the public eye and displays our self-conscious awareness of being seen with contempt. In 4IR, social media shame manifests as an amplified form of public shaming in virtual space with life-altering consequences beyond Facebook or Twitter, increasing the impact on its victims. Their wrongdoing may be a bad joke, a vulgar comment, eating on the underground or a hasty picture on Instagram, but it was witnessed, posted and broadcast. This behaviour on social media can also have a positive impact, if shame is used as an adaptive strategy for moderating online content and supporting vulnerable persons. Aristotle's account of shame addresses the relation of shameful and shameless behaviours diffused in social groups and impact us on a personal level. How does that work, since Aristotle is far removed from the Internet and social media? The answer lies in two common denominators: the socially embedded self and self-esteem as a function of how we see ourselves as being seen.

[3] Cairns (1993, p. 2, 13, 14), Liddell and Scott (2007)

Virtual communities and ancient Greek society both involve our social self—a self which is embedded in and defined by our community. Psychologist Michael Lewis (1992 p. 214) calls the social self the *we-self*, focused on social relationships rather than on separation and individuation. Although it may not be typical for Western society, preoccupied with the individual or "I-self", the "we-self" thrives on social media, where it depends on the opinions and reactions of its audience. *Aiskhyne* and *aidos* occur in interpersonal relations and manifest in someone's community, on their Facebook page or Twitter account. As Lewis (1992, pp. 215–8) remarks, "[s]hame occurs around the we-self. [. . .] Shame appears when the self [. . .] violates core standards and accepts blame for its failure".

Aristotle makes a detailed analysis of *aiskhyne* and *aidos* in the *Rhetoric* (1383b-85a), showing that shame is elicited in our "we-self" when it is linked to failure and disgrace. Aristotle enquires what causes shame [*aiskhyne*], what sort of things people are ashamed of [*aiskhynontai*] or shameless about [*anaiskhyntousin*], before whom they are ashamed and in what state of mind they are when they feel ashamed.[4] He argues that shame [*aiskhyne*] means feeling disgraced when our failings are witnessed:

> Now since shame [*aiskhyne*] is a mental picture [*phantasia*] of disgrace [*adoxia*], in which we shrink from the disgrace itself and not from its consequences, and we only care what opinion is held of us because of the people who form that opinion, it follows that the people before whom we feel ashamed [*aiskhynesthai*] are those whose opinion of us matters to us. (*Rhet* 1384a25–28)

5 The Semiotic Square of Shame, Showing How Shame Dwells in the Eyes (Fig. 17.1)

Psychiatrist Léon Wurmser (2019, pp. 42–43) parses shame into two negatives and one positive, while Aristotle advances a fourfold conception. Wurmser distinguishes between (1) *shame anxiety* or the fear of exposure and disgrace, paralleling Aristotle's *negative aidos*: we are afraid we may be looked at with contempt and seen as worthless. (2) *Shame affect* or wanting to hide and disappear from view mirrors Aristotle's *negative aiskhyne* or painful shame. (3) Shame as a *reaction formation* or protective attitude is a character trait equivalent to Aristotle's *positive aidos*, denoting modesty and respect or feeling a preference for moderation. Aristotle adds (4) *positive aiskhyne*: choosing to feel ashamed and consenting to feel responsible.

[4]Aristotle analyses emotions "under three headings. [. . .] for example, in speaking of anger, we examine (1) the state of mind of angry people, (2) with whom they are angry, and (3) on what grounds they get angry" (*Rhet* 1378a25–26). Wurmser (2015, p. 96) refurbished Aristotle's division of shame in psychoanalytic terms: an objective pole (of what we are ashamed), a subjective pole (before whom we are ashamed) and shame affect (our state of mind).

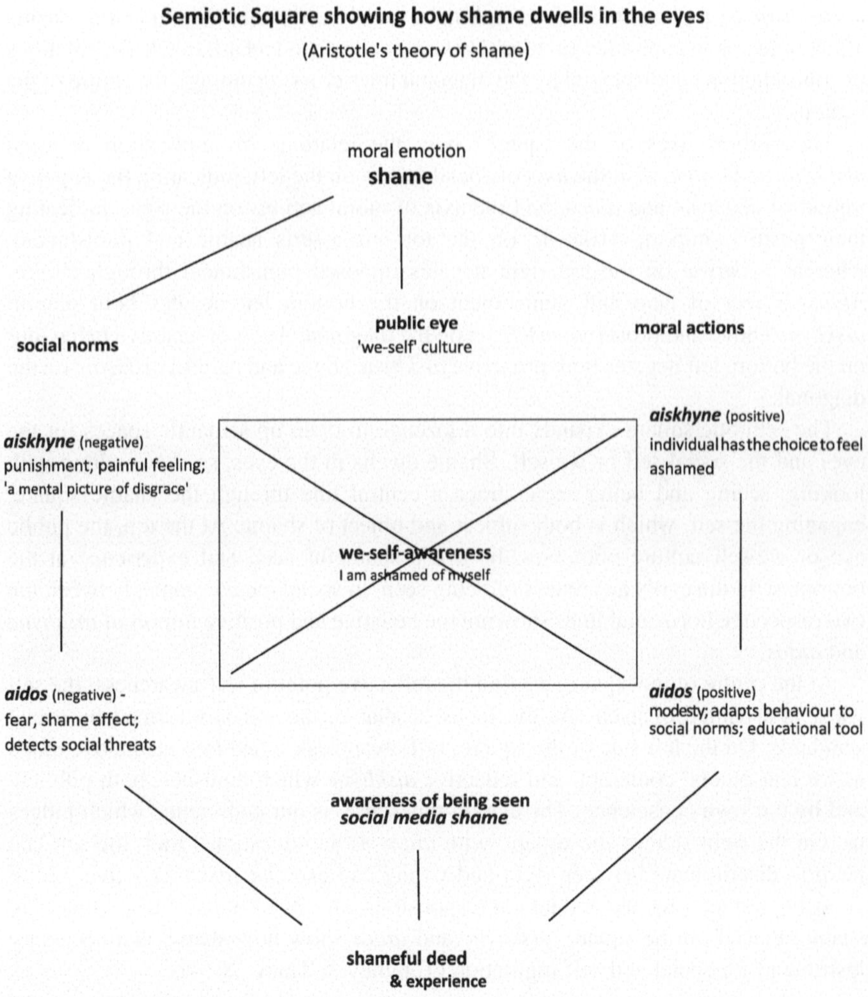

Fig. 17.1 Semiotic square showing how shame dwells in the eyes

Aristotle's account of shame and his use of *aiskhyne* and *aidos* can be displayed in the semiotic square adapted by Algirdas Greimas (1966) from the logical square of oppositions (Chandler, 2017, pp. 124–128). I have modified it as a hexagon to model Aristotle's conception of shame. Here the semiotic square/hexagon shows how the Aristotelian meaning of shame can be mapped through semantic relations of opposition and implication. *Aiskhyne* and *aidos* each have a positive and a negative import, shown on the horizontal axes of the square. The contrast between *aiskhyne* as a painful feeling and punishment for breaking a social norm and *aiskhyne* as a moral choice to feel ashamed on the upper horizontal axis is reflected in the secondary opposition between *aidos* as a fear of disgrace or shame affect and *aidos* as habituating one's behaviour to social norms. The latter is in contradiction to *aiskhyne* as a punishment for breaking a social norm. Likewise, *aidos* as shame affect or fear is in contradiction to *aiskhyne* as a choice to feel ashamed. The relations of contradiction are displayed by the diagonal lines crossing through the centre of the square.

The vertical axes of the square show the relations of implication between *aiskhyne* and *aidos*, with the axis of social norms on the left, indicating the negative import of *aiskhyne* and *aidos*, and the axis of moral actions on the right, indicating their positive import. *Aiskhyne* on the top-left asserts shame and punishment, whereas *aiskhyne* on the top right negates imposed punishment through choice. *Aidos* or fear of pain and punishment on the bottom left negates both painful *aiskhyne* above and proactive *aiskhyne* on the diagonal. *Aidos* or adaptive behaviour on the bottom left negates both proactive *aiskhyne* above and painful *aiskhyne* on the diagonal.

The semiotic square expands into a lozenge to open up semantic spaces for the eyes and the social self or we-self. Shame dwells in the eyes, so they—along with looking, seeing and being seen—trace a central line through the shame square, engaging the self, which is both subject and object of shame. At the top, the public eye or we-self culture witnesses the self's shameful deed and experience at the bottom, with the ego's awareness of being seen, in social media shame, between the two respective horizontal lines showing the negative and positive import of *aiskhyne* and *aidos*.

At the centre of the square, we find the reflective point of self-awareness: the self who? is ashamed of itself. As the focus of shame, the self is informed by social standards. On the left side of the square, self-awareness is tied into instinctive *aidos* as we fear others' contempt, and reflective *aiskhyne* which punishes, both publicly and by our own conscience. The eye, in this sense, is our conscience which judges us. On the right side of the square, with *aidos* as an educational tool, the self can learn to discriminate between right and wrong and exercise *aiskhyne*—free will in choosing to feel ashamed and taking responsibility for its response when witnessing shame. Placed on the square, *aiskhyne* and *aidos* show how shame is a necessary instrument for social and self-regulation (Tangney & Tracy, 2014).

6 *Aiskhyne*: A Mental Picture of Disgrace

Some European languages divide shame into prospective and retrospective shame, such as the French words *pudeur* and *honte*, the Spanish *pudor* and *vergüenza* or the German *Scham* and *Schande*. This distinction between an inhibitory affect and a painful feeling directed towards the self has been highlighted by psychologists (Balick, 2019; Lewis, 1992; Tangney & Tracy, 2014; Wurmser, 1987, 2015, 2019). While the latter is a feeling of mortification and humiliation due to perceived failure and public disgrace, the former is a self-conscious awareness of one's individuality and a defence against losing public esteem. Aristotle, however, does not divide the concept of shame into prospective and retrospective (Konstan, 2006:

99). Rather, he distinguishes between a dual notion comprising an inhibitory affect and a sense of modesty [*aidos*]—corresponding to the old word *shamefastness*—and *shame* [*aiskhyne*] as a painful emotion experienced in regard to *evils* or *misdeeds* [*ton kakon*] causing disrepute.[5]

Aristotle's notion of *aiskhyne* comprises prospective and retrospective shame, for it denotes our perception of evils or misdeeds. Evils can occur at different times, but feeling shame is triggered by our perception [*phainomena*] of them, insofar as these evils affect our sense of self and our reputation. "Shame [*aiskhyne*] may be defined as pain or uneasiness in regard to bad things, past, present, or future, which seem likely to involve us in discredit [*adoxia*]" (*Rhet* 1383b14–16).

Current evils are perceived, past evils are remembered, and future evils are imagined and anticipated. In all of these cases, we feel painful shame [*aiskhyne*] when we remember, see or contemplate wrongdoing, especially when we remember, see or contemplate being seen as having done something wrong or indecent. That is why we feel shame before those whose opinion of us matters to us while, at the same time, feeling ashamed of ourselves [*aiskhynesthai*]. This is a particularly vicious form of shame because it is felt before others and is also reflexive: directed both inwards and outwards.

Aiskhyne happens when our shameful behaviour is witnessed and our reputation is destroyed as these acts are made public. Aristotle does not divide shame into *before* and *after* because he connects both aspects to the eye: we show a sense of shame by veiling ourselves to be protected from other people's gaze (or glare), and, when feeling shame, we want sink into the ground or hide from the public eye. On one side, we wish to avoid exposure to humiliation due to shameful [*aiskhros*] deeds, and on the other side, we feel the pain of humiliation when a shameful deed is exposed. These evils can be present, past or future: *aiskhyne* can evoke them at present, recollect or anticipate them. We feel the pain of *aiskhyne* by remembering, seeing or imagining that our public image is ruined, regardless of when it occurred. In addition, these ills can be done by us or to us, since we also experience *aiskhyne* when we are a victim of shaming.

This aspect of *aiskhyne* is particularly relevant to social media shame in 4IR, which has radically increased an anonymous individual's chances of gaining online infamy. Her onlookers are also mostly anonymous, but they choose to remain hidden while exposing their victim's perceived wrongdoing and ruining her reputation. While anonymity shields from shame, it also shields online shamers from being held accountable for inflicting disproportionate punishments on individuals who violated a social norm. "Anonymity fosters deindividuation—the loss of an individual sense of self—which lessens self-restraint and increases one's willingness to go along with the mob" (Lukianoff & Haidt, 2018 p. 73).

---

[5]A similar distinction occurs in the Bulgarian conceptualization of shame: *svyan* (modesty, bashfulness), *sram* (a painful feeling directed towards the self) and *pozor* (disgrace). *Pozor* combines *shame* and *sight*, being derived from the Slavonic word *zrak* (look, view, sight, vision).

Charity worker Lindsey Stone's reputation was ruined when a picture of her breaking a norm went viral on Facebook, and she suffered *aiskhyne* because an online crowd had seen the post and shamed her. "Overnight, everything I loved was gone". Lindsey pretended to yell while holding up her middle finger at a cemetery, in front of a sign that said: "Silence and Respect". She lost her job, received death and rape threats and fell into a severe depression, barely leaving her house for a year. Nearly 2 years later, she still feared her new employers would find out about the incident (Ronson, 2015, pp. 202–3). *Aiskhyne* is also felt by imagining future damage to one's reputation, though it can be reduced once our community forgets about us. Lindsey's reputation improved when a digital reputation management firm reverse-engineered Google's algorithm by blasting it with positive information (Ronson, 2015, pp. 260–1).

Aristotle explains *aiskhyne* as a social threat detector connected to reputation (the opinion of others) and our concern for their opinion. "Shame is [*phantasia*] about loss of reputation [*adoxia*]". Unlike *aidos*, which is a fear of being disgraced, we feel *aiskhyne* because we see or imagine ourselves as disgraced. *Aiskhyne* is the pain and unease we feel when we see ourselves through others' eyes and detect their disapproval. It expresses a self-reflective perspective on our perceived misdeeds that may diminish the good opinion which others have of us.

Shame meshes with our perceived disgrace, when we see ourselves as discredited or when we are "connected with actions or things that entail disgrace" (*Rhet* 13585a25). As Aristotle says: "We feel more shame [*aiskhynontai*] about a thing done openly, before other people's eyes" (*Rhet* 1384a35-6). The "thing done openly" can be something we have done or was done to us and which was then publicly exposed, to create a lethal effect of double shame. Aristotle's list includes vicarious shame, incurred through acts of a family member or someone close to us, so that we feel shame by association. "Men also feel shame when they are connected with actions or things which entail disgrace [*kataiskhynousin*], for which either they themselves or their ancestors, or any others with whom they are closely connected are responsible" (*Rhet* 1385a25). He insists that feeling shame involves being under the eyes of others: "we feel more shame when we are seen and go about under the eyes of those who know of our disgrace" (ibid).

Aristotle also provides a scenario of future shame or imagining shameful consequences of a possible action. Future shame is included in his definition of shame [*aiskhyne*] as a *phantasia* of disgrace. After the conquest of the island of Samos, Cydias, an Athenian politician, asks his haggling fellow-citizens "to imagine the Greeks to be standing all around them, actually seeing the way they voted and not merely hearing about it later" (*Rhet* 1384b32–35). Imagining the Greek people witnessing how they argued about allocating the conquered territory would make the Athenians feel ashamed [*aiskhyntheien*] and stop them from appropriating the Samians' land. Envisioning shame can thus act as a deterrent and result in a positive change. This is an example of the preventive function of shame, similar to the "pre-mortem" strategy in which project team members imagine scenarios where their project has failed and then work out how to prevent it from failing.

The idea that "shame shrinks from disgrace itself" also suggests that *aiskhyne* can help us avoid disgrace. The preventive function of shame is expressed by *aidos* which kicks in as a defence against shame when we sense a potential threat to our social well-being. However, unlike *aiskhyne*, *aidos* does not involve cognition. When we feel *aiskhyne*, we know why. "We are ashamed when we suffer or have suffered or are about to suffer things which involve us in dishonor and reproach" (*Rhet* 1384a17). *Aiskhyne* involves the possibility to feel remorse or regret for past shame and correct our behaviour to prevent future shame. *Aidos*, however, is a sensitivity to shame, a reaction of embarrassment. "And we feel shame about a thing if it is done openly, before all men's eyes. Hence the proverb, '*shame [aidou] dwells in the eyes*' [. . .] we feel more ashamed [*aiskhynontai*] before those who will always be with us and those who notice what we do, since in both cases eyes are upon us" (*Rhet* 1384a18–19).

7 *Aidos* Dwells in the Eyes

English has several words for the Greek noun *aidos* which covers fear, embarrassment and shame, as well as modesty, respect and awe.[6] Positive *aidos* is personified in Greek mythology: *Aidos* is the goddess of modesty, respect, humility and a sense of shame. The companion of *Nemesis*, *Aidos*, restrains people from doing wrong. Both senses of *aidos* denote a feeling for adapting our behaviour to social convention, a fear of public criticism or public humiliation: one shrinks from appearing naked in public and incurring disgrace by falling short of social standards. Aristotle and Euripides, whom he quotes, use *aidos* in both senses.

Aidos is the "shame that dwells in the eyes"—the physical organ which expresses and feels shame. "[T]he eye is the organ of shame *par excellence*", since to feel ashamed means "I do not want to be seen" (Wurmser, 1987 p. 67).[7] We hide ourselves or turn away from those who see our shame because we are afraid of their condemning glare and of being looked at, or into. We see our shame in their eyes and fear that they may see our guilt in our eyes. Unlike current usage, the ancient Greek notion does not divide feeling shame from feeling guilt, as *aidos* relates to being seen and to fall short of a social standard.

Aristotle cites a proverb from a lost play by Euripides who explores *aidos*. Euripides' Orestes shrinks from facing his grandfather after murdering his mother: "Tyndareus approaches us, the man I am most ashamed [*aidos*] to face, because of the deed I have done. For he nursed me when I was small, [. . .]. What darkness can I

[6]Cairns (1993 p. 2) defines *aidos* as "an inhibitory emotion based on sensitivity to and protectiveness of one's self-image". Von Erffa (1937) distinguishes between a positive and a negative sense of *aidos*.

[7]Wurmser (2019 p. 157) explores the psychological relation between shame and the evil eye and the archaic need to shield from it. If a subject interiorizes the evil eye, she will judge and punish herself. Yet the eye also has an awe-inspiring divine power used in blessings.

find to hide my face? Behind what cloud can I hide to escape the eyes of that old man?" (*Eur*, *Orest* 460–470). In Euripides' *Hippolytus*, Phaedra makes a famous speech about the two senses of *aidos* which are not easily discernible.[8]

> we understand and we can discern what is right, but we don't always accomplish it [...] *aidos*, of which there are two kinds: one not evil, the other a curse to families. But if propriety were always clear, there would not be two things designated by thesame word. (*Hipp* 380–385)

Phaedra is afraid her passion for her stepson will be exposed and she will lose her good reputation, bringing disgrace to her family. She is ashamed of herself, and she is afraid of getting caught (*Hipp* 420). Here *aidos* is both "good" and "bad". Phaedra has an inner sense of shame, and she wants to cover herself because she is aware of having done something wrong: "I am ashamed (*aidoumetha*) of my words. Veil me: the tears stream down from my eyes and my gaze is turned to shame [*aiskhynen*]. For to be right in my mind is grievous pain [...]. Best to perish in unconsciousness" (*Hipp* 244–5). Phaedra is doubly ashamed: of herself and her passion (of what she said) and before society (of what others will say). So the "good" *aidos* is almost indiscernible from the "curse to families"—the "bad" *aidos* which is akin to *aiskhyne*—since the criteria for distinguishing between the two kinds of *aidos* are not clear-cut, as reflexive verb forms *aideisthai* and *aiskhynesthai* indicate, referring to shame as an emotion the subject feels about herself (von Erffa, 1937, pp. 157–8).

Euripides questions the social standard for what is morally good or virtuous and what is shameful, by showing that the two kinds of *aidos* are virtually indiscernible, although Phaedra's suicide is inevitable. She is mortified once her secret is out, because she can no longer avoid public disgrace [*aiskhron*]. The double shame—of her own passion and before society—is unbearable and incites her suicide because death was considered preferable to dishonour (*Hipp*. 503). However, the nurse questions this social norm when she suggests preparing a medicine that would have freed Phaedra of her illicit passion, saving her reputation—and her life.

Aidos as related to keeping something secret and hidden from public view—or *aidos* as a fear of getting caught—raises the question of accountability: if our sense of shame relates to being found out rather than to what we have done, we are not recognizing our responsibility. In this case good reputation—and accountability—depends on secrecy. That is why the *aidos* has to be double, external and internal, entangled with a mindfulness of others' opinion and an awareness that we can be judged, because it arises from living with others and how our community sees us.[9] To be seen and regarded by one's community can be a sign of either respect or disrespect and disgrace, depending on how we are seen. Shame impacts our self-awareness or how we see ourselves when we are aware that we have failed to meet our community's standards. This is how *aidos* regulates our behaviour. However, the community is also accountable, as shown by Aristotle's example of incurring future shame.

[8]See Kasabova (2017).

[9]See von Erffa (1937, p. 9, 131, 156).

For Aristotle, *aidos* relates to the way we are seen and how it affects us—either positively or negatively—how we see ourselves as being seen by others. Our own inner eye reveals our modesty or our failure to ourselves. Hence shame dwells in the eyes—in our downcast glance, in other people's contemptuous glare which we see and in our own eyes as we look into ourselves and painfully see our own faults.

8 *Aidos* and *Aiskhyne* in the *Nicomachean Ethics*

In the *Nicomachean Ethics*, Aristotle determines *aidos* as comprising both modesty and fear. He considers *aidos* as a preventive affect: a fear of disrepute and a guarded sensitivity to shameful acts [*aiskhra*].

> [T]here are some evils which it is right and noble to fear [...] for instance, disgrace [*aiskhron*]. One who fears disgrace [*adoxian*] is an honorable man, with a due sense of shame [*aidemon*]; one who does not fear it is shameless [*anaiskhyntos*].
> (*Nic. Eth.* 3.6.3.1115a3)

Aidos can only be felt in regard to future behaviour and manifests in physical symptoms, such as blushing or turning pale. If I am ashamed of a potentially shameful action, my prospective *aidos* can motivate me to be virtuous. Similarly, modesty [*aidos*] incurs a good reputation, and being well regarded by one's community is pleasing, although it is not a virtue. Aristotle defines *aidos* in terms of fear, considering it a feeling rather than a virtue.[10] "*Aidos* cannot properly be described as a virtue, for it seems more like a feeling, rather than a disposition" (*Nic. Eth.* 4.9.1128b10). Aristotle writes:

> [*Aidos*] is defined as a kind of fear of disrepute [*phobos tis adoxias*], and in itseffects it resembles the fear of danger, for people who feel shame blush, while those who fear death turn pale. (ibid)

In the same passage, Aristotle also distinguishes between *aidos* and *aiskhyne*: the young can be taught how to distinguish between right and wrong, in order to avoid shameful deeds [*aiskhra*]. He argues that *aidos* is an appropriate feeling for young people because their feelings can be trained and their instincts restrained. They can be habituated to feel a sense of shame for themselves and before others, so that they will not need to feel shame [*aiskhyne*]. Older people should already be familiar with *aidos* and have developed a moral character along with a sense of caution. Ideally, they shouldn't be feeling painful *aiskhyne*:

> The feeling of *aidos* is not suitable to every age, but only to the young. We think it proper for the young to be modest [*aidos*], because they live by feeling and therefore often err, and [*aidos*] may restrain them; and we praise young people when they are modest [*aidemonas*], though no one would praise an older man for being shamefaced [*aiskhyntelos*], since we think he should not do anything of which he need be ashamed [*estin aiskhyne*]. (ibid)

---

[10]Burnyeat (1980, p. 73) famously calls Aristotle's *aidos* "a semi-virtue of the learner".

Knowledge of good and bad is key for avoiding shame [*aiskhyne*]. Therefore, says Aristotle, the young should be taught *aidos*, so that they can learn to avoid the humiliation of *aiskhyne*. If they have been taught how to discern between good and bad actions and refrain from the latter, they will not feel the pain of shame [*aiskhyne*]. However, learning how to discriminate between good and bad actions presupposes assimilating the social standard for *aidos* and shameful actions [*aiskhra*]:

> For indeed the virtuous man does not feel shame [*aiskhyne*], if shame is the feeling caused by base actions [*aiskhra*]; since one ought not to do base actions [. . .], and so one never ought to feel shame [*aiskhyne*]. (ibid)

As Phaedra discovered, there are no clear criteria for knowing a good *aidos*, although she is aware of having done something wrong. *Aidos* denotes an awareness or feeling for the right balance between shame and shamelessness.[11] Aristotle says you can develop *aidos* as a habit—an awareness that your actions have consequences which may be painful. Shame [*aiskhyne*] kicks in if we have not developed our preventive *aidos*. Someone who lacks a sense of shame [*aidomenous*] is shameless [*anaiskhyntos*] (*Nic Eth* 2.7.14), and feeling shame [*aiskhyno*] implies that one is not virtuous. Not feeling ashamed [*aidesthai*] of one's wrongdoings is bad, but feeling ashamed doesn't imply that one is virtuous (*Nic. Eth*. 4.9.1128b).

A sense of shame [*aidos*] could be virtuous, if you detect it and think about the consequences of your actions before doing something shameful. However, "*aidos* is not a virtue, although it is praised, and so is the modest [*aidemon*] person" (*Nic. Eth.* 2.7.14). Rather, *aidos* is a feeling for behaving with moderation. As Aristotle says, the man of middle character is modest [*aidemon*], and modesty can be learnt by habituation: "we praise young people when they are modest [*aidemonas*]" (*Nic. Eth.* 4.9.1128b). *Aiskhyne*, by contrast, is learnt the hard way, from painful experience of past events. "Pain is the medium of punishment; for punishment is a sort of medicine" (*Nic. Eth*. 2.3.1104b15–17).

9 *Aiskhyne*, *Aidos* and Social Media Shame

How can *aiskhyne* and *aidos* help us understand social media shame? *Aiskhyne* is tied to public opinion and the "we-self", since it is caused by losing one's reputation. It signals our knowledge that "we suffer or have suffered or are about to suffer things which involve us in dishonor and reproach" (*Rhet* 1384a17–20). *Aiskhyne* not only denotes the painful humiliation we feel when we are exposed to the public eye—regardless of whether we have done or will do something wrong. *Aiskhyne* also indicates that feeling ashamed can be a choice, since it allows us to consider the

[11] In the *Eudemian Ethics* Aristotle defines *aidos* as the golden mean between impudence and shyness (*Eud. Eth.* 3.7.28).

consequences of our actions when contemplating a future misdeed which may cause us disgrace or review our response to a shameful incident.[12]

4IR social media technologies are neither good nor bad; they collect data and facilitate communication. They do not make moral judgements on whether the data is good or bad. As users, we become social media's instruments in spreading the data, and we need to reflect on how we use social media. As a new report by the UK's Royal Society of Psychiatrists makes clear, the risks and benefits of social media are not sufficiently understood. The report calls for social media platforms to share their data with researchers in order to shed light on how young people use social media (Dubicka, 2020). Here the positive sense of *aidos* and *aiskhyne* comes in which allows us to raise our awareness and "implicitly consent to a new 'small value hierarchy' involving a personal disposition to act, perceive, judge in new ways - [. . .] when [acquiring] the sentiment of shame" (De Monticelli, 2015, pp. 152–153). Social networks depend on how we use them: if used badly or without considering the consequences, they can ruin lives and reputations, but if used with discernment, they may trigger the kind of self-awareness leading to individual responsibility.

When experiencing *aiskhyne* in a positive sense, we feel a preference for assuming responsibility. Thus *aiskhyne* can make us sensitive witnesses or it can be used to target people and corporations violating moral norms. When experiencing *aidos*, we may sense a need to limit our posts and a preference for moderating our online activity. *Aidos* can be used for habituating us to be mindful of our tweets and how we respond to online posts. *Aidos* is felt involuntarily; it lacks self-reflection. As we saw in section 1, *aidos* is an inhibitory affect allowing us to anticipate shame and social disgrace, for it denotes a fear of disrepute and a sensitivity to social threats. A specific feature of *aidos* is the fear of being seen as having broken a social norm. *Aidos* therefore involves respect of others' opinion and an awareness that we can be judged, because it arises from living with others and how our community sees us. If we have not behaved in accordance with social norms, we will feel *aiskhyne*. If, however, we heed our *aidos*, we could adapt our behaviour to social rules (or at least not break them), and not suffer *aiskhyne*.

In the *Rhetoric*, Aristotle prefigures shame on social media when he designates gossip and loss of reputation as causes of *aiskhyne*: we are on social media because we want to be seen—we want an audience and to be admired, preferably by those whom we admire, as Aristotle notes (*Rhet.* 1384a15–16). Consequently, we feel *aiskhyne* before those whose opinion we admire and in response to gossip, for when gossipmongers spread tales about us, they think it casts us in a shameful light. We suffer from slander, even if we have done nothing wrong and more so if we are at fault (*Rhet.* 1384b20).

[12]See Coakley (2014).

10 Social Media Shame in 4IR

As we have seen, the self on social media is a we-self, embedded in and defined by other we-selves. "The self that fails in a we-self culture has more to do with group than with individual standards" (Lewis, 1993 p. 218). Social media shame and shaming in 4IR is related to crowd mentality and group-think because, in a we-self context, individual values shift to a shared social identity and its standards—and when these standards are violated, hundreds or thousands of Facebook or Twitter users may respond by throwing virtual stones. "When the 'tribe-switch' is activated, we bind ourselves more tightly to the group, we embrace and defend the group's moral matrix and we stop thinking for ourselves. A basic principle of moral psychology is that 'morality binds and blinds'" (Lukianoff & Haidt, 2018 p. 58). At the same time, the we-self is more vulnerable to experiencing shame because it is defined by its community's standards.

Jon Ronson (2015) published a collection of interviews with people who were shamed online and whose life has been altered because they violated a social norm. Justine Sacco was a PR woman who tweeted little jokes to her 170 followers, until one tweet blew up her life. "Going to Africa. Hope I don't get AIDS. Just kidding. I'm white!" (Ronson, 2015 p. 69). A shaming tweet storm descended on Justine, and she lost her job and her sense of self. "I had a great career and I loved my job and it was taken away from me and there was a lot of glory in that. People were *happy* about that. [. . .] It was incredibly traumatic. You don't sleep. You wake up in the middle of the night forgetting where you are. All of a sudden, you don't know what you're supposed to do. You've got no schedule. You've got no ... purpose" (Ronson, 2015 p. 75). Social media seems to have an authority bias: users attribute more credibility to the opinion of a reputable figure. According to Ronson (2015 p. 73), Justine's story went viral after a journalist received a tweet from one of Justine's followers and retweeted it to his 15,000 followers. Rather than following the target, Justine, the tweet storm followed a trend: Justine's public disgrace—and the more it trended, the worse her defamation became.[13]

In 4IR, social media platforms blurred the division between "public" and "private". Facebook claims its users "have no expectations of privacy on their posts" while promising "that users' information 'will only be seen by who they want to see it'" (Mance, 2019). In other words, by using social media, we—knowingly—forfeit our privacy and tacitly consent to our data being used. Facebook pages and Instagram platforms are windows for social approval and disapproval or shame. Here "we-selves" interact with their audience and feel the effects of praise or punishment (*aiskhyne*). We are also more aware that on social media, we are no longer private selves and have become sensitive to social threats (*aidos*) and more cautious about what we post, for fear of being called out and publicly shamed. However, a recent UK report suggests self-regulation may not be enough and that

[13]See Kasabova (2017).

harmful content on social media platforms should be regulated to safeguard children and young adults (Dubicka, 2020).

As Lindsey's and Justine's cases show, social media shaming causes harmful *aiskhyne*, shame felt before others, and of ourselves, because it involves us in disgrace (*Rhet* 1383b14–18). We see ourselves as disgraced and feel ashamed of being exposed for something we may or may not have done. At its worst, *aiskhyne* causes death because it destroys the self. Rehtaeh, a teenage girl, was raped at a party, and the incident was photographed and shared online. She was bullied on Facebook and via text. Rehtaeh committed suicide after suffering the double shame of sexual abuse and social media shame as a reaction to her abuse. Her mother is quoted as saying, "She became the target, and once that happens it basically tears you down to the core of your being. In a time when you are forming who you are as a person, the social destruction of your very being is at stake" (White & Kral, 2014 p. 127).

More recently, an 11-year-old Parisian schoolgirl committed suicide when her harassing classmates continued to shame her on social media after she had changed schools.[14] De Tarlé (2019) highlights the teacher's role in dealing with social media shaming of schoolchildren. Since the teacher is in a position of authority, she can effectively reverse engineer a social media shaming by providing guidance and support to students. As Aristotle suggests, the young can learn to feel *aidos* "because they live by feeling and therefore often err, and *aidos* may restrain them" (*Nic. Eth.* 4.9.1128b).

There are two sides to *aidos* and *aiskhyne* in education. On one side, children and young people can be habituated to feel a sense of shame, think about the consequences of their posts on social networks and help raise awareness of social media shame. To this effect, secondary school students throughout France have been appointed "ambassadors against harassment". However, the system is still in its infancy, and, according to the French Ministry of Education, 55% of students are affected by online shaming (de Tarlé, 2019). In addition, teachers can be "guardians of spaces where children [...] can show up and be seen" (Brown, 2019). Shame researcher Brené Brown (2019) developed an online hub for educators with guidelines for building awareness of shame and vulnerability in the classroom and tools for helping young people move through shame. Yet teachers also use shaming as a disciplinary tool. A 14-year-old Kenyan girl, who had her first period during school, took her own life after being "period-shamed" by her teacher.[15] In more traditional cultures, periods are still considered shameful and subject to negative *aiskhyne*. By contrast, 4IR social media culture here typifies the positive side of *aiskhyne*: *Buzzfeed media* and *Teen Vogue* helped raise awareness of such stigma by creating a space for women to share their experience and change the narrative (Armitage, 2019; Papisova, 2019). When *aiskhyne* is used to give priority to individual

[14]https://etudiant.lefigaro.fr/article/victime-de-harcelement-scolaire-une-eleve-de-sixieme-se-suicide-dans-sa-chambre_d52f12e2-9724-11e9-bf4f-065c3bd6e928/.

[15]https://www.bbc.co.uk/news/world-africa-49661658.

responsibility and showing support, it becomes a resource-oriented aspect because it is experienced as a positive value-feeling. By addressing the shame stigma on social media platforms, a space is created where women are motivated to change the conversation about menstruation, for example, by redefining "the curse" as a symbol of femininity.

11 Concluding Remarks

This paper aims to explore how an Ancient Greek notion of shame could be relevant today. When reading old texts, we use and interpret past meanings in a contemporary context and invest them with our current understanding, so it is not far-fetched to apply them to current situations.

In my view, reconstructing Aristotle's theory of shame and his use of *aiskhyne* and *aidos* not only provides an insight into their various meanings. We can also extract a toolkit for addressing a current issue: shame culture on social networks in 4IR. The call-out culture on social media causes *aidos* or fear of being publicly shamed, either for putting a foot wrong or for defending someone who is being shamed. Or perhaps we are tempted to join a gleeful audience in witnessing someone else's shaming or *aiskhyne*, because our own bias puts us on the other side. These concerns are not new, although their amplitude is, owing to 4IR technologies. Yet *aidos* and *aiskhyne* also have a positive import when they are experienced as an appropriate emotional response on social media platforms, which can modify the social behaviour of an entire group. When *aidos* is experienced as a preference for moderating one's online content or *aiskhyne* is felt as a choice to support a vulnerable classmate or by envisioning a future shame scenario, a group can be habituated and motivated to stop online shaming. This paper shows how Aristotle's notions can contribute to providing a framework for the ongoing discussion, using the negative and positive import of two old words for different aspects of shame.

References

Aristotle. (1924). *Rhetorica* (W.R. Roberts, Trans.). Oxford: OUP.

Aristotle. (1926). *Art of rhetoric* (J. Freese, Trans.) Cambridge, MA: Harvard University Press. http://www.perseus.tufts.edu/hopper/text?doc=Aristot.+Rh.+2.6.&fromdoc=Perseus%3Atext%3A1999.01.0060. Accessed 09/01/2020.

Aristotle. (1934). *Nicomachean ethics* (H. Rackham, Trans.). Cambridge, MA: Harvard University Press. http://www.perseus.tufts.edu/hopper/text?doc=Perseus%3Atext%3A1999.01.0054%3Abook%3D3%3Achapter%3D6%3Asection%3D3. Accessed 09/01/2020.

Armitage, S. (2019). This is what period-shaming looks like around the world. *Buzzfeed*. https://www.buzzfeed.com/susiearmitage/this-is-what-period-shaming-looks-like-around-the-world. Accessed 30/09/19.

Balick, A. (2019). "*Shame*" in *the digital human* (BBC series 12). https://www.bbc.co.uk/sounds/play/b09cylyp. Accessed 30/10/2019.

BBC News. (11.09.2019). *Kenyan schoolgirl takes her own life after 'period shaming'*. https://www.bbc.co.uk/news/world-africa-49661658. Accessed 12/09/19.

Brown, B. (2019). *Dare to lead # Daring classrooms*. https://brenebrown.com/daringclassrooms/. Accessed 03/08/19.

Burnyeat, M. (1980). Aristotle on learning to be good. In O. Rorty (Ed.), *Essays on Aristotle's ethics* (pp. 69–92). Los Angeles: University of California Press.

Cairns, D. (1993). *Aidos*. Oxford: OUP.

Chandler, D. ([2002] 2017: 128). *Semiotics, the basics*. London: Routledge.

Coakley, M. (2014). *Aeschyne in Aristotle's conception of human nature*. https://pdfs.semanticscholar.org/ef4d/c0012759b7381ffca4f3fdb0183fe58b54d9.pdf?_ga=2.149538227.448172397.1572371877-1161419633.1572371877. Accessed 29/10/2019.

De Monticelli, R. (2015). *The sensibility of reason. Outline of a phenomenology of feeling*. http://rivista.thaumazein.it/index.php?journal=thaum&page=article&op=view&path%5B%5D=46. Accessed 17/01/2020.

de Tarlé, S. (2019). *Harcèlement scolaire: l'ampleur du phénomène*. http://video.lefigaro.fr/figaro/video/harcelement-scolaire-l-ampleur-du-phenomene-decrypte-par-sophie-de-tarle/6056876984001/. Accessed 31/07/19.

Dubicka, B. (2020). *Technology use and the mental health of children and young people*. https://www.rcpsych.ac.uk/docs/default-source/improving-care/better-mh-policy/college-reports/college-report-cr225.pdf. Accessed 17/01/2020.

Euripides. (1996). *Hippolytus* (D. Kovacs, Trans.). Cambridge, MA: Harvard University Press. http://www.perseus.tufts.edu/hopper/text?doc=urn:cts:greekLit:tlg0006.tlg005.perseus-eng1:373-418. Accessed 09/01/2020.

Figaro Etudiant. (2019). *Victime de harcèlement scolaire, une élève de sixième se suicide dans sa chambre*. https://etudiant.lefigaro.fr/article/victime-de-harcelement-scolaire-une-eleve-de-sixieme-se-suicide-dans-sa-chambre_d52f12e2-9724-11e9-bf4f-065c3bd6e928/. Accessed 31/07/19.

Higgins, N. (2015). Shame on you: The virtuous use of shame in Aristotle's Nicomachean ethics. *Expositions, 9*(2), 1–15.

Kasabova, A. (2017). From shame to shaming. *Open Cultural Studies, 1*, 99–112.

Konstan, D. (2006). *The emotions of the ancient Greeks*. Toronto, ON: University of Toronto Press.

Lewis, M. (1992). *Shame: The exposed self*. New York: The Free Press.

Lewis, M. (1993). Self-conscious emotions: Embarrassment, pride, shame, and guilt. In M. Lewis & J. M. Haviland (Eds.), *Handbook of emotions* (pp. 563–573). The Guilford Press.

Liddell, H., & Scott, R. (2007). *An intermediate Greek-English Lexicon*. http://www.perseus.tufts.edu/hopper/. Accessed 29/10/2019.

Lukianoff, G., & Haidt, J. (2018). *The coddling of the American mind*. London: Penguin.

Mance, H. (2019). Is privacy dead? *Financial Times* https://www.ft.com/content/c4288d72-a7d0-11e9-984c-fac8325aaa04. Accessed 31/07/2019.

Papisova, V. (2019). How social media and positivity are ending period stigma. *Teen Vogue*. https://www.teenvogue.com/story/period-shaming-stigma-menstruation-body-positivity. Accessed 30/09/19.

Ronson, J. (2015). *So you've been publicly shamed*. London: Picador.

Scibona, S. (2019). The industrial revolution of shame. *The New York Times*. https://www.nytimes.com/2019/03/09/opinion/sunday/internet shaming.html?searchResultPosition=3. Accessed 18/09/19.

Tangney, J., & Tracy, J. (2014). Self-conscious emotions. In M. R. Leary & J. Tangney (Eds.), *Handbook of self and identity* (pp. 446–478). New York: Guildford Press.

von Erffa C.E.. (1937). *"Aidos" und verwandte Begriffe in ihrer Entwicklung von Homer bis Demokrit*. Leipzig: Dieterich'sche Verlagsbuchhandlung.

White, J., & Kral, M. (2014). Re-thinking youth suicide. *Journal for Social Action in Counseling and Psychology, 6*(1), 122–142.

Wurmser, L. (1987). Shame: The veiled companion of narcissism. In D. L. Nathanson (Ed.), *The many faces of shame* (pp. 64–91). New York: Guilford Press.

Wurmser, L. (2015). Primary shame, mortal wound and tragic circularity. *The International Journal of Psychoanalysis, 96*(6), 1615–1634.

Wurmser, L. (2019). *Scham und der böse Blick.* Stuttgart: Kohlhammer.

Anita Kasabova, PhD, teaches philosophy at CityLit, London, UK. She has published a monograph, On Autobiographical Memory (Cambridge Scholars Publishing, 2009), and numerous articles on topics in the history of philosophy and various aspects of memory. Her research interests include memory theories and moral emotions.

Chapter 18
Naming and Shaming in Cyberspace: Forms, Effects and Counterstrategies

Claude-Hélène Mayer and Elisabeth Vanderheiden

1 Introduction

From an evolutionary point of view, shame is primarily a social regulator (Gilbert, 2019; Scobel, 2017) which serves to adhere to socio-cultural rules and to ensure social cohesion. Historically it also ensures the survival of a group (see also Chaps. 25 in this book), but at the same time represents a resource for individual and collective development (Briegleb, 2014; Mayer & Vanderheiden, 2019, pp. xix–xxxiii; Vanderheiden, 2019; Vanderheiden & Mayer, 2017, pp. 1–43). In evolutionary terms, shame occurred mainly as a temporary exclusion and as a group reaction to an actual or supposed norm violation. If the norm violation was admitted, reintegration into the group usually took place.

However, contemporarily, the Internet has fundamentally changed the mechanisms of shaming with regard to their function as well as their scope, depth and sustainability. The social and cultural group boundaries in connection with online shaming have changed dramatically, and boundaries regarding new peer group formations are being shifted and expanded (Frevert, 2017, 2019, 2020; see Chaps. 25 in this book).

Frevert (2017, 2019, 2020), for example, points this out in her work on the history of public humiliation and shaming, when she emphasises that the historical responsibility for public shaming, in the form of infamous punishments as a social regulator in the Western world, traditionally belonged to the church or the state, until, with the

C.-H. Mayer (✉)
Department of Industrial Psychology and People Management, University of Johannesburg, Auckland Park, Johannesburg, South Africa

Kulturwissenschaftliche Fakultät, Europa Universität Viadrina, Frankfurt (Oder), Germany

E. Vanderheiden
Global Institute for Transcultural Research, Römerberg, Germany
e-mail: ev@keb-rheinland-pfalz.de

C.-H. Mayer et al. (eds.), *Shame 4.0*, https://doi.org/10.1007/978-3-030-59527-2_18

developing civil society, the state increasingly renounced this privilege and, at the beginning of the nineteenth century, the press appropriated the power of public shaming. In the meantime, the Internet, especially the social networks, has taken over this function of institutions such as the state or the church. In addition to the differences in reach and sustainability already mentioned above, there are other noteworthy differences, such as the "immortality" of these shaming practices which cannot be easily wiped out or changed in the memory of the Internet (see Chap. 16 in this book). Solove (2007a, p. 96) describes the situation as follows: "It ceases to be a temporary mark of disgrace and becomes a lasting inscription of stigma".

Further, the inadequate and nationally varying and divergent ethical and juridical procedures make it difficult to deal with naming and shaming in the new, virtual world (see, e.g. de Vries, 2015). Additionally, shameful experiences usually draw on holistic experiences in situations of social engagement and are often moderated through non-verbal gestures and face-to-face interactions to limit social damage of the person in the focus of shame (Vallverdú, 2014). However, a holistic form of communication, taking relevant information of verbal, non-verbal and paralinguistic aspects into account, differs in virtual and face-to-face interactions and might therefore have different impacts on the shamed person (Jaffe, Florez, Gomes, Rodriguez & Achury, 2014). Online shaming appears to be relatively direct by showing photographs or videos and directly spelling out the shameful situation without any mediating effect.

In this chapter, the authors aim to provide a theoretical insight into the topic of online shaming and present a clear idea of what online shaming means, the forms it takes and how to effectively deal with online shaming to transform it from a toxic emotional experience into a useful resource of self-development and inner growth. The authors' perspectives are anchored in the view that the experience of online shame can have a positive and transformational effect on the individual, if a person works through the experienced pain and suffering towards seeing shame as a marker for personal growth and development (Mayer & Vanderheiden, 2019; Wong, 2019).

This chapter falls into the broad perspective of positive psychology (PP) and particularly the positive psychology wave two (PP2.0) movement which highlights the importance of balancing negative and positive views on emotions experienced, as well as their transformational energy (Wong, 2019).

2 What Is Online Shaming?

Online shaming has been described in different ways during the past; it is also referred to as cyber-harassment, cyberbullying and trolling (Packiarajah, n.d.). What all of these terms have in common is what Braithwaite (1989, p. 100) refers to as "societal processes of expressing social disapproval". As with other kinds of shaming, online shaming is linked with the idea of established social norms and the breaking of such norms (Klonick, 2016). Skoric, Chua, Liew, Wong and Yeo (2010) also point out that individuals who use technology to police others, use so-called shaming transgressions to shame others virtually.

The term is defined as the shaming of individuals using social media platforms, websites, blogs or messenger services, based on an alleged or actual violation of norms or a failure to comply with etiquette. This can be related to appearance, a specific physical characteristic or membership of a particular group. Online shaming is defined as a form of public shaming which has its roots in different socio-cultural contexts and has always been used to punish individuals through social exclusion (Vanderheiden & Mayer, 2017).

Online shaming has far-reaching consequences for those affected, especially because toxic shame is such a profound emotion. It can lead to a reduction in social self-esteem, traumatisation, feelings of inadequacy, fear (Tangney, Miller, Flicker & Barrow, 1996; see Chaps. 8 and 11 in this book) and also withdrawal from social life and even to suicide (Gruenewald, Kemeny, Aziz & Fahey, 2004; Mayer & Vanderheiden, 2019, pp. xx–xxii; Vanderheiden & Mayer, 2017, pp. 1–43).

Through technologisation, online shaming has become a global phenomenon in the 4IR context. However, shame is experienced and managed in many different and new, virtually adjusted and digitalised ways, always being influenced by socio-culturally specific determinants, such as those described, for example, for the Japanese society (see Doi, 1973; see Chap. 8 in this book). As shown for the Japanese society, online shaming practices can have several effects on individuals, their families and specific group members.

Kalra and Bhugra (2013) point out that the far-reaching consequences of sexual and sexualised violence can be very shameful in culture-specific ways. They stress that, for example, in sociocentric societies where shame is a dominant emotion, victims of sexual violence may keep their trauma secret, which not only has a negative impact on themselves but also affects their understanding of the true nature of the trauma and the frequency of these acts, thereby influencing policy-making. Kalra and Bhugra (2013) attribute this to the fact that in sociocentric cultures, relationships between people are central, and individual identity is subordinated to family or kinship. In so-called egocentric cultures, the relationship to the self is emphasised, and independence is given more importance than "interdependence". Sociocentric and egocentric cultures supposedly have different emotional expressions and experiences of shame and guilt. Sociocentric cultures, which are more socialised, tend to generate a more social sense of shame, while egocentric cultures are more individualistic and may lead to a more private sense of guilt in the victim (see Chaps. 3, 4, 7, 8, 14, 15, 19 and 20 in this book). The emotions of a victim of sexual violence are thus shaped by the victim's culture. Shame in this context has been reported, across cultures as being associated with violence and aggression (Teyber & Teyber, 2017). In sociocentric cultures where the dignity of the family comes before that of the individual, the damage caused by sexual violence is more likely to be shared by the family members, whereas in egocentric cultures, the damage from sexual violence is more likely to be concentrated on the dignity and identity of the individual (Kalra & Bhugra, 2013) (see Chaps. 3, 8 and 15 as well as Chaps. 4 and 14).

Röttger-Rössler (2020, p. 232) also stresses that although the emotional capacity for shame is pan-human and can be found universally, it is weighted and evaluated differently depending on the cultural context. This offers new insight when we explore the new cultures of online shaming as part of the 4IR movement.

Although the consequences of online shaming are so obviously dramatic and far-reaching, many people nonetheless consider it legitimate, deliberately distinguishing it from cyberbullying, as Amy de Vries (2015) was able to prove in a qualitative study in the UK. She interviewed 30 participants (21 female, 9 male) aged 18–25 years. Analysis of the data revealed that many of the young people interviewed associated the term "online shaming" with "duty"—possibly even as a friendly obligation—in order to justify its use, as a reaction to socially unacceptable behaviour, as a deterrent to similar behaviour, and to punish the person concerned. The author of this study comes to an interesting conclusion:

> This aligns with the historical literature on the function of public shaming, and social media potentially reverses the effects of more urbanised societies on the utility of shaming. (de Vries, 2015, p. 2059)

The discussants delimited their behaviour from cyberbullying by arguing primarily in terms of the merit of the behaviour in question, but also by pointing out that shaming is associated with a goal and produces a positive effect.

However, studies with victims of such cyberattacks paint a completely different picture. For example, Huffman's (2016) study of 321 respondents aged 18–24 years and residing in the USA showed that 78% of people who experienced online shaming via social media said that they felt terrible, worthless, helpless, embarrassed or overwhelmed. Only a small group of 9% described thinking about themselves, realising they had made a mistake or said something inappropriate, while another 8% said they were unaffected by the experience. However, more than a quarter of respondents who experienced online shaming described the behaviour of those responsible and the events themselves as traumatic. Huffman's survey also found that women were twice as likely as men to reduce their social media posts after witnessing online shame on social networks, with 77% of women in particular reducing their posts, or who were even willing to delete their account as a result (Huffman, 2016, p. 40).

This willingness to exercise self-control or "self-censorship" could in turn also be observed among the perpetrators, as de Vries (2015) was able to demonstrate in the first-mentioned study. de Vries (2015) emphasises how dialectically the justification for online shaming was approached in relation to the discussions about behavioural contexts: on the one hand, shaming was presented as justified on the basis of the "evidence" of the exposed actions, but on the other hand, it was also recognised by the shamed persons that each of the actions in question could also have been taken out of a certain context (and declared suitable for shaming, especially on the assumption that people act differently when they believe they are being observed) (de Vries, 2015).

In the Spanish context, Bonavia and Brox-Ponce (2018) deal with precisely this question. In a study of 165 people between 20 and 24 years of age, they investigated whether potentially unethical decisions caused by shame turn out differently if they can be made public to others. However, their findings suggest that people are more likely to avoid unethical decisions if they are made public to others than if they remain private. The authors therefore suggest that the main factor in avoiding unethical decisions is related to the need to avoid exceeding one's own moral standard of behaviour and that the role of the public is less relevant than expected.

3 Forms and Causes of Online Shaming

In the literature, different forms of online shaming have been described. Klonick (2016), for example, refers to online shaming as a form of social norm enforcement which is framed in new ways and is based on newly created social and cultural conditions. Therefore, instead of online shaming being seen as public shaming which is technologised and applied through a new medium—it should rather be seen as a new form of shaming which enforces new morals, ethics, social and cultural values and norms.

While previous forms of public shaming have often taken governmental views and laws for the implementation of public shaming into account, as, for example, described in the context of crime, crime punishment and law enforcement (Braithwaite, 1989; Mayer, 2019), the new forms of online shame do not necessarily refer to a specific source of morality, ethics or law, but rather use new creations of moral, ethical and lawful perspectives which are enforced by the online community itself. Often, forms of online shaming tackle specific members of groups, for example, women, or individuals with specific sexual orientation, nationality, culture or social background. Skoric et al. (2010) highlight that there are different forms of online shaming in terms of the ways in which the recording and sharing of the perceived violation of the social norm or standard through digital devices and technology takes place.

Online shaming has probably become popular because it allows anonymity and provides a split identification in the sense that there seems to be a dissociation of real and online identities (Morio & Buchholz, 2009, p. 298). Norlock (2017) emphasises that online shaming addresses primarily the "imaginal relationships" people entertain when they engage in social media or activity in cyberspace. Online activities usually result in more relationships than one previously had, entailing new and more responsibilities, and a relational behaviour allows for ethical assessment. The anonymity of the real identity supports the ease of the shaming, as does the fact that often the shaming and naming stays unpunished owing to the lack of law enforcement in the online reality (Norlock, 2017).

Laidlaw (2017) highlights that particularly the right of privacy is under attack in online shaming which can be found, according to the author, in vigilantism, bullying, bigotry and gossiping. Online shaming is clearly linked to a decrease in privacy and dignity on one hand, but it can also be viewed as a tool to enforce rules of civility in online communities (Solove, 2007b).

In the current chapter, the authors focus particularly on online shaming which reduces the dignity of human beings (online and offline) by highlighting, presenting and/or judging specific behaviour. According to de Vries (2015), several websites exist contemporarily which are dedicated to shaming individuals and groups for different kinds of behaviour online. These websites usually tackle topics such as racism, cruelty against animals, sexism, inappropriate behaviour or homophobia. Other websites further use privately taken pictures or videos and upload them on specific Facebook groups, for instance, thereby shaming the person photographed or video-recorded (e.g. women eating on public transport, individuals being secretly filmed while having sex or committing self-injuring behaviours). However, at the time of writing, the authors note that some of these websites have been closed down—which shows that the Internet is not only a place where there is a lack of law enforcement, but that it is also a space where law enforcement takes place.

In the following sections, the authors discuss three often occurring online-shaming strategies: "slut-shaming", shaming in the context of eating (including eating disorders) and self-injuring behaviour. These are very common areas in which shame interlinked with disgracing individuals.

3.1 Slut-Shaming

Slut-shaming is a recently coined term for what is currently considered one of the fastest growing forms of cyberbullying (Hill & Kearl, 2011). Turnbull (n.d., p. 4) provides the following definition:

> 'Slut-shaming' is when the term slut (and numerous synonyms) is used in a derogatory way that is meant to shame women and police their sexuality.

According to Sweeney (2019), slut-shaming refers to:

> deliberate efforts to discredit people by associating them with sexual deviancy, especially sexual immodesty and promiscuity. Victims of slut shaming, who are disproportionately girls and women, may attain a poor reputation, experience social isolation and a loss of social status, as well as feel negative, painful emotions such as embarrassment, humiliation, regret, and sadness.

Slut-shaming usually manifests itself by posting explicit photos or videos or sending text messages on social media or websites, often in conjunction with inappropriate, embarrassing, insulting or sexualised comments about the body of the person concerned. These photos and videos are usually taken without the knowledge of the target person and without the consent of the photographed or filmed person to display it publicly online. Further,

> Slut-shaming is telling a girl to be ashamed of her body. It's supporting the idea that men are superior to women. [reemhassan277, 2020]

However, it can also involve photos or video recordings which, for example, were taken during a consensual sexual encounter in the course of a relationship without the knowledge of the person concerned and then also posted on the Internet without that person's consent. "Sexting" can also lead to slut-shaming if, for example, sexually explicit or naked photos which were shared in the course of a relationship are then shared online by one of the (former) partners.

Here, however, the fact that different sexual scripts apply to men and women plays a decisive role (Garcia, Reiber, Massey & Merriwether, 2012; Kågesten et al., 2016; Vanderheiden, 2020), which finds expression in specific culturally dependent gender role assignments. The concept of sexual scripts describes the idea of an individual culture-specific gender-related spectrum of behaviour, combined with corresponding role specifications and schemes for gender role behaviour in the sexual sphere. Sexual scripts also include ideas about gender identity, sexual orientation with regard to sexual behaviour and the manifestation of sexual activities. Simon and Gagnon (1986, 1999, p. 29) emphasise the great importance of cultural contexts and imprints in regard to sexuality and sexual behaviour:

> Scripts are a metaphor for conceptualizing the production of behaviour within social life. Most of social life most of the time must operate under the guidance of an operating syntax, much as language is a precondition for speech. For behaviour to occur, something resembling scripting must occur on three distinct levels: cultural scenarios, interpersonal scripts, and intra-psychic scripts. (Simon & Gagnon, 1999, p. 29)

Garcia et al. (2012, p. 164) point out not only that social roles and sexual scripts have a decisive influence on how adolescents in a certain socio-cultural context move, but also that media play a decisive role in this context (Garcia et al., 2012, p. 167). Perryman and Pohto (2018) were also able to demonstrate these differences in their studies in the USA. These authors showed that more women than men experienced different types and methods of slut-shaming and that the women who were called "sluts" were more likely to describe a sexual double standard, i.e. that women were harshly condemned for their sexual activities, while men were praised for the same behaviour (Perryman & Pohto, 2018, p. 2). Almazan and Bain (2015) could also prove in studies in the US college context that slut-shaming is strongly influenced by factors such as class affiliation, culture, media, gender, feminism, ethnicity, religion and sexuality. These sexual double standards apply to ratings of real friends and acquaintances, as demonstrated in a recent study (Marks, Young & Zaikman, 2019). The participants ($n = 4455$) rated a single, randomly assigned friend or acquaintance whose sexual history was known to them, with women being rated more negatively if the number of sexual partners increased, while men were not rated correspondingly negatively.

There are no valid statistics on the extent of slut-shaming and on gender shares in terms of perpetration available to date. But Armstrong, Hamilton, Armstrong and Seeley (2014) were able to demonstrate in their research that women also participate in slut-shaming. These authors see women's participation in slut-shaming as an internalised form of oppression, because women here apply disadvantageous sexual double standards set by men. Women with high social status obviously used slut-shaming in the college context to assert their class advantage, while women with low status expressed class contempt towards women with supposedly more exclusive status. At the same time, their high status allowed them to engage in more extensive sexual experimentation because their definitions dominated the dominant social scenes and secured them certain sexual privileges. In contrast, women with supposedly low status risk public shame when they try to enter this dominant social world (Armstrong et al., 2014).

This can also be observed as a phenomenon in other cultural contexts. For example, Willem, Araüna and Tortajada (2018) describe the double standard of *choni* and *pija* for Spain. Here two concepts of femininity are constructed and put in competition with each other: The supposedly tasteless and sexualised *choni*, which is meant to symbolise the female incarnation of the failed underclass in Spain, is contrasted with the stylish *pija*, which is attributed with high moral standards. Online contexts are crucial for the manifestation and transmission of these constructs.

In certain contexts, slut-shaming can lead to slut-shaming being used as an instrument of power against women or men who oppose or are accused of opposing common gender scripts or the political mainstream (Ayyub, 2019; Kaczynski, 2019; Pascoe, 2019). At the same time, however, social media, websites and blogs increasingly offer opportunities to organise or experience solidarity in cases of slut-shaming, for instance, in a public sphere with "slut walks" (Carr, 2019) or to open up educational spaces (Hill & Kearl, 2011; Sills et al., 2016). Slut walks are demonstrations that speak out against so-called victim blaming. They protest against the fact that victims of sexual violence are made partly responsible for the assaults because of the way they are dressed. Slut walks in particular have developed into a global phenomenon and are an expression of female awareness of life, usually with a feminist orientation. They were originally created in Toronto in 2003 in response to a statement made by police officer Michael Sanguinetti during a lecture on everyday security:

> Women should avoid dressing like sluts so as not to become victims. (Volkery, 2011)

This statement spread rapidly through the social media and some women called for a demonstration, which they called a "slut walk". Their aim was to make it clear that the victims are not to blame for sexual assault.

However, shame can also be a resource in digital contexts, because a

> very important aspect of shame is of course also that it protects intimacy, the innermost core of the soul, protects integrity. The feeling of shame also makes sure that we don't venture too far out, which is more important today than ever, because especially young people are seduced to expose themselves and are then often confronted with disastrous consequences, so the feeling of shame is an aid to protect one's own integrity and not to exclude others in such situations. (Köhler, 2017)[1]

In other words, in the context of slut-shaming, shame becomes a resource when it protects the individual from more behaviour which could be detrimental to them, when the feelings help the individual to reflect upon their own behaviour as well as on the behaviour of others and the standards, values and norms of self within the

[1]Translated from German by Elisabeth Vanderheiden.

embedding socio-cultural context. Shaming can also be seen as a resourceful act when members of a group which is shamed—such as women—become active and respond, for instance, with slut walks or when the shaming leads to new, open and transparent discourses (verbally, non-verbally or in action). If these discourses can lead to new institutional changes, such as educational courses, trainings, workshops, awareness days or weeks, or new curricula formation, the experienced shame has led to participation, activities, new group formations and the placement of the individual standing in terms of values, needs and norms. It then becomes a resource on individual, organisational, societal and maybe even global levels.

3.2 Glorifying Eating Disorders, Body Image and Shame

Eating disorders are among the most common chronic diseases experienced by adolescents, which now increasingly affect more children, adolescents and younger adults (Jugendschutz.net, 2019). Studies estimate that about 16 million people worldwide were affected by eating disorders in 2017, i.e. a 0.2% share of the global population, of whom 0.13% are males and 0.29% females (Ritchie & Roser, 2018). The most affected countries are Australia (0.94%), Italy (0.63%), Spain (0.73%) and Austria (0.68%), followed by the USA, Canada and other Western European countries, Scandinavian countries, Argentina, Chile, Japan and South Korea (between 0.4 and 0.5%). Figure 18.1 presents on overview of eating disorders.

The trend of eating disorders is rising, with around one fifth of 11–17-year-olds in Germany showing signs of an eating disorder (Bundesministerium für Familie, Senioren, Frauen und Jugend, 2011, p. 6). The consequences are dramatic, as eating disorders have the highest mortality rate among psychiatric illnesses (Ritchie & Roser, 2018). Figure 18.2 provides an overview of death rates based on eating disorders.

With anorexia nervosa and bulimia, the most serious eating disorders, those affected deliberately starve themselves to be underweight or suffer from bulimia. They emulate a pathological ideal of slimness, for which they also take radical, life-threatening measures. In 2017, for example, 50 people died in Japan as a result of eating disorders, 42 in the USA and 40 in China (Ritchie & Roser, 2018).

In Germany, 15% of anorexic people die from the consequences of their eating disorder (Bundesministerium für Familie, Senioren, Frauen und Jugend, 2011, p. 6). Nasser, Katzman and Gordon (2001) and Nasser (2006) point out that eating disorders are no longer limited to Western cultures, but have rather taken on a global dimension. This can be attributed to the influence of the media, the market economy and urbanisation. Particularly in connection with veiling—a new form of body regulation that reacts to the forces of cultural change—Nasser and di Nicola (2001) also recognise a search for self-definition in relation to the needs of others or, in a broader sense, similarities to the culturally determined phenomena of self-mutilation.

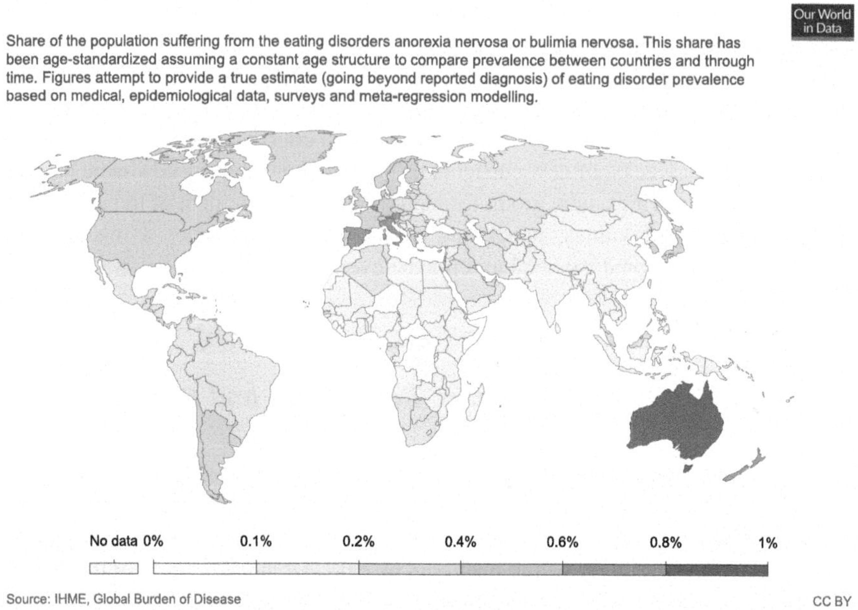

Fig. 18.1 Share of population with an eating disorder, 2017

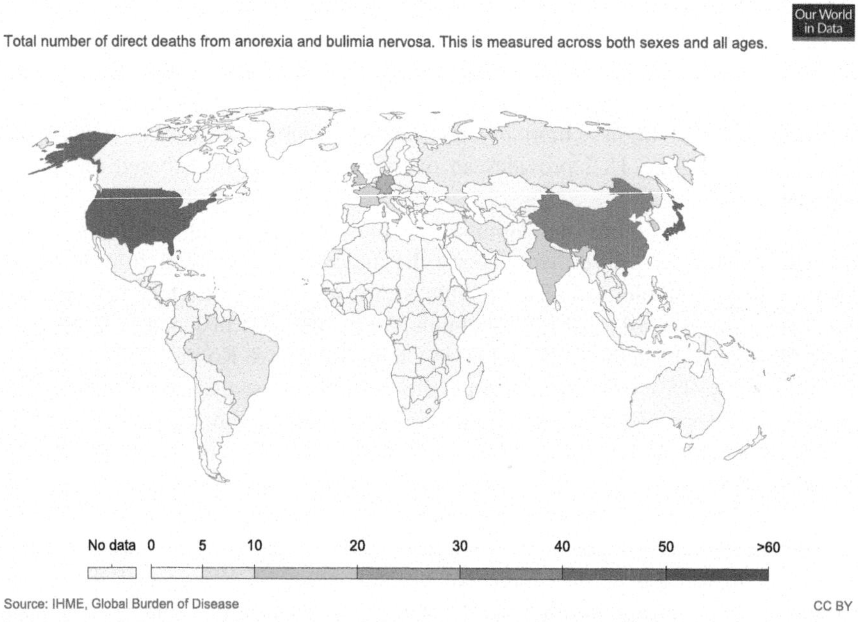

Fig. 18.2 Death from eating disorders, 2017, across both sexes and all ages

Gordon (2001) believes that eating disorders are on the rise in regions of the world outside Western Europe and the USA. Until the 1960s, only Japan reported eating disorders outside the US and Western Europe (Gordon, 2001, p. 9). Since the 1990s, increases have been reported from Hong Kong, Mainland China and South Korea, with Singapore and India added to these (Gordon, 2001, pp. 10–11). The number of studies has also been increasing since the late 1990s, in African and South and Central American countries. Gordon (2001) suspects there are various commonalities here, for instance, that these countries are highly developed economies (such as Hong Kong and Singapore) or that they are experiencing rapid market changes with social upheavals and their associated effects on gender relations, especially on the position of women. Gordon (2001) also discerns a strong link between a global consumer culture and the cultivation of a certain body ideal. In the discussion of eating disorders, he recognises the influence of changing patterns of food consumption and production, as well as new eating fashions, which may be in stark contrast to traditional eating habits (Gordon, 2001, p. 12).

Social media platforms such as Facebook, YouTube, Instagram, Snapchat and TikTok play a decisive role in the spread of eating disorders by giving them a new global and virtual dimension. On websites and in forums, anorexia and bulimia are deliberately glorified or else played down and presented as a desirable lifestyle. These eating disorders are often accompanied by shame and social anxiety, as Grabhorn, Stenner, Kaufhold, Overbeck and Stangier (2005) were able to prove in a study of 104 patients. Patients with anorexia and bulimia nervosa achieved significantly higher global shame values than patients with anxiety disorders and depression in this study. In contrast to anorexia patients, bulimic patients also achieved higher values in the area of social performance anxiety compared to the two anxiety disorder groups, and they also differed significantly from anxiety disorders in the area of interaction anxiety. These results led the authors to conclude that not only shame but also social anxiety is an important influencing factor, especially in bulimia nervosa. With regard to social anxiety, Grabhorn et al. (2005) suggest that it could possibly be the result of a shift of shame to the body. This could be relevant in the context of digital viewing contexts. Other authors such as Sipos, Bohus and Schweiger (2011) assume that shame manifests itself differently depending on the stage of the disease, but it can be assumed that patients with eating disorders usually perceive pronounced body-related shame. In their opinion, body-related shame is caused by experiences of offending peer groups, or family members, or it has cultural influences. This shame is further intensified by eating fits and weight gain. Vomiting, fasting and social avoidance can be shame strategies of those affected in order to weaken the effect of shame.

Teenagers who do not conform to an overly slim body image, or want to emulate it, are shamed accordingly. The eating disorders themselves are not perceived as diseases, but are declared as lifestyle, vilified and trivialised: the affected ones call themselves pro-Ana (= anorexia nervosa, anorexia) and pro-Mia (= bulimia nervosa, eat-break addiction).

Current studies show an obvious connection between social media use and eating disorders. For example, Sidani, Shensa, Hoffman, Hanmer and Primack (2016) have shown that frequent logging on to social media sites during the week or following different social feeds for hours during the day is associated with a greater risk of young adults developing eating and body image concerns. Tiggemann and Slater (2013) also demonstrated a significant link between Facebook use and the internalisation of a thin body ideal, body control and the pursuit of slimness in a study of over 1000 girls aged between 13 and 15 years.

Fardouly, Diedrichs, Vartanian and Halliwell (2015) emphasise the very direct connection between Facebook use and increased body dissatisfaction with one's own appearance and the immediate emergence of a corresponding negative mood or a positive relationship. Facebook usage and concerns about body image, such as increased comparisons of appearance in general, the frequency of comparisons with close friends and distant peers and so-called upward comparisons (judging one's own appearance as worse) with distant peers and celebrities are closely related (Fardouly & Vartanian, 2015) (see also Chap. 11 in this book).

This is not limited to Facebook. For example, in a Twitter study by Cavazos-Rehg et al. (2019), tweets with eating disorder references or body image-related keywords ($n = 3000$) showed that 2584 of peers were not aware of the fact that had similar experiences. Of the 3000 tweets related to an eating disorder, 65% said that they were concerned with body shape, 13% reported problems related to eating and calorie intake and 4% said that body weight was important to them.

Particular dangers arise from platforms such as TikTok, which appeal in particular to young people aged 13 and over who are essentially challenge-orientated. TikTok is a social media offering from China that is particularly popular with children and younger teenagers because of its playback music videos that users can easily create and upload themselves. Another special feature is the so-called challenges or compilations. TikTok users face these challenges in their videos. In the "Waist Challenge", for example, girls uploaded videos in which they presented their buttocks and the narrowest possible waist. The hashtag #waistchallenge alone was called 67 million times in 2019. This is an extremely significant range, as 35% of all TikTok users participate in challenges, and 16% of all TikTok videos are created in response to challenges. The app is extremely successful, with 800 million monthly users to 1.5 billion users (Mediakix, 2019) depending on the source; TiKTok has its largest European markets—in Germany, France, the UK, Spain and Italy—with around 17 million monthly users worldwide, who spend an average of 39 min using the app.

By comparison, Facebook advertised in 2016 that its users spend 50 min on Instagram, Messenger and Facebook together (Handelsblatt, 2019). It must be kept in mind that this target group is extremely vulnerable. In France, for example, 40% of all 11–14-year-olds use TikTok accounts, while in Germany over four million young people are registered (Fuest, 2019). The largest user group of TikTok is based in India with about 120 million users. In India, in April 2019, TikTok was banned by the highest Indian court on suspicion of encouraging paedophilia and prostitution. However, the ban was lifted shortly afterwards. Easy access to these sites is also a problem, as shown by a 25-country survey by EU Kids Online (Livingstone,

Cagiltay & Ólafsson, 2015), which found that 10% of children between the ages of 9 and 16 had viewed pro-eating disorder sites online.

Interestingly enough, the online initiatives for the dissemination of such social media accounts originate from adolescents (especially girls and young women) who have fallen ill themselves, but who do not show any interest in a cure or therapy. They use these sites to post photos of their weight loss progress, to ask others to join the pro-Ana or pro-Mia movement or to distribute "Letters From Ana" (e.g. Detroit Metro Times, 2019) or from "Mia" ("Letter From Mia", 2019). Personal self-shaming and shaming of others plays a central role, as the following quotations show:

> God, you are such a fat cow!!!! . . .if you eat, all the control will be broken . . . do you WANT that?? To revert back to the fat COW you once were?? I force you to stare at magazine models. Those perfect-skinned, white-teethed, waifish models of perfection staring out at you from those glossy pages. I make you realize that you could never be them. You will always be fat and never will you be as beautiful as they are. When you look in the mirror, I will distort the image. I will show you obesity and hideousness. I will show you a sumo wrestler where in reality there is a starving child. But you must not know this, because if you knew the truth, you might start to eat again and our relationship would come crashing down. (Detroit Metro Times, 2019)

or

> Only you will know when I'm around. You will know when you eat something, you will know when you see that chocolate cake on the counter, because I will in the back of your mind telling you things. Sometimes I will tell you not to eat it, and you will listen. Other times, you will disobey me and devour the entire cake. Then I will really make you feel guilty. You should have followed my orders! Now go and throw that cake up you FAT COW! How could you do that to yourself? You will take my comments to heart, and go into the bathroom, turn on the faucet, and force yourself to vomit. You will spend hours vomiting at times. Your face will be red, snot will pour, your eyes will be bloodshot, you jaw will hurt of swollen glands...serves you right! If you want to be my friend and get the full effect of what I can give you, you must follow my orders. You will soon learn that I am in control. Even when you don't do as I say, you can still hear me, screaming at you, telling you to work harder, telling you to take diet pills, telling you how fat you are, telling you what those people across the room are really whispering about. ("Letter from Mia", 2019)

Characteristic of these websites is that they propagate extreme underweight and glorify eating disorders as a lifestyle; anyone who does not follow the appropriate "ideal" and standards is a failure, a "fat cow". Especially for children and adolescents who are not yet consolidated in their personality and body image, pro-Ana and pro-Mia websites can have a particularly strong and dangerous influence because, for example, it prevents them from developing a positive and healthy relationship with their body or makes them experience normal food intake as punishable. The fact that the debate about one's own appearance and the attainment of the ideal of beauty takes place in the quasi-public space of the Internet aggravates the general conditions. Food intake and the slightest weight gain can lead to public loss of face and possible embarrassment and shame.

Shaming the body consequently leads to poor health-related decisions which are based on massively impaired understandings of what is a healthy, desirable appearance, as confirmed by two recent studies by Lamont (2019). This leads to serious and lasting changes in body image, which according to Williams and Currie (2000) refers to the physical characteristics of an individual and the perception of these characteristics in comparison to those of the person's environment. Attitudes and representations of physical characteristics often influence the body image of adolescents, which is of central importance for their still developing self-concept and is likely to significantly influence adaptation (Williams & Currie, 2000). Borzekowski and Bayer (2005) point out that the body image must be regarded as a multidimensional construct that is influenced by biological, psychological and social factors. This is supported by Manzoor and Shahed (2015), who stress that body images can form perceptual attitudes in individuals, often influenced by historical, civilisational, social, individual and genetic factors in a population. Continued and internalised embarrassment and negative manifestations of one's body image and internalised body shame can therefore have serious physical and psychological consequences (see Chap. 11 in this book).

4 Counterstrategies to Transform Shame in the 4IR Context

Based on the above discussions, the authors have shown that shame—as an age-old phenomenon—has made its way into the virtual and digitalised world. Shame in the virtual world differs in forms and effect from face-to-face interactions by being expanded in terms of extreme body shaming, access to a huge number of social groups and global imagined relationships as well as split online and offline identities. Thereby, boundaries have shifted, and it appears that counterstrategies to deal with online shame and transformation are needed. These strategies need to be developed individually, but can take social, organisational and global aspects into account. Before focusing on the different levels of online shaming counteraction, it needs to be highlighted that the first step is to create awareness in children and adolescents and also in adults about new trends of shaming and naming online. This awareness needs to include the knowledge that online shaming is a global phenomenon with culture-specific nuances. It is constantly changing and poses a serious threat to mental, physical, socio-cultural and spiritual well-being.

On an **individual level**, individuals need to become aware, conscious and mindful of the influence of the virtual world on their life and well-being. Interdependences and overlaps of virtual and natural realities need to be understood, and the influence the virtual world has on the natural world needs to be consciously defined and vice versa. Further, individuals should become conscious of their real and their imaginal virtual relationships and of the ways in which individuals communicate with each other. Additionally, every individual should remember that the extent of public online shaming cannot be controlled (see also Norlock, 2017) by the person who shames, nor by the shamed one. The shame experienced by the shamed can only be transformed within the self. This seems to be a challenge particularly in online shaming situations, since the individual who is shamed online often sits in a remote (online) space which does not necessarily provide access to trustful offline and non-virtual relationships which might be used as a resource to overcome online shaming. The person experiencing this felt loneliness through online shaming needs specific individual skills and tools, as well as attitudes of mindfulness, consciousness and transformational competencies to turn the pain, suffering and negative virtual experiences into personal growth and development in the offline space. The individual also needs to reassess identity, self-responsibility with regard to cyberspace communication and relationship-building in the online and offline worlds.

In this regard, online campaign platforms such as change.org, campact.de and https://avaaz.org are also becoming increasingly important as a digital resource in the transformation of shame (see Chap. 12 in this book) either as a starting point for preventive awareness campaigns or for presenting alternative voices and perspectives for victims of discrimination. These platforms also address stereotypes, cultural myths, clichés and prejudices that often correlate with experiences of shame on the part of those affected. Alternatively, such platforms can provide the basis for so-called obstructive campaigns, which are more likely to fight against various manifestations of different forms of discrimination (European Action Week Against Racism, 2019). There is still a lack of valid data in many cases which could demonstrate, especially in a global context, how successful and sustainable these campaigns really are, but it seems that active online participation also promotes offline participation in this context (Christensen, 2011). Initiating or participating in such campaigns can therefore be an important addition to the purely mental or emotional level and can also take into account the social system and action levels in the virtual and non-virtual worlds.

On a **social and cultural level**, different strategies can be used in the 4IR context. On one hand it appears that online shaming needs to be recognised as a new way of defining new social and cultural, as well as global boundaries, which are clearly obvious to regulate through law and ethical standards. Therefore, it might be important that individuals take the online experiences of shame into their face-to-face world to evaluate, reassess, transform and reduce the negative effects of the experiences. This process of working through the pain and suffering of the online shaming in the virtual world and placing it into new discourses in the natural socio-cultural surrounding might provide individuals with new worldviews and perspectives which derive from their natural environment and help them to anchor themselves in a more supporting and socially comforting context, reconnecting them with their natural reality.

With regard to the socio-cultural group membership, individuals can switch in and out of memberships of groups online and offline and seek new memberships which better suit their individual values, norms and ethics. The digitalised world provides individuals with a choice of various transcultural memberships which can become an advantage in terms of acceptance into specific socio-cultural groups online and offline, such as anti-discrimination or support groups. However, taking the easy way out of or into a socio-cultural group can also bring risks and insecurities. Particularly individuals with a weak sense of coherence, orientation, understanding and belonging might be caught up in group memberships which are not healthy for them. Online and offline support groups for these individuals might help them to cope with and overcome stress and strain online.

Further, counselling and therapeutic contexts will have to develop new ideas, concepts and practices regarding how to work with experiences of negative emotions which either are initiated through digital devices and mediated through technology or are anchored in the digital realm and in technologised communication and imaginal identities and relationships. Making use of digitalised tools, such as counselling apps, virtual reality chatbots and 24/7 connections to online coaching, counselling and therapists might also be a way to counteract the 24/7 online-shaming experiences. Social support can no longer be limited to the natural world alone, but needs to be taken into the virtual world—is that your intended meaning. This gap between the online experience and the offline counteraction support will in the future need to be closed in a way that victims of online shaming might gain quicker access to supporting systems in the online community and online shame transformation forums might be further developed to support individuals on all levels and with different socio-cultural backgrounds. Although supportive social groups and platforms online do exist, they might appear to have such a strong influence as that of the discriminating and shaming groups on the individual and on social cultural groups—which could also depend on the social background and culture of origin.

As the transformation of shameful experiences is usually anchored in a specific socio-cultural value set, the virtual world might hold, on **a global level**, new options and alternatives to deal with shame in a transformational and constructive way, as, for example, shown in the globally occurring slut walks. Slut walks can certainly be seen as a resource-orientated international and global counterstrategy to transform shame in this context and has meanwhile found global support and acceptance:

> SlutWalks are demonstrations against sexism, sexualised violence, rape myths and trivialisation. ... People protest for their right to self-determination regarding body, gender and sexual desire. (Humanistischer Pressedienst, 2011; translated by Vanderheiden)

The first slut walk in Toronto went viral very quickly, and others have emerged in 75 cities in the USA, Canada, Sweden and South Africa within a short time (Valenti, 2011). Slut walks are now also taking place in Brazil, Nicaragua and Honduras, Germany and Australia (Völkel, 2020). In this respect, they are a global form of expression, which allows for far-reaching experiences of transformation and self-efficacy on all levels.

Because the new virtual worlds provide access to various socio-cultural arenas, new cultural contexts and a variety of groups based on values differing from one's own socio-cultural background, the Internet provides the individual with new global perspectives. This global access might be a key to developing new perspectives, new concepts for dealing with personally experienced shame and new platforms to educate oneself and move towards new world views. However, in order to transform in this way by using access to new socio-cultural perspectives, the individual needs the ability to self-reflect at a deep level and at the same time to value openness, stimulation and active learning so as to be able to use new ways to transform oneself and grow in a world which is expanding to new heights of complexity.

5 Conclusion

It might be concluded that shame—in the context of the 4IR—shows itself to be risky, challenging, toxic and problematic rather than positive one per se. It might be assumed that responsibility lies with the individual, the socio-cultural group and the global community of online users and offline entities to create a new consciousness regarding the effect of online and offline communication in online and offline settings. Individuals need to take self-responsibility and action into account to counteract shame and public (online) shaming and to develop counterstrategies to act against it.

Figure 18.3 provides an overview of strategies to counteract and transform online shaming.

However, legal and censorial interventions can only be part of the answer, because ethical questions—and these are the issues at stake here—must indeed be controversially discussed in public political discourse. This includes questions about who a society grants the right to judge others morally, on the basis of which criteria and standards, and how a society wants to behave when individuals or groups take the right to publicly shame and punish other individuals or groups. Since the Internet knows virtually no national borders, a global dialogue is necessary for this purpose, which includes diverse cultural perspectives.

Finally, it is essential to explore the development of pedagogical and psychological concepts that transform and further develop knowledge about shame as a resource, which has developed in recent decades, especially in positive psychology 1.0 and 2.0 and indigenous psychology, in the context of the 4IR.

In the following section, suggestions are made concerning future theory development and practice and the issues that might need to be clarified in this context on individual, social-cultural and global levels.

6 Outlook Regarding Future Theory and Practice

With regard to future theory and practice of transforming shame, scientists need to take previous shame theories and public-shaming theories into account and validate whether these theoretical approaches are effective and valid for the relatively new phenomenon of online shaming. Further, research should assess how, on the individual level, shamed individuals deal internally and externally with the experience of shaming and being shamed in offline and online contexts and evaluate if there are differences and/or similarities in the experiences of shaming and being shamed in virtual and non-virtual contexts.

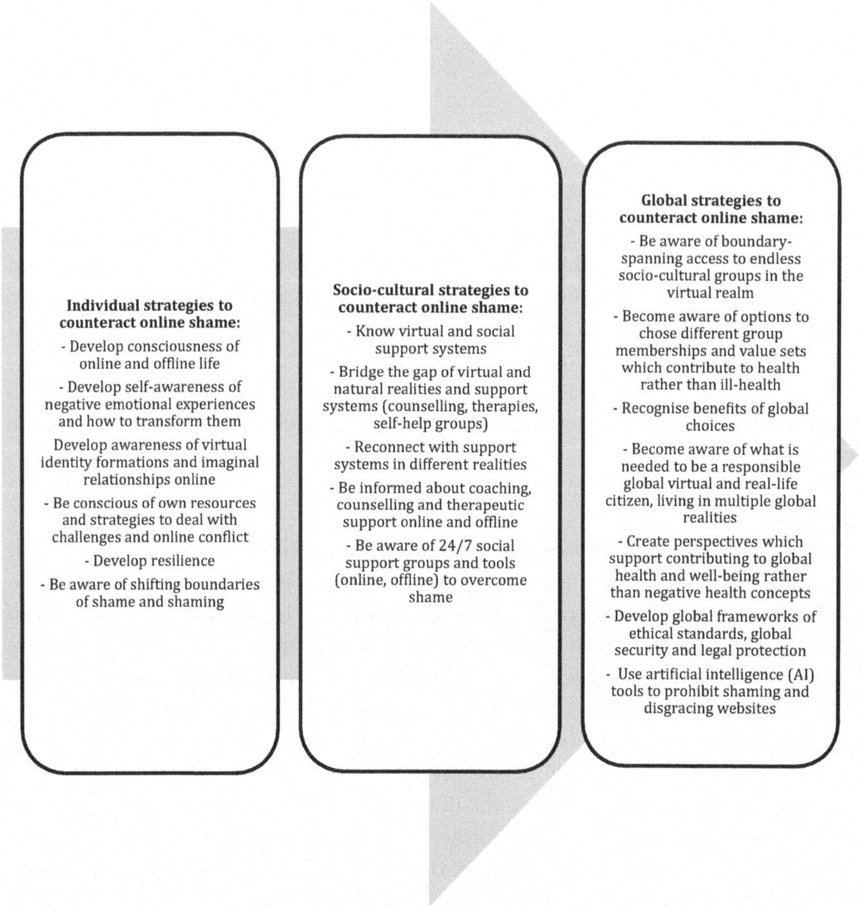

Fig. 18.3 Strategies to counteract and transform online shame (Mayer)

The ways in which the creation of identity and formation of imaginal relationships online and offline differ should be explored, as well as how previous theories on identity and relationship construction and shame in offline settings adhere to the new technologised and digitalised online contexts. On global levels, scientists should further explore how individuals from different cultural and social contexts transform the mainly negative experiences of online shaming, which resources they use and how resilient they are with regard to online shaming. Here, cross-cultural and transcultural studies are needed concerning strategies to counteract toxic online shame and to transform it on the different levels at which it presents.

There is another new and exciting need for research: if, for example, an app like TikTok spreads so rapidly in the most diverse cultural contexts as described above, what effects can be observed here regarding the understanding of shame or the development and handling of shame and embarrassment in the various cultural contexts? Additionally, scientists have to ask what effects online shaming has on gender roles, gender scripts and gender-related concepts of shame in various cultural contexts and on a global level. What does shame do to the actors in the online and offline field and in terms of new gender dynamics?

In practical terms, it is important to question—at individual, socio-cultural and globally level—if and how to implement juridical standards which might protect individuals from becoming perpetrators and victims of online shaming while promoting private and civil rights and human dignity online and offline. Or which legal frameworks would be useful, in particular to enable victims to seek redress, appropriate compensation or even the deletion of websites and/or identity constructs and imaginary relationships related to online shaming.

Irrespective of the legal question, it would be desirable to succeed in enforcing global ethical standards for social media, website providers and the like, which would prevent such online attempts of embarrassment and shame in advance. A large part of this could be reliably prevented automatically via an AI solution, while the majority of these attempts currently still have to be securely deleted by human employees.

References

Almazan, V., & Bain, S. (2015, May). College students' perceptions of slut-shaming discourse on campus. *Research in Higher Education Journal, 28*.

Armstrong, E., Hamilton, L., Armstrong, E., & Seeley, J. (2014). Good girls. *Social Psychology Quarterly, 77*(2), 100–122. https://doi.org/10.1177/0190272514521220.

Ayyub, R. (2019). *Slut-shaming women all around the world*. Retrieved February 10, 2021, from https://umdgenderandglobalization.wordpress.com/2018/08/20/slut-shaming-women-all-around-the-world/.

Bonavia, T., & Brox-Ponce, J. (2018). Shame in decision making under risk conditions: Understanding the effect of transparency. *PLoS One, 13*(2), E0191990. https://doi.org/10.1371/journal.pone.0191990

Borzekowski, D. L. G., & Bayer, A. M. (2005). Body image and media use among adolescents. *Adolescent Medicine Clinics, 16*, 89–313. https://doi.org/10.1016/j.adme-cli.2005.02.010.

Braithwaite, J. (1989). *Crime, shame and reintegration*. Cambridge: Cambridge University Press.

Briegleb, T. (2014). *Die diskrete Scham*. Frankfurt: Insel Verlag.

Bundesministerium für Familie, Senioren, Frauen und Jugend. (2011). *Gegen Verherrlichung von Ess- störungen im Internet. Ein Ratgeber für Eltern, Fachkräfte und Provider.* [online] Bmfsfj.de. Available at: https://www.bmfsfj.de/blob/93692/96f2606252083cf6c5017bd9673ae466/essstoerungen-ratgeber-pdf-data.pdf . Accessed 27 Dec 2019.

Carr, J. (2019). The SlutWalk movement: A study in transnational feminist activism. Retrieved December 30, 2019, from https://digitalcommons.uri.edu/jfs/vol4/iss4/3/?utm_source=digitalcommons.uri.edu%252Fjfs%252Fvol4%252Fiss4%252F3&utm_medium=PDF&utm_campaign=PDFCoverPages

Cavazos-Rehg, P., Krauss, M., Costello, S., Kaiser, N., Cahn, E., Fitzsimmons-Craft, E., et al. (2019). "I just want to be skinny.": A content analysis of tweets expressing eating disorder symptoms. *PLoS One*, *14*(1), e0207506. https://doi.org/10.1371/journal.pone.0207506

Christensen, H. (2011). Political activities on the Internet: Slacktivism or political participation by other means?. Retrieved February 21, 2020, from https://www.researchgate.net/publication/223956345_Political_activities_on_the_Internet_Slacktivism_or_political_participation_by_other_means

Detroit Metro Times. (2019). A letter from Ana. Retrieved December 28, 2019, from https://www.metrotimes.com/detroit/a-letter-from-ana/Content?oid=2174214

de Vries, A. (2015). The use of social media for shaming strangers: Young people's views. In *48th Hawaii international conference on system sciences*. Retrieved from https://doi.org/10.1109/HICSS.2015.24

Doi, T. (1973). *The anatomy of dependence*. Tokyo: Kodansha.

Eating Disorder Statistics United Kingdom. (2019). *Eating Disorder Statistics UK | Priory Group*. [online] Priorygroup.com. Available at: https://www.priorygroup.com/eating-disorders/eating-disorder-statistics. Accessed 27 Dec 2019.

European Action Week Against Racism. (2019). *Tips for online activism*. [online] European Action Week Against Racism 2019. Available at: http://weekagainstracism.eu/join-the-campaign/tips-for-online-activism/. Accessed 20 Feb. 2020.

Fardouly, J., Diedrichs, P., Vartanian, L., & Halliwell, E. (2015). Social comparisons on social media: The impact of Facebook on young women's body image concerns and mood. *Body Image, 13*, 38–45. https://doi.org/10.1016/j.bodyim.2014.12.002.

Fardouly, J., & Vartanian, L. (2015). Negative comparisons about one's appearance mediate the relationship between Facebook usage and body image concerns. *Body Image, 12*, 82–88. https://doi.org/10.1016/j.bodyim.2014.10.004.

Frevert, U. (2017). *Die Politik der Demütigung. Schauplätze von Macht und Ohnmacht*. Frankfurt/Main: S. Fischer.

Frevert, U. (2019). *Scham und Beschämung*. [online] https://www.history-of-emotions.mpg.de/de/texte/scham-und-beschaemung. Available at: https://www.history-of-emotions.mpg.de/de/texte/scham-und-beschaemung. Accessed 27 Dec 2019.

Frevert, U. (2020). The power of humiliation. Retrieved January 2, 2020, from https://www.mpg.de/11993269/W001_Viewpoint_010-015.pdf

Fuest, B. (2019). TikTok: Jetzt bekommen Eltern ein Problem - WELT. Retrieved December 28, 2019, from https://www.welt.de/wirtschaft/webwelt/article189584913/TikTok-Jetzt-bekommen-Eltern-ein-Problem.html

Garcia, J., Reiber, C., Massey, S., & Merriwether, A. (2012). Sexual hookup culture: A review. *Review of General Psychology, 16*(2), 161–176. https://doi.org/10.1037/a0027911.

Gilbert, P. (2019). Distinguishing shame, humiliation and guilt: An evolutionary functional analysis and compassion focused interventions. In C. Mayer & E. Vanderheiden (Eds.), *The bright side of shame. Transforming and growing through practical applications in cultural contexts* (pp. 413–431). Cham: Springer.

Gordon, R. (2001). Eating disorders East and West: A culture-bound syndrome unbound. In M. Nasser, M. Katzman, & R. Gordon (Eds.), *Eating disorders and cultures in transition* (pp. 1–24). New York: Taylor and Francis.

Grabhorn, R., Stenner, H., Kaufhold, J., Overbeck, G., & Stangier, U. (2005). Scham und soziale Angst bei Anorexia und Bulimia nervosa. *Zeitschrift Für Psychosomatische Medizin Und Psychotherapie, 51*(2), 179–193. https://doi.org/10.13109/zptm.2005.51.2.179

Gruenewald, T., Kemeny, M., Aziz, N., & Fahey, J. (2004). Acute threat to the social self: Shame, social self-esteem, and cortisol activity. *Psychosomatic Medicine, 66*(6), 915–924. https://doi.org/10.1097/01.psy.0000143639.61693.ef.

Handelsblatt. (2019). TikTok: Wie eine chinesische App deutsche Jugendliche und Werber begeistert. Retrieved December 28, 2019, from https://www.handelsblatt.com/unternehmen/it-medien/tiktok-wie-eine-chinesische-app-deutsche-jugendliche-und-werber-begeistert/24035480.html?ticket=ST-37430261-jOoeEQU4IjfD20Av2ngs-ap6

Hill, C., & Kearl, H. (2011). *Crossing the line. Sexual harassment at school*. Washington, DC: AAUW.

Huffman, E. (2016). *Online shaming's impact on social media participation call-out culture: How online shaming affects social media participation in young adults.* (MA). Faculty in Communication and Leadership Studies School of Professional Studies Gonzaga University.

Humanistischer Pressedienst. (2011). *"SlutWalk - Was soll das Ganze?"*. [online] Hpd.de. Available at: https://hpd.de/node/11829. Accessed 20 Feb 2020.

Jaffe, K., Florez, A., Gomes, C. M., Rodriguez, D., & Achury, C. (2014). On the biological and cultural evolution of shame: Using internet search tools to weight values in many cultures. *arXiv* preprint arXiv:1401.1100.

Jugendschutz.net. (2019). *Wer ist Ana? • Veränderungen im Essverhalten • ständige Gewichtskontrolle • Ausreden, um nicht zu essen oder das gemeinsame Essen zu verpassen Verherrlichung von Essstörungen im Internet.* [online] Jugendschutz.net. Available at: http://www.jugendschutz.net/fileadmin/download/pdf/Faltblatt_Pro-Ana.pdf. Accessed 27 Dec 2019.

Kaczynski, A. (2019). A GOP congressman once lamented not being able to call women 'sluts' anymore. Retrieved December 30, 2019, from https://www.cnn.com/2018/07/18/politics/kfile-jason-lewis/index.html

Kågesten, A., Gibbs, S., Blum, R., Moreau, C., Chandra-Mouli, V., Herbert, A., et al. (2016). Understanding factors that shape gender attitudes in early adolescence globally: A mixed-methods systematic review. *PLoS One, 11*(6), e0157805. https://doi.org/10.1371/journal.pone.0157805.

Kalra, G., & Bhugra, D. (2013). Sexual violence against women: Understanding cross-cultural intersections. *Indian Journal of Psychiatry, 55*(3), 244. https://doi.org/10.4103/0019-5545.117139.

Klonick, K. (2016). Re-shaming the debate: Social norms, shame, and regulation in an internet age. Shame, and regulation in an internet age. *Maryland Law Review, 75.4*, 1029–1065.

Köhler, A. (2017). Die Rolle der Scham - Vom Pranger auf dem Marktplatz zu dem im Netz. Retrieved December 31, 2019, from https://www.deutschlandfunk.de/die-rolle-der-scham-vom-pranger-auf-dem-marktplatz-zu-dem.1148.de.html?dram:article_id=406077

Laidlaw, E. (2017). Online shaming and the right to privacy. *Laws, 6*(1), 3. https://doi.org/10.3390/laws6010003.

Lamont, J. (2019). Effects of body shame on poor health decisions: The mediating role of body responsiveness. *Current Psychology*. https://doi.org/10.1007/s12144-019-00528-y.

Letter from Mia. (2019). Retrieved December 28, 2019, from https://yourfriendana.weebly.com/letter-from-mia.html

Livingstone, S., Cagiltay, K., & Ólafsson, K. (2015). EU Kids Online II Dataset: A cross-national study of children's use of the Internet and its associated opportunities and risks. *British Journal of Educational Technology, 46*(5), 988–992. https://doi.org/10.1111/bjet.12317.

Manzoor, H., & Shahed, S. (2015). Gender differences in young adults' body image and self-esteem. *Pakistan Journal of Women's Studies, 22*, 107–117.

Marks, M., Young, T., & Zaikman, Y. (2019). The sexual double standard in the real world. *Social Psychology, 50*(2), 67–79. https://doi.org/10.1027/1864-9335/a000362.

Mayer, C.-H. (2019). Crime and shame: Reflections and culture-specific insights. In: C. -H. Mayer & E. Vanderheiden (Eds.), *The bright side of shame. Transforming and growing through practical applications in cultural contexts* (pp. 117–130). Cham: Springer.

Mayer, C., & Vanderheiden, E. (2019). *The bright side of shame. Transforming and growing through practical applications in cultural contexts*. Cham: Springer.

Mediakix. (2019). 13 TikTok stats for marketers: TikTok demographics, statistics, & key data. Retrieved December 31, 2019, from https://mediakix.com/blog/top-tik-tok-statistics-demographics/

Morio, H., & Buchholz, C. (2009). How anonymous are you online? Examining onlie social behaviours from a cross-cultural perspective. *AI and Society, 23*(2), 297–307.

Nasser, M. (2006). Eating disorders across cultures. *Psychiatry, 5*(11), 392–395. https://doi.org/10.1053/j.mppsy.2006.08.008.

Nasser, M., & di Nicola, V. (2001). Changing bodies, changing cultures: An intercultural dialogue on the body as the final frontier. In M. Nasser, M. Katzman, & R. Gordon (Eds.), *Eating disorders and cultures in transition* (pp. 171–194). New York: Taylor and Francis.
Nasser, M., Katzman, M., & Gordon, R. (2001). *Eating disorders and cultures in transition.* New York: Taylor & Francis.
Norlock, K .J. (2017). Online shaming. Pre-publication draft of accepted copy, Social Philosophy Today. https://philpapers.org/archive/NOROS.pdf
Packiarajah, T. S. (n.d.). Online shaming. Exploring factors behind online shaming perpetration as well as its prevalence in adults. Tilburg University. http://arno.uvt.nl/show.cgi?fid=143336
Pascoe, A. (2019). Senator Sarah Hanson-Young on sexism and slut shaming. Retrieved December 30, 2019, from https://www.marieclaire.com.au/sarah-hanson-young-on-sexism-in-politics
Perryman, M., & Pohto, P. (2018). Slut shaming perceptions and experiences among college students. In *Arts, humanities, social sciences & education. 2018 Hawaii University International Conferences.*
reemhassan277. (2020). Slut-shaming is global. Retrieved February 22, 2020, from https://reemhassa.wordpress.com
Ritchie, H., & Roser, M. (2018). *Mental health.* [online] Our world in data. Available at: https://ourworldindata.org/mental-health. Accessed 27 Dec 2019.
Röttger-Rössler, B. (2020). Die kulturellen Facetten der Scham. In: H. Kappelhoff, J. Bakels, H. Lehmann, & C. Schmitt (Eds.), *Emotionen. Ein interdisziplinäres Handbuch* [online] (pp. 230–235). Berlin: J. B. Metzler. Springer. Available at: https://doi.org/10.1007/978-3-476-05353-4. Accessed 20 Feb 2020.
Scobel, G. (2017). Scham und Schuld. Retrieved October 4, 2019, from https://www.3sat.de/wissen/scobel/scham-und-schuld-100.html
Sidani, J., Shensa, A., Hoffman, B., Hanmer, J., & Primack, B. (2016). The Association between social media use and eating concerns among US young adults. *Journal of the Academy of Nutrition and Dietetics, 116*(9), 1465–1472. https://doi.org/10.1016/j.jand.2016.03.021.
Sills, S., Pickens, C., Beach, K., Jones, L., Calder-Dawe, O., Benton-Greig, P., et al. (2016). Rape culture and social media: Young critics and a feminist counterpublic. *Feminist Media Studies, 16*(6), 935–951. https://doi.org/10.1080/14680777.2015.1137962.
Simon, W., & Gagnon, J. H. (1986). Sexual scripts: Permanence and change. *Archives of Sexual Behavior, 15*, 97–120.
Simon, W., & Gagnon, J. H. (1999). Sexual scripts. In: R. Parker & P. Aggleton (Eds.), *Culture, society and sexuality: A reader* (pp. 29–38). London: University College London Press.
Sipos, V., Bohus, M., & Schweiger, U. (2011). Dialektisch-behaviorale Therapie für Essstörungen (DBT-E). *Ppmp - Psychotherapie · Psychosomatik · Medizinische Psychologie, 61*(02), 87–91. https://doi.org/10.1055/s-0030-1265972.
Skoric, M. M., Chua, J. P. E., Liew, M. A., Wong, K. H., & Yeo, P. J. (2010). Online shaming in the Asian context: Community empowerment or civic vigilantism? *Surveillance & Society, 8*(2), 181–199.
Solove, D. (2007a). *The future of reputation: Gossip, rumor, and privacy on the Internet.* New Haven, CT: Yale University Press.
Solove, D. J. (2007b). 'I've got nothing to hide' and other misunderstandings of privacy. *San Diego Law Review, 44*(2007), 745–772.
Spiegel Online. (2017). *Zeitgeist: Und raus bist du - Der Spiegel 39/2017.* [online] Spiegel.de. Available at: https://www.spiegel.de/spiegel/print/d-153305008.html. Accessed 27 Dec 2019.
Sweeney, B. (2019). The SAGE encyclopedia of psychology and gender. Retrieved December 30, 2019, from https://doi.org/10.4135/9781483384269.n530
Tangney, J. P., Miller, R. S., Flicker, L., & Barrow, D. H. (1996). Are shame, guilt, and embarrassment distinct emotions? *Journal of Personality and Social Psychology, 70*, 1256–1269.
Teyber, E., & Teyber, H. F. (2017). *Interpersonal process in therapy: Integrative model.* Boston: Cengage Learning.

Tiggemann, M., & Slater, A. (2013). NetGirls: The Internet, Facebook, and body image concern in adolescent girls. *International Journal of Eating Disorders, 46*(6), 630–633. https://doi.org/10.1002/eat.22141.

Turnbull, C. (n.d.). *The power of 'slut': The construction of 'slut' and 'slut-shaming' in contemporary youth culture* (MA). Brock University St. Catharines, Ontario.

Valenti, J. (2011). *Washington Post.* [online] Slut walks and the future of feminism. Available at: https://www.washingtonpost.com/opinions/slutwalks-and-the-future-of-feminism/2011/06/01/AGjB9LIH_story.html. Accessed 20 Feb 2020.

Vallverdú, J. (2014). *Artificial shame models for machines? Psychology of shame: New research.* New York: Nova.

Vanderheiden, E. (2019). "Nothing I accept about myself can be used against me to diminish me"—Transforming shame through mindfulness. In C. Mayer & E. Vanderheiden (Eds.), *The bright side of shame. Transforming and growing through practical applications in cultural contexts.* Cham: Springer.

Vanderheiden, E. (2020). "I have a friend with benefits, whom off and on I see." - Friends with benefits relationships. In C. Mayer & E. Vanderheiden (Eds.), *International handbook of love.* Cham: Springer.

Vanderheiden, E., & Mayer, C.-H. (2017). *The value of shame—Exploring a health resource in cultural contexts.* Cham: Springer.

Völkel, J. (2020). [online] Hinterland-magazin.de. Available at: http://www.hinterland-magazin.de/wp-content/uploads/2016/12/hinterland-magazin-18-78-nein-heisst-nein-pdf.pdf. Accessed 20 Feb 2020.

Volkery, C. (2011). *Frauenprotest: Schlampen an die Front.* [online] Spiegel.de. Available at: https://www.spiegel.de/panorama/gesellschaft/frauenprotest-schlampen-an-die-front-a-767985.html. Accessed 20 Feb 2020.

Willem, C., Araüna, N., & Tortajada, I. (2018). Chonis and pijas: Slut-shaming and double standards in online performances among Spanish teens. *Sexualities, 22*(4), 532–548. https://doi.org/10.1177/1363460717748620.

Williams, J. M., & Currie, C. (2000). Self-esteem and physical development in early adolescence: Pubertal timing and body image. *The Journal of Early Adolescence, 20*, 129–149. https://doi.org/10.1177/0272431600020002002.

Wong, P. T. P. (2019). Foreword: From shame to wholeness: An existential positive psychology perspective: Foreword. In C. -H. Mayer, & E. Vanderheiden (Eds.), *The bright side of shame. Transforming shame in cultural contexts* (pp. v–ix). Cham: Springer.

Claude-Hélène Mayer (Dr. habil., PhD, PhD) is a Professor in Industrial and Organisational Psychology at the Department of Industrial Psychology and People Management at the University of Johannesburg, an Adjunct Professor at the European University Viadrina in Frankfurt (Oder), Germany, and a Senior Research Associate at Rhodes University, Grahamstown, South Africa. She holds a PhD in Psychology (University of Pretoria, South Africa), a PhD in Management (Rhodes University, South Africa), a Doctorate (Georg-August University, Germany) in Political Sciences (socio-cultural anthropology and intercultural didactics) and a Habilitation (European University Viadrina, Germany) in Psychology with focus on work, organisational and cultural psychology. She has published several monographs, text collections, accredited journal articles and special issues on transcultural mental health and well-being, sense of coherence, shame, transcultural conflict management and mediation, women in leadership in culturally diverse work contexts, constellation work, coaching and psychobiography.

Elisabeth Vanderheiden is a pedagogue, theologian and intercultural mediator. She is the president of Catholic Adult Education in Germany and CEO of the Global Institute for Transcultural Research. Her publishing activities focus on pedagogy, in particular on the further education of teachers and trainers in adult education, vocational and political education, but also on the challenges of digitalisation. She has also edited books on intercultural and transnational issues. Her most recent publications deal with shame as a resource as well as with mistakes, errors and failures and their hidden potentials in the context of Culture and Positive Psychology 1.0 and 2.0. Current research projects deal with love in transcultural contexts, with life crises as well as humour in the context of Positive Psychology 2.0. Another focus of her work is Design Thinking in transcultural contexts.

Chapter 19
Body Shame and Social Media for Chinese International Students in the United States

Zixuan Wang, Wei Gabriel Qi, Leila Z. Wu, and Xiaochen Luo

1 Introduction

1.1 The Concept of Shame

Shame plays a powerful role in our living experience, yet it is also one of the last emotions that researchers studied in the recent decade (Shermer, 2010). Brene Brown (2006) argued that shame is "one of the most primitive and universal human emotions" (p. 43). Shame can be defined as "the intensely painful feeling or experience of believing that we are flawed and therefore unworthy of love and belonging — something we have experienced, done, or failed to do makes us unworthy of connection" (Brown, 2013). This is a concept that is often mistaken with other distressing emotions, such as guilt and embarrassment. While guilt and embarrassment can be adaptive and helpful for individuals by acknowledging that

Z. Wang (✉)
Quince Orchard Psychotherapy, Gaithersburg, MD, USA

W. G. Qi
School of Psychology, Fuller Theological Seminary, Pasadena, CA, USA

Department of Psychiatry, Stony Brook University, Stony Brook, NY, USA
e-mail: gabrielqi@fuller.edu

L. Z. Wu
The Pennsylvania State University, Department of Psychology, 361 Moore Building, University Park, Pennsylvania, PA, USA

X. Luo
Department of Counseling Psychology, Santa Clara University, Santa Clara, CA, USA
e-mail: xluo@scu.edu

C.-H. Mayer et al. (eds.), *Shame 4.0*, https://doi.org/10.1007/978-3-030-59527-2_19

their actions caused discomfort in self or others, shame can be maladaptive and destructive when it is connected to the belief in a flawed self (Pivetti, Camodeca, & Rapino, 2016).

Despite of shame existing in all cultures, studies have shown that there is no universal expression of shame across cultures (Jack, Garrod, Yu, Caldara, & Schyns, 2012). Previous research has mapped out the comparison of the shame experience in Western[1] versus Confucian cultures,[2] including how shame needs to be conceptualized on both relational and individualistic levels (Bedford, 2007) (see also Wong and Hwang in this book, see also Kotera et al. in this book, and see Takano in this book). More specifically, individualistic theories uphold the idea that all human beings are created equal, and thus boundaries around the individual self are believed to be worthy of protection. In contrast, Confucian cultures emphasize the continuity of life, meaning that individuals are the inheritance from their ancestors as to progress the flow of life. Therefore, boundaries of group, such as a family unit, should be protected in addition to the self. These different understandings of the self may impact one's proneness of shame, as a self-conscious emotion in a cultural context (Furukawa, Tangney, & Higashibara, 2012). Furthermore, for people who have cross-culture living experience, such as those who have lived in both Confucian and Western cultures, there are complicated sociocultural factors that should be taken into account in the understanding of individual's experience of shame, as immigration and acculturation process brings a series of complicated transformations on one's identity (Akhtar, 2015).

1.2 Shame and Self-Identity in Cultural Contexts

The collective self-identity is often defined by the system of relationships in which an individual is involved. This means that this person's other personal relations (family, friends, romantic partners, colleagues, etc.) may also be treated as part of the self. Many researchers labeled it as the "relational identity" as opposed to the conceptualization of an individualistic identity. By comparison, there is a higher degree of freedom, autonomy, and a sense of uniqueness in the traditional individualistic self-concept (Roland, 1996).

Shame can serve different functions in collective cultures versus individualistic cultures in the development of self-concepts. Gerlach (2016) indicated that in collective cultures such as the Chinese culture, shame relates less to the conduct of one's private life and more to the protection of the social form, which was shown in

[1]Western culture, which is equated with Western civilization, Western lifestyle, or European civilization, is defined as a term that broadly refers to a heritage of social norms, ethical values, traditional customs, belief systems, political systems, and specific artifacts and technologies that have some origin or association with Europe.

[2]Confucian culture is defined as a system of thought, ethical values, rationalistic religion, philosophy, a way of governing, or a way of living, originated from ancient China.

high levels of compliance with formalized social relation structures and deeply rooted rituals and rules. One example is the concept of *filial piety* or children's reverence and duty of care toward their parents. Any violation of this system of rules and commitments creates the risk of "losing face" for not only the individual but also the family, which incurs shame among the whole family and is therefore avoided at all costs. Unlike in the individualistic cultures where shame is construed as a private and self-conscious experience, in historically Confucian societies, shame is more likely induced by prosecution and humiliation from a group, which has resulted in one compensating for the humiliation by working hard and performing according to strict social rules and norms.

As Salman Akhtar (2015) summarizes, self-conscious emotions like shame glue identity and morality across cultures, but their developmental realms diverge across the adult life span. In Confucian cultures, when group harmony is disrupted by one person, individual's feelings of responsibility for the loss of group status conflict with one's core self-identity, hence producing the experience of shame. Because of the close connection between affective experience and one's concept of self, one can internalize shame through anger and blaming toward self, generalize shame from a behavior to an aspect of self-concept, which in turn generates more painful and maladaptive experience (Roos, Salmivalli, & Hodges, 2015).

1.3 Social Media and Body Shame in the Fourth Industrial Revolution

We are currently living in the era of the Fourth Industrial Revolution, where technologies like artificial intelligence, big data, and computing power are affecting and merging in our lives at an exponentially increasing speed (see Mayer and Vanderheiden on The Meaning of Shame in Cultures of the fourth Industrial Revolution; see Oosthuizen). One critical part of it is the almost ubiquitous usage of online social media, which has led to a monumental shift in how we live our daily lives. As social media rapidly gain popularity over traditional media (e.g., TV channels, newspapers, magazines, mail fliers, etc.), researchers started to look into the possible effects and consequences of new social media platforms on individuals' mental health. Many have found that the unique features of online social media have impacted body image and raised concerns about body shame (Fardouly & Vartanian, 2016; Holland & Tiggemann, 2016). Some of these features include the focus on the users themselves, the desire to present an idealized version of themselves, and the purpose of interacting with different people while allowing posting of comments or using the "like" function to provide feedback on one's appearance (Fardouly & Vartanian, 2016). Studies have found that greater social media usage was associated with greater body image concerns, higher tendency to make appearance comparisons to peers, more eating concerns, more shame, and more self-esteem issues especially among teenagers and young adults (Fardouly & Vartanian, 2016; Rodgers &

Melioli, 2016). In addition, issues of body objectification, sexualization, and misrepresentation have also been pervading online social media usage (Deighton-Smith & Bell, 2018; Davis, 2018).

From a cross-cultural perspective, Chinese people are often represented differently in Western social media (e.g., Facebook, Instagram, Twitter, YouTube, etc.) from native Chinese social media platforms (e.g., WeChat, Weibo, Zhihu, TikTok, etc.) (Cheng & Youngju Kim, 2018; Pang & Hill, 2018). It remains unclear how cultural contexts moderate the impacts of social media on individual's perception of self, social relationships, and affective experience. In Pang and Hill (2018)'s article, they addressed the role social media plays in Chinese young adults' identity formation process. They suggested that the ideal body image represented by social media is associated with the internalization of the dominant values and norms of appearances, resulting in negative psychological outcomes, such as body dissatisfaction, anxiety, and shame. These idealized images presented "norms" for masculinity, femininity, career success, and physical and psychological well-being.

For Chinese young adults who have been exposed to the American culture, such as Chinese international undergraduate students, their years of living experience in the United States (many would stay for at least 4 years to complete college) often comes with multifaceted stress and issues with cross-cultural adjustment (Li, Marbley, Bradley, & Lan, 2016). The adjustment process is partly complicated by the differences between the dominant ideal body image discourses in Chinese versus American social media (Jackson et al. 2016). In their study, Jackson and Chen concluded that there has been increased pressure for young Chinese women from comparing their physical appearance to that is depicted in Chinese/Asian media and more disturbances in body image concerns than it is associated with American social media. However, there is dearth knowledge about how specifically the cross-cultural media exposure has an impact on one's affective experience and self-identity.

In our study, we want to take a closer look at how the social media usage contributes to a specific group—Chinese international students living in the United States, their self-awareness and shame experiences. With the focus on body shame in the cross-cultural social media contexts, we hope to shed light on how technologies play a role for this understudied group experience from a newly developed angle.

2 Method

2.1 Participants

Three Chinese international undergraduate students were recruited through recruitment messages posted on social media. Two of the participants were male and one was female. They were between sophomore and senior years in an American college and have living experience in both the United States (2–3 years) and China. Purposeful sampling was employed to ensure that participants have had experiences relevant to our research questions.

2.2 Procedures

After receiving approval from the university's Institutional Review Board (IRB), a recruitment message written in Chinese describing the study purposes and target populations was sent out to several social media platforms that Chinese international students usually use (e.g., WeChat) as well as students' information bulletin at three large universities in the Midwestern and Northeastern United States. Participants were asked to email the primary investigator to confirm their intent to participate and were then assigned to one of the researchers for an hour-long interview through Zoom. Informed consent was obtained orally at the beginning of the interview. They were notified that the interviews would be recorded for transcription purposes. The recordings and transcripts were stored on a secure cloud storage service provider that was approved by the IRB.

We conducted semi-structured interviews with questions designed to ensure that the topics of interest were covered in the interview. Sample questions covered both the Chinese and American social media platforms that the interviewees use, including their frequency and purposes; the interviewees' understanding and definition of shame and body shame experiences; and their experience on how social media use has impacted their body image. All interviews were conducted in Mandarin Chinese. Due to the interviewees' familiarity with English use, there were rare occasions during interviews that English terms were used. Researchers tried to refrain from initiating the use of English.

2.3 Phenomenology Approach

The current study used a scientific phenomenological approach described by Giorgi (1997). According to Giorgi, three modified steps are required in this approach: (a) phenomenological reduction, (b) description, and (c) search for essence.

First, phenomenological reduction includes two major components: adopting a natural attitude and bracketing past knowledge. In this scientific method, phenomenological reduction is not expected from the research participants, but researchers should adopt the attitude by a) "withhold[ing] past knowledge about the phenomenon he or she is researching in order to be fully present to the concrete instance of the phenomenon as presented by the subject's description" and b) making no existential claim for the description (Giorgi, 1997).

Secondly, Giorgi (1997) defined "descriptions" as "the use of language to articulate the intentional objects of consciousness within the constraints of intuitive evidence." In scientific phenomenology, "descriptions" of phenomenon by the participants are seen from the perspective of the natural attitude and are not held against the criteria of phenomenological reduction. "The details, biases, errors, and prejudices" that the participants carry are what are to be scrutinized and understood.

The third component of scientific phenomenology is the search for "essences." Giorgi (1997), citing Husserl, defined essences as "the most invariant meaning for a context" or "the articulation, based on intuition, of a fundamental meaning without which a phenomenon could not present itself as it is." He pointed out that scientific essences differ from the philosophical essences, as scientific perspectives are normally narrower and more specified. Therefore, psychological essences in the current study were sought for with sensitivity to psychological science. This search was still characterized by phenomenological reduction, but within a limited context of psychological science.

2.4 Data Analyses and Credibility

As was suggested by Giorgi (1997), the steps of analyzing the transcripts include the following: (a) thorough reading of the data by each researcher; (b) breaking the data into "meaning units"; (c) organizing and summarizing the "meaning units" as themes, consistent with psychological theories; (d) the themes were categorized as major clusters, representing various components of the participants' experience; and (e) synthesizing the themes by cross-validation among researchers, where different opinions or interpretations of meanings were discussed and reconciled, in an effort of achieving phenomenological reduction by bracketing individual presumptions.

3 Results

We organized our findings according to themes that surfaced in content analyses of the interviews in three categories: experiences of body shame, body shame in a cross-cultural (Chinese versus American) context, and body shame in social media.

3.1 Experiences of Body Shame

3.1.1 Theme 1. Shame as a Challenging Feeling to Communicate

Explicitly or implicitly, all interviewees indicated that shame is difficult to describe, disclose, and discuss. Two out of the three participants explicitly reported such struggles in regard to their feelings of shame. One participant even defined shame as "a feeling that is hard to mention.[3]" Participants often took long pauses, asked

[3]All quotes from the interviewers and interviewees were originally in Mandarin Chinese and were translated by the authors in the current article.

clarifying questions, and needed further redirections when they attempted to define their experiences of shame. It seemed that discussing shame may evoke feelings that resemble the experience of shame itself, which involves the urge to avoid the painful feeling. Additionally, the experience of "not wanting to communicate" or "not knowing how to communicate about it" constitutes the core experience of shame, according to its definition.

The level of discomfort in shame discussions also varied among interviewees. One interviewee easily identified "feeling hot" as one physical sensation when feeling ashamed and also defined shame as feeling that she is responsible for something that she has done wrongly (e.g., not controlling her body weight appropriately).

3.1.2 Theme 2. The Various Focuses on the Body

The three interviewees reported body shame experiences with a variety of focuses on their bodies. Regarding body dissatisfaction, multiple participants reported dissatisfaction regarding body height (i.e., feeling "not tall enough"), facial appearance (i.e., emphasis only in the face rather than body shape), and muscle tones (i.e., wanting to have more muscles). Skin (wanting to have smoother skin without acnes) and weight (feeling "not thin enough") were mentioned once as sources of body dissatisfaction. Among these aspects, dissatisfaction regarding body height, facial appearance, and body weight were mentioned as the main reasons for body shame (see Mayer and Vanderheiden on Naming and Shaming; see Koops et al.).

3.1.3 Theme 3. Body Shame as Comparisons to Real or Imaginary Others and the Norm

All interviewees highlighted the role of others or the norm in body shame experiences. One female interviewee recalled memories of people commenting on her appearance in a negative manner (e.g., "you became fatter"). This interviewee thus cited her peers as a major source of pressure for her to focus on her appearance.

Other interviewees mentioned frequent comparisons with others that are part of their body shame experience. One interviewee mentioned comparisons with imaginary others while knowing that this person may or may not even be better-looking than him.

> *Interviewee 1: I will compare myself to my ex-girlfriend's male friends. I do not know why she broke up with me and whether there was a better person around her. Therefore, I was afraid, and I was guessing – I would go look for clues on social media. Perhaps this person (the imagined boyfriend of the ex-girlfriend) may be less attractive than me physically; but at the time, I thought I'm less than him.*

Another interviewee reported that he compared himself with his ex-girlfriend's current partner, feeling that the other person is more handsome and taller, even though this person "may not be as warm and considerate" as he is.

In both cases, the interviewees reported that they were aware that these comparisons may lack actual basis. They also reported that they have never received direct negative feedback, judgment, or comments on their appearance. In fact, when they thought about others' attitudes, they usually received positive or neutral feedback. They reported little influences from their parents and indicated that the pressure regarding appearance originated more from themselves. Nonetheless, they engaged in these comparisons as ways to inflict pain and shame on themselves. For these interviewees, their self-criticism seemed to not directly come from opinions from others but come from comparisons with their internal "templates." For example, one interviewee mentioned that he perceived a template of "the ideal body" that most people would like, and he would feel ashamed when he perceives his appearance as far away from the ideal norm. Overall, frequent social comparisons by others or by oneself seemed to be a central cognitive piece in the experience of body shame.

3.1.4 Theme 4. Body Shame is a Major Contributor to Low Self-Esteem

All interviewees reported that their body shame experience directly leads to low self-esteem. Some interviewees reported that they perceived themselves as flawed individuals that people would not like and that they have no way to fix the issue (e.g., not tall or attractive enough). For others, body shame regarding weight triggered their self-judgment of "not having enough self-control." One interviewee highlighted the pervasiveness and generalizability of body shame experience and described the experience as "if you felt ashamed about this one thing (height), you felt ashamed about everything regarding yourself."

3.1.5 Theme 5. Consequences of Body Shame: Romantic Relationship Barrier, Social Isolation, and Urges for Compensatory Behaviors

All interviewees perceived body shame as a major barrier to pursuing romantic relationships. All interviewees reported past or current experience of feeling hesitant to pursue romantic relationships because they perceived their appearance as not attractive enough and believed that few people would be romantically interested in them. Furthermore, body shame also influenced how people understood their relationship failure. Two interviewees who have had romantic relationships attributed the end of the relationship to their appearance, indicating that perhaps their ex-partners found someone who was more attractive physically and thus ended the relationships. It seems that body shame is directly connected to the imagined or perceived failure of romantic relationships when appearance is one of the top considerations for romantic pursuits.

The interviewees also reported tendencies of isolating themselves socially when they felt ashamed of their bodies: two interviewees reported that they tended to withdraw socially, and they would not leave home or interact with others for reasons other than classes. Furthermore, the interviewees reported various "compensatory" behaviors or urges in association with their body shame: one male interviewee reported having thoughts of going to do plastic surgery at least once a week due to his body shame experience. Another interviewee reported that if she felt like she ate too much 1 day, she would do exercises on that day even at midnight. Interestingly, multiple interviewees expressed concerns regarding "getting addicted" to doing plastic surgeries or to using photography filters to adjust their appearances. These concerns demonstrated the interviewees' insight into both the rewarding and dangerous aspects of efforts to pursue ideal physical appearance and alleviating body shame.

3.2 Body Shame in the Cross-Cultural Contexts

3.2.1 Theme 1. Different Internalized Cultural Norms/Values

All interviewees shared their lived experiences growing up in China and coming to the United States to attend college. The three interviewees all reported their perception of the different aesthetic values and norms between the Chinese and American cultures. Interestingly, the aspects they emphasized and compared between the two cultures were all different from each other. One male interviewee reported that while he believes *height* is a dominant aesthetic value in both cultures, the ideal male height is higher in the United States than it is in China, which is associated with increased insecurities in his own height when he came to the United States. The other male interviewee emphasized the differences in the dominant values of ideal *facial appearance* in the two cultures, including the softness versus the toughness of facial characteristics that are applauded in Chinese versus the American cultures. The female interviewee reported her experience of being subjected to values of more strict female *body shape* in China than it is in the United States, including lower body weight and slimmer physique. The only dominant value that all three agreed on in terms of its cross-cultural difference is that the ideal beauty in Chinese culture has more emphases on the feminine qualities (e.g., pale skin, lean body shape), whereas there are more masculine qualities emphasized in the description of ideal beauty in American culture (e.g., muscular body shape, firm face contours), which is applicable to both the male and female genders.

These internalized values of ideal body image were reportedly associated closely with body dissatisfaction and body shame. The interviewee who discussed height being a dominant aesthetic value expressed dissatisfaction in his own height and how it could be a source of his shameful experience. The interviewee who discussed facial appearance also emphasized dissatisfaction in this part of his self-image. The female interviewee described the salience of female body shape in both cultures' ideal beauty standard, which had negative impacts on her self-image and was related to increased insecure feelings toward her body image. The overall theme of negative perceptions of body image seems to be related to the internalization of these dominant ideal beauty values that occurred in their cross-cultural experiences.

3.2.2 Theme 2. Earlier Body Shame Experience in the Cultural Context

The three interviewees shared their earlier body shame experience growing up in China. Interestingly, all interviewees recalled interactions with peers from middle or high school when they were prompted to discuss earlier memory of their body image. The two male interviewees associated their confidence or dissatisfaction in body image with their assumed judgment from peers, whereas the female interviewee reported receiving more frequent direct feedback from their peers. One interviewee recalled this experience in high school:

> ***Interviewee***: *I felt somewhat unconfident about my height…in my (high school) class, there were about 20 boys, and my height was around 5 to 6 to the last.*
>
> ***Interviewer***: *What did it mean personally to you that you were not as tall as some of your peers?*
>
> ***Interviewee***: *I think it partly impacted my self-esteem and made me feel that in some aspects, I was not as good as others. I understand that I cannot change it, but it only made me feel more inferior. Like when I was attracted to a girl, I'd be embarrassed…because the norm was that a girl would only like a guy who is taller than her, or a guy with a certain height, which could give her a sense of security. That value was ingrained in my mind.*
>
> ***Interviewer***: *Have you ever received any feedback from others [about your body image]?*
>
> ***Interviewee***: *In my impression, very little. I had pretty good relationships with my peers, and they never intentionally commented on my height. The most was to make a joke or such…*

Another interviewee reported similar experience of dissatisfaction in his facial appearance and recalled comparing it to his peers in middle school whom he perceived as being more handsome than he was. This interviewee described attributing his interpersonal difficulties (e.g., breakup with his girlfriend) to the flaws of his appearance, despite the lack of direct negative feedback from his peers. When the assumption of judgment from others is discussed, this interviewee stated that "I would not share with my friends about my dissatisfaction with the way I look, because they would never tell me that I am ugly, which I wouldn't be able to take in anyways. Then I got myself into a vicious cycle."

The female interviewee shared receiving negative feedback from her high school peers about her weight: "when I went to visit my friends, there was a mirror in the house. She told me, 'look at you, how much weight have you gained?' That was the earliest experience of when I felt that I became fat." This interviewee also recalled receiving similar judgment from her family members. However, when her experience of feeling satisfied with her weight is discussed in the context of comparing to the dominant values in China, she did not report receiving any positive feedback from her peers.

When prompted to share their body shame experience, the interviewees tend to trace back to their earlier experience living in China. This suggests a strong connection between their adolescent years of living and emotional experience, potentially moderated by the dominant values and norms in the Chinese cultural context.

All of the interviewees also highlighted how the aspects of their body shame experience were reinforced by the cross-cultural experience, in a sense that the parts of the body that were perceived as "flawed" in their lived experience in China are subjected to a new norm in American culture. Higher salience of these norms was reported by interviewees when they returned to a Chinese cultural context, either through online social media platforms, with their Chinese social groups in the United States, or when they went back to the home country. Overall, the interviewees reported that shameful experience and higher emotional disturbance occurred predominantly in contexts related to Chinese culture rather than in the American cultural context.

3.2.3 Theme 3. Positive Lifestyle Changes in Cultural Adjustment

In addition to perceiving different norms and predominant values of ideal beauty between the two cultures, the three interviewees also shared their positive changes in their lifestyle during the process of the cross-cultural adjustment. For example, the interviewees all reported increased adherence to the values of fitness and exercise living in the United States and reported higher body satisfaction and improved self-confidence as they prioritized these values over the parts of their body that used to provoke dissatisfaction, inferiority, and shame.

It is also noteworthy that despite experiencing positive influence from her American peers who value healthy diet and exercise over a thin body, the female interviewee reported receiving concerns from these peers of her being "underweight":

> ***Interviewee:*** *My personal experience has been that my American friends would think of me as being too skinny and they would tell me to eat more, whereas my Chinese friends, including those on social media, they are very, very, thin.*
>
> ***Interviewer:*** *Sounds like there are two different sets of standards between China and the United States. What kind of feedback have your American friends given you about your appearance?*
>
> ***Interviewee:*** *So far they have been pretty positive. They tend to be more concerned about how much I eat and have told me that they are concerned that I don't eat at all. They often tell me that I'm "too thin."*
>
> ***Interviewer:*** *How did that make you feel?*
>
> ***Interviewee:*** *Umm...confused. Because my friends in China like to say that I have gained weight, yet my friends in America tell me that I'm thin. It makes me wonder what exactly I am?*

In contrast, neither of the male interviewees reported similar experience of receiving such direct feedback from their peers, either in China or in the United States. While positive lifestyle changes can be a positive outcome of cultural adjustment, there seems to be a gender factor as well in how explicit they are.

3.3 Body Shame and Social Media

3.3.1 Theme 1. Social Media Influences Ideal Body Image

Though the three interviewees reported various focuses on their bodies, all of them discussed how social media influences the formation of their ideal images. The interviewees reported that they did not develop their ideal body images directly from social media, as they all recalled that the concept of body images started to develop in their early adolescence through comparison with their peers, when social media was not yet very popularly used among them. However, the three interviewees all discussed how their frequent social media use further shaped their ideal images as they grew older. The three interviewees reported different reasons to use social media: connecting with friends, following celebrities or influencers, inquiring information, sharing personal life, etc. There was a shared similarity, though, on the tendency to collect information about the popular trend of ideal body images.

The female interviewee specifically talked about the distortion of ideal body images on social media, which was by adjusting and filtering the actual, real-life body appearances. Though she reported that social media had little impact on her life due to the awareness of this distortion, she still reported having an ideal body image exemplified by a thinly shaped body due to the influence of social media. Both of the male interviewees mentioned developing their ideal male images by referring to comments made by females on social media platforms. One male interviewee talked about how he started to pay attention to his body shape after using social media in the United States, and before his primary focus is on his facial appearance in his adolescent years when he lived in China. Another male interviewee discussed how he used the social norm learned on social media as references and adjusted his ideal image to follow the social norm.

3.3.2 Theme 2. Social Media Triggers Negative Emotions and Enhances Body Shame

The three interviewees recalled how social media triggered their negative emotions on various degrees. The female interviewee reported feeling angry when her old friends commented negatively on her posted pictures, specifically about her gaining weight. She also reported feeling guilty for not keeping up to her ideal body image when she referred to the ideal beauty norm, especially when she ate more than expected in 1 day. She also reported feeling frustrated about the phenomenon of self-image adjustment on social media. One male interviewee described feeling envious of others on social media, which was associated with lower self-esteem and insecurities in a romantic relationship. He also reported feeling the need to improve his self-image, both via exercising and seeking plastic surgery for better facial appearance.

The female interviewee and one of the male interviewees both talked about how they have negative emotions toward the ideal images frequently seen on social media. The female interviewee complained about the lack of diversity and tolerance in the ideal norm of beauty on social media. For example, she noticed that people with wider faces are seldomly considered as beautiful. She described it as the explanation for using beautifying tools (e.g., Photoshop) to adjust her face before posting on social media. The male interviewee expressed strong criticism toward male images with makeups presented on social media, which he considered as "too feminine."

Overall, having their earliest experience of body shame in the context of peer relationships rather than social media is a common theme among the interviewees. However, they agreed that social media use has continued to enhance their shame or dissatisfaction in their body images.

3.3.3 Theme 3. Peer Comparison and the Interaction on Social Media

All interviewees reported that using social media increased their comparison with peers on social media. Each of them talked about how the comparison generated stronger dissatisfaction in their body image and how they coped with the increased negative feelings. The male interviewee who never posted any pictures of himself on social media reported that he would judge his appearance based on the pictures that his peers posted on social media. He reported that he will try to avoid thinking about appearance to reduce his feelings of shame and vulnerability. For the two interviewees who had experience posting their own pictures on social media, both talked about the desire to present an idealized version of self on social media through photo enhancement/adjustment techniques. They also shared the experience of comparing horizontally with other peers' pictures and thinking about how much affirmation (e.g., receiving "likes") they would receive for these posts. Both interviewees reported posting less frequently on social media when they feel less satisfied with their pictures or their appearance.

The female interviewee reported that she would not post the photoshopped picture if it looked better than her real appearance. She also reported deleting her old friends from her social account due to their negative comments on her pictures. Similarly, one male interviewee reported feeling more self-conscious about his picture. In general, the three interviewees adopted reducing interaction on social media as their copying mechanism when they experienced stronger body shame through peer comparison.

3.3.4 Theme 4. Shifting Focus Away from Social Media

Both two male interviewees reported changed perceptions in the use of social media as their age increases. They shared the belief that one's appearance becomes less important in the later stages of life, and the attention is shifted toward one's ability and achievement. They both described the maturity of understanding social media's influence and becoming more selective with information that they received on social media, which is also associated with reduced body shame experience. One interviewee reported that he still cares about his body image and appearance strongly, but he knows that he will not prioritize it in the future. He explained that "good looking is very important to younger people, at least I think so, as you don't have much more to compare with others when everyone is similar in school, but there will be many more important aspects to make evaluation of a person later in life."

4 Discussion

The results of our phenomenological study illustrate how the self-conscious emotion, shame, manifests in specific cross-cultural contexts and how it interplays with social media use. We focused on inviting the participants to reflect on and describe their body shame experience in their native language, and our findings support that body shame experience can be more deeply rooted in one's earlier cultural context and can be enhanced by social media use, both through the means of peer comparison. While the participants' reported experience demonstrated the difficulties of communicating shame, the curiosity, observation, and insight into their body shame experience have shown the value for continued research on this powerful yet challenging to verbalize emotion. Through the phenomenological approach, the psychological essence of shame can be more effectively studied in a nonmanipulative way.

One of the major limitations of our study is its generalizability, given the small sample size and the very specific contextual factors. Our narratives were restricted to Chinese international students attending colleges in the United States, and their experience with body shame, perception of ideal beauty norms in the two cultures, as well as social media use are likely to be very different from others who do not fall in this group. Needless to say, the generalizability within this group is also limited by the sample size, gender, and the participants' individual acculturation process. As this is a preliminary phase of the study on body shame experience in Chinese adults who migrated to the United States, we aim to further our work by focusing on a wider age range of participants and their experiences on this issue.

5 Conclusion

The Fourth Industrial Revolution facilitates globalization, which not only increased human's mobility, such as the example of increased number of international students who travelled abroad to study, but also enhanced cross-cultural exchanges of images, ideas, and values. Our paper discussed how the Fourth Industrial Revolution plays a role in how cultures and technologies shape the way we view ourselves and our bodies.

Our paper indicates that on one hand, the Fourth Industrial Revolution blurs the lines between the digital, physical, and psychological worlds: our interviewees have access to visual and verbal sources of ideas about ideal body image easily, and their shame experiences can come from more comparisons with imagined peers or judgments from social media than receiving direct feedback in real relationships. Future studies can focus on how the Fourth Industrial Revolution influences the social process of forming and shaping our identities and our bodies.

On the other hand, the increased digital connection is not equated with increased psychological connection and openness. It seems that body objectification is one of the most dominant ideas that all of the interviewees have encountered. The abundant digital information did not produce more diverse ideas regarding ideal body, mind-body relationship, and body's role in identity. The interviewees all described experiences where they could not fit into the finicky "template" of the ideal body, which decreased their senses of self-worth, and more importantly, it negatively impacted their sense of connections with others. In this case, shame is the key mediator component linking the digital world where people connect more *and* the physical world where people choose to be more isolative.

Our paper further illustrated the complex picture and the need for future research to explore the role of culture in our emotion and identity in an increasingly globalized world. Our interviewees, who lived physically in American culture, raised in Chinese culture, socialized with people from both cultures off-line and were exposed to both cultures online and exhibited awareness of cultural variation in ideal body and potentially ideal identity. However, these cross-cultural experiences and awareness seemed to have little impact on how they continued to internally compare themselves to ideal body norms only in their native culture. It would be interesting for future studies to examine how cross-cultural experiences influence the stability of values regarding body image in this increasingly digital world.

References

Akhtar, S. (Ed.). (2015). *Shame: Developmental, cultural, and clinical realms*. London: Karnac Books.

Bedford, O. A. (2007). *Guilt, shame, & identity: A cultural perspective*. Seoul: Kyoyook-Kwahak-Sa.

Brown, B. (2006). Shame resilience theory: A grounded theory study on women and shame. *Families in Society, 87*(1), 43–52.

Brown, B. (2013, January 14). *Shame vs. Guilt [Blog post]*. Retrieved from https://brenebrown.com/blog/2013/01/14/shame-v-guilt/

Cheng, H. L., & Youngju Kim, H. (2018). Racial and sexual objectification of Asian American women: Associations with trauma symptomatology, body image concerns, and disordered eating. *Women & Therapy, 41*(3–4), 237–260.

Davis, S. E. (2018). Objectification, sexualization, and misrepresentation: Social media and the college experience. *Social Media+ Society, 4*(3).

Deighton-Smith, N., & Bell, B. T. (2018). Objectifying fitness: A content and thematic analysis of# fitspiration images on social media. *Psychology of Popular Media Culture, 7*(4), 467.

Fardouly, J., & Vartanian, L. R. (2016). Social media and body image concerns: Current research and future directions. *Current opinion in psychology, 9*, 1–5.

Furukawa, E., Tangney, J., & Higashibara, F. (2012). Cross-cultural continuities and discontinuities in shame, guilt, and pride: A study of children residing in Japan, Korea and the USA. *Self and Identity, 11*(1), 90–113.

Gerlach, A. (2016). Psychoanalysis and the understanding of Chinese life experience. *Psychoanalysis and Psychotherapy in China, 2*, 51–59.

Giorgi, A. (1997). The theory, practice, and evaluation of the phenomenological method as a qualitative research. *Journal of Phenomenological Psychology, 28*, 235.

Holland, G., & Tiggemann, M. (2016). A systematic review of the impact of the use of social networking sites on body image and disordered eating outcomes. *Body Image, 17*, 100–110.

Jack, R. E., Garrod, O. G., Yu, H., Caldara, R., & Schyns, P. G. (2012). Facial expressions of emotion are not culturally universal. *Proceedings of the National Academy of Sciences, 109*(19), 7241–7244.

Jackson, T., Jiang, C., & Chen, H. (2016). Associations between Chinese/Asian versus Western mass media influences and body image disturbances of young Chinese women. *Body Image, 17*, 175–183.

Li, J., Marbley, A. F., Bradley, L. J., & Lan, W. (2016). Attitudes toward seeking professional counseling services among Chinese international students: Acculturation, ethnic identity, and English proficiency. *Journal of Multicultural Counseling and Development, 44*(1), 65–76.

Pang, B., & Hill, J. (2018). Representations of Chinese gendered and racialised bodies in contemporary media sites. *Sport, Education and Society, 23*(8), 773–785.

Pivetti, M., Camodeca, M., & Rapino, M. (2016). Shame, guilt, and anger: Their cognitive, physiological, and behavioral correlates. *Current Psychology, 35*(4), 690–699.

Rodgers, R. F., & Melioli, T. (2016). The relationship between body image concerns, eating disorders and internet use, part I: A review of empirical support. *Adolescent Research Review, 1*(2), 95–119.

Roland, A. (1996). The influence of culture on the self and selfobject relationships: An Asian-North American comparison. *Psychoanalytic Dialogues, 6*(4), 461–475.

Roos, S., Salmivalli, C., & Hodges, E. V. (2015). Emotion regulation and negative emotionality moderate the effects of moral (dis) engagement on aggression. *Merrill-Palmer Quarterly, 61*(1), 30–50.

Shermer, V. L. (2010). Between shame, death, and mourning. In *The Shame of death, grief, and Trauma* (pp. 33–57). New York: Routledge.

Zixuan Wang, Psy.D., is a licensed clinical psychologist who is currently working in a group practice in Rockville, Maryland. She completed her graduate study at the George Washington University's Professional Psychology program and earned her B.A. in Psychology at New York University as an honored student. She completed her postdoctoral fellowship at the Kennedy Krieger Institute's Child and Family Therapy Clinic, and her doctoral internship at Pennsylvania Hospital. She has specialized interests in self-conscious emotions, intersecting identity issues, as well as adjustment/acculturation issues.

Wei (Gabriel) Qi received his PhD in clinical psychology with a major area of study in clinical neuropsychology in the Graduate School of Psychology at Fuller Theological Seminary, California, USA. He completed his pre-doctoral internship at Baylor College of Medicine and TIRR Memorial Hermann in Houston, Texas, USA. His research interests include neuropsychological tool development (esp. in Chinese languages and in indigenous perspectives) and rehabilitation psychology. He practices psychotherapy and counseling with patients/clients of wide diversity and specializes in neuropsychological evaluations and rehabilitation psychological interventions.

Leila Z. Wu, M.A., is a Ph.D. candidate in clinical psychology at Pennsylvania State University. She holds a B.A. in psychology as a Schreyer honor student at Pennsylvania State University and continues her graduate study there. Her research interests are broadly focusing on personality disorders, personality assessment, interpersonal functioning, and cross-cultural clinical application, especially on Chinese population.

Xiaochen Luo, M.A., M.S., is a doctoral candidate in clinical psychology at Michigan State University. She is currently doing her clinical internship at SUNY Upstate Medical University. She earned her B.S. in psychology and B.A. in philosophy from Peking University and her master degree in Clinical and Psychosocial Epidemiology from the University of Groningen. She has specialized interests in treatment outcomes and interpersonal processes in psychotherapy, as well as the interactions between body shame, eating, and cultural identity.

Chapter 20
Shaming in the Internet Era: Evaluating the Reintegrative Function of Shame in Digital Spaces

Grace Maria Jochan and Trina Banerjee

The more things a man is ashamed of, the more respectable he is.

1 Defining the Concept of Shame

Shame is one of the oldest self-blaming emotions that encouraged people to engage in pro-social and constructive behavior. Shame and guilt are often considered synonymous with one another, but shame is identified as a self-related emotion that motivates one to hide and escape, whereas guilt is identified as the emotion that motivates one to repair (Bastin, Harrison, Davey, Moll, & Whittle, 2016; Keng & Tan, 2017). Shame is one of the grimmest emotions to comprehend as it vaguely borders between the personal and social contexts of an individual (Nash & Kilday, 2010). In shame, the focus is usually on the individual, and it can often be painful (Schalkwijk, Stams, Dekker, & Elison, 2016). Shame helps one to compare the "real self" with the "ideal self," and any discrepancy in that can bring about embarrassment. Hence, it can also be called a self-conscious emotion (see Mayer and Vanderheiden on The Meaning of Shame in Cultures of the fourth Industrial Revolution–An Introduction). Shame can bring about a concept of being exposed to real or imagined audience, and more than the external judgment, the internal self-flagellation is what brings about the distress. The sense of self is stigmatized and unfavored. Although shame assumes the function of the reintegration of an individual to the mainstream society, the process of shaming can be an unpleasant experience for the shamed. Therefore, shame can also be categorized as a problem emotion, either as generating conformity or inhibiting non-conforming opinions (Stearns, 2017). In this context, shaming is considered as an age-old technique of

G. M. Jochan (✉) · T. Banerjee
Department of Psychology, Mount Carmel College, Bangalore, India

C.-H. Mayer et al. (eds.), *Shame 4.0*, https://doi.org/10.1007/978-3-030-59527-2_20

denunciation, a process where two groups of people, the ones expressing shame and ones receiving shame, converse with each other where the later tells the other that they are "dishonorable and unworthy of respect as an equal person" (Trottier, 2017).

A central concept to experience shame is the presence of an audience to watch the act of shaming. The idea of being observed by another makes the experience of shame very unpleasant and creates feelings of inferiority regarding the standards they hold for themselves. Some research also suggests that most of the time, shame occurs when people fail to meet the norms that they expect for themselves (Maibom, 2010). However, this idea might not hold, especially when the victims of abuse or racism experience feelings of shame (see Vanderheiden on The Terror of being Judged). On the other hand, shame does assume pro-social functions that help in maintaining the social fabric together. Adaptive pro-social shame encourages individuals to maintain social decorum and regulate their behavior according to social and cultural norms (Tignor & Colvin, 2017). When the social regularity function of the shame creates appeasement in the one who is ashamed, the reintegrative function non-stigmatizes shame and integrates the appeased individuals back into the social circle (Braithwaite, 1993; Maibom, 2010).

2 Historical Notions About Shame and Shaming

The concept of shaming dates back to the history of humankind. Historical examples of doxing and shaming can be traced back to the middle ages like the phrase "Shamed be the one who thinks evil of it" which made its way to the British royal coat of arms, to colonial practices of public lettering to maintain shame, as recorded in many fictions (Stearns, 2017). For a long time in history, religious institutions used the concept of shame to promote cooperative behavior. Public penances and penitential practices in religions like Christianity played an essential role in reforming unwanted behaviors and were later adopted to political doctrines in the eighteenth and nineteenth centuries in Europe and America (Wettlaufer, 2012). Transgressors of norms during this period often were inflicted with ignominy and humiliation as a torture method, a practice that was stigmatizing rather than reintegrating (Braithwaite, 1993). Norbert Elias gave one of the classic studies on shame in Western history. He proposed that the social transformation from the knighthood and nobility to courtly structure happened based on the feelings of shame. The magnanimous number of changes brought in by the education of the proletariat and losing the power of church combined with the thirst for democratic doctrines brought in feelings of shame among the noble classes. However, this theory is criticized for being more or less a unilinear evolution. As we moved toward modernity, the power vested with religious institutions diminished, and social systems like families became more accepting and adaptive, thereby promoting the reintegrative functions of shame (Braithwaite, 1993; Wettlaufer, 2012).

2.1 The Culture of Shame

Every emotion has a unique way of expression and response in every culture. The feeling and expression of shame-related emotions for a long time were compartmentalized into two significant distinctions: the guilt culture and the shame culture. Guilt cultures focused on repairing the infarction, whereas shame cultures emphasized on the inner conscience of ethics and etiquette (Creighton, 1990). Traditionally, individualistic school of thought aligned with the guilt culture perspective, and the oriental thoughts encompassed the shame culture. Debates on which model of emotion is better than the other had brought in the concept of cultural relativity in understanding shame, which states that each culture needs to be understood in its unique coherence rather than in comparison with some other value system. However, with the changing phase of development, the coming of the Fourth Industrial Revolution of digitization, the fission ideology of the occidental, and the fusion ideology of the oriental have fused among themselves to create a more inclusive model of globalist cosmopolitanism (Rousell, 2016; Tuo, 2017).

2.2 Shame and *lajjA*

Since the study primarily focused on participants from the Indian subcontinent, it is essential to understand the concept of *lajjA*, unique to the Indian culture. *lajjA* derives its etymology from a Sanskrit word *lajj*, meaning shame. It is considered as a virtue that allows one to be aware of the social appropriateness and expression of the same. Although not a part of the nine prominent *rasas* or emotional expressions, shame is considered as 1 of the 33 prominent subsidiary *bhavas* in the *rasa* theory. This emotion is very synonymous with shame or modesty or bashfulness and is considered as noble emotion to possess (Bhawuk, 2017) (see also Bhawuk in this book; see Puttaraju and D'Souza in this book). In the Indian psychological context, life is considered as a sacrifice that desires the benefit of others. It determines intergroup dynamics and instills a conscious force where the well-being of the other is considered equally valuable as the well-being of self, an inner thought in collectivistic cultures. Western thoughts contemplate shame and guilt as synonymous, of which guilt is regarded to be more useful than shame as it employs learning and growth. In the Indian context, shame is a transient emotion leading to reintegration, and doSa is the sin that needs *prayazcitta*, an act of atonement. Unlike guilt, which can stay repressed and dormant, prayazcitta takes away the doSa and thereby the lajjA associated with it (Bhawuk, 2017, 2019). The concept of *lajjA* often appears as a gendered construct, more associated as a desirable quality embarking femininity and female beauty. In men, *lajjA* is the emotion denoting their fall from their stereotypical masculine roles (Sinha & Chauhan, 2013).

The first mention of this word comes in Vishnu Purana, as the name of the daughter of King Daksha and Prasuti. An alternative storyline considers *lajjA*

Gauri as an incarnation of Goddess Parvati, who covers her face in embarrassment when sages appear as she and her husband Lord Shiva was procreating. In the Vedic times, female nudity was not associated with shame but was regarded as auspicious. Reminiscents from this thought can be observed in many religious shrines, where the female genitalia are worshipped. The following eras of dynastic rule brought in more stringent boundaries to the concept of *lajjA*, and it became more and more associated as a desired virtue of the female. With Westernization, women became vehicles of *lajjA*, confined into the purity of their homes, espousing feminine and spiritual qualities (Sinha & Chauhan, 2013). However, strong women, who proved their might in different areas, were not expected to follow the norm of *lajjA* to showcase their femininity.

Contrary to its counterpart shame, *lajjA* is experienced at times of praise as well as criticism. *lajjA* is equally likely to be aroused when an individual is tempted to engage in forbidden activities as well as when he engages in a rightful behavior making *lajjA* a complex emotional state to decipher. *lajjA* also mediates infamy, thereby making people adhere to cultural norms to avoid *lajjA* and subsequently infamy. The concept of *lajjA* can also appear as a gendered construct, more associated as a desirable quality embarking femininity and female beauty (Bhawuk, 2019; Sinha & Chauhan, 2013). When shame is the falling short of aspirations, *lajjA* is a virtue that helps one to live up to the standards through a sense of awareness and regard for society. The subtlety and indirectness of this expression make it a desirable virtue of modesty. From a sociological viewpoint, *lajjA* plays a significant role in the maintenance of social and power structures, but from a psychological point of view, *lajjA* can sometimes become a challenge to one's mental well-being. In modern times, where cultures have become more inclusive and cosmopolitan, where gender roles and gendered concepts are diminishing, the concept of *lajjA* requires careful study and scrutiny.

2.3 The Industrial Revolution and Digital World

The history of the Industrial Revolution is vast and dynamic. It was a phenomenon that was highly popularized in the late sixteenth century, and humanity continues to contribute to it even today. The advent of the phenomenon started with a shift in the industry, which was primarily based on agriculture and handicraft to a system dominated by machine manufacturing (Industrial Revolution, 2019). The period from 1760 to 1830 witnessed some significant changes as a result of the Industrial Revolution. The agricultural improvements enhanced food productivity. The growth of cities and urbanization was also one of the significant social changes that were observed. However, the Industrial Revolution also left psychological scars. Studies have revealed that people belonging to former industrial regions in Great Britain and the USA have shown more considerable psychological morbidity revolving around neuroticism, conscientiousness, life satisfaction, and life expectancy than people in other regions. Regions like Blaenau Gwent in the UK and the Rust Belt in the USA had industry workers who reported unhappy personality traits (Obschonka, 2018).

From the late nineteenth to early twentieth century, the world witnessed the advent of technology in the field of industry and commerce. This phase is popularly known as the "Second Industrial Revolution" (Niiler, 2019). The technology made rapid production of factory goods possible, which perhaps made people busier. More and more workers were now required with specialized skills to utilize technology. Among the many sociological changes, child labor became prominent around this time. Children were exposed to long hours of hard labor in the factories involved in production work. In 1889, Jane Adams, a social activist, had planned a Christmas party in a group home she founded in Chicago slums. At the party, she had offered candy to impoverished children who refused to have them. The explanation was that they were sick of the constant smell of candy from working long hours in a candy factory. The children were found to work from seven in the morning to nine at night for 6 weeks (Niiler, 2019).

As the aftermath of the Second World War, the world was introduced to a new kind of energy resource: nuclear energy. The invention of the microprocessor and the implementation of telecommunication devices opened a new era of connectivity. With the increased use of telecommunication devices, individuals were able to remain more connected to each other than before (Rifkin, n.d.).

India was ruled by the British at the time of the Industrial Revolution. With all the upheaval happening in Great Britain during this time, India also received a noteworthy impact. The effect of the Industrial Revolution in India happened much later than the sixteenth century. Around the time of the Second Industrial Revolution, after the nineteenth century, the Indian economy started witnessing major changes. The onset of the revolution started with a rapid decline in the production and sale of handicrafts, something that was a specialty of Indian culture and was a primary source of income for many Indian artisans (Gandikota & Rao, 1955). India, around 1820, had started building ships and making textiles for the British market (Kumarappa, 1945). The Lancashire cotton goods made considerable destruction to the status of the handloom and the Indian spinning wheel (Gandikota & Rao, 1955). The introduction of the Indian Railways also marks a milestone in the impact of the Industrial Revolution in India. With the railways becoming an easier means of transport for the citizens, there was increased connectivity and enrichment of trade and commerce. Common men affiliated power structures to the British and their mechanisms of living, causing a sense of inferiority about anything that was locally produced.

In the current socio-political situation, there is an increase in technological advancement, which brings us to the Fourth Industrial Revolution, where boundaries between the physical, biological, and digital world are blurred (McGinnis, 2018). Artificial intelligence and newer computational technologies have gained popularity. The connectivity from the third phase of the Industrial Revolution expanded to the digitization of the whole phenomenon. The concept of digital identity has come into being, and individuals have been successful in creating a virtual existence of themselves. This digital identity, just like a real identity, can be subject to criticism and shaming. In the era of digitization, the criticisms of the virtual self can also be made virtually, which might equally impact the real person behind the virtual identity.

India has also not been spared from the effect of the fourth stage of the Industrial Revolution. With the rise of digitization and technological advancement, there has been a real change in the dynamics of Indian society. The *Economic Times* (2020) has explained that with automation adoption, the cost of labor and skill level has changed. The primary concern of this age seems to be data privacy. Controversies against social networking sites have been brought, stating they may not be safe after all, and anyone and everyone can get access to the data (Ariffin, 2018). India is aiming toward becoming a hub of artificial intelligence, with the government declaring a national program on AI to encourage AI-related technologies (Ariffin, 2018). Press Trust of India (2018) reports that the Prime Minister of India, Narendra Modi, also opinioned that artificial intelligence, machine learning, blockchain, and big data have the potential to take India to new heights of civilization. However, there is a growing concern about the status of jobs after automation.

Online activities can control one's health and well-being. Digital shaming can invade a person's privacy and ferment distrust among individuals. With the power residing in our fingertips, the civility of individuals in the online platform can be witnessed through social media activity. Many a time, the power is wrongfully channelized giving rise to trolling and Internet bullying. The Internet or digital vigilantes take matters into their own hands, and their simple act of expressing their views becomes an act of shaming in itself.

Sometimes, digital shaming comes as a disguised form of Internet activism. Digital activism, also known as cyber-activism, has proved to be a powerful means of political mobilization. Digital networks all over the world have been used for action, protests, affirmation, and opposition of thoughts and expression. In this process, vigilantes often end up shaming the opposite viewpoint, and the theme becomes more of an aggressive exchange of information.

The digital world acts more or less like a microcosm of the real world, and our social identities have branched out into virtual identities. The connectedness, diversity, and spontaneity of the digital spaces have made our virtual interactions more efficient. Nevertheless, at the same time, it has also made it irrevocable to erase our digital footprints. Shaming in traditional societies allowed an individual to distance himself from the transgressors physically. However, the virtual web not only makes this escape impossible but also allows easy and excruciating breach of privacy. The metaphorical analogy of Foucault, panopticon, can no longer be considered a metaphor, with the Internet being the medium of digital surveillance and privacy, a questionable possession (Goodlad, 2003). The uses and gratification theory by Blumler and McQuail (1969) explain the silence of the audience, as appearing in shame act. The theory suggests that the silence acts like an incentive to further shame the person who has or has been perceived to have violated a cultural norm.

3 Significance of the Study

This chapter attempts to understand the concept of shaming in the context of digital spaces and questions if virtual spaces have become a space of stigmatization and ostracism of the transgressors rather than being reintegrative in nature. The concept of the irreversibility of shame information and accessibility to breach the privacy of the transgressed makes the ignominy irrevocable. Shame is indisputably quintessential in regulating deviant behaviors in any society and provides us with the liberty to feel pride at respecting others and shame when trampling on the rights of others (Braithwaite, 1993). However, when propelling this emotion through the medium of the Internet, we often engage in medieval methods of shaming that allows little room for reintegration and social regulation but stigmatization and ostracism. Since digital media and shaming are a newly found construct developed only in the last two decades, there is a dearth of information that we can find concerning how people experience vigilantism and subsequent shame in a virtual space. We are yet to explore the disadvantages of this fast-paced technological growth, and therefore long-term mental health consequences of online shaming are likely to be explored only shortly.

4 Methodology

4.1 Participants

The population for this study included 24 participants, 6 males and 19 females, from India within the age range of 18–29, since this population accounts for the maximum social media usage, and the same population has witnessed the complete life cycle of social media (Huffman, 2016). Participants were recruited using a convenience sampling method due to skimpy availability of consent for participation.

Inclusion Criteria Participants should have at least one active social media account. Participants should give consent to participate in the study. Participants should be a resident of India.

Exclusion Criteria Participants who were unable to associate with the sociocultural context of India were excluded from the study.

4.2 Research Paradigm

The researchers attempted to understand and interpret the notion of young adults about shaming in digital spaces. A qualitative analytical approach allows in-depth interaction with the data and therefore aids in the inductive process of understanding notions of shame. The approach involved thematic analysis of content obtained through a survey questionnaire. The rhetorical assumption was that the informal and personal voices of the participants were considered essential in constructing the formulated thematic framework.

4.3 Procedure

A brief about the purpose of the study was circulated among different online chat groups, and those who consented and fit the inclusion criteria were provided with the online survey questionnaire. They were ensured about their rights to be a research participant, especially regarding confidentiality and their right to withdraw. Their responses were recorded as text through a survey questionnaire and were further analyzed.

4.4 Survey Questionnaire

The survey questionnaire was constructed to collect the data online using the chat groups available on social media. The first part of the questionnaire contained sociodemographic details of the participants like age, gender, highest educational qualification, and nationality. The second part of the questionnaire contained the main section with questions directly inquiring about digital shaming. There were ten questions directly focusing on the concept of "digital shaming" and its effect on the participants.

4.5 Method of Data Collection

Data was collected using a survey questionnaire prepared by the researchers using themes derived from the conceptual map. It mostly included the idea of digital media, the breach of privacy, and the irreversibility of information, the concept of shame as witnessed and experienced in the digital world. Different facets of these constructs were conceptualized to obtain a framework. It was further validated by two academicians from the discipline of psychology. The survey questionnaire contained open-ended questions to which participants expressed their thoughts, opinions, and experiences in digital spaces. Table 20.1 shows the lines of inquiry and sample questions in the survey questionnaire.

Table 20.1 Showing the lines of inquiry and sample questions in the survey questionnaire

Domain	Lines of inquiry	Sample questions
The idea about digital media and online shaming	To understand notions of privacy and irreversibility of info, online shaming	What do you think about privacy online? What is your opinion about online shaming?
Shame	Experiencing or witnessing shame	Have you ever experienced online shaming? Describe the experience Have you ever witnessed online shaming? Describe the experience
Consequence of shaming	Actions following the act of shaming	What steps would you take if you are shamed (trolled) in social media for one of your actions? What do you think is the future of individuals once shamed in social media?
Apology	The reaction toward apology if any	If you had been shamed publicly in social media, what would you feel if people apologize privately for shaming you? If you had been shamed publicly in social media, what would you feel if people apologize publicly for shaming you?

4.6 *Analysis*

The data obtained were manually coded for repeated words, phrases, or ideas. Similar codes were clustered to form themes and were then corroborated with overarching themes. Organizing and global themes were derived, and the patterns within the data were represented in a conceptual framework.

4.7 *Ethical Considerations*

The proposal was presented at the research committee of the affiliated institution for ethical clearance. The consent for participation was obtained from all the participants. They were briefed about the objectives of the study and possible implications. Pseudo names respective to their gender and age were used in the analysis to quote relevant themes. They were assured confidentiality of the information shared, and the personally identifiable data (mail address) collected was assured to be deleted 1 year after the study by October 2020.

5 Findings

The data received from the survey questionnaire was subjected to the process of qualitative research using the procedures of coding, categorizing, and deriving relevant themes while maintaining a connection with the raw data. An inter-subjective validation procedure, where both the authors coded the data separately, was performed to ensure maximum engagement with the data.

The preliminary categories of grouping after coding were considered as the basic themes, and the grouping of sub-themes resulted in the four main themes (Table 20.2).

5.1 Notions About Online Shaming

This chapter attempted to understand the concepts of online shaming in young adults. Online shaming refers to the act of engaging in shaming the behavior of a group or of an individual who have or is perceived to have violated a cultural norm through blaming, inducing guilt, assigning blame, sharing their identity or hate content, and calling in for a similar action from the members of the social group (Huffman, 2016). From the data received, the authors identified four major themes regarding the notions of online shaming among young adults: encountering shame, perceived sentiments on shaming, perceived consequences of shaming, and characteristics assigned to the vigilante (Fig. 20.1).

5.2 Characteristics Assigned to the Vigilante

With respect to shaming behavior, two groups converse with each other, one that shamed and the other that shames. In the process of shaming, the latter tells the other that they are not worthy enough and instill feelings of inadequacy. The data suggested that there are some common characteristics for those in the latter group, like feelings of inferiority, concept of policing, use of anonymity, and ingenuity (Fig. 20.2).

Table 20.2 Showing an illustration of the process of theme construction

Text	Code	Sub-theme	Main theme
Once shamed, it stays in your conscience forever	Experience of shaming	Fear of being infamous	Perceived sentiments on shaming
I just took the simplest step out of it. I deleted my online account walked out of it	Reaction to online shaming	Limiting activity	Encountering shame

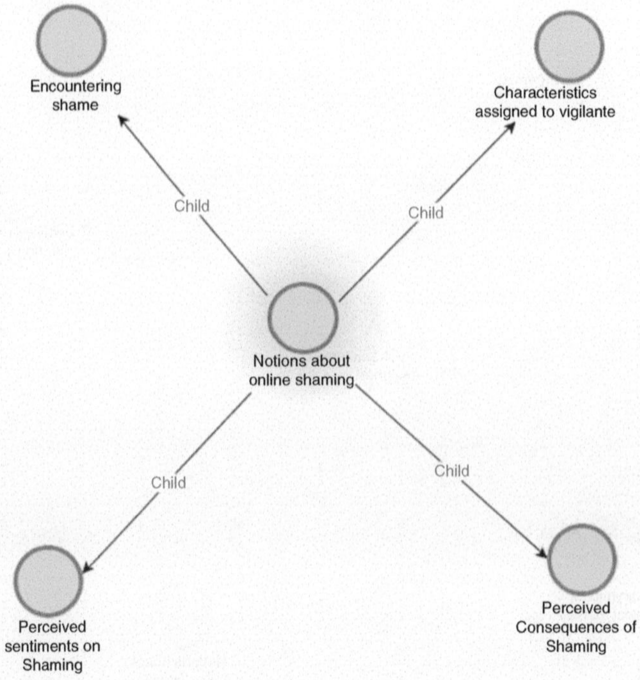

Fig. 20.1 Pictorial representation of the main themes derived from the data

5.2.1 Feelings of Inferiority

Most participants considered that people engage in shaming others because they potentially had a dearth in themselves. Many considered that these people were inferior in their intellect that they could not take another perspective and therefore assumed that the best option to deal with shaming was ignoring the shaming behavior. According to the data, people who engage in vigilante behavior often considered themselves to be cultural warriors and therefore have a need to monitor the actions of others. According to the survey results, a participant, Joseph, a 29-year-old student from South India, commented, "And ignored if the standard and intellectual capacity of the commenters were well visible. I don't respond to people who don't deserve it" (Personal Communication, October 25, 2019).

5.2.2 Anonymity of Physical Identity

In a digital space, an individual is identified by his digital profile, and therefore his physical identity remains anonymous. Often vigilante behaviors root from anonymous profiles, where the vigilante is at his comfort behind a screen and has little physical contact or knowledge about the victim.

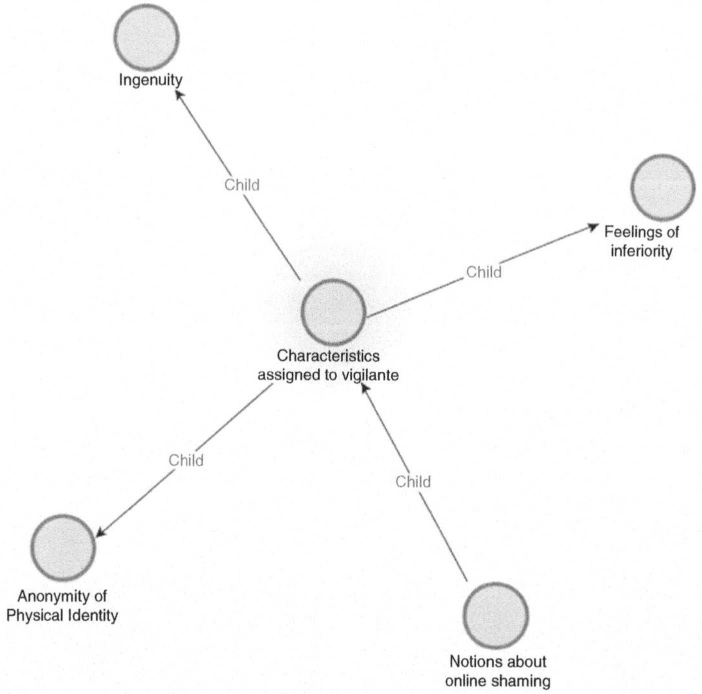

Fig. 20.2 Pictorial representation of organizing theme – characteristics assigned to vigilante

> The social media society consists of a mass of people who have found comfort behind the comparatively safer side behind the phone or laptop. Sharing their thoughts have become easier and with it the control they exercise over their thoughts have drastically reduced. So, I see it as nothing lesser than an utter spineless, misdemeanor that should have been rooted out at a younger age (Rishit, 19 years of age, male participant, Personal Communication, November 13, 2019).

5.2.3 Ingenuity

The data suggested that those who engage in vigilante behavior are less likely to be genuine even when they made an apology when some considered their behavior to be attention-seeking and gaudy; others opine that they do things to avoid trouble for themselves. "Somewhat relieved with public apology though if the apology was only for show then of course it won't sit well with me" (Hiya, 21 years of age, female participant, Personal Communication, November 23, 2019).

5.3 *Encountering Shame*

Although not many participants were comfortable to disclose their personal experiences of shaming in the digital space, there was a consensus about the excruciating commonness of online shaming and its consequences on the victim. When the participants witnessed or experienced shaming in the digital space, most of them reported having altered some fragments of their behavior online to cease the effects of shaming. Some limited their activity or contact, whereas some others resorted to their feelings of agitation and uneasiness and suffered in silence. The sub-themes derived revolved around the reaction of the victim toward the shaming situation and the vigilante (Fig. 20.3).

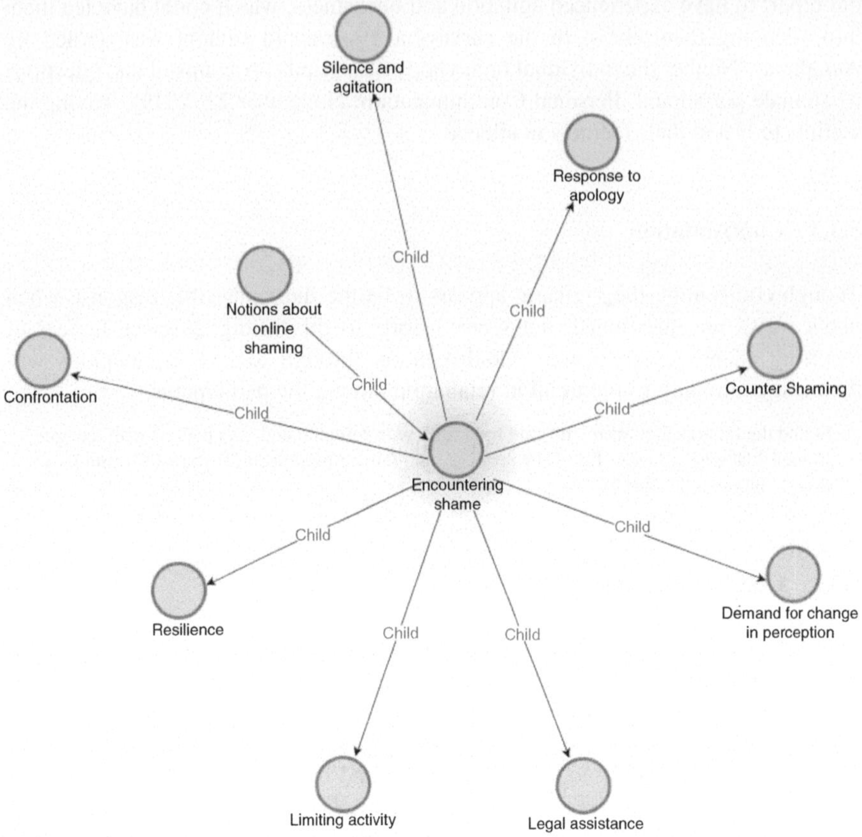

Fig. 20.3 Pictorial representation of organizing theme – encountering shame

5.3.1 Limiting Activity

One of the most common responses was to limit their activity online. Few responded that they would "deactivate" their accounts or at least "remove" the controversial material (Alex, Mahika, Aaradya & Shaiza, Personal Communication). One of the participants even attempted to explain the reduced activity from a gendered perspective in shaming behavior:

> I have seen and experienced it especially when a woman come out and speak there is a group of men and women who starts abusing you on the basis of gender, religion etc. Most of the women do not comment on social media to avoid conflicts even if they want to support someone. (Hiya, 21 years of age, female participant, Personal Communication, November 23, 2019)

5.3.2 Silence and Agitation

Though there was not any explicit mention of fear of consequences, few participants did report to have experienced agitation and uneasiness, which could have led them into silencing themselves. In the survey, a 19-year-old student was quoted by Aaradhya, "Neither the individual or anybody else stands up against it and questions it" (female participant, Personal Communication, November 23, 2019), leaving the victims to brood their feelings in silence.

5.3.3 Confrontation

Though confronting the vigilante appears to be the most plausible response when one's views are questioned, not many resorts to this in digital space in fear of recurring shaming experiences. Confrontation through logical explanations was the most commonly found trend in retaliation among the participants.

> Stated the facts as they were, the cold hard truth with research and stats backed with receipts in their blabbering faces (Tanvi, 19 years of age, female participant, Personal Communication, November 13, 2019).

5.3.4 Counter Shaming

The data advocates that people sometimes engage in shaming the vigilante for his shaming behavior. It is found to be shared mainly when the shaming is not inflicted on self but someone close to self. Rishit had strongly opinionated about the same as below "If it calls out only to me, I'd feel free to ignore it. But if it is raised against my kin or friends, I am going to take it personally and make sure he feels ashamed for what he did" (Rishit, 19 years of age, male participant, Personal Communication, November 13, 2019). When interpreted with the collectivistic notion of blending with one's in-group, an other-promoting self can be observed in the above lines.

5.3.5 Legal Assistance

Since digital space is a relatively new interactive space, the legal systems have not adequately defined and structured the behavior expectations in this space. However, many participants reported having sorted legal assistance at the face of shaming and believed that shaming could be controlled and regulated with legal systems in place. Participants like Hem, 22-year-old male participant, showed their belief in systems "I would immediately take a screenshot and take it up with the cyber wing of the police and see to that the culprit is caught and punished" (Personal Communication, November 13, 2019), whereas, for participants like Aaradhya, 19-year-old female participant, seeking legal assistance was a valor that they had to develop as interpreted from lines below "I think now I am confident about myself I would complain about it" (Personal Communication, November 23, 2019).

5.3.6 Resilience

Resilience is the ability to be positive about the experiences and therefore strive toward better outcomes rather than brooding on past downfalls. Although scarce, data suggested that resilience is one key element that helps the victims of online shaming to revert to their previous selves. Most of the data had an empathetic approach toward the victim, as in the excerpt from the response of a 21-year-old Hiya, "Some overcome it some never come out of it. It's sad and bad" (Personal Communication, November 23, 2019).

5.3.7 Demand for Change in Perception of Vigilante

The data suggested that when people encountered shaming experiences, they wanted to either prove the vigilante wrong or make them understand that their perception is not the only truth. Although both are more or less similar in the functionality, it was found that data excerpts for proving the vigilante wrong were found to be more aggressive as in "I will ask them to post the same publicly, in the same platform they have made the negative comments and also withdraw their initial posts" (Joseph, 29 years of age, male participant, Personal Communication, November 25, 2019), whereas when data suggested changing the perception of the vigilante, participants took a more cordial tone. An example of the same is given below "It would be a great relief not that I got an apology but because at least one person changed his/her ugly perspective" (Hiya, 21 years of age, female participant, Personal Communication, November 23, 2019).

5.3.8 Response to Apology

When enquired about the response to the apology, many demanded that anything less than a public apology is a farce. An example of a demanding apology is "If people shame you in front of everyone, they should have the courage to apologize that way too" (Shaiza, 20 years of age, female participant, Personal Communication, November 23, 2019). A small proportion of the participants responded that they are ready to forgive the vigilante as in "I would forgive them. Everyone deserves a second chance" (Saloni, 22 years of age, female participant, Personal Communication, November 13, 2019) or in "I will forgive them but no further interaction" (Navya, 21 years of age, female participant, Personal Communication, November 13, 2019). Further probing and analysis are required to understand if forgiveness comes from the idea of supremacy over the vigilante with respect to intellect.

5.4 Perceived Consequences of Shaming

When individuals face shaming in digital spaces, responses are many ranging from silence to counter shaming the vigilante. However, the data suggests a few long-term consequences of shaming – stunting of creativity, self-doubt, and the irreversibility of shame (Fig. 20.4).

5.4.1 Stunting Creativity

Digital spaces are often areas of expression and creativity of oneself. However, when a person is shamed for his opinion or creativity, self-doubt is likely to occur, which leads to the stunting of creativity. "Online shaming does take a toll. This would make us think twice before speaking out again. Then again, that's what these people want" (Hem, 22 years of age, male participant, Personal Communication, November 13, 2019).

5.4.2 Self-Doubt

It is the most common and excruciating consequence of shaming as perceived by the participants. Individuals, once shamed, enter a vicious cycle where their experience of shaming makes them doubt their opinions, thereby stopping them from making further expressions online. It can be considered in conjunction with the fear of judgment. A fragment of this fear can be observed in the excerpt, "Consider if what I did was really worthy of being shamed, was it really wrong?" (Tanvi, 19 years of age, female participant, Personal Communication, November 13, 2019).

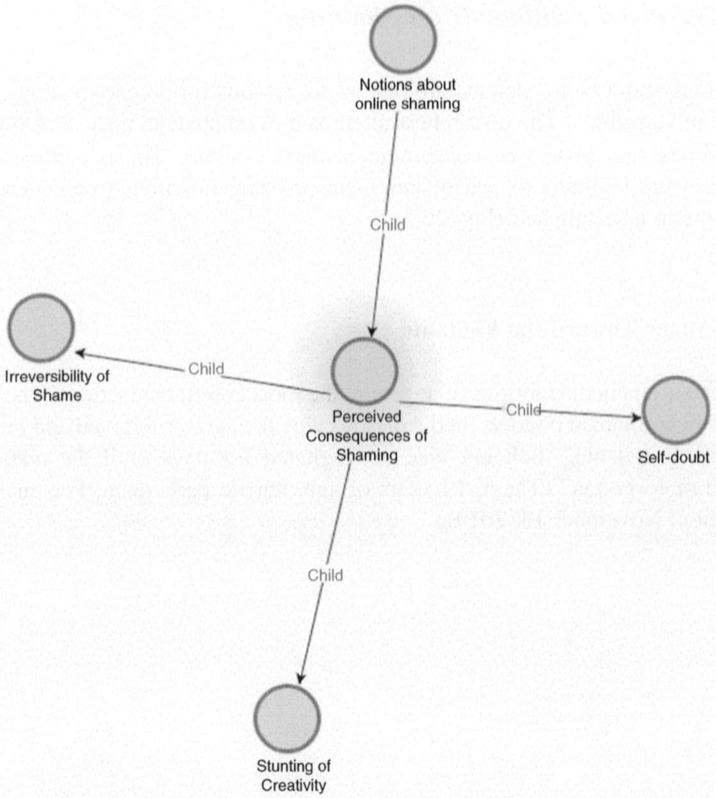

Fig. 20.4 Pictorial representation of organizing theme – perceived consequences of shaming

5.4.3 Irreversibility of Shame

Digital spaces are closed spaces where any information, once let out, cannot be contained. This property of irreversibility of the Internet makes it difficult for victims of shaming to distance themselves from the shamed content. A quote from Shaiza that "Once you are publicly shamed nothing changes the fact that everyone's seen it and is probably making a joke about it" (20 years of age, female participant, Personal Communication, November 23, 2019) represents this fear for irreversibility. Some data even proposed that even apology at any length would not ease the situation for the person who has been shamed. Therefore, the fear of irreversibility of shame alone is strong enough to limit one's activity online.

5.5 *Perceived Sentiments on Shaming*

Perceptions about being shamed are one of the reasons for people to avoid shame-related conversations. The researchers attempted to understand these different fears and feelings one possesses concerning shamed content. Those included anger directed at the vigilante to fear of judgment or being infamous to embarrassment and shame in asserting self (Fig. 20.5).

5.5.1 Anger Toward the Vigilante

When one is shamed, emotions of anger are the most common reactions. The person who has been shamed ponders on the reasons why he/she was targeted and felt anger toward the vigilante. "Felt not nice and agitated for days until the matter was resolved or forgotten" (Tanvi, 19 years of age, female participant, Personal Communication, November 13, 2019).

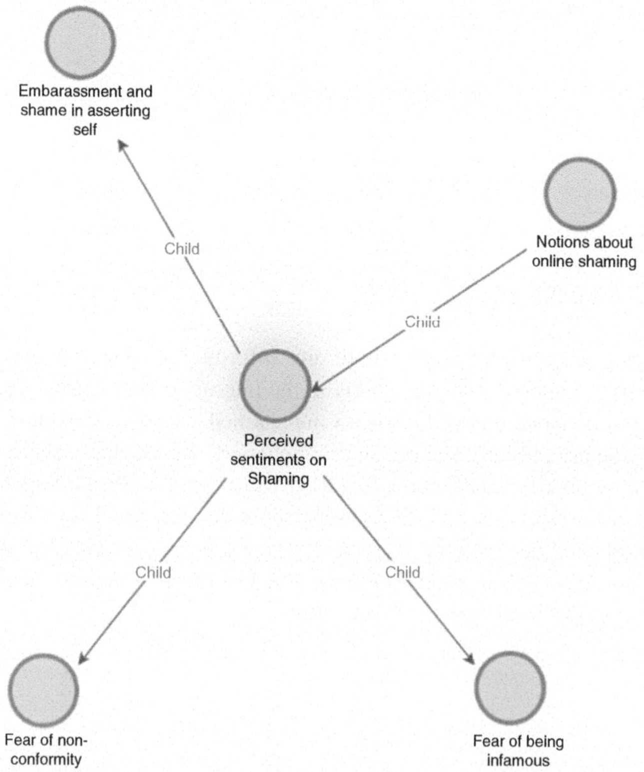

Fig. 20.5 Pictorial representation of organizing theme – perceived sentiments on shaming

5.5.2 Fear of Non-conformity and Judgment

Most people choose to conform to societal systems and rules in their fear of judgment from others. This fear of judgment due to non-conformity needs curbs his creativity and also contributes to self-doubt. An excerpt from the data is as below "I would not consider expressing my opinions on any online platform which can be assessed by anyone" (Aarav, 28 years of age, male participant, Personal Communication, November 25, 2019).

5.5.3 Fear of Being Infamous

Shame-related conversations are sometimes avoided due to the fear of becoming infamous. It should be considered in conjunction with the irreversible nature of data online. As in the excerpt below, "Being known for a bad thing is not a very good thing. These individuals surely have a lot to face which they actually shouldn't be facing" (Hiya, 21 years of age, female participant, Personal Communication, November 23, 2019); the fear of being infamous can also curb one's creativity and growth.

5.5.4 Embarrassment and Shame to Assert Self

Most of the time, participants were accepting of the vigilante when the self was targeted. However, when a close friend or kin was shamed, the response was more outrageous. Although the reason for this self-sacrificing behavior is quite grimmer, it can be assumed that the collectivistic cultural outlook and its ingraining with the ideology of promoting self only after the other have contributed to the feelings of embarrassment and shame to assert one's self. An example of the expression can be seen below.

> If it calls out only to me, I'd feel free to ignore it. But if it is raised against my kin or friends, I am going to take it personally and make sure he feels ashamed for what he did (Rishit, 19 years of age, male participant, Personal Communication, November 13, 2019).

6 Discussion

Shaming has been an age-old technique of denunciation to ostracize or reintegrate outliers into the mainstream line of thought. Often this has helped us in maintaining values and harmony within the communities. With the dawn of the Internet and instant connectivity in the early 1990s, many people have tried to conquer the digital spaces with their expressions and ideologies. The Internet, more or less, became a second space where we assumed an identity very similar to our physical identity, but unlike the physical identity, this new face in the virtual world has the advantage of instant connectivity and vast opportunity for exploration. The Internet brought with it a virtual society where ignominy became much more comfortable to inflict than ever before due to the easy accessibility of the other. In this chapter, we attempted to explore the notions of online shaming among young adults from a predominantly collectivistic culture who had been more or less part of the Internet throughout its life cycle.

In cases of social surveillance and associated shaming, people had a choice to distance themselves from the transgressors by maintaining a physical distance, whereas, in the virtual world, it is nearly impossible to distance oneself from the effects of surveillance. The metaphorical analogy of Foucault, the panopticon, has become more or less a reality than a metaphor with the Internet being the medium of digital surveillance and privacy, a questionable possession. Individuals, therefore, become "carefully fabricated" in the social order of the virtual space rather than being devoid of repression (Mason, 2019). However, surveillance need not necessarily be immoral or unjustified always, as in the case of a mob surveilling the tyrannies.

The Internet allows many conveniences, which we cannot avail in social spaces like the ones of anonymity, connectivity, and spontaneity. Anonymity is like a double-sided sword that allows people to express freely without being publicly identified but, at the same time, undermining privacy by allowing easy invasion into other's privacy (Wehmhoener, 2010). Connectivity and spontaneity have eased our access with the world and, on the contrary, facilitate shaming behavior to be spread like wildfire. Shaming behavior is essential in any societal order to maintain conformity to rules and for reintegrative purposes in cases of violation. However, the paper questions to what extent this can be performed when shaming behaviors are adopted to virtual spaces. The profound breach of privacy and irreversibility of the shame or shaming content are the two significant characteristics that make online shaming maladaptive. Online spaces allow easy access to one's information, therefore making it easier for the vigilante groups to target and shame the individual in all spheres of his/her life. From the data on online notions on shaming, there was a broad consensus on the idea of the irreversibility of shame. When the concept of the irreversibility of information is paired with the profound breach of privacy, it becomes a vicious cycle, where the victim is subjected to experience shame for an enduring and incessant time leading to mental health consequences in many.

Being the victim of shaming for whatsoever reason is not a pleasant experience. Especially when one's privacy has been invaded, and shaming content has become viral, victims of shame generally undergo an exceptional level of stress. Data suggests that silence is to be considered as one of the most common reactions to shaming. This silence can include distancing themselves from virtual spaces by limiting activity or limiting contact. The concept of organizational silence by Morrison and Milleken (2000) can be observed among the audience of shaming. Although they experience cognitive dissonance with the vigilante, the social contagion creates a "climate of silence," and they remain silent instead of being the next victim. The spiral of silence theory by Noelle-Neumann (1974) can also be applied in this context where people superficially agree to the vigilante by maintaining silence but do not believe the same internally (Huffman, 2016). This silence is assumed to be a product of the fear that people possess, the fear of judgment or non-conformity. Often when one falls prey to shaming behavior, either witnessing or experiencing it, a sense of self-doubt can arise, especially concerning the rightness of one's thoughts and actions. The cultural context of shame induction through etiquette and ethics, which is common in collectivistic cultures through concepts like lajjA, can also aggravate the situation. lajjA assumes silence as a modest method of retaliation and often is faced with more shaming from the vigilante. It can lead to severe mental health complications that might require clinical assistance to come out. Another critical finding derived from the data is that individuals were very reluctant to assert themselves, but when they supported someone close to them, they were actively confronting the vigilante. This concept needs further probing, and the authors assume that this behavior can be correlated with the notions of collectivistic culture. The authors assume that the fusion ideology of the east, especially the embodiment of concepts like lajjA, enables people to support one another, increasing in-group loyalties and demarcating out-groups as unknown. An alternate explanation could also be the concept of empathy. The fact that individuals can support someone else comes from the concept that they may feel empathetic toward their plight. The first step of empathy is about feeling the same emotion that the other victim is going through. It is possible mostly when the former has experienced prior shaming but was helpless to take a stand for themselves.

Shaming or doxing as a method aimed at reintegrating individuals back into the community, and it is this very emotion of shame that keeps us away from engaging in unlawful or harmful behaviors. However, when shaming behavior occurs in digital spaces, the same reintegrative function might not be a consequence for many. The irreversibility of the shaming content interweaved with the invasion of privacy most times only leads to ostracism. Therefore, it would be unjust to consider that shaming on the Internet has a reintegrative function making it an ideal example of maladaptive shaming. The concept of cultural relativity can well enumerate the reason for individuals engaging in consequent self-conscious activities like limiting contact, maintaining silence, and so on and so forth.

The idea of who is a vigilante and what characteristics he can be associated with was an interesting finding. When people who engaged in vigilantism considered themselves to be warriors of culture, many on the other side of the act considered that they had an inferior intellect, and that is the reason for their inability to accept another perspective very different from theirs. The supremacy that the victim feels through this characterization could be interpreted as a method of dealing with the shame that they had been inflicted. Also, the idea of reverse shaming, where the vigilante is shamed by the victim, leading to a role reversal, was an unexpected finding. It can be assumed that those who engage in reverse shaming could become vigilantes of their ideologies under adequate circumstances, thereby contradicting their association of vigilante with the feelings of inferiority.

7 Summary

The chapter attempted to understand the notion of shaming in virtual spaces in a predominantly collectivistic culture through a phenomenological approach. Online shaming was assumed to be a common phenomenon experienced by young adults in the Indian context, and therefore a convenient sampling method was adopted to understand the same. The data derived from the survey questionnaire was thematically analyzed to create a comprehensive understanding of the concept in the peculiar cultural context of India, where shame, *lajjA*, is an ambivalent emotion of shame experienced both at times of not doing what is expected and at times of doing what is expected. The concepts of reverse shaming, who qualifies to be a vigilante, and how the property of irreversibility in virtual spaces contributes to the experience were key findings of the study. Shame is an ambivalent emotion, and the peculiar notions of Indian culture make the experience of shame both pleasant and unpleasant at the same time. Digitization and the advent of networking websites have exponentially improved connectivity and spontaneity of communication. At the same time, this also brings in the challenge of dealing with excruciating shaming patterns. As we embrace the fast-paced technological advancements, we also need to inculcate novel practices of safety and data protection to reap the benefits of shame.

8 Limitations and Future Directions

The data recommend a few future directions that need to be further probed and inquired in order to understand the concept of shame and shaming in digital spaces more comprehensively. The chapter was a preliminary approach to understand the experience and observations on shame in digital spaces. It did not emphasize on gendered expressions of shame in virtual spaces. The concept of reverse shaming requires further inquiry to have a comprehensive understanding of shaming in digital spaces. Future research should explore the different in-group dynamics within the virtual space, which might be different from physical geographical boundaries and corroborate the same with that in a social space. It should also question the notion of vigilante being the very dynamic nature of virtual spaces as well as the socioeconomic and political nature of society; its inculcation of cosmopolitan globalism and the subsequent effects on ignominy require elaborate phenomenological approaches.

References

Ariffin, E. (2018, October 15). *India's new fourth industrial revolution* centre. The Asean Post. Retrieved from: https://theaseanpost.com/article/indias-new-fourth-industrial-revolution-centre

Bastin, C., Harrison, B. J., Davey, C. G., Moll, J., & Whittle, S. (2016). Feelings of shame, embarrassment and guilt and their neural correlates: A systematic review. *Neuroscience and Biobehavioral Reviews, 71*(1), 455–471. https://doi.org/10.1016/j.neubiorev.2016.09.019.

Bhawuk, D. P. (2017). lajjA in Indian psychology: Spiritual, social and literary perspectives. In E. Vanderheiden & C.-H. Mayer (Eds.), *The value of shame- exploring a health resource in cultural contexts* (pp. 109–134). Cham: Springer Nature.

Bhawuk, D. P. (2019). lajjA: Learning, unlearning and relearning. In C. H. Mayer & E. Vanderheiden (Eds.), *The bright side of shame transforming and growing through practical applications in cultural aspects* (pp. 35–49). Cham: Springer Nature.

Blumler, J. G., & McQuail, D. (1969). *Television in politics: Its uses and influence*. Chicago: University of Chicago Press.

Braithwaite, J. (1993). Shame and modernity. *The British Journal of Criminology, 33*(1), 1–18. Retrieved January 14, 2020, from www.jstor.org/stable/23637738

Creighton, M. R. (1990). Revisiting shame and guilt cultures: A forty-year pilgrimage. *Ethos, 18*(3), 279–307. Retrieved from:. https://doi.org/10.1525/eth.1990.18.3.02a00030.

Gandikota, V., & Rao, S. (1955). The impact of industrialization on indian society. *Columbia Journal of International Affairs., 4*(2), 50–60.

Goodlad, L. (2003). Beyond the Panopticon: Victorian Britain and the critical imagination. PMLA, 118(3), 539–556. Retrieved January 18, 2020, from www.jstor.org/stable/1261525

Huffman, E. M. (2016). *Call-out culture: How online shaming affects social media participation in young adults* (Order No. 10120833). Available from ProQuest Dissertations & Theses Global. (1795577817). Retrieved from https://search.proquest.com/docview/1795577817?accountid=38885

Industrial Revolution. (2019). In A. Augustyn, P. Bauer, B. Duignan, A. Eldridge, E. Gregersen, A. McKenna, M. Petruzzelo, J. P. Rafferty, M. Ray, K. Rogers, A. Tikkanen, J. Wallenfeldt, A. Zeidan, & A. Zelazko (Eds.), *Encyclopaedia Britannica*. Retrieved from: https://www.britannica.com/event/Industrial-Revolution

Keng, S. L., & Tan, J. X. (2017). Effects of brief mindful breathing and loving-kindness meditation on shame and social problem solving abilities among individuals with high borderline personality traits. *Behaviour Research and Therapy, 97*(1), 43–51. https://doi.org/10.1016/j.brat.2017.07.004.

Kumarappa, J. C. (1945). *Public finance and our poverty*. Ahmedabad: Navajivan Publishing House.

Maibom, H. (2010). The descent of shame. *Philosophy and Phenomenological Research, 80*(3), 566–594. Retrieved January 14, 2020, from www.jstor.org/stable/20722807

Mason, L. (2019). The self & political possibilities in dewey & foucault: comparative implications for school & society. *Journal of Thought, 53*(2), 3–20. https://doi.org/10.2307/26727282.

McGinnis, D. (2018). *What is the fourth industrial revolution?* Retrieved from: https://www.salesforce.com/blog/2018/12/what-is-the-fourth-industrial-revolution-4IR.html

Morrison, E. W., & Milliken, F. J. (2000). Organizational silence: A barrier to change and development in a pluralistic world. *Academy of Management Review, 25*(4), 706–725. Retrieved from:. https://doi.org/10.5465/amr.2000.3707697.

Nash, D., & Kilday, A. M. (2010). The history and theory of shame — Then and now. In *Cultures of shame*. London: Palgrave Macmillan. https://doi.org/10.1057/9780230309098_1.

Niiler, E. (2019). *How the second industrial revolution changed Americans' lives*. Retrieved from: https://www.history.com/news/second-industrial-revolution-advances

Noelle-Neumann, E. (1974). The spiral of silence a theory of public opinion. *Journal of Communication, 24*(2), 43–51. https://doi.org/10.1111/j.1460-2466.1974.tb00367.x.

Obschonka, M. (2018). *The industrial revolution left psychological scars that can still be seen today*. Retrieved from: https://hbr.org/2018/03/research-the-industrial-revolution-left-psychological-scars-that-can-still-be-seen-today

Press Trust of India. (2018, October 11). Modi sees India making a big contribution to '4th industrial Revolution'. *The Hindu*. Retrieved from: https://www.thehindu.com/news/national/4th-industrial-revolution-to-change-nature-of-jobs-modi/article25193154.ece

Rifkin, J. (n.d.). *Welcome to the third industrial revolution*. Retrieved from: https://magazine.wharton.upenn.edu/issues/summer-2015/welcome-to-the-third-industrial-revolution/

Rousell, J. H. (2016). Cross cultural expressions of pathological narcissism. In *International conference on counselling, psychotherapy and wellness*. Bangalore: Christ University.

Schalkwijk, F., Stams, G. J., Dekker, J., & Elison, J. (2016). Measuring shame regulations: Validation of the compass of shame scale. *Social Behavior and Personality, 44*(11), 1775–1791.
Sinha, M., & Chauhan, V. (2013). Deconstructing lajjA as a marker of Indian womanhood. *Psychology and Developing Societies, 25*(1), 133–163. https://doi.org/10.1177/0971333613477314.
Stearns, P. (2017). The impact of modernity: Some possibilities. In *Shame: A brief history* (pp. 49–56). Urbana, Chicago; Springfield: University of Illinois Press. Retrieved January 9, 2020, from www.jstor.org/stable/10.5406/j.ctt1vjqrq8.8.
The Economic Times. (2020, September 22). From finance to healthcare, India is adopting automation at a global pace: ET-ILC members. *The Economic Times*. Read more at: https://economictimes.indiatimes.com/tech/ites/from-finance-to-healthcare-india-is-adopting-automation-at-a-global-pace-et-ilc-members/articleshow/78251041.cms?utm_source=contentofinterest&utm_medium=text&utm_campaign=cppst; https://economictimes.indiatimes.com/tech/ites/from-finance-to-healthcare-india-is-adopting-automation-at-a-global-pace-et-ilc-members/articleshow/78251041.cms?from=mdr.
Tignor, S. M., & Colvin, C. R. (2017). The interpersonal adaptiveness of dispositional guilt and shame: A meta-analytic investigation. *Journal of Personality, 85*(3), 341–363. https://doi.org/10.1111/jopy.12244.
Trottier, D. (2017). Digital vigilantism as weaponization of visibility. *Philosophy & Technology, 30* (1), 55–72. https://doi.org/10.1007/s13347-016-0216-4.
Tuo, C. (2017). New perspective of cosmopolitanism: From individualism to globalism. World Economics and Politics, 9, 156–157. Retrieved January 18, 2020 from http://jtp.cnki.net/bilingual/detail/html/SJJZ201709003
Wettlaufer, J. (2012). Neurohistorical and evolutionary aspects of a history of shame and shaming. *RCC Perspectives, 6*, 49–54. Retrieved from: http://www.jstor.org/stable/26240405.

Grace Maria Jochan considers herself as a zealous professional in psychology, currently working as an Assistant Professor at Mount Carmel College, Bangalore, India. She has completed a master's degree in clinical psychology from Christ University, Bangalore, and has qualified the National Eligibility Test for Assistant Professorship. She is keen on qualitative research and has made a publication on self-expression and entitlement among individuals high on narcissism in the International Journal of Indian Psychology. Research areas that she would like to focus include self, personality, digital media, women, and health. She had ample internship experiences at various mental health institutions in South India and looks forward to challenging and rewarding tasks that would help her harness her personal research, clinical, and teaching skills.

Trina Banerjee is a licensed clinical psychologist, behavior analyst, and a psychotherapist currently working as a lecturer in psychology at Mount Carmel College, Bangalore. She has a clinical experience of 4 years and has practiced as a psychotherapist in government hospitals. She also works in the industry as an organizational psychologist. Trina completed her masters in psychology from the University of Calcutta, followed by an MPhil in clinical psychology from the Institute of Psychiatry – Centre for Excellence, Kolkata. She has received a certification of Applied Behavior Analysis from Board Certified Behavior Analyst (BCBA) in 2013. She has presented papers at national and international conferences. She was the winner of "Saugata Basu Memorial Award" for receiving the highest score in clinical psychology in 2014. Trina takes interest in an eclectic approach to psychotherapy. She believes in integrating the various therapeutic approaches to deliver what is best for the present situation. She values art and tries to integrate art and music into a therapeutic framework. She has been trained in behavior therapy, cognitive behavior therapy (CBT), and psychoanalysis. She has experience in couples' therapy, mostly involving marital discord. Trina's area of interest involves neuropsychological profile of developmental disorders of children. She has worked extensively with specific learning disability, autism, and communication disorders. Her work constituted of neuropsychological assessment and neurorehabilitation of children and adolescents.

Chapter 21
Real-World Consequences of Devirtualization from Online to Offline Spaces: The Role of Shame as a Resource in the Honor Killing of Qandeel Baloch

Paul A. Wilson and Barbara Lewandowska-Tomaszczyk

1 Introduction

There are many instances of the role of shame in protest campaigns conducted within the space of social media. For example, activists on social media have recently employed the tactic of "flight-shaming" in an attempt to reduce aviation carbon dioxide emissions (Calma, 2019). Walter Palmer, a Minnesota dentist, received a barrage of online criticism in 2015 in an attempt to shame him for killing Cecil the lion while he was on safari in Zimbabwe (Molloy, 2018). Given the global presence of such online protests, it is important to understand that as the meaning of shame differs across cultures (Lewandowska-Tomaszczyk & Wilson, 2017), the role of this emotion in these campaigns is also likely to depend on cultural variation. In recent years women in Pakistan have employed the use of social media to campaign against the oppression of women in their patriarchal, honor-based society. The present study investigates the role of shame in the honor killing of the Pakistani woman, Qandeel Baloch, by her brother, Waseem, following her online protest against such treatment.

P. A. Wilson (✉)
Institute of English Studies, University of Lodz, Lodz, Poland
e-mail: paul.wilson@uni.lodz.pl

B. Lewandowska-Tomaszczyk
State University of Applied Sciences in Konin, Konin, Poland
e-mail: barbara.lewandowska-tomaszczyk@konin.edu.pl

C.-H. Mayer et al. (eds.), *Shame 4.0*, https://doi.org/10.1007/978-3-030-59527-2_21

1.1 Background to the Honor Killing of Qandeel Baloch

Qandeel Baloch (real name Fouzia Azeem) was born into a modest family about 130 km from Multan in the traditional village of Shah Sadar Din in the South Punjabi district of Dera Ghazi Khan (Gabol & Subhani, 2016). She described her marriage at the age of 17 as her parents' enforcement of an uneducated husband upon her. She gave birth to a son and initially attempted to raise him on her own in Darul Aman after she fled there to escape the physical abuse by her husband. However, she was forced to transfer legal guardianship of her son to her husband after the child became seriously ill as she knew that she would be punished if the child died. After that she completed her bachelor's degree and had various jobs before modelling in photo shoots and fashion shows (Chaudhry, 2016).

Qandeel adopted her pseudonym and became a well-known social media celebrity who posted controversial comments, images, and videos in her feminist stance against the unequal treatment of women in the patriarchal society that dominates Pakistan. Her expression of her feminine sexuality, which she expressed through her scanty attire and provocative poses, as well as her verbal attacks on political and religious leaders (see Sect. 5), offended traditionalists in Pakistani society, but it also generated an online following of over 700,000 (Habiba, 2018). As Habiba (2018) further observes, it appears that Qandeel responded to her maltreatment in Pakistani patriarchal society by using her social media presence to call for women to empower themselves to oppose such gender inequality. She further called for women in Pakistan to become independent and support each other in this mission.

A key turning point in the demise of Qandeel was a scandal with Abdul Qavi, a famous cleric *Mufit* who is a member of the Religious Council in Pakistan. Qandeel posted a video and selfies of a meeting she had with Qavi on her online social media, in which she was dressed in a manner that could be deemed provocative in Pakistan and behaved inappropriately, for example, by posing playfully in Qavi's religious cap (Tahir, The Guardian, 2017). As a result of this, she appeared in talk shows on television in which the *Mufit* criticized her behavior as inappropriate. From this moment the mainstream media criticized the impropriety of her online actions. As Qandeel became the focus of further media scrutiny, one media outlet managed to obtain her passport and thus revealed her true identity. On 16th July, 2016, her brother, Waseem, sedated her and then strangled her to death. He stated that he did not regret murdering her as he felt compelled to do it to uphold the honor of his family (BBC Stories, 2017; The Guardian, 2017).

1.2 Aims

The overarching aim is to analyze a number of issues pertaining to the role of shame in the murder of Qandeel by her brother. It is initially important to note that an understanding of the underlying reasons for killing requires an analysis of both the actions of the victim and the perpetrator. From the viewpoint of shame as a social threat, it is necessary to attempt to determine how Qandeel and Waseem responded to this threat at different points. The role of audience is crucial in this respect, as identified in its potential to devalue the protagonists, their ability to replace a critical audience by forming new relationships, and their capacity to withstand devaluation on the basis of social status. Furthermore, these dynamic features of shame proneness need to be assessed from the perspective of Pakistani honor culture in terms of its relative influence on both the space of online social media and the offline space of the real world, as well as the boundary between them. Within this dynamicity, we further explore how Qandeel, through the online space that she created, transformed the resource of shame that was imposed on her as a woman in Pakistani honor culture into a vehicle of protest.

2 Shame

One of the major eliciting features of shame is negative criticism of the global self and is therefore related to evaluations of self-worth and self-esteem (Lewis, 1971). The central elements pertaining to this global self include acceptance or rejection by others, self-regulation, and self-evaluation. It is clear that such criticism involving the global self is more likely to be more threatening as damage to the very essence of one's being is at stake. Shame is further characterized by fear of this damage or criticism to the global self (Kam & Bond, 2008). Such involvement of the global self can be seen more clearly when one compares it with guilt, which is another self-conscious emotion, but one that is typically less hurtful than shame as the main focus is on behavior, not one's core self, and hence one's self-worth and self-esteem are less threatened (Tangney & Tracy, 2012). Ogarkova, Soriano, and Lehr (2012) observe that shame is elicited in response to the violation of an important social standard in which the transgressor is concerned with others' actual or imagined evaluations, which might lead to external sanctions. This highlights the social embeddedness of shame, which pertains to the major concern of social evaluation, namely how one perceives how one is viewed through the eyes of others rather than just negative assessment per se (Lewis, 1971). In this sense, audience is central to the experience of shame.

With respect to the effects of shame, the feeling of being small and the desire to avoid being seen by others lead to avoidance and withdrawal behaviors. Shame is more of an intense emotion than guilt and is associated with feelings of weakness, powerlessness, and helplessness. The tendency to hide, withdraw, and disappear, feelings of powerlessness, negative focus on the global self, and failure to meet one's standards and accomplish one's aspirations are consistent with approaches to shame outlined by Fontaine et al. (2006). Shame, unlike guilt, is also not characterized by an emphasis on reparations or penance (Ogarkova et al., 2012). Finally, shame can lead to aggressive behavior (Scheff, 2014).

2.1 Shame as a Master Emotion

The prominence of shame as one of the most, if not *the* most, important emotion in our lives can be witnessed in its unique function in social relationships due to its psychological and social importance, which has led to it being labeled a master emotion. To gain an understanding of the possible mechanisms underlying the influence of shame on emotions in its closest proximity, one needs to understand how physical threats and the threat of social exclusion are both associated with affective pain. MacDonald and Leary (2005) argue that "the aversive emotional state of social pain is the same unpleasantness that is experienced in response to physical pain" (p. 203). They further propose that one is motivated to avoid possible situations that threaten social exclusion through the feelings of pain that they are often coupled with in a similar way in which one learns to avoid physical threats. The role of shame in socially threatening situations is highlighted by Dickerson, Gruenewald, and Kemeny (2004), who identify shame and the physiological activity that accompanies it as a fundamental underlying emotional response to such threats in the same way that, for example, fear and its physiological responses occur when one is physically threatened. To summarize, shame can be viewed as an emotional response to social pain that is equivalent to unpleasant emotional states that are elicited by situations involving physical pain and threat.

The emotions that derive from the affective pain that accompanies threats to the preservation of one's social self, and hence shame, are similar to those emotions that have been widely documented to arise from the affective pain associated with physical threat. Furthermore, the social pain that underlies shame and physical pain elicit the same mechanisms to defend against such threats, namely the responses pertaining to *fight* (active opposition), *flight* (avoidance or withdrawal), and *fright* (immobility or freezing) (Elison, Garofalo, & Velotti, 2014).[1] These responses are directly relevant to the central proximity of shame to other emotions, with *flight* characterizing the prototypical fear response, opposition being a salient feature of *fight* and anger, and *fright* having close conceptual propinquity with depression due to the common feature of entrapment.

There are a number of factors that might determine which response, *fight*, *flight*, or *fright*, is more likely to be elicited in a certain situation. In this respect, contextual influences in the case of physical threat are likely to be equivalent to those present in the case of shame. The type of response elicited is determined by the proximity of threat. A moderately close threat induces fleeing, with fighting occurring in response to a more imminent danger and *fright* deployed in cases in which the source of danger is the closest (Bracha, 2004; Gallup, 1974; Ranter, 1977). MacDonald and Leary (2005) further contend that *fight* is the least preferred option with *flight* being preferred if there is an escape route and *fright* another alternative when escape is not possible. It is also important to note that *fright* is elicited in cases in which *fight* or

[1]Elison et al. (2014) prefer to use the term *freeze* instead of *fright*. However, these are equivalent and the term used in the present paper is *fright*.

flight is not likely to be effective (Schmidt, Richey, Zvolensky, & Maner, 2008). The fluidity that characterizes the deployment of these different types of strategies in response to threat is consistent with the observation by Elison et al. (2014) that, rather than being dependent on stable neurological architecture, these action tendencies are flexible and dependent on the situation and experience of similar incidents in the past.

2.2 *The Information Threat Theory of Shame*

The dynamics of protest within the online space of social media differ to that characterizing offline space in a number of ways. The information threat theory of shame (Sznycer et al., 2012) is relevant in this respect as it proposes that shame proneness is dependent on the following three variables: the opportunity to develop new relationships; the potential that an audience has to engage in devaluation; and the value of one's social status. Sznycer et al. (2012) further argue that a key feature in one's potential to reduce harmful effects of devaluation is *relational mobility*, which is the extent to which one is able to terminate old social relationships and develop new ones. This becomes clear if one considers the case in which an individual's established relationships constitute an audience that devalues them and are hence elicitors of shame. In the past, if that individual came from a society which was restricted in terms of mobility they would have less opportunity to replace such threatening relationships with more supportive relationships than an individual living in a more mobile society. However, with the development of online media, the fluidity regarding relationship termination and development is less restricted to geographical location. Specifically, it is possible to shift the emphasis of one's social engagement on new relationships within social media that are more supportive in favor of devaluing relationships in one's offline space. In these terms, the development of an online space can be viewed as an opportunity to increase *relational mobility* to transform the shame that can be used by society as a resource to coerce an individual to follow imposed norms into a protest platform that reaches a more supportive audience.

3 Shame and Honor Killing in Pakistan

The majority of honor killings are committed in Pakistan, India, and the Middle East, with the usual victims being females who are murdered by male family members because of their behavior that is perceived to be a source of family shame and dishonor. There were 1957 honor killings in Pakistan between 2004 and 2007 (Nasrullah, Haqqi, & Cummings, 2009), and although Patel and Gadit (2008) observe that the more remote areas of Sindh in Pakistan have a particularly high incidence, such murders have been reported in all four provinces of this country (Shah-Davis, 2011).

To understand the concept of honor killings, one needs to initially appreciate the role that women play in the honor of families and the wider community. As Shah-Davis (2011) observes, Pakistan is a typical collectivistic culture in the sense that honor, rather than being a feature of the individual, is a fundamental value of the family and the wider community. Specifically, honor in Pakistan underscores moral structure pertaining to rules, norms, and behavior, and is also the basis of respect toward one's family and social standing in one's community. Furthermore, in patriarchal cultures such as Pakistan it is male family members who have the role of protecting the honor that is seated in female members. Women can bring dishonor to the family by having, or allegedly having, an extramarital sexual affair. More recently, dishonor has been judged to include expressions of independence and autonomy such as choice with respect to whom to marry or divorce. Such autonomy is a key feature of dishonor that is relevant to our case study of Qandeel Baloch (see below), as is the expectation of modest behavior on the part of women, which is viewed as another source of dishonor.

It is additionally important to understand the motives of the, usually male, perpetrators of honor killings. From a social point of view, such murderers can be seen as victims of society, which exerts pressure on them to commit what is generally judged as an act of courage and honor (Habiba, 2018). With respect to the relevant debate concerning legitimacy and extenuating circumstances, however, many welcomed the change in Pakistani law in 2016 that imposes a mandatory 25-year prison sentence for honor killings and no longer allows pardons from family members (Boone, 2016). At the heart of the complex relationship between victim and perpetrator are shame and honor. A woman who engages in behavior deemed improper loses her social position and is shamed, which has a direct impact on the manliness and reputation of the male members of her family as they have lost ownership of the honor that resided in their female relative. In this sense, it is the woman's behavior, alleged or otherwise, that determines the honor status of the male family members. To regain honor that is lost and remove the shame, men need to punish the female transgressor, often violently. The sense of shame that underscores lost honor is evident in the disgrace and ridicule that can not only affect the family but the entire community. In terms of the significance of audience in the experience of shame that was outlined above, it is important to highlight that if a man fails to restore honor through killing the woman who is deemed dishonorable, he loses the respect and honor of other male family members and the community, who question his masculine status. The key point to note with respect to audience is that a potentially shameful act that is committed by a female family member only becomes a matter of honor to her male relatives if it becomes public knowledge.

4 Blurred Boundaries in Social Media Communication

A prototypical communicative act involves two participants: an author and an addressee engaged in a face-to-face spoken interaction. Computer-mediated communication provides a prototypical instance of the *interchangeability* design feature of language and human communication: the speaker interchanges his/her role with the addressee, and the exchanges develop dynamically during an interaction. However, what is observed in this form of communication is blurring the boundaries between the author and audience with the new concept of "audiencing," that is active authoring and exchanging the messages and massive user-generated content (Lewandowska-Tomaszczyk & Zeller, 2012). What is witnessed in contemporary situations is a further extension of the prototypical communication act, of a dialogic face-to-face character, toward multiple authors and multiple addressees, *produsers* (Bruns, 2008; Toffler, 1980), who are the active content producers and, simultaneously, the audiences/users. Social media enable more massive participation with larger groups of active participants, entirely or partly anonymous. The users, to a larger or lesser extent, shape and construct their Internet identities, more or less congruent with their authentic selves. One only has to look at the massive scale of social media use to gain an understanding of the extent to which social media and mobile technologies have changed the landscape of our platforms of communication. For example, as reported by the Pew Research Center (2019), 69% of Americans build connections with one another and share and monitor information through the use of social media technologies such as Facebook and Twitter, which means an average of 4.2 million daily social media exchanges across Facebook and Twitter only in the United States (Delello and Mokhtari 2017: 1).

The digital revolution has changed the landscape with regard to a number of communicative properties: ordinary language and behavior combine with both popular and elite forms in what Turner (2010) calls the "demotic turn," in which fiction merges with reality in reality shows. Also, while in the more distant past a distinction between the public and the private used to be respected more rigidly, the blurring of private and public spaces becomes a rule, and privacy now seems an aberration in the context of social media. As observed by Mike Sachoff (2010, quoted after Carruthers (2010), slide 13) we are turning into "ambient broadcasters who disclose a great deal of personal information in order to stay connected and take advantage of social, economic, and political opportunities." There are different reasons for this state of affairs. Social media users want to find and form communities, build reputation, and possibly make money. All of this is possible by the social media *amplification effects* in terms of numbers of comments and responses. This context also facilitates building a desired self-projected identity (Herring, 2004).

Nevertheless, the possibility of constructing a projected identity is a double-edged sword. Facts that are considered to be a source of fame and satisfaction in some countries in Europe or North America will be considered inconvenient, unflattering, or even disgraceful, blameworthy, and condemned by members of other cultures. In the context of less intensive communication links, they may be concealed and largely constrained to smaller groups, which can reduce the threat of public shame in face-to-face, offline contexts. However, as shown in the discussion of Pakistani honor culture in the present chapter, the social media amplification effect at present allows increased access to and spread of the content. This makes a potentially very large audience aware of the acts and highlights their possible honor-threatening conditioning in the communities of honor value.

4.1 Social Media Versus Real-World Protest

Social media offer the possibility of a voice in an online space that is radically different to a contained, offline spatial environment connected to a certain culture. Within our current focus on shame, it is important to understand how gender equality protests within such offline spaces differ to online social media spaces and the nature of the interaction between these (see Shaw and Silverio on Transcending Shame Through Rebellion: The Modern Arab Woman, Sexual Suppression, and the Will to Break Free; see Mayer and Vanderheiden on Naming and Shaming; see Vanderheiden on The Terror of being Judged).

However, it is important to understand the differences that online versus offline spaces offer in terms of the potential opposition to devaluation that underscores the information threat theory of shame. In the traditional sense, *relational mobility* offers the opportunity, especially for those who are in more mobile environments, to deal with the threat of shame by potentially improving their social status through the development of new, relatively more permanent relationships that might constitute a more positive audience. Although social media also present an opportunity for *relational mobility* in terms of the potential to immerse oneself in such online spaces to varying degrees, this social engagement tends to run parallel to one's offline social relationships and can interact with these at both private and professional levels. For example, Newsom (2012), commenting on online feminist activity in the revolutions in Tunisia (December, 2010 to January, 2011) and Egypt (January to February, 2011), observes that because "online activism occurs in a liminal 'third space', a place where traditional rules governing society can be set aside" (p. 32), it only constitutes contained empowerment. This means that although it has the potential to attract global attention and hence encourage involvement, the potential power gained from this is constrained within local, traditional power structures that need to be negotiated with if such global support is to be recognized and accepted in this offline space.

5 Case Study: The Honor Killing of Qandeel Baloch

It appears that Qandeel was a typical teenager living in the patriarchal, honor culture of rural Pakistan. However, she did not accept the societal norms that dictated how she was treated at that time. Habiba (2018) reports that Qandeel stated on her Twitter account in 2016 that she ran away from her husband to Darul Aman as he was physically abusing her and that she did not receive support from her family.

The role of shame in this event is consistent with womens' "potential for shame" in Pakistan observed by Shah-Davis (2011, p. 193), which restricted Qandeel's options in her attempts to deal with her husband's abuse. In fact, in the patriarchal, honor culture of Pakistan, the options available for countering such abuse are limited. A decision to separate and file for divorce is likely to elicit a sense of shame, disgrace, and dishonor and possibly murder at the hands of male family members. On the basis of viewing shame as a resource, the threat of shame underscoring Pakistani rules imposed on women meant that while Qandeel was subjected to follow these oppressive rules to ensure she did not bring shame to her family, her husband and other family members, including Waseem, benefitted from her obeyance by the respect afforded to them by the community as "shame-free", honorable men.

Referring back to our discussion of *fight*, *flight*, and *fright* outlined above, the employment of a *fight* strategy by Qandeel in this sense would not appear to offer a successful outcome. A second option, remaining in the relationship and suffering further abuse, would be tantamount to entrapment, which, as noted above, is equivalent to *fright* and can lead to depression. A possible outcome of this is suicide, as evidenced by Khan and Reza (1998) who report that there is a disproportionately large number of married females admitted to hospital for parasuicide in Pakistan, with many of these citing their relationship with their husband or in-laws as the reason. The option taken by Qandeel was clearly based on *flight*, as she fled to Darul Aman. In terms of the information threat theory of shame (Sznycer et al., 2012), Qandeel managed to remove herself, if not permanently, from the devaluation that was directed at her by her current social audience. In this respect, she managed to exercise a certain degree of relational mobility and formed new social relationships within the spheres of studies, work, and modelling, which clearly offered her a higher social status.

However, it is crucial to point out that the new social sphere that Qandeel developed was still situated in Pakistani culture, which was not conducive to the campaign that she sought to launch. Recall that rather than just being restricted to incidences, or accusations, of marital infidelity, honor in Pakistan can be threatened by female expressions of autonomy and immodest behavior.

It was clear that Qandeel needed a new space to launch her feminist offensive that was not restricted by the hegemonistic, patriarchal rules imposed by Pakistani society. The nature of the online space that she created on social media platforms allowed her to achieve these goals. In a sense, by establishing an online social media identity Qandeel transformed her *flight* response to both physical abuse and the social threat of shame into a *fight* response that was directed at the very heart of the source of shame, namely the patriarchal, honor-based belief system that oppressed women. Furthermore, it can be deduced that this reduced her shame proneness. To comprehend this more fully one needs to understand the key features of the online space that Qandeel created. First, it transcended the borders of Pakistani society. On the basis of the information threat theory of shame (Sznycer et al., 2012), this meant that she had acquired a new audience that was not only relatively much larger but had the potential to include those from non-honor cultures who were more likely to be more sympathetic to her cause. With respect to her online audience in Pakistan, there is evidence that her controversial stance tended to polarize support and opposition. Second, again with reference to the theory of Sznycer et al. (2012), it can be surmised that Qandeel's online activity improved the value of her social status, at least online. Third, her online space allowed her to operate with some degree of anonymity, which was important as it created further distance between her potentially shameful online activities and the offline, honor-based community inhabited by the male members of her family who had the potential to avenge her feminist campaign. Within the constraints of this virtual space, such anonymity can increase *relational mobility* as the individual can respond to possible harmful online devaluation relatively easily by withdrawing their online identity from that space and possibly establishing another anonymous identity in a new space. However, this assumes that anonymous online identities have distinct social spaces from offline spaces, which, as outlined below, was not the case with Qandeel and played a major role in her death.

Although Qandeel's actions were judged by many in Pakistan to be obscene and offensive, she gained 750,000 followers (Marszal, 2016). The main accusations of indecency centered on her scantily clad presence in sexually provocative videos that she posted on social media such as Facebook and Twitter. She also stated that she would perform a striptease live online if the Pakistani cricket team beat India, and in a separate video, she asked the former captain of the Pakistan cricket team and prominent politician to marry her (The Guardian, 2017). Many Pakistanis also considered it unacceptable for a woman to exercise autonomous expression of political views in the rebellious way that Qandeel did. For example, on the 14th of February, 2016, Qandeel, in response to Pakistani President Hussain's message that Pakistani people should not celebrate St. Valentine's Day as it is a Western tradition, stated in a video "happy Valentine's Day to everybody. You cannot stop people from loving. Only lazy and idiot politicians use such antics. I hate it" (The Guardian, 2017).

As long as Qandeel operated her campaign anonymously within the online social media space that she had created, she had a position of strength as the patriarchal, honor-based rules had little influence. At this stage of her online campaign, both her controversial means of expressing her message and opposition to this were contained within the space of online social media. Analyzing her messages, we can see a number of distinct elements. First, her *fight* strategy against her previous treatment by her family and husband can be clearly seen in a statement made in a video: "I was only 17 years old then. My education was not complete. I wanted to do so much. My parents married me off to this backward man . . . But this man was violent, he would beat me, torture me, burning my neck with cigarettes. These people are so dangerous" (The Guardian, 2017). Therefore, this can clearly be viewed as a *fight* strategy against her previous treatment by her family and husband. Second, the nature of the online space that she occupied allowed her to reach a wider audience and direct her opposition toward the heart of Pakistani society. Her statement promoting St. Valentine's Day was clearly directed against the Pakistani authorities. Third, Qandeel "became the voice of all the women who want to control their sexuality" (Nighat Dad, The Guardian, 2017), and "people saw her as a kind of an unlikely sort of beacon for progressive ideas" (Ahmed, The Guardian, 2017). Her aim to represent women in their struggle against oppression is witnessed in her social media statements where she referred to herself as a powerful female symbol and called for women to stand up for themselves against the oppression in society (Habiba, 2018). The resilience in her leadership of this struggle is clear in her video statement: "I'm 99% sure that you guys hate me. I'm also 100% sure that I don't give a damn" (The Guardian, 2017).

Qandeel's online campaign and the conflict it generated were initially contained in the online space of social media. With reference to the term *produser*, outlined above, Qandeel was able to use this space to construct an Internet identity that afforded her a degree of anonymity and was more congruent with her beliefs pertaining to the injustice that women face in Pakistani honor culture. Furthermore, her message was received by a massive audience, as evidenced by the more than half a million followers on Facebook and being one of the top ten Google searches in Pakistan (The Guardian, 2017). In terms of the information threat theory of shame (Sznycer et al., 2012), there are elements that reduce her shame proneness. Although she was attacked and criticized online, and therefore devalued, she also was supported by her followers. Indeed, she was regarded as a media star (Tahir, The Guardian, 2017), which meant that her social status within this space was high. The decision by the authorities to block Qandeel's Facebook page for dishonoring the national name of Baloch (The Guardian, 2017) is significant in that it shows that such opposition to her campaign at that moment was restricted to the online social media space.

To understand why Qandeel's online protest permeated the boundary of that space and became an issue in the offline society of Pakistan, one needs to analyze Qandeel's relationship with Abdul Qavi. Their first meeting was on one of the most popular TV chat shows in Pakistan, during which Qavi suggests that they meet up when he next visits Karachi. During their meeting in a hotel room in Karachi on 20th June, 2016, Qandeel dressed immodestly in jeans and t-shirt and took photos and videos of her provocative behavior in the presence of Qavi, which she posted online. These went viral and became headline news in the mainstream media. Qandeel's behavior has been assessed by some as a direct attack on the authenticity of his piety: "I think what she was trying to do there was to obviously expose him as being someone who was not perhaps as pious he would like people to think" (Ahmed, The Guardian, 2017). As a consequence of this, Qavi faced the humiliation of being suspended from the nation religious council (BBC Stories, 2017). Qandeel was invited on TV shows in which, when asked about the incident, she continued her offensive against Qavi, alluding to a possibility that he had developed a romantic interest in her: "He was sharing my tea, my Coca-Cola, even the cigarettes I was smoking. He said it would increase our love. What kind of love does he want to grow?" (The Guardian, 2017). Considering the patriarchy in Pakistani society and its strength of religious conviction, it is not surprising that the media supported Qavi in favor of Qandeel. As Tahir (The Guardian, 2017) states, "the mainstream media made it legitimate to establish a divide between what is respectable and ought to be protected and what is not respectable and ought to be caricatured, laughed at, berated, and dismissed." Furthermore, the mainstream media leaked private information about Qandeel, such as her passport information and hence her real name and where she was from, which meant that she lost her anonymity. In a press conference she stated that after the incident with Qavi the many death threats that she had been receiving had caused her to lose peace in her life and that she could not sleep at night. On 23rd June, 2016, she stated on social media "I'm Literally Feeling Alone In The Fight" (The Guardian, 2017). As she fled to her parents from these threats she attempted to conceal her identity. She told her mother "ma, I'm coming home. I'm restless, the media is after me". Her mother further stated that "she was scared, had covered her body and face with a niqab and loose clothes so no one could recognize she was Qandeel Baloch" (Qandeel's mother, The Guardian, 2017).

It is important to understand how Qandeel's position of strength in the online space was transformed into a weaker presence in her offline reality. It is clear that by posting her meeting with Qavi online her intention was to attack him within the confines of that online space. However, the amount of online interest that it generated, which was not surprising due to its relevance to the very heart of Pakistani society, namely religion, meant that it caught the attention of the mass media. Another reason for the interest and attention of the mass media was the suspension of the famous cleric, Qavi, from the Religious Council. On the basis of the information threat theory of shame, one can surmize that Qandeel's transition from her online to offline activity increased her shame proneness. First, her main audience had become the mass media, which took the opportunity to devalue her. From her own words, we know that Qandeel felt threatened by this. Furthermore, from her attempt to be anonymous during her journey to her parents, it can be deduced that the source of this threat extended to the wider public domain. Second, her attempt at anonymity at this point is significant in terms of *relational mobility* as it clearly shows that she was restricted in her ability to form new, supportive relationships. One can imagine, given the negative coverage in the mass media with respect to the Qavi affair, that a greater degree of physical mobility in the sense relocating to another region of Pakistan would not have allowed Qandeel to improve her *relational mobility*. Third, her mocking at the hands of the mass media reduced her social status. Furthermore, Qandeel had lost control over her persona in the online space as a consequence of the blurred boundaries that exist in social media communication. Alternatively, in a more traditional sense, it was the mass media that were in control of the image of her, and they projected it to Pakistani society. Losing her online space, Qandeel was subjected to the influence of the offline, honor-based Pakistani society. The patriarchal audience that constitutes this society dictated that Qandeel's actions were shameful, and as she had no means to *fight*, she engaged in *flight* and returned to what she thought was the safety of her childhood home.

If audience was important in the shame proneness of Qandeel that governed her sense of weakness, it seems to have been even more of a decisive factor in Waseem's sense of shame and his actions. Recall that the key factor determining whether a female relative's shameful act has an effect on the honor of a man is the extent to which it is public knowledge. The important point to note with respect to the potential dishonor experienced by Waseem is that he was also the beneficiary of the degree of anonymity gained by Qandeel as a result of her adoption of a pseudonym. Specifically, the anonymous, online social media space within which Qandeel operated her campaign against Pakistani society was separate to Waseem's offline community in the area of Shah Sadar Din. Likewise, the transition of Qandeel to her offline space as a consequence of the media coverage of the Qavi affair meant that the actions of Waseem's sister that were judged as shameful in the public eye were common knowledge in the social community of his public space. A better understanding of the relatively little effect that Qandeel's online social media campaign had on Waseem in comparison to the reports of the Qavi affair in the traditional media can be gained from figures showing much higher television viewing figures than Internet usage in Pakistan (89% versus 6%, respectively, as defined by use in the past 12 months) (Yusuf & Scoemaker, 2013). The effect of the role of audience in Qandeel's transition on the shame and dishonor experienced by Waseem is demonstrated in the confession of his sister's murder. He stated that he killed her because "she was doing videos on Facebook and dishonoring the family name of the Baloch." In response to the challenge why he had not killed his sister earlier considering that Qandeel had been active on media and Facebook for many years, Waseem said that "there were many other issues as well . . . the issue with the cleric—our house was besieged by the media. Before it wasn't like that" (The Guardian, 2017). As Taha (BBC Stories, 2017) explains, "the personal details (about Qandeel, exposed by the mass media) added nothing to the story, but they brought a level of shame that embarrassed the family. In Pakistan, everyone knows where that can lead."

Indeed an analysis of Waseem's murder of his sister reveals the central role of shame and honor following the shift in Qandeel's campaign to offline Pakistani society. In terms of the information threat theory of shame (Sznycer et al., 2012), his shame proneness increased as a consequence of the devaluation imposed on him by his audience. From his confession, we know that this audience took the form of the media invading his private space in his home and the general public in his community and Pakistan society in general who received the mass dissemination of this information. This would have clearly limited his *relational mobility*. With his social status being significantly harmed by an audience he could not escape from, the option of *flight* in the face of such a shame-eliciting social threat would therefore not appear to have been possible. To understand his decision to murder his sister, one needs to consider his remaining options, namely that of *fight* and *fright*, from the perspective of Pakistani culture. From the severity of the social threat, one might expect many individuals to experience a *fright* response and the resultant manifestation of hopelessness or depression. However, in Pakistani culture such inactivity would lead the immediate audience to accuse the individual of dishonor. From this perspective, one can gain some insight into why he chose the *fight* strategy that he did. Specifically the honor culture of Pakistan dictated that Waseem needed to kill his sister to restore the honor that was lost through Qandeel's behavior, to himself, his family, and the wider community. It can therefore be argued that it was not only Qandeel but also Waseem who was a victim of Pakistani honor culture in this tragic case.

6 Conclusions

The fundamental elements in the understanding of the honor killing of Qandeel are the nature of her online versus offline realities and the border between them. The upper part of Fig. 21.1 depicts Qandeel's online social media campaign against Pakistani honor culture, and the lower part shows her offline presence in this culture following the Qavi affair. With reference to the former, Qandeel's anonymous presence on online social media platforms meant that she was able to launch her campaign from this space that was detached to some extent from the real-world space of the patriarchal, honor-based society that she was opposing. Specifically, her anonymity meant that the distance between her online space and the real-world space in Pakistani society was enough to make her feel less threatened and hence allow her to employ a defiant *fight* strategy comprising raunchiness and direct opposition to those in authority who were responsible for imposing a sense of shame on women. On the basis of the information threat theory of shame (Sznycer et al., 2012), although she received criticism from the online community, the space that she created afforded her a great deal of *relational mobility* as she had millions of followers, and her status as a social media star increased her social standing in that community, which meant that her shame proneness was low. In terms of "audiencing" within computer-mediated communication, Qandeel was able to construct an online identity that was much closer to her real identity – her opposition of Pakistani honor culture. It is crucial to understand at this point that the opposition from the authorities, which is shown by the arrow labelled "opposition" from the offline to the online space, was contained within Qandeel's online space as her Facebook page was shut down.

It is important to understand how Qandeel utilized shame as a resource in the online space that she created to launch her campaign against the very source of the shame-based oppressive rules that she was subjected to, namely Pakistani honor culture. Specifically, in a similar way that FEMEN[2] protest against religious and

[2]A solely female, international feminist protest group that uses controversial tactics (Hungerford, 2015).

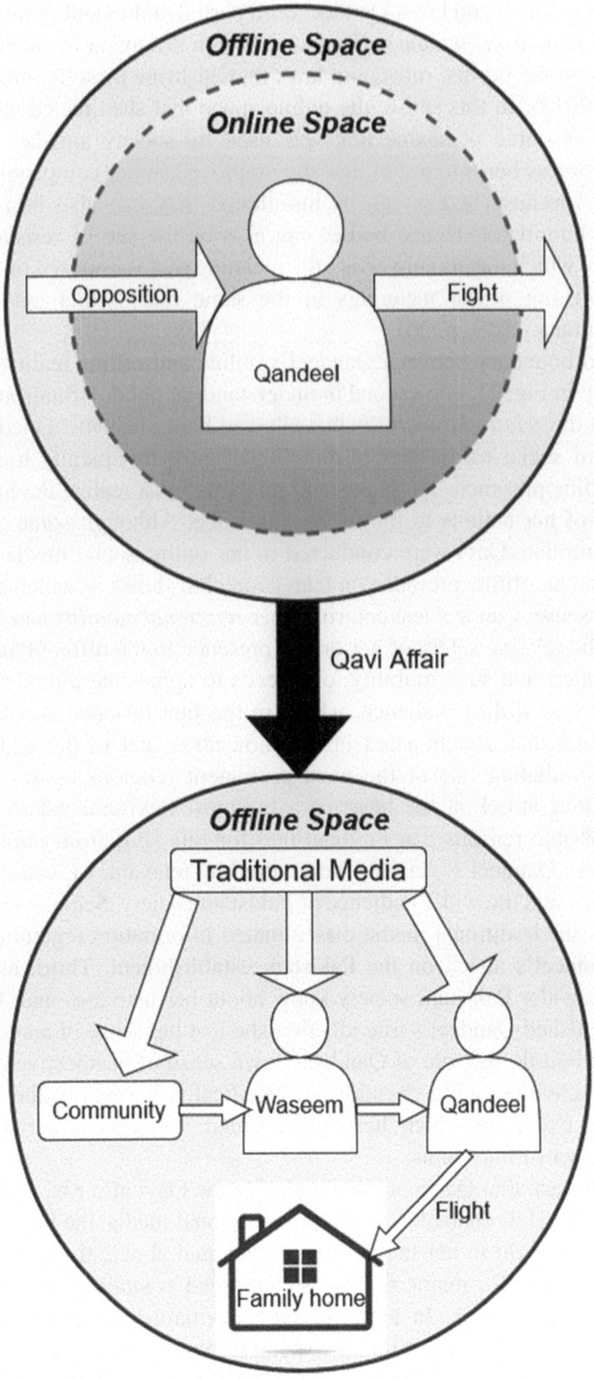

Fig. 21.1 Qandeel's devirtualized mobility from online to offline space

political cultural norms and laws, Qandeel used partial nudity and unruly behavior to transform and undermine female body shame, which is a major element of Pakistani honor, to oppose the norms, rules, and laws that enshrine these feminine standards (Hungerford, 2015). In this sense, the online space that she created allowed her to transform the resource of shame that was used by society and her male family members to oppress her into a tool that she employed in her campaign and protest. To conclude, "because bodies can be humiliated they can also be resignified to humiliate the humiliator. Hence bodies can also be the site of resistance through resignification, which means subverting the meaning that is imposed on a humiliated body and investing newer meanings in the same body which renders it more powerful" (Sultana, 2013, p. 36).

The blurred boundary between Qandeel's online and offline realities (shown by the dashed line in Fig. 21.1) is crucial in understanding her devirtualization. It could be argued that the *relational mobility* that allowed her to become a media star in the online space of social media was bi-directional and subsequently transported her back to an offline presence. To understand this, one must realize the importance of the relevance of her actions to the offline audience. Although some of Qandeel's attempts to humiliate Qavi were conducted in her online social media space, these attacks also had an offline presence on television chat shows in which she appeared with him. In a sense, Qandeel lost control of her *relational mobility* and involuntarily moved from the relative safety of her online presence to the offline Pakistani honor culture. To understand such mobility, one needs to appreciate the relevance of her actions to her new offline audience, which in the first instance was the Pakistani traditional media that disseminated information about her to the wider Pakistani society. By humiliating one of the most prominent religious clerics in Pakistan, Qandeel's actions struck at the heart of a foremost Pakistani value—religion. A number of possible reasons can be identified for this shift from online to offline presence. First, Qandeel's actions were directly relevant to real-world issues concerning Qavi and the wider audience of Pakistani society. Second, understanding this relevance, the traditional media disseminated information regarding what they viewed as Qandeel's attack on the Pakistani establishment. Third, media reports meant that the wider Pakistani society knew about her activities and, furthermore, when they published Qandeel's true identity, she lost her sense of anonymity in her offline reality. Fourth, the role of Qandeel's own sense of perspective in her online versus offline activities can be questioned. Specifically, it might be the case that she misjudged the extent to which her online social status as a social media star translated into her offline status.

The offline space that Qandeel inhabited after the Qavi affair is, as shown in the lower part of Fig. 21.1, characterized by the traditional media, the local community, Waseem, and her *flight* to her family home. As noted above, the traditional media appear to have played a major role in her enforced *relational mobility* from the online to the offline space. In terms of the information threat theory of shame (Sznycer et al., 2012), it is clear that the social threat of shame directed at Qandeel from the media following the Qavi affair reduced her social status.

Also, her negative portrayal by the media meant that she became well-known in Pakistani society. Compared with the degree of *relational mobility* that she displayed when she fled from her oppressive husband to create a new life for herself in Darul Aman, her infamy in Pakistani society meant that her *relational mobility* was now restricted, and this explains her attempt to engage in the *flight* strategy of retreating to her family home in secret. Quandeel's transition from her *fight* stance in her online space to *flight* in her offline space is reflected in the change in the relative use of shame as a resource by Qandeel vis-à-vis the traditional media and Pakistani society in general. By losing her online space, Qandeel was no longer able to use her activities in that environment to shame Pakistani political and religious authorities. Conversely, it could be argued that the traditional media took the stance of defending religious and other cultural values in Pakistan by humiliating Qandeel.

It is crucial to understand the role that Qandeel's devirtualization had on Waseem and on his audience in particular. The effect of the social threat of the traditional media on Waseem is clear from his murder confession, which he referred to as an invasion of his personal space in his home. Such mass communication of information would have meant a higher degree of shame proneness due to his lowered social status in the eyes of his immediate audience, namely his local community. With his *relational mobility* limited due to Qandeel's media attention, it would appear that Waseem was restricted in terms of employing the *flight* strategy to escape to an environment unaware of his sister's case. Also, inactivity or *fright* would not have allowed him to regain his lost honor. It is clear that the *fight* strategy that Waseem chose conformed to what his local Pakistani culture expected of him, and in this sense he can be viewed as a victim of this culture. From the point of view of shame as a resource, by imposing a sense of shame on Waseem, Pakistani society judged him to be dishonorable and not worthy of respect as he had allowed his sister to disobey and challenge its rules. He killed his sister to restore the honor that had been lost and free himself of the shame imposed on him as a consequence of her acts that were deemed to be shameful.

The crucial element that stands out in our case study analysis of the honor killing of Qandeel is that devirtualization, as a consequence of the fluidity of the border between online and offline spaces, can have tragic consequences in the offline, real world. Our analysis further identifies a number of possible factors that facilitate such an enforced transportation from an online to an offline space. There is a clear need for further research to explore these more fully. First, *relational mobility*, which is a key feature of audience, appears to have the potential to be very fluid between the two spaces. Second, social status, which is related to *relational mobility*, also has the capacity to change dramatically between one's presence in online versus offline environments. Third, one's immersion in the online space could create an illusion whereby the individual might lose a sense of perspective, leading them to misjudge the appropriateness of their behavior in the reality of their offline environment. Fourth, highlighting the role of culture, the relevance of the online actions of an individual to offline cultural norms is likely to influence boundary fluidity. Fifth, the ability to maintain one's anonymity in the online space is likely to influence boundary permeability. Sixth, traditional, online media coverage is likely to be a particularly powerful means of enforcing an offline presence. The real-world consequences of such an enforced presence in one's offline space are dependent on various situational and personal factors that determine the efficacy with which one can employ *fight*, *flight*, or *fright* strategies to counter social threats.

References

BBC Stories. (2017). Qandeel Baloch Murder: One year on (full documentary). In: *YouTube*. https://www.youtube.com/watch?v=ptVjXHgsal4&list=PLDoNdwvEa9nF5UgoFwWPgIcvcUL4j67bo&index=2. Accessed 12th November, 2019.

Boone, J. (2016). *Pakistan makes 'honour killings' punishable by mandatory prison time*. The Guardian. https://www.theguardian.com/world/2016/oct/06/pakistan-honor-killing-law-prison-sentence

Bracha, H. S. (2004). Freeze, flight, fight, fright, faint: Adaptationist perspectives on the acute stress response spectrum. *CNS Spectrums, 9*, 679–685.

Bruns, A. (2008). *Blogs, wikipedia, second life, and beyond: From production to produsage*. New York: Lang.

Calma, J. (2019). *When it comes to the environmental costs of flights 'we need to figure out how to turn that shame into action': The battle between convenience and conservation*. The Verge. https://www.theverge.com/2019/9/26/20872267/flight-shame-nyc-united-nations-climate-change-environmental-costs

Carruthers, K. (2010). *Social media: Blurring the boundaries*. www.katecarruthers.com | © Kate Carruthers 2010 10.

Chaudhry, H. (2016). No one gives me any credit for speaking about girl power: Qandeel Baloch. *Images Dawn*, July 14, pp. 1–9.

Delello, J. A., & Mokhtari, K. (2017). Blurring the boundaries: The impact of social media in the higher education classroom. *International Journal of Interactive Communication Systems and Technologies (IJICST), 7*(1), 1–14. https://doi.org/10.4018/IJICST.2017010101.

Dickerson, S. S., Gruenewald, T. L., & Kemeny, M. E. (2004). Psychobiological responses to social self threat: Functional or detrimental. *Self and Identity, 8*, 270–285.

Elison, J., Garofalo, C., & Velotti, P. (2014). Shame and aggression: Theoretical considerations. *Aggression and Violent Behavior, 19*, 447–453.

Fontaine, J. R. J., Luyten, P., De Boeck, P., Corveleyn, J., Fernandez, M., Herrera, D., Ittzės, A., & Tomcsányi, T. (2006). Untying the Gordian knot of guilt and shame: The structure of guilt and shame reactions based on situation and person variation in Belgium, Hungary, and Peru. *Journal of Cross-Cultural Psychology, 37*(3), 273–292.

Gabol, I., & Subhani, T. (2016, July 16). Qandeel Baloch murdered by brother in Multan: Police. *Dawn*. https://www.dawn.com/news/1271213

Gallup, G. G. (1974). Animal hypnosis: Factual status of a fictional concept. *Psychological Bulletin, 81*, 836–853.

Habiba, U. (2018). Honor killing in Pakistan: A case study of Qandeel Baloch. *International Journal of Social Sciences and Humanity, 8*(9), 247–254.

Herring, S. (2004). Online communication: Through the lens of discourse. In M. Consalvo, N. K. Baym, J. Hunsinger, K. B. Jensen, J. Logie, M. Murero, & L. R. Shade (Eds.), *Internet research annual* (pp. 65–76). New York, NY: Peter Lang.

Hungerford, K. (2015). FEMEN's grotesque transformation of female body shame. *Women's Studies in Communication, 38*, 361–366.

Kam, C. C.-S., & Bond, M. H. (2008). Role of emotions and behavioral responses in mediating the impact of face loss on relationship deterioration: Are Chinese more face-sensitive than Americans? *Asian Journal of Social Psychology, 11*, 175–184.

Khan, M. M., & Reza, H. (1998). Suicide and parasuicide in Pakistan: Time for a change? *The Journal of the Pakistan Medical Association, 48*(10), 292–293.

Lewandowska-Tomaszczyk, B., & Wilson, P. A. (2017). Shame and guilt across cultures. In Y. Y. Kim (Ed.), *International encyclopedia of intercultural communication*. Malden, MA: Wiley & Sons.

Lewandowska-Tomaszczyk, B., & Zeller, F. (2012). The media in transforming audiences and societies. In P. Pezik (Ed.), *Corpus data across languages and disciplines* (pp. 127–148). Frankfurt am Main: Peter Lang.

Lewis, H. B. (1971). Shame and guilt in neurosis. *Psychoanalytic Review, 58*(3), 419–438.

MacDonald, G., & Leary, M. R. (2005). Why does social exclusion hurt? The relationship between social and physical pain. *Psychological Bulletin, 131*(2), 202–223.

Marszal, A. (2016). Pakistani social media star 'murdered by her brother' in apparent honour killing. *The Telegraph*. https://www.telegraph.co.uk/news/2016/07/16/pakistani-social-media-star-murdered-by-her-brother-in-apparent/

Molloy, M. (2018, 25 June). Online shaming: The dangerous rise of the internet pitchfork mob. *The Telegraph*. https://www.telegraph.co.uk/news/2018/06/25/online-shaming-dangerous-rise-internet-pitchfork-mob/

Nasrullah, M., Haqqi, S., & Cummings, K. J. (2009). The epidemiological patterns of honour killing of women in Pakistan. *European Journal of Public Health, 19*(2), 193–197.

Newsom, V. A. (2012). Arab women, social media, and the Arab spring: Applying the framework of digital reflexivity to analyze gender and online activism. *Journal of International Women's Studies, 13*(5), 31–45.

Ogarkova, A., Soriano, C., & Lehr, C. (2012). Naming feeling: Exploring the equivalence of emotion terms in five European languages. In P. A. Wilson (Ed.), *Dynamicity in emotion concepts. Lodz studies in language* (Vol. 27, pp. 253–284). Frankfurt am Main: Peter Lang.

Patel, S., & Gadit, A. M. (2008). Karo-Kari: A form of honour killing in Pakistan. *Transcultural Psychiatry, 45*(4), 683–694.

Pew Research Center. (2019). *Social Media fact sheet*. https://www.pewresearch.org/internet/fact-sheet/social-media/

Ranter, S. C. (1977). Immobility in invertebrates: What can we learn? *Psychololological Review, 1*, 1–14.

Sachoff, M. (2010). webpronews.com 13/07/2010.

Scheff, T. J. (2014). The ubiquity of hidden shame in modernity. *Cultural Sociology, 8*(2), 129–141.

Schmidt, N. B., Richey, J. A., Zvolensky, M. J., & Maner, J. K. (2008). Exploring human freeze responses to a threat stressor. *Journal of Behavior Therapy and Experimental Psychiatry, 39*(3), 292–304.

Shah-Davis, S. (2011). A woman's honour and a nation's shame: 'Honour killings' in Pakistan. In J. Jones, A. Grear, R. A. Fenton, & K. Stevenson (Eds.), *Gender, sexualities and law* (pp. 188–200). New York: Routledge.

Sultana, P. (2013). Nakedness and resistance: Understanding naked protests of women. *Meridian Critic, 20*(1), 31–43.

Sznycer, D., Takemura, K., Delton, A. W., Sato, K., Robertson, T., Cosmides, L., & Tooby, J. (2012). Cross-cultural differences and similarities in proneness to shame: An adaptionist and ecological approach. *Evolutionary Psychology, 10*(2), 352–370.

Tangney, J. P., & Tracy, J. L. (2012). Self-conscious emotions. In M. R. Leary & J. P. Price (Eds.), *Handbook of self and identity* (2nd ed., pp. 446–478). New York: The Guilford Press.

The Guardian. (2017). Qandeel Baloch. In: *YouTube*. https://www.youtube.com/watch?v=jUVyz2OQjbc&list=PLDoNdwvEa9nF5UgoFwWPgIcvcUL4j67bo&index=1 Accessed 11 November, 2019.

Toffler, A. (1980). *The third wave*. Bantam Books. Bruns 2008,

Turner, G. (2010, January). *Ordinary people and the media: The demotic turn*. Los Angeles, CA: Sage. https://doi.org/10.4135/9781446269565.

Yusuf, H., & Scoemaker, E. (2013). *The media of Pakistan: Fostering inclusion in a fragile democracy?* (p. 9). BBC Media Action: Policy Briefing.

Paul A. Wilson (PhD) holds the post of professor in the Department of Corpus and Computational Linguistics at the University of Lodz, Poland. He completed his PhD on the interplay between cognition and emotion at Birkbeck (University of London) in 2000. His main research interests include the conceptual representation of emotions from a cross-cultural perspective. More recently he has focused on the role of shame in educational and conflict contexts.

Barbara Lewandowska-Tomaszczyk (Dr. Habil.) is a full professor of English and applied linguistics at the State University of Applied Sciences in Konin, Poland, Department of Language and Communication and for many years served as head of the Department of English Language and Applied Linguistics at the University of Lodz. She is also an author and editor of numerous books and papers in cognitive and corpus linguistics, emotion studies, and translation and was invited to read papers at conferences and give workshops at European, American, and Asian universities.

Chapter 22
Transcending Shame Through Rebellion: The Modern Arab Woman, Sexual Suppression, and the Will to Break Free

Shereen H. Shaw and Sergio A. Silverio

1 Introduction

Shame has been often been argued as a culturally bound emotion, which can affect a country's citizens to varying degrees. Arab societies are often regarded as being heteronormative, masculinist, and patriarchal. These cultures are themselves in turn often synonymous with shame narratives associated with the suppression of women and sexuality. Arab women have therefore been gazed upon as objects or chattel among Arab societies and Arab men, leading to heavy critique being delivered by the Western World against the lack of emancipation and sexual freedom Arab women are seemingly able to have agency over. Having been suppressed and also having been viewed as suppressed subjects of society, we may question how authentically Arab women may lead their lives, and truly fulfil their sexual desires. The Arab World has, however, recently experienced huge political, economic, and social upheaval, most notably recognisable as the 'Arab Spring'. Decades of political stagnation caused by petulant and immovable dictatorships came to an end across much of the Arab World, fuelled by violent uprisings by the public. Generally, it was younger members of these societies who grew frustrated with the lack of future thinking by their governments. They communicated their dismay and organised themselves for demonstrations via social media, whilst also using it as a platform to reach the Western World's mass media. After the uprisings, new governments were formed across much of the Arab World, but Arab women found themselves with little extra freedom, but a greater hunger to rebel. This chapter will explore the

S. H. Shaw (✉)
Department of Secondary and Further Education, Edge Hill University, Ormskirk, UK
e-mail: Shereen.Shaw@edgehill.ac.uk

S. A. Silverio
Department of Women and Children's Health, King's College London, London, UK
e-mail: Sergio.Silverio@kcl.ac.uk

C.-H. Mayer et al. (eds.), *Shame 4.0*, https://doi.org/10.1007/978-3-030-59527-2_22

reclamation of sexuality by Arab women and how their rebellion against centuries of suppression is tackling the culture of shame in which they continue to exist.

In a world where women were once confined to the home and dedicated to raising a family and carrying out household chores, Arab women in the last decade or so have *invaded* the public domain, claiming their identity and breaking free with a new feminist ideology. Certain countries struggled to maintain order and prevent chaos, whilst others swiftly fell with very little hope to recover. Women, however, seem to have found a once lost identity and a glimpse of optimism to transcend domestic isolation and anonymity in a much more contemporary context. This reclamation of identity is not a foreign idea to many women in the Arab world. In the final decades of the nineteenth century, women from middle-class Syrian and Egyptian origins were publishing books and periodicals, acting as founders and editors who often signed their real, *female* names, deliberately. This phenomenon showed intellectual women, Muslim, Christian, and Jewish, in the public domain as contributors to a form of feminist expression. As a result, we saw a rise of women writers under the women's awakening (al-Nahda al-Nisa'iyah), a renaissance in the Arab world (Badran, 1996). One would imagine that this period (1922–1938) saw women participating in public life as their ideas were published. This, unfortunately, was not the case; rather on the contrary, *'women, as publishers or contributors, need not have stepped far outside their houses (most published their journals from their homes), [only] their voices, names, and ideas penetrated the public domain'* (Badran, 1996, p. 61). Women such as Aisha al-Taymuriyah, Zaynab Fawwaz, Malak Hifni Nasif, Huda Sha'arawi, and Nabawiyya Musa (the latter founders of the Egyptian Feminist Union) and many more have introduced Arab women to a new and dynamic culture which gave women the freedom to partake in rallies around certain political issues. Arab women have evolved with the change in education and in the political landscape, nationally and internationally. Education and politics, together, continue to play a key role in the shaping of Arab women's identity today. Not only did the Arab Spring (a 2-year spate of anti-government protests across much of the Islamic world which commenced in late December 2010) encourage women to assert themselves as free agents and their voices be heard, but also women saw opportunities to rise beyond the limitations of shame and the patriarchal mould whose imperatives and symbols, at times, they could not easily overlook or discard. Although educated women, for whom teaching was the most common vocation, found in journalism another scope for political engagement which may have nurtured their ideas, skills, and knowledge, since the Arab Spring, the debate between national identity, modernisation, and the will to break free continues to be overlooked and, within society, not acknowledged.

1.1 Defining 'Arab' Women and the 'Arab' World

Defining Arab women in contemporary literature has long been problematic and debated. After the Arab revolution, Ghannoushi (2011) wrote *the stereotype of the submissive, repressed victim has been shattered by female protestors in Egypt, Tunisia and Yemen'*. This chapter focuses on how the Arab revolutions have shaken many decades of long myths, silence, invisibility, and perceptions of women in the Arab world today. The term 'Arab world' often perpetuates a phantom identity of 'Arabs', namely, those who speak a dialect of Arabic. It is used with no consideration to the 35 dialects of Arabic language spoken or the slight cultural differences, across the Middle East and North Africa [MENA] regions (Barakat, 2018). For this reason, in this chapter, the use of the term 'Arab' is both convoluted and politically charged. The chapter aims to showcase what has inspired women across the MENA regions to thrust themselves into the heart of protest as an act of rebellion and a yearning for change. It is a calling for political freedom as it sweeps the lands '*...as revolt turns into hiatus and stalemate from Yemen to Tunisia, Egypt and Libya, Bahrain and Syria, one thing is clear: for all their organising, marching, rabble-rousing, blogging, hunger-striking, and, yes, dying, Arab women are barely one small step forwards on the road to greater equality with their menfolk. Women may have sustained the Arab spring, but it remains to be seen if the Arab spring will sustain women'* (Rice et al., 2011).

The Fourth Industrial Revolution [4IR] has shaken many parts of the world, especially leaving many countries in a state of flux. Several stereotypes of the feminine ideology were being dismantled, and narratives were challenged. Protestors in Tahrir Square expressed: *'if you ask someone if they want gender equality, that's a loaded term here. Do you mean all women should be like men? Most would say no. If you mean women have choice and equal protection under the law, most would say yes'* (Rice et al., 2011). For example, the association of the Islamic headscarf (hijab) with segregation and oppression was challenged by women activists wearing the hijab marching in the streets side by side with unveiled women and men. At the same time, anxieties around sexual purity, honour, and women's status as condemned to a life of confinement and childbearing at the mercy of patriarchal societies were openly and, perhaps more importantly, politically debated. Stereotypes imposed by a Euro-American neoliberal view of Arab and Muslim women were scrutinised in the process. Women were seen through the narrow prism of victimhood: *'as objects of pity in need of their benevolent intervention—intellectual, political, even military—for deliverance from the dark cage of veiling to a promised garden of enlightenment and progress. Arab women are rebelling against both narratives. They refuse to be treated with contempt, kept in isolation, or be taken by the hand, like a child, and led on the road to emancipation. They are taking charge of their own destinies, determined to liberate themselves as they liberate their societies from dictatorship. The emancipation they are shaping with their own hands is an authentic one defined by their own needs, choices and priorities. There is, and will be, resistance to this process of emancipation'* (Ghannoushi, 2011).

The dynamics unleashed by the revolution was irreversible. In the aftermaths, the assumption, Ghannoushi (2011) writes, was that *'those who have led the struggle to dismantle the old regimes will no doubt remain at the forefront in rebuilding the new order on its ruins'*. However, this was not the case as women were expected to return to shying away from the public domain. Egyptian-American journalist Mona

Eltahawy is an Arab woman who wrote a provocative cover story for *Foreign Policy* on how 'misogyny' has become so endemic to Arab societies. Eltahawy, regardless of the merit of her ideas, was subject to criticisms for attempting to expose some of those anxieties related to the exploitation of women in relation to Arab economies and societies' dynamics. Her piece showed that *'the struggle was about much more than just gender'* (Fisher, 2012). The backlash against Eltahawy was because she is an Arab woman who is living in the West and who speaks American-accented English. The scrutiny she received showed her background has complicated her position and limited the reach of her ideas and authenticity of her voice. The scrutiny, ironically, predominantly came from Arab Muslim feminists living in various parts of the Arab world where the mass literature tiptoe around the use of the term 'Arab' and cultural anxieties in relation to anything that is seen or dubbed as Western-imposed values.

2 Unconscious Dynamics of Shame in the Context of Arab Culture

To identify the key discussions on the conceptualisation of shame, it has been useful to turn to psychoanalytic literature; however the focus on shame in the Arab world is somewhat more limited. More specifically, that which focuses on *shame* and Arab *women* is usually bound up with literature on sexualisation of women's bodies, honour culture, and the concept of modesty (see Abu-Lughod, 2016). There is therefore a lacuna in the literature base which foregrounds shame in public Arab life and, particularly, the impact of shame on gender discourse in patriarchal societies. Having said that, however, psychoanalytic literature on shame has grown over the past years (Benedict, 1934; DeYoung, 2015; Lewis, 1995; Margherita & Troisi, 2013; Mayer & Vanderheiden, 2019; Nathanson, 1994; Pettigrove & Parsons, 2012; Shweder, 2003; Vanderheiden & Mayer, 2017). These works are key in contesting the assumption that the meaning and impact of *shame* are the same from culture to culture and experienced in the same way by men or by women. In these years of writing on shame, it has come to be known as *'the Cinderella of the unpleasant emotions'* as coined by psychoanalyst Charles Rycroft (1972, p. 152) and has *'received much less attention than anxiety, guilt and depression'*. Certainly, Freud and those he influenced, including Lacan, thought little of the concept of shame, and others, such as Laplanche and Pontalis (1967/1973), included no entry for 'shame' in their seminal works. Although the conceptualisation of shame has been more pronounced in American psychoanalysis, experiencing a resurgence in recent years, it appears and remains *'strangely unmoored there'* (Ivy, 2008, p. 1).

2.1 Conceptualising Shame

Anthropology has seemingly had a very different relationship with the concept of shame, however. In 1934, Ruth Benedict, an American anthropologist, wrote a now-lauded work in anthropology: the *Patterns of Culture.* This text emerged as a leading authority on culture as Benedict drew comparison between the culture of shame and the culture of guilt in Western societies. Generally speaking, *'All cultures manage to get people to internalize their social norms, and also to internalize psychological mechanisms for holding unacceptable thoughts and behaviors in check. Thus, it is argued, some cultures put more emphasis on guilt to regulate behavior, while others put more emphasis on shame. Cross-cultural psychologists often describe cultures as falling along an individualism-collectivism continuum'* (Fish, 2016).

The culture of shame is the culture of several societies around the world and has its characteristics that distinguish it from the culture of guilt. These two concepts, shame and guilt, were explored by Benedict in *The Chrysanthemum and the Sword: Patterns of Japanese Culture* (first published in 1946) as she compared the American culture as one based on feelings of guilt and Japanese culture as one based on feelings of shame (which also resembles the culture found in the Arab world). As a result of the study, societies were divided into two types: those predicated on shame and honour (usually found in Asia and some of Africa, including the Middle East) and those which were based on a culture of guilt (which is mostly depicted in Western societies). Ivy (2008, p. 3) perhaps best translates Benedict's work on the differences between *guilt* and *shame*:

> In this story of Japan (and the United States), shame plays a central role. Shame has a twin, too, in Benedict's story: guilt. In her para-Freudian anthropology, Japan is a shame culture, America a guilt culture: "A society that inculcates absolute standards of morality and relies on men's developing a conscience is a guilt culture by definition. ... In a culture where shame is a major sanction ... a man does not experience relief when he makes his fault public even to a confessor. So long as his bad behavior does not 'get out into the world' he need not be troubled. ... True shame cultures rely on external sanctions for good behavior, not, as true guilt cultures do, on an internalized conviction of sin. ... [Shame] requires an audience or at least a man's fantasy of an audience. Guilt does not.

The characteristics, as Benedict shows, of the two cultures are based upon various factors such as in a culture of shame, often families are of larger numbers, such as tribes or clans or extended families, whereas in a culture of guilt, families are of smaller sizes and nuclear in span and have values driven by social norms and customs, whereas for the former, the values are driven from religion, tradition, and heritage. In both cultures, the individual's ability to self-govern and to conform plays a key role. In shame-based cultures, shame occurs when an individual is exposed to others or to the community (external), whereas in guilt culture, the emotion is of intrinsic value.

In other work, the word shame has been explored in relation to being a destructive manifestation of the self. Léon Wurmser (1981) in *The Mask of Shame* provides an insightful analysis of clinical manifestations of shame from birth and sheds light on the most self-destructive patterns in personality disorders where he prescribes their origin to shame. He states: *since by and large 'shame' is evoked by weakness and 'guilt' by strength, it is evident that the person who defends against aggression by passivity is consequently more disposed to manifest shame than the one who turns his aggression into activity. That is, the primarily passive person tends to feel 'ashamed', the primarily active one 'guilty'.* (Wurmser, 1981, p. 77)

Establishing a link between shame and guilt is profound when looking at the gender discourse of Arab women from birth and the manifestation of shame as a result of an 'inherent inferiority'. In his article 'Toward a Deep Cultural Psychology of Shame', Shweder asks *'can one hope for more than just a frequency account of cross-cultural variations in emotional functioning, something a bit more "meaning centred"?'* (Shweder, 2003, p. 1110). Shame, unlike guilt, alters one's self-conception; it *'can be considered a more archaic and more destructive affection than guilt because it has no admittance to atonement and deals with a total failure of the identity of the individual forced to face [one's] impotence'* (Margherita & Troisi, 2013). Post-revolution, Arab women found themselves with little extra freedom, but a greater hunger to rebel. The reclamation of sexuality and how their rebellion against centuries of suppression manifested during the Arab Spring has tackled the culture of shame in which they continue to exist. Through rebellion, Arab women found new avenues that potentially gave them the form of liberation they eagerly sought.

2.2 Shame and the Arab Context

To understand the theoretical underpinnings in psychoanalytic thinking regarding shame and its meaning, we delineate the phenomenon of shame and describe its various forms and the socio-cultural slant which can be readily given to its perception and even its existence in the Arab world. The conception of shame in the Arab world is negative and, taken culturally, is at polar opposites to honour which many of the Arab cultures pride as the core value intertwined with the context of *home* and *family*. Women for decades witnessed and experienced ills as daughters, wives, and mothers: *'women are expected to marry at a young age and yet all efforts to secure a suitable match are frowned upon. It is a mystery as to how women find suitable men to marry if all efforts are restricted by family, culture and religion'* (Shaw, 2018). The restrictions are often imposed out of fear of shame which may be brought upon the family by the female body. This fear contributes to the self-inherent inferiority which resides in how the structure of the family manipulates women's choices and dictates their future at a very early age under the pretence of protecting the family's 'honour' (*al-sharraf*).

In the Arab world, *honour* is predominantly used as a word which refers to a high moral worth. The word itself can be prescribed to men and women alike: a man of honour or a woman of honour means a person who holds a high moral worth of the self and identity and perhaps so much so that any potential cause for shame will be avoided. For example, rape is seen as a primary cause for shame as it is an invasion and humiliation of the body and, thus, causes extreme shame to the victim, whether emotions of self-shame or a shame imposed by society and culture. According to Freud, shame is linked directly to the 'ideal of Ego' and to the narcissistic expansion (and 'guilt' to the super ego). Shame involves the *self* and identity, and it is the affectation that reflects a sense of *deficit* of self, meaning that shame is a 'failure' of the self, felt as an emotion system (Margherita & Troisi, 2013).

Women's sexuality is one of many taboo topics in the Arab world (see Abu-Lughod, 2016; Shaw, 2018). This is a result of fear of questioning one's honour. A young woman who hits puberty is seen as a potential 'threat' to the family's honour, and, thus, men with patriarchal privileges feel the need to swiftly enforce excessive protection and restrictions on her freedom (see Abu-Lughod, 2016). Puberty for young females in the Arab world is usually an unwelcomed traumatic experience, and mothers or other female family members are known to manage the event and ensure the conversation around it is kept to a minimum, and certainly away from any males (Deeb et al., 2018).

The female body becomes subject to emotions that cannot be spoken about, explored, or acknowledged with significant others. It becomes a young female's secret, only discussed by the parents amongst themselves and female family members only; often the discussions continue to revolve around the necessity of resolving a problem by finding a suitor. This secrecy continues as a normal part of young Arab woman's upbringing from puberty to adolescence. Poverty, ignorance, and lack of education are factors which contribute to young Arab women's insecurities and struggles, but also, more importantly, the failure to have key discussions around sexuality out of shame and fear enslaves and continues to haunt women. As the female body develops, in the process, the changes in the body causes a huge sense of shame that a young female, for example, feels obliged to hide from the *male gaze* (see Silverio, 2019). This is reflected in simple mundane tasks such as the change of dress and style (see Abu-Lughod, 2016). What a young female would have been able to wear prior to puberty, she can no longer wear after puberty in fear of attracting attention and being 'seen', a euphemism for being sexualised or sexually objectified (Silverio, 2019). Similarly, stepping out of the family home becomes a chaperoned activity with restrictions, and social interactions begin to be governed by boundaries and limitations. One may argue this objectification of the female body runs deep in the Arab culture from the age of ignorance *(al-Jahiliyyah)* and persists to exist, contrary to common beliefs, after the arrival of the Islamic revelation because it is ingrained into Arab cultures and traditions than a religious issue. Young females, thus, grow to adapt mechanisms to overlook the changes in the body, to cover and to hide as a result of fear of the male gaze, and to struggle to fit into a societal mould with its attributes which call for a portrayal of all young females as 'honourable'. *'The term "Jahiliyah" is familiar to most Muslims. It is derived from the Arabic verb "jahala", meaning to be ignorant. "Jahiliyah" therefore refers to the "Days of Ignorance", which is used in Islam to describe pre-Islamic Arabia'* (Askoul, 2015). The threat to which the female body is exposed in patriarchal societies has almost paved the way for female genital mutilation [FGM] practices. FGM is seen as a solution to restrict and cease sexual desires and *'in the Arab World, FGM is concentrated in poorer Arab countries on the African continent: it is frequent in Somalia, Djibouti, Egypt and Sudan. According to UNICEF, Somalia has the highest prevalence of FGM of any predominantly Arab country, with an estimated 98% of females between 15 and 49 years having undergone the practice. In Egypt, an estimated 87% of girls and women 15 to 49 have also undergone FGM. Egypt has the highest population of any country in the Arab world, with 95 million people. Among girls 0 to 14 years, Mauritania has the highest percentage of FGM practice, with 54% having been circumcised. Yemen then follows, with 15%, and Egypt afterward with 14%'* (Dockery, 2018).

Expression or discussion of sexuality or sex, as topics, are strictly frowned upon (see Chap. 11 in this book). Egyptian feminist, Nawal El Saadawi, campaigned against FGM between 1979 and 1980 as the United Nations advisor for the Women's Programme in Africa and the Middle East, and, also in her capacity as a physician working in deprived areas of Upper Egypt, she wrote: *I was fighting against the very limited conception of virginity; at that time in upper Egypt, when a girl was supposed to marry not virgin, her parents could kill her.; the father killed the daughter because on the wedding night there is no blood of virginity. Almost 30% of women were born with no 'hyman' they were non-virgins. And some of them were killed while they were innocent. I was obliged as a physician to write about sexual problems, illegal abortion; some village women died because they tried to abort themselves in very bad conditions.* (El Saadawi, 2000)

El Saadawi, who was circumcised as a child, presented to the Egyptian Organization for Human Rights an estimate that at least 90 per cent of girls in Egyptian villages had been victims of female genital 'circumcision'. She went on to claim that this is part of *'the punishment for being born a woman'*. This conviction led to El Saadawi's dismissal from her position as Director of Education for Egypt's Ministry of Health and as Editor of *Health* magazine (see Shaw & Silverio, 2019, for a detailed description of El Saadawi's work). In addition, El Saadawi was also prevented from practising as a doctor, but this did not stop her from advocating against FGM as an experience of encroachment in a very physical and violent way. Thus, she referred to it as 'psychological circumcision'. Shame is amongst the repressing forces acting against the sexual instinct according to Freud. This, he states, *'occurs in little girls earlier and in the face of less resistance than in boys; as a result, the tendency towards repression of sexuality is greater in the former. This difference becomes more prominent in puberty when girls are seized by sexual repugnance and boys by sexual desire'* (Freud, 1905/2017, p. 219). Marriage is ultimately seen as a sacred institution that should be honoured and cherished. For Arab women, all expressions of sexuality are restricted to monogamous marriage whereas men can fulfil certain conditions to engage in polygamy and are, through Islamic ideologies, able to take up to four wives at one time. Certain observations of course can be made about the interpretations of the *Shar'iah* law regarding marriage, sexuality, and gender.

2.3 (Arab) Women in (Arab) Society

Families have a great power in all Arab society. They interfere in directing the life of individual members, as the parents, for example, determine a child's education, career trajectory, marriage, and other key aspects of life. One can argue these guidance and support, though may appear at a glance as a welcomed expectation and an integral characteristic of close-knit family ties in the Arab world, often limit the child's self-expression and the margin of freedom is very narrow and sometimes non-existent. Strict familial expectations further narrow these children's field of expectation and freedom as they reach the age of puberty. The interference often also includes, for females specifically, childbearing and the number of children to be born as communities greatly influence individual decisions. Those who may not wish to marry, or 'secure' a husband, or perhaps do not possess the desire to carry and bear children, as well as those who experience fertility issues, will often be made to feel a great sense of shame due to their inability to satisfy familial and community expectation. One must note that regardless of social progression and modernisation of the state and society, the patriarchal family has not relinquished control, nor would the state exact it. The expectations from Arab women, not just at a young age, but at *all* ages, are submission, an unquestionable chastity until marriage, and conformity to patriarchal laws and governance. For this reason, early marriages in the Arab world are seen by the likes of Huda Sha'arawi, as *'the first obstacle to the development of the young woman'* (Badran, 1996, p. 127). Sha'arawi's motive was to stop early marriages from truncating young women's education, and hence, the minimum marriage age for girls was set at 16, and 18 for males. This law, however, in many parts of the Arab world, was not implemented because it was not taken seriously.

Many prominent Arab women wrote to protest forced marriages of young girls to old men or forcing the marriage of a woman without her consent. El Saadawi was one of those who continued to lobby and campaign. She also wrote about the very fact that losing one's virginity before marriage is *shameful* and *socially unacceptable* in the eyes of those who keep to the word of their religion. The act brings dishonour to the family, and shame is brought upon individuals because the act was committed outside of the sacred institution of marriage. Arab women are, thus, subject to what is referred to as so-called *'honour* killings*'*. These killings occur throughout several regions and amongst diverse ethnic populations and are not restricted to Muslims. A crime of honour is *'the killing of a woman by her father or her brother for engaging or being suspected of engaging in sexual practices before or outside marriage'* (Abu-Odeh, 2010; see Chap. 21) A lack of sexual education, ignorance, and conversations around sex impact and determine the lives of many young Arab women who are born with a fear of failure in the eyes of the patriarchy and society (and perhaps God in some religious communities). In some rural areas in upper Egypt, failure to satisfy husbands', families', and communities' expectations can lead a young woman to feeling a great sense of shame and endangering her life. This, however, is not common in urban areas of Arab societies, but rather often restricted to areas of deprivation and poverty in many rural regions. Sadly, regardless of the campaigns to implement the law and to call for change in societies with regard to women, their well-being, and health, the discrepancies between areas and countries continue regardless of the request for birth certificates as proof of age that were introduced by many countries as a requirement by law. Simply put, this law in many parts of the Arab world is overlooked and ignored.

These attitudes and those associated with sexual violence against women have continued to fester due to weak laws, many of which shun and dismiss the victims in favour of their male attackers. Laws across the Arab world, or lack thereof, see many victims lose out on, while perpetrators escape true justice. As Margherita and Troisi (2013) state, *'Some affections related to the body prevail, above all the shame which expresses itself in characteristics which reinforces the element of trauma. The loss of a capacity to represent and symbolise is not only a psychic dynamic, but it also reproduces itself in the social systems, shaping that zone of "silent concealment", that drives the phenomenon of gender violence'*. When young Arab women are betrothed by the family to an old man, the family celebrates this opportunity which is often seen as a privilege bestowed about the family and the young woman. Often it is said to the young woman, *'this man will make of you an honourable woman'* (see also Abu-Lughod, 2016). This implies that without a man, the female is *not* honourable; perhaps more so, she is seen as, biologically, self-*deficient: Families who marry off their daughters at such a young age may believe that it is in the girls' best interest, not realizing that they are violating their daughters' human rights. Early marriage often means an end to the girls' schooling, forced sexual relations, and early childbearing. Moreover, girls who marry at a younger age are generally more vulnerable to spousal violence than girls who wait longer to marry.* (Kharboush et al., 2010)

The ingrained emotions of duty and obligation imposed by the family at a very young age contribute to the sense of inferiority and 'shame'. When the young female has negative experiences as a result of an early marriage, shame is felt *'as a failure to live- up to one's cherished self-image'* (Shweder, 2003, p. 96). Shame can also be felt when young women are expected to bear children at a young age and experience severe health complications during childbirth or lose a pregnancy due to the unreadiness of her body. The trauma of these experiences is unacknowledged by families and by husbands and is manifested in shame and disappointment. Shame *is*, thus, a monitor of personal responsibility which informs one's sense of duty, morality, and ethics. Shame embodies a loss of self-appraisal. According to Shweder (2003), it is perceived implications of the emotional response for personal identity, agency, social standing, and self-regard. There is a huge societal consequence and higher risk of perpetuating inter-generational cycles of poverty.

3 Women and the Culture of Psychosocial Shame

In exploring the dynamic change in perceptions of the Arab subject in an unstable political scene (such as that of the Arab Spring), one can highlight some of the most debatable accounts from individual cases which suggest, according to Shweder (2003), that cross-cultural variation in emotional functioning may explain and shed light on the idea there is a lot of shame in the East, certainly more than there is in the West. In the Arab world, *shame* is often used alongside the word *forbidden*; the use of these words is interlinked. The latter implies that there are key principles (i.e. honour, respect, and loyalty) which govern the structure of Arab societies and their functions. In this respect, a forbidden act, for example, is a shameful act which signifies non-conformity and the breaking of such principles. Furthermore, the individual is held responsible by society for acting not only against social norms (and expectations) but also against religious doctrines, the notion of family, and the 'benefit of all'. In fact, one can argue that failure to conform is the main cause which underlies shame-based cultures in the Arab world. The Arab world is made of collectivistic societies whereby identity is defined by the group to which one belongs. When individuals meet, the conversation is often to figure out which group, family, village, or area the other individual is from. This goes back to a deep-rooted 'clan-mentality' within Arab history where 'honour' is a shared commodity and individuals are held responsible for bringing honour into disrepute and, therefore, shame upon the community of which they belong.

3.1 *Arab Women and Shame*

Arab male and female children alike are taught from an early age to bring honour to the family and to avoid shame even at personal cost. On the other hand, for many Western cultures, family is a voluntary association where at the age of 18 or so, young adults can leave to find or build their own lives independently with minimal expectations. The freedom that comes with this fundamental difference in cultures contributes to an individual's conception of the self, identity, and emotional functioning with regard to shame. Women's participation in the Arab world is heavily regulated. Although a glimpse of rebellion and non-conformity can be seen in the works of women who dared to be seen and heard whilst bearing grave consequences (from the community, families, or government), one can assert that the role of women is debatable today, a work in progress which requires breaking new frontiers in many contemporary Arab societies. This is due to how women are continuously seen within patriarchy as a mass-detrimental tool for devaluing the Arab self which obstructs individuals and collective social, emotional, and intellectual progress. They are seen as having the power to be detrimental due to women's history being linked to the ability to give life and preside over death—something which men have not been able to do, cannot currently do, and will not ever do; and something which is feared and therefore controlled in masculinist societies (see Silverio (2019) for more detailed discussion). This view of course is contested in the works of contemporary Arab female writers and activists such as Syrian author Samar Yazbek; Palestinian human rights activist and writer Susan Abulhawa; Iraqi author and journalist Inaam Kachachi; Saudi Arabian writer and novelist Badriah Al-Beshr, who continues to write novels focusing on strong female themes despite the pushback from the Saudi state at times; and Egyptian author and activist Nawal El Saadawi.

Arab women continuously experience a culture of mental and emotional shame as main factors that drive behaviour. The disclosure of an act of non-conformity within societies is in an act that brings emotions like shame, disgrace, and violence towards women. Women have been so controlled over time that their transgressions are met more harshly than their male counterparts in order to keep the patriarchal structure in balance. When they do something 'shameful', they are imprisoned by the act, such that, when it has been exposed, they are unable to use any defence to justify the action or even to restore self-image. Arab men, on the other hand, can justify an action that has the potential to bring shame. The defence and justification also can rectify self-image. For example, men who commit adultery often justify their act by expressing their dissatisfaction with their marriages and, perhaps also, the lack of sexual fulfilment from their wives. Hence, their marriages have failed to meet their needs, and in which case, these reasons (which are commonly used by patriarchal societies, families, and communities), are socially acceptable. Another example that can cause potential shame and yet is justified and accepted within Arab societies is the use of illegal substances and drugs. Their use is justified within societies as a normalised act that is often unspoken about or discussed and yet an act of wrongdoing which is committed in 'secrecy'. If exposed, men resort to claiming that other members influence or sway one's behaviour or admit to stress or feeling a sense of shame for drug using, and ultimately, societies as well as families do very little to condone this individual act and behaviour. Shame *'leads to hiding and to concealment and its antidote is either the desire for revenge, or the acceptance of the inadequate and faulty Self'* (Margherita & Troisi, 2013, p. 172).

3.2 The Rise of Arab Women

In shame-based cultures, social capital can be a key to growth and development in the sense that it requires the ability to maintain intricate networks of relationships which are an important asset to the individual. The constant strive for an Arab subject is to maintain social networks and protect one's reputation, respect, and status in society. The necessity to vigorously defend one's honour is a trait of shame-based cultures as they are antagonistic, meaning individuals compete for honour. When an Arab woman is shamed, male members of the family are dishonoured and ashamed and appear weak for failing to 'protect' her honour. The cultures' response is to defend the family's name with aggression, either against the woman herself (i.e. shunned by society and punishment) or against the aggressor (i.e. by the law or other means determined by involved members), though often both are enacted. This method of intimidation was born out of several sources of fear: fear of being exposed to others; fear of being disgraced amongst others, shunned by societies, punished by the law, and frowned upon by families; and, finally, within several communities, fear of God.

The Arab Spring undoubtedly gave contemporary Arab women a position of strength in a national and global context. The instability in the Arab world encouraged women to be at the heart of a dynamic national and international movement, economically, socially, and, more importantly perhaps, *politically*. The Arab Spring has awakened a sense of national pride and brought to light key contemporary issues that face progressive nations and leaders with regard to identity, freedom (and freedom of speech), sovereignty and power, human rights, political activism, and citizenship. This also awakened a necessity for many women to enter forcefully the public domain and to take to the streets to voice their demands and express their national identity. It was unthinkable that women who did so would be subject to violence, mistreatment, beating, physical and moral abuse, humiliation, and forcing into silence. These actions against Arab women activists and participants were *'legitimated by cultural assumptions, that adolescents embodied immoral desire; therefore it was possible to annihilate their bodies, their maternity, their dignity, and their female identity'* (Margherita & Troisi, 2013, p. 177). Violent actions against protestors were met by a counter-response from angry citizens—male and female—who marched the streets in objection to tyrannical governments. The message was one all over the Arab world: people demanded the overruling of tyranny once and for all. The atmosphere was portrayed by news channels and social media outlets as 'electrifying' in every country which experienced such political and social upheaval and contributed to what we now refer to as the 'Arab Spring'. This movement has not only brought to light in a contemporary and global context the issues that face Arab citizens in the last decade nationally and internationally, but also awakened deep-rooted social, psychological, and cultural emotions around identity, self-regard, duty, agency, status loss or threat to one's social appraisal, and shame-based cultures. The questions which many Arab citizens suddenly had to consider were the following: Who is the Arab subject in today's contemporary context? Can this subject think of him-/herself in terms and language that is organic to his/her history? Can Arabs have an authentic existence, and is it possible for Arabs to become modern on their own terms? The answers to these questions situate Arab citizens at the heart of an ontological exploration of identity and its meaning and perspectives. It was a time in history, in such context, where change was much needed. The demands of the people were seemingly the same from one Arab country to another: social justice; a demand for a fair and equal society between men and women, and the rich and poor; better education and health services; basic human rights and freedom of speech; and an end to corruption, to name only a few.

4 Transcending Shame Through the Fourth Industrial Revolution

The role of young Arab women has been a fundamental trait of the Arab Spring which marked the beginning of social and political change. The act of revolt had swept across the Arab world and caught the attention of many countries and organisations from a security and civil society standpoint; however, the global health community has lagged behind overlooking the well-being of many Arab women who were subject to violence and abuse in the process. *During the police repression of the Tunisian revolution, they were beaten by security thugs, and in rural areas around Kasserine some were raped by police after demonstrations. There were several reports of rape in Egypt amid the hurly burly, and a South African reporter for the US network CBS was sexually assaulted. In a notorious case in Tripoli, a woman, Iman al-Obeidi said she was raped by about 15 pro-Gaddafi militia. Scores of women across the region have also been detained or disappeared. A number of Bahraini women have been seized by the authorities, including at least nine doctors and four nurses. In Yemen, Karman was detained for 48 hours, though the outrage caused was largely a function of the 'shame' of male soldiers seizing a woman from her car in the night.* (Rice et al., 2011)

The role of technology has gradually, but steadily, dominated many debates with regard to the Arab Spring. It is fair to say that its role, specifically that of the Internet's role, has evolved over the past years, and, more recently, it is seen as a tool for empowering the people in response to it being used to build walls around which has become increasingly unwelcomed (Shaw, 2015).

The events in the Arab world show us several key statements: Firstly, that technology has aided the people, to a great extent, to overcome a set of various obstacles that have been endured over many years such as poverty, social injustice, and inequality. Secondly, and perhaps more importantly, in the aftermaths of the Arab Spring, technology has asserted itself as an integral feature of contemporary Arab societies with its advancements and as a tool which enables innovative ideas to become reality. This also means it is a tool for individual and social liberation, a powerful tool in which people can use it to voice their views, fears, and demands at any time, especially at times of turmoil or instability. This continues to assert the premise that technology, when put to good use, has a positive influence over our lives and, more generally, can drive Arab societies specifically towards progress. The role of technology as liberating the Arab subject from own predicaments is key in the sense that it gave the Arab subject a social, economic, and political stance on several issues from education, politics, citizenship; to well-being, and health-related issues. At the same time, however, during the events leading to the Arab Spring, technology has also revealed the restrictions on the Arab subject posed by shame-based cultures which chain the emotional and intellectual domain.

4.1 *The Rise into Rebellion*

'Revolution' is a commonly used word today, used to describe a specific period in the history of contemporary Arab societies. One revolution after another has swept rapidly the Arab world and evidently reshaped citizens' views on technology and its importance.

In Egypt, for example, technology has been used to mobilise citizens' protests, to upend what seemed like an everlasting regime and to give voice to the Egyptian people. Edward Said reiterated the 'speaking truth to power' mantra in his works, but, in the context of Egypt, one wonders what this 'power' is. Is it the government? Or is it the public which is let loose neither respected sufficiently to be spoken the truth to nor sufficiently cared for to deliver from its shackles which have become its own most dangerous enemy? What gave the Egyptian people hope in the events leading to 2011 revolution was *technology*. It is said that *'A grainy cell phone video of a Tunisian street vendor's self-immolation helped spark the massive protests that toppled longtime ruler Zine El Abidine Ben Ali, and Egypt's "Facebook revolution" forced the ruling regime out of power and into exile'* (Diamond & Plattner, 2012). The role of technology suddenly became integral in overthrowing the invulnerable authoritarian regimes in Tunisia and, equally, in Egypt. People's realisation and knowledge that technology can have, or can give, such power extended to reach different parts of the world linking events to one another and forming a wider global culture which transcended shame through rebellion. *From the earliest rumblings of discontent in Tunisia at the turn of the year, it was clear that old images of Arab women as deferential, subservient and generally indoors would have to be revised. From the highly-educated Tunisian female elite of doctors, barristers and university professors to the huge numbers of unemployed female graduates, women were key players in the uprising that launched the Arab spring. In Cairo, they were instrumental not just in protests but in much of the nitty-gritty organisation that turned Tahrir Square from a moment into a movement. Women were involved in arranging food deliveries, blankets, the stage and medical help. In Yemen, it was a young woman, Tawakul Karman, who first led demonstrations on a university campus against the long rule of Ali Abdullah Saleh. Karman emerged as one of the leaders of a revolution still yet to run its course. In Bahrain, women were among the first wave that descended on Pearl Square in the capital—some with their children—to demand change. And the Bahraini movement has latterly found a figurehead in Zainab al-Khawaja, the woman who went on hunger strike in protest at the beating and arrest of her father, husband and brother-in-law. 'Women have played a hugely influential role this time and put themselves in danger,' said Nabeel Rajab, president of the Bahrain Centre for Human Rights. 'They treated the injured in the streets and nursed them in their homes when they were too afraid to go to hospital'.* (Rice et al., 2011)

The instrumental role that technology has played in enabling the planning and organising of protests led to people's liberation but also revealed the shackles posed by authoritarian regimes who control means of communication and have strong surveillance of everything that links the countries to the outer world. Citizens, male and female, were politically aware and better informed which undermined the authorities of governments who feared losing grip on power.

4.2 Liberation and Control

In discussing the popular dichotomy of 'liberation' versus 'control' with regard to the Internet and the socio-political dimensions of such controls, information and communication technologies [ICT] have generated a pluralistic flow of ideas and information within authoritarian contexts. On the one hand, these contexts have been challenged by individuals, citizens, who feel empowered by technology (i.e. internet and mobile phones) to an extent where they call for freedom and expand pluralism. And on the other hand, authoritarian states continue censoring, constraining, monitoring, and punishing the use of ICT for that purpose. Leading to the Arab Spring, one may argue, citizens and organised groups have developed techniques to circumvent authoritarian censorship and control of these technologies. For example, *Ushahidi* is a platform developed to document human rights abuses in the wake of Kenya's 2007 elections, whilst, for example, in the Middle East, *Alkasir* (meaning *The Underage*) is a tool which has been used widely throughout Middle Eastern countries to circumvent cyber-censorship and discuss issues that are considered taboo (e.g. circumcision, sex, etc.). The thriving debates in the Arab world on the intersection of information and communications technology and the global struggle for democracy assert that people are no longer hostile to unfamiliar ideas such as the possibility of a 'revolution'. *The term 'liberation technology' has been widely used to highlight technology's ability to defend the rights of the people, to empower them, to lobby with governments and to promote change and to present a new pursuit of a variety of social goods. As history shows us, the route to liberation is one that is full of obstacles. These can be legal, political, cultural or social obstacles from individuals, from groups or from governments.* (Shaw, 2015)

An Internet that builds walls around people, cuts the lines of global communication, and revokes the right of every citizen to be heard freely without fear of prosecution is an Internet that is unwelcomed in the Arab world. And yet, according to a list compiled in 2015 and again in 2019 by the Committee to Protect Journalists (2019) research, it is revealed that access to the Internet in several Arab countries continues to be subject to restrictions and social media channels are banned.

Non-conformity to such laws may lead Arab citizens to be subject to the use of tactics ranging from imprisonment, repressive laws, and surveillance. Viral videos which have been censored or blocked altogether in Turkey allegedly insult 'Turkishness', and those in Egypt evidently are either against certain political ideologies, government initiatives, or the current regime. This is not to mention social networking sites which are blocked or restricted from countries like Saudi Arabia, Iran, and the United Arab Emirates to prevent what is believed to be the *corruption* of the people, *indecent* content, and general *immorality*. This is to an extent where the Internet has been referred to as *the work of the devil* by clergymen across the Arab world. In 2011, telecommunication companies have cut off the broadband networks and telephone lines to prevent further communications and obstruct organised revolts. Governments in many Arab countries have encouraged companies to provide or maintain poor service as a means of censorship. The question, however, of who has the right to censor what citizens see and what information is received is one that continues to be long debated and is equally a vital question in many contemporary Arab societies today.

5 Conclusion

The Arab spring has, undoubtedly, given Arab women the opportunity to be seen and heard; however, the Arab Spring was not about gender equality. Many women who were involved hold that view. El Saadawi, and many others, journalists and activists, wrote about how many women are alarmed that their efforts during the revolution were unrewarded and that men who were keen to encourage them to march and cry freedom are not so happy to have women in parliament, government, and in senior positions within societies. *'Women smell freedom at Change Square where they feel more welcomed than ever before. Their fellow [male] freedom fighters are showing unconventional acceptance to their participation and they are actually for the first-time letting women be, and say, what they really want'* (Rice et al., 2011). The increasing concerns regarding women's participation in contemporary Arab societies today, and since the collective aftermath of the Arab Spring, should continue to be at the very heart of every investigation into gender in relation to Arab shame-based cultures. The hope for many Arab women was that when the dust has settled, they could hold strategic positions within their communities and societies, and to continue to play a dynamic and important role, in what would have been a dramatic shift forward in these otherwise patriarchal societies. However, the Arab Spring led many women to realise that the gender divide and the equity gap were so ingrained into the very fabric of Arab identity, that their contributions were diminished as they returned from the fires of revolution to the hearths of their households. *'Through protesting, organising, blogging and hunger-striking, women have taken a central role, but it remains to be seen whether their rights will improve'* (Rice et al., 2011). The Arab Spring although may not have led to true gender equality across much of the Arab world, it certainly allowed Arab women to transcend shame through rebellion, transcend sexual suppression through self-expression and discovery in protest to the old regimes, and gave many women the will to break free. The time to break free may not have been at the dawn of the Arab Spring, and may not be now, but the desire was certainly awakened, and the technological future brings with it endless possibilities.

References

Abu-Lughod, L. (2016). *Veiled sentiments: Honor and poetry in a Bedouin society*. California: University of California Press.

Abu-Odeh, L. (2010). Honor killings and the construction of gender in Arab societies. *The American Journal of Comparative Law, 58*(4), 911–952.

Askoul, R. (2015, April 14). *Women are treated as if they were in 'Jahiliyah'*. The National. https://www.thenational.ae/opinion/women-are-treated-as-if-they-were-in-jahiliyah-1.637738

Badran, M. (1996). *Feminists, Islam, and nation: Gender and the making of modern Egypt*. Princeton, NJ: Princeton University Press.

Barakat, N. (2018, April 18). Let's banish the term 'Arab world'. *What does it mean anyway?* The Guardian. https://www.theguardian.com/commentisfree/2018/apr/18/lets-banish-the-term-arab-world-what-does-it-mean-anyway

Benedict, R. (1934). *Patterns of culture*. London: Routledge.

Benedict, R. (1946). *The chrysanthemum and the sword: Patterns of Japanese culture*. Boston: Houghton Mifflin Harcourt.

Committee to Protect Journalists. (2019). *10 most censored countries*. New York: Committee to Protect Journalists.

Deeb, A., Akle, M., Al Zaabi, A., Siwji, Z., Attia, S., Al Suwaidi, H., Al Qahtani, N., & Ehtisham, S. (2018). Maternal attitude towards delaying puberty in girls with and without a disability: A questionnaire-based study from the United Arab Emirates. *BMJ Paediatrics Open, 2*(1), 1–5.

DeYoung, P. A. (2015). *Understanding and treating chronic shame: A relational/neurobiological approach*. New York: Routledge.

Diamond, L., & Plattner, M. F. (Eds.). (2012). *Liberation technology: Social media and the struggle for democracy*. Baltimore: The Johns Hopkins University Press.

Dockery, W. (2018, February 6). *Where does the Arab world stand on female genital mutilation?* Made for minds. https://www.dw.com/en/where-does-the-arab-world-stand-on-female-genital-mutilation/a-42472991

El Saadawi, N. (2000, March 01). *Nawal El Saadawi – A creative and dissident life*. [interview with B. Belton & C. Dowding]. Infed archive. http://infed.org/mobi/nawal-el-saadawi-a-creative-and-dissident-life/

Fish, J. M. (2016, September 20). *Guilt and shame. Psychology today*. https://www.psychologytoday.com/gb/blog/looking-in-the-cultural-mirror/201609/guilt-and-shame

Fisher, M. (2012, April 25). *The real roots of sexism in the Middle East (It's not Islam, race, or 'hate')*. The Atlantic. https://www.theatlantic.com/international/archive/2012/04/the-real-roots-of-sexism-in-the-middle-east-its-not-islam-race-or-hate/256362/

Freud, S. (2017). *Three essays on the theory of sexuality: The 1905 edition*. Verso Books. Original work published in 1905.

Ghannoushi, S. (2011, March 11). *Perceptions of Arab women have been revolutionised.* The Guardian. https://www.theguardian.com/commentisfree/2011/mar/11/arab-women-revolutionised-egypt-tunisia-yemen

Ivy, M. (2008). Benedict's shame: Translating the *Chrysanthemum and the Sword*. *Cabinet, 31*, e1–e10.

Kharboush, I. F., Roudi-Fahimi, F., Ismail, H. M., Mamdouh, H. M., Muhammad, Y. Y., Tawfik, M., El Sharkawy, O. G., & Sallam, H. N. (2010). *Spousal violence in Egypt*. Washington, DC: Population Reference Bureau.

Laplanche, J., & Pontalis, J.B. (1973). *The language of psycho-analysis*. (Trans. D. Nicholson-Smith). Original work published in 1967.

Lewis, M. (1995). *Shame: The exposed self*. Simon & Schuster: New York.

Margherita, G., & Troisi, G. (2013). Gender violence and shame. The visible and the invisible, from the clinical to the social systems. *La Camera Blu: Journal of Gender Studies, 10*, 166–185.

Mayer, C.-H., & Vanderheiden, E. (Eds.). (2019). *The bright side of shame: Transforming and growing through practical applications in cultural contexts*. Cham: Springer.

Nathanson, D. L. (1994). *Shame and pride: Affect, sex, and the birth of the self.* New York: W.W. Norton & Company.

Pettigrove, G., & Parsons, N. (2012). Shame: A case study of collective emotion. *Social Theory and Practice, 38*(3), 504–530.

Rice, X., Marsh, K., Finn, T., Sherwood, H., Chrisafis, A., & Booth, R. (2011, April 22). *Women have emerged as key players in the Arab spring*. The Guardian. https://www.theguardian.com/world/2011/apr/22/women-arab-spring

Rycroft, C. (1972). *Critical dictionary of psychoanalysis.* Pennsylvania: Penn State University Press.

Shaw, S. H. (2015, June). *The age of technology: Freedom and choice.* Paper presentation at the annual meeting of the Caribbean philosophical association, Riviera Maya, Quintana Roo, Mexico.

Shaw, S. H. (2018). Gender and sexual health post the Egyptian revolution. *British Mensa's: ANDROGYNY, 2*(3), 14–20.

Shaw, S. H., & Silverio, S. A. (2019). A critical reflection on Egyptian feminism and psychology: Nawal El Saadawi, the best loved, most hated and best-known feminist in the Arab world. *Psychology of Women and Equalities Review, 2*(1), 82–86.

Shweder, R. A. (2003). Toward a deep cultural psychology of shame. *Social Research: An International Quarterly, 70*(4), 1100–1129.

Silverio, S. A. (2019). Reconstructing gender to transcend shame: Embracing human functionality to enable agentic and desexualised bodies. In C.-H. Mayer & E. Vanderheiden (Eds.), *The bright side of shame: Transforming and growing through practical applications in cultural contexts* (pp. 149–165). Cham: Springer.

Vanderheiden, E., & Mayer, C.-H. (2017). An introduction to the value of shame – Exploring a health resource in cultural contexts. In E. Vanderheiden & C.-H. Mayer (Eds.), *The value of shame: Exploring a health resource in cultural contexts* (pp. 1–39). Cham: Springer.

Wurmser, L. (1981). *The mask of shame.* Baltimore: The Johns Hopkins University Press.

Shereen H. Shaw is an academic lecturer, course leader, and researcher within the Edge Hill University's Further Education and Training programme. She is also a lecturer in existential philosophy at the University of Liverpool's Continuing Education Department. Shereen's inter-disciplinary research interest is in philosophy, literature, and gender. In 2015, she received a doctorate in philosophy from the University of Liverpool. Shereen read for a master of philosophy and literature at the University of East Anglia. She subsequently went on to complete a postgraduate certificate in education and training at the University of South Wales as well as teaching within various academic departments. She first read for a double honour bachelor in arts in English and comparative literature and philosophy at the American University in Cairo where she graduated with a *magna cum laude*. Most notable amongst her academic posts is her appointment as a programme leader in further education and training at Edge Hill University and her nomination for a staff students' award in 2017. Since her appointment at Edge Hill, Shereen has received a research investment fund for an interdisciplinary research project on 'Britishness, Identity, and Belonging'. Her early work in this area explored Arab women's gender identity, sexual health, and the ontology of being, post the Arab Spring. Shereen adapts an existential lens in her comparative research and focuses on various ontological questions on meaning and purpose. This enables her to philosophically explore critical discourses on Arab women, identity, gender and social, cultural, and political debates

Sergio A. Silverio is an academic Psychologist whose work can be best described as falling within the field of 'Medical Psychology', that is, the application of psychological knowledge to both health and healthcare services. His work in this area aims to understand both personal experiences of psychopathology and health system policy and practice regarding public health priorities. Specifically, the main focus of Sergio's work has been women's mental health and psychological well-being over the life course and through key life transitions (i.e. pregnancy, birth, ageing, and widowhood). His early work which explored older never married women's gender identity and social networks attracted critical acclaim from The British Psychological Society. Later work, using hospital ethnography to explore anxiety relating to early pregnancy and antenatal clinic visits, received international acclaim from The Society for Reproductive and Infant Psychology. Methodologically, Sergio specialises in qualitative methods and analysis, and he has particular expertise in conducting in-depth interviews on sensitive topics. This has led to the development of a theoretical interest into the ethics of qualitative inquiry. Sergio's work involves—at one end—embracing critical psychology perspectives to contribute new theoretical bases for research and—at the other—adopting formal evaluative frameworks to influence, adapt, and transform policy. He is currently employed at the Department of Women & Children's Health, King's College London, and holds honorary fellowships at the Elizabeth Garrett Anderson Institute for Women's Health, University College London, and the Department of Psychological Sciences, University of Liverpool. He is an associate fellow of The British Psychological Society, a Life Fellow of The Royal Anthropological Institute, and a fellow of the Royal Society for Public Health.

Chapter 23
A Place for 4IR in Transforming Shame in Returning Migrants

Gillian McKay

1 Introduction

The sophistication of digital technology is having an extensive impact on humanitarian and development sectors, and with no signs of slowing down—or giving us time to catch up—we need to embrace the changes it brings. This Fourth Industrial Revolution (4IR) is going to change the way we live and work and how we interact with each other at the individual, societal and global levels. Indeed, it is undoubtedly disrupting the way we live our lives, and most of us are now more interconnected than ever before. On the one hand, the digital age has given rise to many freedoms, whilst many others view these changes as a means for governments to exert power over their citizens: through Internet blackouts, for example (Selva, 2019). For Schwab (2017), the 4IR goes beyond previous revolutions for a number of reasons, including the exponential speed at which technological advances are progressing. Despite the tremendous speed with which the 4IR is changing our lives, globalisation has actually shown us that humanity is able to effectively adapt to changes that each revolution brings (see Mayer and Vanderheiden on The Meaning of Shame in Cultures of the fourth Industrial Revolution—An Introduction).

Having said that, this revolution does have the potential to cause greater destruction and inequality by facilitating widespread job insecurity where digital technology has the capacity to take their place. Economists have been predicting unemployment as a result of technological advances as far back as 1931 (Schwab, 2017), though this time these warnings may have substantial merit that they once lacked. Indeed, more recent studies have ranked the jobs most likely to be replaced by automation, with administrators and hospitality workers amongst the most susceptible to these changes (Frey & Osborne, 2013). Emphasis has shifted towards roles with greater reliance on creativity and the development of new ideas, such as positions in the field

G. McKay (✉)
Department of Politics and International Studies, University of Leeds, Leeds, UK

C.-H. Mayer et al. (eds.), *Shame 4.0*, https://doi.org/10.1007/978-3-030-59527-2_23

of psychology or in management more generally, with this idea echoed by others who think that philosophy degrees will be more useful in the digital age than computing qualifications (Montag, 2018). Although the long-term impacts of the 4IR on the labour market are still largely unknown, it will have an indubitably significant impact on migration—whether this is because people can use technology to work remotely from anywhere in the world (Lee, 2016) or because it has left them unemployed and, in many cases, destitute (see Worth in this book; see Mayer on Shame 4.0—Empirical Evidence of the Importance of Emotions in a Technologising World of Work).

Although the 4IR is now often considered to be a driver of migration, it may also offer solutions within displaced populations. Technology now plays a significant role in managing humanitarian data, for example. First, social media allows individuals to mark themselves safe during natural disasters, and by following and/or sharing updates, we can all understand more about crises worldwide – though this may be based more on opinion than fact (Miller, 2017). Of course, all of this assumes that everyone has access to this technology—which is simply not true (yet).

Second, systems exist in the humanitarian sector that can facilitate more rapid and effective responses. For instance, the Humanitarian Data Exchange (HDX) provides a platform for organisations to share data on population statistics, development progress and migration movements; the Signal Code published by the Harvard Humanitarian Initiative facilitates the translation of human rights into humanitarian action; the International Committee of the Red Cross' *Handbook on Data Protection in Humanitarian Action* supports staff to understand and apply relevant standards in collecting and processing data; the Humanitarian Unmanned Aerial Vehicle Network's Code of Conduct provides guidance for organisations in ethical and responsible use of autonomous drones; and Monitoring, Evaluation, Research and Learning Tech provides a platform for humanitarian and development actors to understand the value and impact of digital technology in their roles (World Economic Forum, 2019).

Data in migration has also improved vastly over the years, with many organisations referring to artificial intelligence and satellite imagery to inform their programming (Garber & Carrette, 2018). For instance, in using historical data to predict trends and outcomes, the placement algorithm piloted by the International Rescue Committee is able to recommend areas in which refugees are most likely to thrive (World Economic Forum, 2019). Similarly, The Hive uses satellite imagery to provide more rapid response to refugee crises by counting the number of shelters in camps and facilitating a more streamlined flow of aid (Ibid). SpaceKnow is also working with humanitarian organisations to promote the use of satellite imagery analysis in mapping and responding to migration crises (IOM, 2018).

None of this is to say that migration is a new phenomenon in need of monitoring, but with an estimated one billion migrants worldwide, including 763 million internal migrants (UN DESA, 2013), 272 million international migrants (IOM, 2019a) and 70 million displaced persons (Edwards, 2019), the situation is the worst it has ever been. According to these statistics, every seventh person on our planet is a migrant. Furthermore, the World Bank (Rigaud et al., 2018) has estimated that 140 million more people are expected to migrate as a result of climate change in the coming years; almost the entire population of Russia. Not only are people still migrating under more 'traditional' characteristics trends are now surfacing that demonstrate a number of new reasons behind these recent migration surges. Thanks to the digital age, it is now possible for us to develop a greater understanding of these specific characteristics (Bartolucci, Villosio, & Wagner, 2018), including drivers and impacts of migration, and the emotional and psychosocial effects of returning to a country of origin.

Shame is just one of these many emotions experienced by migrants—from a pressure to flee the shame of living in poverty, to the shame experienced in the undignified treatment or conditions on their journey or even upon arrival at their destination country. Less explored is the experience of shame in returning migrants, whether these are migrants who have been forcibly returned or those who have returned voluntarily. This chapter seeks to explore the role of 4IR in transforming this experience of shame in returning migrants and empowering them to catalyse more positive change in their communities.

2 Shame as a Driver of Migration

People migrate for a myriad of reasons: some may be trying to flee conflict, persecution or natural disasters, whilst others may be seeking better employment or other economic opportunities. These migrants may travel short distances or make longer journeys in search of greater commerce and industry and where their earning potential is up to 70 times higher than at home (Mohieldin, 2019). Indeed, many migrants have these economic motives, but many others simply have an inherent desire to 'better themselves' through material assets and will take on any opportunity to showcase their worth in society (Lee, 1966). For Schwab (2017), beyond a remapping of the labour market, the primary reasons behind migration include an individual's want to realise their life aspirations and to redefine both their individual and familial identity.

Of course, it is difficult to identify specific factors which may encourage an individual to migrate, particularly since the reasons for migration inherently depend on *who* is migrating: whether they are large groups escaping conflict zones or prosperous individuals with diasporic potential (Bartolucci et al., 2018). Factors which may influence an individual's decision to migrate include those which arise in their home country or at their intended destination, or personal circumstances more generally. These push and pull factors can ultimately place these migrants at greater risk of violations and/or abuse—a risk many are still prepared to take.

Advances in technology have also played a pivotal role in driving migration. Thanks to previous industrial revolutions, we are now living in a more fast-paced world than ever before, leaving developing countries behind and driving entire communities to seek opportunities elsewhere. This globalisation has also left many developing nations exposed to the devastating impact of climate change, causing further displacement and migration. Furthermore, the 4IR will indubitably impact the probability and nature of conflict, and just as lines are becoming blurred between the physical and the digital, international humanitarian law may no longer provide a distinction between war and peace or combatants and non-combatants (Schwab, 2017). Indeed, the 4IR can only add to the already dangerous catalogue of weapons that can, and undoubtedly one day will, cause irreparable harm to thousands, if not millions, of people. On the other hand, innovative technology can also offer protection, and access to 24-h media means we are also more aware of global events and, in turn, more prepared to react (Weidman-Grunewald, 2017).

Socioeconomic pressures also continue to influence more people than ever to migrate and send money back to their families (Bolzman, Gakuba, & Guissé, 2011) (see also Vanderheiden on life crises in this book), with diaspora sending home billions globally every year (World Bank, 2018a). Migrant workers escaping poverty tend to seek opportunities elsewhere in response to household decisions, as opposed to at the individual level. For instance, an individual may feel pressured to leave in order to provide for their family, evoking feelings of shame if they refuse since they may then not be considered 'real men' (Bolzman, Gakuba, & Amalaman, 2017). Indeed, for many communities, unemployed youth or individuals with more 'informal' work are often subject to criticism and are compared to successful migrants (i.e. returning migrants often associated with wealth) who send money home to their families (European Council on Refugees and Exiles, 2005). In fact, some cultures celebrate international migrants as heroes (Dunsch, Tjaden, & Quiviger, 2019), simultaneously increasing pressure for others to follow suit.

In this way, individuals emigrating for work is becoming the norm and almost even a measure of social success in some communities (Tanon & Sow, 2013). This pressure is exerted almost exclusively on young men, with communities maintaining that family responsibility lies with the man and that by taking the risks involved with migration, they are able to (re)affirm their masculinity (Bolzman et al., 2017). Ultimately, if one is afraid of these risks, one should be ashamed of oneself (Heller, 2003), and in this way, shame has the ability to 'regulate ambition—triggered by the failure to live up to expectations' (Ibid).

At their destination, migrants often find themselves living and working in harsh, often deplorable, conditions, and they will hesitate to communicate their hardships with their loved ones back home: Both they and their families have invested too much in getting this far, and they are reluctant to expose their fears since they have been conditioned to feel ashamed if they are unsuccessful. As a result, these migrants often accept degrading work because it enables them to work overseas and maintain a successful facade from afar. Although many labour migrants are young males, migrating women can often find themselves burdened by the shame of survival sex—whether consensual through smuggling or otherwise through trafficking (Pittaway, 2010). Thus, migrants may also experience shame as a result of their journeys or encounters, and what they may have done to survive (Gorman, 2001).

Unrealistic expectations are rarely met amongst migrants, and since returning migrants often reinforce the idea that migration is a gateway to success, this ultimately exerts further pressure on others to follow the same path (Bolzman et al., 2017). Returning migrants will not share their humiliation or degrading experiences as this would tarnish the image of success they feel pressured to paint (Aguilar, 1996), ultimately leading to mixed emotions of guilt and shame, and a residual pressure to promote migration to others. This truth-masking creates a vicious cycle in which returning migrants are almost actively encouraging others to do as they have done.

3 Shame in Returning Migration

In the most basic sense, returning migrants are those who return to their country of origin either forcibly or voluntarily. The latter, as defined by UNHCR, occurs only when the return is dignified, sustainable and without force (Carr, 2014). As migration flows fluctuate globally, return migration continues to increase, with 5.5 million asylum seekers and undocumented migrants having returned from Europe in 2017 alone (World Bank, 2018b).

Voluntary return migration is driven by a number of factors. Just as there are push and pull factors for someone to leave their country, so too are there many reasons to return: they may be destitute or subject to harassment and violence in the destination country; they may return home for personal/family reasons or illnesses; or the security situation may have improved at home, thus allowing them to return (Carr, 2014).

Forced return is a different story. Despite new developments that promise protections for climate refugees (UN Human Rights Committee, 2020), specifically in line with the principle of *non-refoulement*, many migrant workers still find it difficult to claim asylum once they have reached their destination unless they can definitively prove that they are at direct risk of persecution back home. Indeed, the majority of migrants who successfully make it to Europe do not have appropriate legal status to stay and/or work (Bolzman et al., 2017), resulting in many forced returns.

Managing these returns comes with its own challenges, but managing the emotional and psychosocial support required is one challenge in and of itself. Indeed, 'psychosocial assistance' is listed as one of the means to achieve Objective 21 of the Global Compact for Safe, Orderly and Regular Migration: specifically, to achieve sustainable reintegration (UN General Assembly, 2018). The European Parliament has also argued that '[s]uccessful reintegration is highly dependent on . . . psychosocial health' (Latek, 2017). However, as yet, efforts have been unconvincing, and the experience of shame specifically has been largely unexplored.

Migration is complex—returning migration even more so—so it is imperative to acknowledge that shame is just one of many emotions experienced by returning migrants (Castles & Miller, 2003). Shame itself is an emotion found at the intersection of social and individual dimensions (de Gualejac, 1996) and emerges from a problematic relationship with others, whereby an individual will internalise external judgements (Heller, 2003). Many theorists have described shame as an attack on the self and the experience of losing face (Goffman, 2003). If this inferiority complex persists, it can often give rise to more permanent vulnerability. Indeed, one study found that shame was correlated with post-traumatic stress disorder (PTSD) in refugee minors (Stotz, Elbert, Müller, & Schauer, 2015), and others have also demonstrated that young people aged 11–20 at the time of migration are at greater risk of a range of 'affective, cognitive, and behavioural disorders' (Nidorf, 1985). With the median age of migrants decreasing worldwide (UN DESA, 2017), this is somewhat concerning.

Many returning migrants have experienced significant trauma on their journeys—in fact, they may have been returned home before they even had a chance to receive psychosocial support of any kind (Dunsch et al., 2019). Others may be overwhelmed by the shame that accompanies the recruitment agencies or smugglers who come to collect their payments after the fact (Schuster & Majidi, 2015). The literature on managing psychosocial support for these groups is sparse, and with some cultural taboos restricting dialogue about suicide, for example, many instances go unreported (Ibid).

Returning home empty handed is just not an option for many of these migrants. Some will in fact return to their home country but never actually return to their families, simply as a consequence of shame (Whewell, 2019); they would rather live in extreme poverty than admitting their 'failure' or defeat. This has been echoed in research conducted by Amalaman (2016), who demonstrated that 64% of unsuccessful asylum seekers in his study said that they would not go home if they had to return empty handed. A failure to migrate is seen by many as a social failure (Bolzman et al., 2017), with many migrants returning home only to be branded as such because they have tried to migrate but ultimately failed those 'whom [they] had promised a better future' (IOM, 2019b). For instance, migrants returning to Afghanistan have commented on the shame of coming back empty handed (European Council on Refugees and Exiles, 2005), whilst those returning to Sierra Leone have faced comparable humiliation (Carr, 2014). Families have often made huge sacrifices for the migrant to leave so they can feel disappointed and unsupported by failed migration attempts and can shut out their returning loved ones as a result (IOM, 2019b). In order to avoid disappointing their families, some migrants will delay reunions for as long as possible, whilst others may contemplate never returning home or they may even let their families believe that they are no longer alive (Searcy & Jaime, 2017).

Return is not necessarily the end of the migration process either (European Council on Refugees and Exiles, 2005), and reintegration provides yet another struggle for returnees—particularly for those who have been forcibly returned, but also for those who choose to return voluntarily and whose expectations may actually be higher. '[T]he reality is that often people return to face poverty and continuing persecution, some are detained, tortured by the authorities and/or go missing' (Ibid). For others, it may be difficult to reintegrate into a community that they so strongly felt the need to leave in the first place (Ghanem, 2003). Psychological preparation is therefore required to minimise the negative impact of return: first and foremost, people need to be prepared for the fact that life will not necessarily be the same.

This suppression is unsurprising and echoes a *spiral of silence* theory which would suggest that returning migrants are reluctant to share their experiences because they are conditioned to feel ashamed of being an unsuccessful minority (West & Turner, 2017). Thus, returning migrants are in unique need of psychosocial support insofar as they experience the need to integrate twice during their migration journey: first, if and when they arrive in their destination country and again when they return home (Fonseca, Hart and Klink, 2015). Overwhelming experiences of shame can disrupt an already difficult reintegration process, and without feeling able to talk to anyone about their experiences, some fail to cope at all.

4 What's the Need?

For Schwab (2017), the four most important kinds of knowledge required to harness the 4IR include *contextual*, *emotional* and *inspired* intelligence. In other words, emotionally intelligent leaders across academia, governments, civil society and the private sector should seek to collaborate in order to achieve sustainable and inclusive change. Returning migrants themselves also hold responsibility: they must take care of their own physical and mental health.

Having largely been ignored in public health discussions, people are now beginning to acknowledge some of the links between shame and a number of different behaviours, including violence and depression (Brown, 2006). With this growing sense of importance, shame has been described as 'the preeminent cause of emotional distress in our time' (Karen, 1992). Migrants are particularly vulnerable to the experience of shame, especially given the complex and often competing expectations that lead them to migrate (Brown, 2006) or, indeed, return. Thus, there is a need to understand the specific experience of shame in returning migrants in order to provide effective psychosocial support that facilitates full reintegration to their home country. Brown (2012) has acknowledged that although shame is a universal phenomenon, the experience of shame differs across genders, with men feeling particular pressure to 'climb their way to the top or die trying': a sentiment echoed in research that identifies shame as a driver to migration (e.g. Bolzman et al., 2017).

Studies have also shown that shame more often than not leads to avoidance (Leach & Cidam, 2015) and is often associated with our vulnerabilities, since it is our awareness of societal expectations that forces us to do things that make us feel ashamed or that cause us to experience shame in the first place (Brown, 2006). In one particular study, Brown found that participants with little to no awareness of this connection between our personal experience and societal issues often lacked the ability to deconstruct or contextualise their experience of shame. Instead of framing their experience within a wider picture, they tend to focus on the individual experience, thus heightening the perceived sense of shame. The same study demonstrated that talking about (and understanding) shame allows us to develop something known as *shame resilience* (Ibid).

Shame resilience theory describes the coping mechanisms through which an individual can challenge the negative experience of shame. Brown (2012) argues that researchers have been unable to correlate shame with any positive outcomes and that it is in fact 'more likely to be the cause of destructive and hurtful behaviours'. Indeed, studies have found that social rejection can induce emotional turmoil that hurts much in the same way as physical pain would (Kross, Berman, Mischel, Smith, & Wager, 2011). Meanwhile, other studies have shown that suppressing negative thoughts and emotions can take a physiological toll on our bodies but that outward expression of these thoughts and emotions can lead to improved physical health (Petrie, Booth, & Pennebaker, 1998).

Shame resilience provides us with the tools 'to come out on the other side of the shame experience with more courage, compassion, and connection than we had going into it' (Brown, 2012). To do this, we need to be able to detach our self-worth from the judgement of others: we cannot let what other people think define our sense of self. In this way, shame resilience is our capacity to recognise disappointment not as defeat but as a drive to overcome and ultimately improve our self (Davidoff, 2002). To do this, however, an important transformation is required that lifts the narrative and transcends from humiliation to dignity (Gorman, 2001): basically, we need to learn to talk about it.

Brown (2012) argues that '[s]hame derives its power from being unspeakable... [and] [i]f we cultivate enough awareness about shame to name it and speak to it, we've basically cut it off at the knees'. For her, in the same 'way exposure to light was deadly for the gremlins, language and story bring light to shame and destroy it'. In this way, '[s]hame resilience is key to embracing our vulnerability'.

5 Current Efforts

Research has demonstrated that humanity does have the ability to overcome shame by empowering indigenous groups to share their stories publicly (Louth, 2012). Much in the same way that the Australian National Curriculum Board has given teachers the responsibility to deliver lessons about indigenous cultures (Ibid), or how emerging technology is reducing marginality experienced by young indigenous groups through music (Warren & Evitt, 2010), so too must organisations be given the responsibility to help returning migrants share their stories.

One such project that is already encouraging such communication methods has been piloted by the International Organization for Migration (IOM): an inter-governmental organisation with specific expertise in the field of migration. The Organization works closely with migrants and governments globally and has nine regional offices which serve as focal points for the coordination of activities in the region, in addition to engagement with government and other UN agencies working in the field. To respond to increasing migration to Europe, IOM wanted to challenge the misperceptions of irregular migration amongst potential migrants, primarily as a means to deter such movements (Dunsch et al., 2019). More specifically, the

Organization implemented a peer-based awareness-raising campaign in Guinea, Senegal and Nigeria. The project, entitled *Migrants as Messengers* (MaM), was piloted between December 2017 and March 2019, and was the first of its kind in the field of migration.

Specifically, the project intended to address the challenges of traditional awareness-raising campaigns, which were more information-heavy, by introducing an emotive dimension to outreach engagement. As irregular migration continues to increase, current information sharing campaigns are proving to be ineffective, and, despite the need for information being clear, migrants are still largely misinformed about the potential dangers of irregular migration prior to departure (Foran & Iacucci, 2017). For instance, MaM participants were either unaware of how many migrants had lost their lives en route to Europe or predicted a number (i.e. <1000) significantly lower than the actual reported number of deaths (i.e. $>22{,}000$). Almost three quarters of participants 'did not know what asylum' was, and of 'those who reported economic reasons for wanting to leave, almost half thought they would be eligible for refugee status'. Beyond this, respondents seemed to think that the journey itself would take far less time (e.g. 1 month) than the majority of most reported journeys (i.e. up to several years).

A total of 80 returning migrants were provided with training which qualified them to volunteer with the Organization and 'capture authentic video testimonies from fellow migrant returnees'. Individual testimonies were shared on social media platforms, though this part of the project was not evaluated. Rather, the documentary *On est Ensemble*, as an amalgamation of each individual clip, was played to a treatment group across various town halls, whilst the control group watched an alternative documentary. A number of themes were covered in the treatment group documentary, including trafficking, modern slavery, detention, conditions on the road and returning.

An in-depth impact evaluation of the project highlighted a number of positive effects, including an increase in awareness of the associated risks of irregular migration and a decrease in likelihood to migrate irregularly in the near future. In addition, communities' 'social perception of returnees' had also been changed as a result of MaM events—from before, when one third of participants felt that migrants who return home empty handed should feel ashamed of themselves. However, there was a lack of 'factual knowledge on the legal context, length and cost of journeys, as well as expected potential earnings at destination' which is unsurprising 'given that the focus of the events was on emotional identification with the personal experience of returnees rather than the dissemination of facts'. Thus, future programming could benefit from a mix of both factual and emotive content.

This is useful: we can see some positive impact of the emotive engagement with someone who has lived experience of migration. However, the primary focus of this particular MaM project was to deter prospective migrants from taking irregular routes, rather than providing specific support to the returning migrants who had volunteered to record the testimonies. Beyond the MaM project, others have created a platform known as 'Migration Conversation' where they encourage returning migrants to share their stories as a means to address and overcome feelings of shame on their return (IOM, 2019c). This is a great start, but the sharing of individual testimonies should also be explored as private engagement may prove more effective than the group context in which participants watched and reviewed the documentary here.

6 Harnessing the 4IR

Digital participation is undoubtedly central to modern life; we are living in a world where technology enables us to do a multitude of exciting and innovative things. This revolution is characterised specifically by advances in artificial intelligence and machine learning, and, although both are very much in their infancy, the trajectory for their development seems almost incomprehensible. Schwab (2017) understands that the 4IR goes beyond previous revolutions for three primary reasons: first, the exponential speed at which this revolution is progressing; second, the apparently infinite depth that new combinations of physical, digital and biological technologies seem to uncover; and third, the impressive transformations observed across structures and societies globally. The latter is perhaps of greatest relevance to our discussion of migration, and Schwab, in encouraging us to think about how we can best harness this revolution to shape and improve our futures, suggests that we should collaborate across sectors and industries in order to benefit from these revolutionary transformations. In addition, increasing cooperation amongst academia, governments, civil society and the private sector will help to challenge the inequalities exacerbated by the revolution itself.

These collaborations will allow stakeholders to regulate innovation and shape both local and global transformations, in addition to an opportunity to simply pause and take a step back at a time when humanity has developed a sense of instant need and urgency in our daily lives. Schwab (2017) makes reference to this when he argues that 'the 24-h news cycle puts pressure on leaders to comment or act immediately to events, reducing the time available for arriving at measured principles and calibrated responses'. Thus, collaboration effectively buys more time and facilitates maximum efficiency.

The first step towards collaborative working requires access to the technology they seek to implement. To date, this has been one of the main barriers to facilitating progress, particularly in less developed countries. However, the World Economic Forum (2015) has estimated that 80% of people are expected to be connected to the Internet by 2025. Additionally, 90% of the population will be using smartphones with regular access to the Internet: 'nearly everyone will soon have a literal supercomputer in their pocket' (Schwab, 2017). Indeed, statistics show that more than half of the global population currently has access to the Internet,[1] with studies estimating that 3.9 billion people will be able to access the web using smartphones by 2023

[1] internetlivestats.com/internet-users; worldometers.info/world-population

(Kumar & Meena, 2019). In no time at all, smartphones have become more available and more affordable than ever before, and the right to this access runs parallel with some of the most fundamental human rights (e.g. the right to access clean safe water or the right to life).

This evidence points to the fact that, if we can embrace the fundamentals of this 4IR, cost efficiency of any innovation can likely be met in a relatively short period. If we can overcome the problems of accessing this technology, the benefits seem unrivalled. Governments, first and foremost, must acknowledge the potential that this digital revolution can have in transforming the 'hyper-connected' society in which we find ourselves (Schwab, 2017). Thus, the first step for them in realising the transformative power of the 4IR is to ensure that no one is digitally excluded from civic life.

Once we overcome the issue of access, these collaborative groups need to consider how technology can be used to overcome some of the problematic issues faced by the affected populations they seek to support. If we can create a platform that alters the way groups (e.g. returning migrants) relate to others (e.g. communities resistant to welcoming them back), then the battle is already half won. In the same way that technologies are being used to facilitate integration into host communities (Duarte, Ataei, Degbelo, Brendel, & Kray, 2019), so too should the digital revolution be harnessed to facilitate successful reintegration for migrants who have returned to their country of origin.

The technology under consideration here needs to go beyond basic story telling or information sharing. We are living in a time where information is available almost instantly to the majority of the population (Schwab, 2017), but evidence suggests that migrants still often pursue irregular journeys in spite of the warnings that they have received (van Bemmel, 2019). Furthermore, the information that is out there does not necessarily lead to acceptance or tolerance, and this is particularly apparent in the field of migration. The news is filled with awful stories of people fleeing terror and conflict and the trauma that they experience on their journeys to safety. Yet, thousands of people want to deny them the right to seek refuge within their borders: evident most recently in Brexit campaigners who framed immigration as a problem in the United Kingdom (Garrett, 2019). It is therefore clear that what is currently being done is insufficient: we are neither able to deter irregular migration nor able to accept those who choose to migrate irregularly.

By harnessing the technological advances of this 4IR, we can simultaneously challenge the destructive impact of the revolution by capitalising on its benefits (Schwab, 2017). Ultimately, giving people a voice enables them to participate fully in civic life and make a positive contribution to society, both locally and globally. More specifically, it offers returning migrants an opportunity to transform their negative feelings of shame into a powerful movement that can help to influence decision-making at all levels.

It may be helpful to reflect on research which has explored the use of artificial intelligence in challenging mental health issues. For instance, artificially intelligent chat bots have improved symptoms of depression in users (Inkster, Sarda, & Subramanian, 2018), and other projects which engage young people to seek mental health support online have had similar success (Naqshbandi et al., 2016). However, these methods are not perfect, and research has demonstrated that a *spiral of silence* theory still persists in technology-based communications where users can openly see the opinions of others, meaning they are still likely to withhold or even withdraw (Lang, 2014).

Creating a more private communications system, whereby prospective migrants can reach out to ask questions of returning migrants, could simultaneously inform decision-making amongst prospective migrants and foster an environment in which returning migrants can both provide and seek useful support that allows them to meet their essential psychosocial support needs. By harnessing the knowledge gained through lived experience, their shame can be transformed into a sense of purpose and ultimately serve to improve their well-being in the long term.

References

Aguilar, F. V. (1996). The dialectics of transnational shame and national identity. *Philippine Sociological Review, 44*(1/4), 101–136.

Amalaman, M. (2016). *Problématique du retour des requérants d'asile déboutés (RAD) et non-entrée en matière (NEM) d'origine ouest-africaine en Suisse romande (Genève, Vaud, Fribourg, Neuchâtel).* Haute École de Travail Social de Genève et Université de Genève, Rapport de stage postdoctoral.

Bartolucci, C., Villosio, C., & Wagner, M. (2018). Who migrates and why? Evidence from Italian administrative data. *Journal of Labor Economics, 36*(2), 551–588.

Bolzman, C., Gakuba, T. O., & Amalaman, M. (2017). Honte et migration: une relation complexe à saisir. *Pensee Plurielle, 44*(1), 129–138.

Bolzman, C., Gakuba, T. et Guissé, I. (2011). *Migrations des jeunes d'Afrique subsaharienne. Quels défis pour l'avenir?* Retrieved January 30, 2020, from http://www.editions-harmattan.fr/catalogue/couv/aplat/9782296550582.pdf.

Brown, B. (2006). Shame resilience theory: A grounded theory study on women and shame. *Families in Society, 87*(1), 43–52.

Brown, B. (2012). *Daring greatly: How the courage to be vulnerable transforms the way we live, love, parent, and lead.*

Carr, H. (2014). Returning 'home': Experiences of reintegration for asylum seekers and refugees. *The British Journal of Social Work, 44*(Suppl_1), i140–i156.

Castles, S., & Miller, M. (2003). *The age of migration* (3rd ed.). New York: Guilford Press.

Davidoff, F. (2002). Shame: The elephant in the room: Managing shame is important for improving health care. Resource document. *British Medical Journal.* Retrieved January 30, 2020, from https://www.ncbi.nlm.nih.gov/pmc/articles/PMC1743562/pdf/v011p00002.pdf.

de Gualejac, V. (1996). *Les sources de la honte.* Paris: Desclée de Brouwer.

Duarte, A. M., Ataei, M., Degbelo, A., Brendel, N., & Kray, C. (2019). Safe spaces in participatory design with young forced migrants. *International Journal of CoCreation in Design and the Arts*, 1–23.

Dunsch, F. A., Tjaden, J., & Quiviger, W. (2019). *Migrants as messengers: The impact of peer-to-peer communication on potential migrants in Senegal.* Impact Evaluation Report. International Organization for Migration. Retrieved January 30, 2020, from https://publications.iom.int/books/migrants-messengers-impact-peer-peer-communication-potential-migrants-senegal-impact.

Edwards, A. (2019). *Global forced displacement tops 70 million. Resource document.* UNHCR. Retrieved January 30, 2020, from https://www.unhcr.org/news/stories/2019/6/5d08b6614/global-forced-displacement-tops-70-million.html.

European Council on Refugees and Exiles. (2005). *Increasing refugee participation in the field of voluntary return. Resource document.* Retrieved January 30, 2020, from https://www.refworld.org/docid/465416e92.html.

Fonseca, A., Hart, L., & Klink, S. (2015). *Reintegration: Effective approaches. Resource document.* Retrieved January 30, 2020, from https://www.iom.int/files/live/sites/iom/files/What-We-Do/docs/Reintegration-Position-Paper-final.pdf.

Foran, R., & Iacucci, A. A. (2017). *Lost in translation: The misinformed journey of migrants across Italy. Resource document.* Interviews. Retrieved January 30, 2020, from https://internews.org/sites/default/files/Internews_Lost_In_Translation_Publication_2017-05-23.pdf.

Frey, C. B., & Osborne, M. A. (2013). The future of employment: How susceptible are jobs to computerisation? *Technological Forecasting and Social Change, 114*, 254–280.

Garber, K., & Carrette, S. (2018). *Using Technology in Fragile, conflict, and violence situations. Resource document.* World Bank Group. Retrieved January 30, 2020, from https://openknowledge.worldbank.org/bitstream/handle/10986/30502/BRI-ntechn-PUBLIC-ADD-SERIES-HNP-Knowledge-Brief-TAG-TO-VC-Knowledge-note.pdf?sequence=1.

Garrett, A. (2019). *The refugee crisis, Brexit, and the reframing of immigration in Britain.* EuropeNow. Garrett 2019. Retrieved January 30, 2020, from https://www.europenowjournal.org/2019/09/09/the-refugee-crisis-brexit-and-the-reframing-of-immigration-in-britain/.

Ghanem, T. (2003). *When forced migrants return 'home': The psychosocial difficulties returnees encounter in the reintegration process.* Refugee Studies Centre. Retrieved January 30, 2020, from https://www.rsc.ox.ac.uk/publications/when-forced-migrants-return-home-the-psychosocial-difficulties-returnees-encounter-in-the-reintegration-process.

Goffman, E. (2003). *Les rites d'interaction.* Paris: Minuit.

Gorman, W. (2001). Refugee survivors of torture: Trauma and treatment. *Professional Psychology: Research and Practice, 32*(5), 443–451.

Heller, A. (2003). Five approaches to the phenomenon of shame. *Social Research: An International Quarterly, 70*(4), 1015–1030.

Inkster, B., Sarda, S., & Subramanian, V. (2018). An empathy-driven, conversational artificial intelligence agent (Wysa) for digital mental Well-being: Real-world data evaluation mixed-methods study. *JMIR mHealth and uHealth, 6*(11), e12106.

International Organization for Migration. (2018). *Monthly update #3. Resource document.* Retrieved January 30, 2020, from https://www.iom.int/sites/default/files/situation_reports/file/somalia_sr_201803.pdf.

International Organization for Migration. (2019a). *World migration report 2020. Resource document.* Retrieved January 30, 2020, from https://publications.iom.int/system/files/pdf/wmr_2020.pdf.

International Organization for Migration. (2019b). *When returning home is a deadly journey, "shame is the returnee's worst enemy".* Press Release. Retrieved January 30, 2020, from https://www.iom.int/news/when-returning-home-deadly-journey-shame-returnees-worst-enemy.

International Organization for Migration. (2019c). *Returnees share harrowing experiences at latest 'migration conversation'.* Press Release. Retrieved January 30, 2020, from https://www.iom.int/news/returnees-share-harrowing-experiences-latest-migration-conversation.

Karen, R. (1992). Shame. *The Atlantic Monthly, 269*(2), 40–70.

Kross, E., Berman, M. G., Mischel, W., Smith, E. E., & Wager, T. D. (2011). Social rejection shares somatosensory representations with physical pain. *Proceedings of the National Academy of Sciences, 108*(15), 6270–6275.

Kumar, S., & Meena, S. (2019). *Forrester analytics: Mobile, smartphone, and tablet forecast, 2018 to 2023 (global). Resource document.* Retrieved January 30, 2020, from https://www.forrester.

com/report/Forrester+Analytics+Mobile+Smartphone+And+Tablet+Forecast+2018+To+2023+Global/-/E-RES145709#.

Lang, K. (2014). *Opinion expression on social networking sites-testing an adapted spiral of silence model for political discussion on Facebook. Resource document*. University of Miami, Coral Gables. Retrieved January 30, 2020, from https://scholarlyrepository.miami.edu/cgi/viewcontent.cgi?article=2361&context=oa_dissertations.

Latek, M. (2017). Reintegration of returning migrants. Resource document. European Parliament, Brussels. Retrieved January 30, 2020, from https://www.europarl.europa.eu/RegData/etudes/BRIE/2017/608779/EPRS_BRI(2017)608779_EN.pdf.

Leach, C. W., & Cidam, A. (2015). When is shame linked to constructive approach orientation? A meta-analysis. *Journal of Personality and Social Psychology, 109*(6), 983–1002.

Lee, E. S. (1966). A theory of migration. *Demography, 3*(1), 47–57.

Lee, J. (2016). Drivers and consequences in transforming work practices. In J. Lee (Ed.), *The impact of ICT on work* (pp. 71–92). Singapore: Springer.

Louth, S. (2012). Overcoming the 'shame' factor: Empowering indigenous people to share and celebrate their culture. In *International conference: Innovative research in a changing and challenging world: Conference proceedings (B)* (pp. 265–275). Tasmania: Australian Multicultural Interaction Institute.

Miller, S. (2017). *The dangers of techno-optimism*. Retrieved January 30, 2020, from https://bpr.berkeley.edu/2017/11/16/the-dangers-of-techno-optimism/.

Mohieldin, M. (2019). *Migration can support economic development if we let it*. Retrieved January 30, 2020, from https://www.weforum.org/agenda/2019/03/migration-myths-vs-economic-facts/ .

Montag, A. (2018). *Mark Cuban says studying philosophy may soon be worth more than computer science – here's why*. CNBC. Retrieved January 30, 2020, from https://www.cnbc.com/2018/02/20/mark-cuban-philosophy-degree-will-be-worth-more-than-computer-science.html.

Naqshbandi, K., Milne, D. N., Davies, B., Potter, S., Calvo, R. A., Hoermann, S. (2016, November). Helping young people going through tough times: Perspectives for a peer-to-peer chat support system. In *Proceedings of the 28th Australian Conference on Computer-Human Interaction* (pp. 640-642).

Nidorf, J. F. (1985). *Mental health and refugee youths: A model for diagnostic training*. Resource document. U.S. Department of Education. Retrieved January 30, 2020, from https://files.eric.ed.gov/fulltext/ED266199.pdf#page=393.

Petrie, K. J., Booth, R. J., & Pennebaker, J. W. (1998). The immunological effects of thought suppression. *Journal of Personality and Social Psychology, 75*(5), 1264–1271.

Pittaway, E. (2010). *Making mainstreaming a reality – Gender and the UNHCR policy on refugee protection and solutions in urban areas: A refugee perspective*. Resource Document. Centre for Refugee Research, University of New South Wales. Retrieved January 30, 2020, from https://www.unhcr.org/4b0bb83f9.pdf.

Rigaud, K., de Sherbinin, A., Jones, B., Bergmann, J., Clement, V., Ober, K., Schewe, J., Adamo, S., McCusker, B., Heuser, S., & Midgley, A. (2018). *Groundswell: Preparing for internal climate migration*. Washington DC: World Bank Group.

Schuster, L., & Majidi, N. (2015). Deportation stigma and re-migration. *Journal of Ethnic and Migration Studies, 41*(4), 635–652.

Schwab, K. (2017). *The fourth industrial revolution*. New York: Crown Publishing Group.

Searcy, D., & Jaime, Y.B. (2017). *Why migrants keep risking all on the 'deadliest route'*. NY Times. Retrieved January 30, 2020, from https://www.nytimes.com/2017/06/22/world/africa/migrants-mediterranean-italy-libya-deaths.html.

Selva, M. (2019). Reaching for the off switch: Internet shutdowns are growing as nations seek to control public access to information. *Index on Censorship, 48*(3), 19–22.

Stotz, S. J., Elbert, T., Müller, V., & Schauer, M. (2015). The relationship between trauma, shame, and guilt: Findings from a community-based study of refugee minors in Germany. *European Journal of Psychotraumatology, 6*(1), 25863.

Tanon, F., & Sow, A. (2013). Unaccompanied young migrants from Africa: The case of Mauritania. *The Annals of the American Academy of Political and Social Science, 648*(1), 189–203.

UN DESA. (2013). *Cross-national comparisons of internal migration: An update on global patterns and trends. Resource document.* Retrieved January 30, 2020, from https://www.un.org/en/development/desa/population/publications/pdf/technical/TP2013-1.pdf.

UN DESA. (2017). *International migration report. Resource document.* Retrieved January 30, 2020, from https://www.un.org/en/development/desa/population/migration/publications/migrationreport/docs/MigrationReport2017_Highlights.pdf.

UN Human Rights Committee. (2020). https://tbinternet.ohchr.org/_layouts/15/treatybodyexternal/Download.aspx?symbolno=CCPR%2fC%2f127%2fD%2f2728%2f2016&Lang=en

United Nations General Assembly. (2018). *Global compact for safe, orderly and regular migration. Resource document.*

van Bemmel, S. (2019). The perception of risk among unauthorized migrants in Ghana. *Journal of Risk Research, 23*(1), 47–61.

Warren, A., & Evitt, R. (2010). Indigenous hip-hop: Overcoming marginality, encountering constraints. *Australian Geographer, 41*(1), 141–158.

Weidman-Grunewald, E. (2017). *How should the humanitarian sector respond to the fourth industrial revolution? World Economic Forum.* Retrieved January 30, 2020, from https://www.weforum.org/agenda/2017/01/what-will-it-take-to-transform-humanitarian-response/.

West, R., & Turner, L. H. (2017). *Introducing communication theory: Analysis and application.* New York: McGraw-Hill Education.

Whewell, T. (2019). *We failed to reach Europe – Now our families disown us.* BBC. Retrieved January 30, 2020, from https://www.bbc.co.uk/news/stories-50391297.

World Bank. (2018a). *Record high remittances sent globally in 2018. Resource document.* Retrieved January 30, 2020, from https://www.worldbank.org/en/news/press-release/2019/04/08/record-high-remittances-sent-globally-in-2018.

World Bank. (2018b). *Migration and remittances: Recent developments and outlook. Resource document.* Retrieved January 30, 2020, from https://www.knomad.org/sites/default/files/2018-12/Migration%20and%20Development%20Brief%2030.pdf.

World Economic Forum. (2015). *Deep shirt: Technology tipping points and societal impact. Resource document.* Retrieved January 30, 2020, from http://www3.weforum.org/docs/WEF_GAC15_Technological_Tipping_Points_report_2015.pdf.

World Economic Forum. (2019). *Civil society in the fourth industrial revolution: Preparation and response. Resource document.* Retrieved January 30, 2020, from http://www3.weforum.org/docs/WEF_Civil_Society_in_the_Fourth_Industrial_Revolution_Response_and_Innovation.pdf.

Gillian McKay is a Human Rights Law graduate currently working with the UN Migration Agency in Somalia where she has developed a keen interest in return and reintegration of migrants. She will shortly be returning to the UK where she will be undertaking PhD study in mass atrocity prevention at the European Centre for the Responsibility to Protect.

Chapter 24
The Terror of Being Judged: Public Shaming as Resource and Strategic Tool

Elisabeth Vanderheiden

> [She] had heard it said that there was only one emotion which, in recollection, was capable of resurrecting the full immediacy and power of the original-one emotion that time could never fade, and that would drag you back any number of years into the pure, undiluted feeling, as if you were living it anew. It wasn't love . . . and it wasn't hate, or anger, or happiness, or even grief. Memories of those were but echoes of the true feeling. It was shame. Shame never faded. *Laini Taylor, Dreams of Gods and Monsters*

1 Introduction: Shame as Political Tool

> The terror of being judged George Eliot (as cited in McDavid, 2015)

Shame is often—especially in Western contexts—perceived as an emotion and usually has negative connotations, but is also increasingly perceived as a resource (see Wurmser, 2007; Vanderheiden & Mayer, 2017; Mayer & Vanderheiden, 2019; Briegleb, 2016; Heil, 2018). This chapter will focus on shame and shaming as a political resource and strategic tool (Jacquet, 2014, 2015a, 2015b, 2020) in response to the experience and perception of discrimination and marginalisation (Jacquet, 2014, 2015a, 2015b, 2020). This chapter will discuss the conditions under which public shaming is considered legitimate and its advantages and disadvantages. A case study from the economic context is presented. This will be analysed and interpreted, and limitations will be identified. Conclusions for future research needs are also proposed.

In dealing with shame as an instrument, US environmental researcher Jennifer Jacquet has been able to prove in various studies published in 2014 that the threat of shame increases the willingness to cooperate by about 50%. In her view, shame is

E. Vanderheiden (✉)
Global Institute for Transcultural Research, Römerberg, Germany
e-mail: ev@keb-rheinland-pfalz.de

C.-H. Mayer et al. (eds.), *Shame 4.0*, https://doi.org/10.1007/978-3-030-59527-2_24

> an instrument, a delicate and sometimes dangerous tool that we can use to solve serious problems. Shame is a form of non-violent resistance that anyone can use and which, unlike guilt, can influence the behaviour of entire groups (Jacquet as cited in Deutschlandfunk, 2020; translated by the author).

In this context, Heil (2019) speaks of shame as a socialisation tactic (Heil, 2019, p. 353). Shame as a political instrument is particularly relevant when no formal punishment is envisaged or possible. In international politics, there are still hardly any possibilities of formal punishment; those that exist are not applied or implemented. For this reason, shame remains one of the most effective means of coercion, especially when other legal means are not available or effective. In many cases, the main concern is to combine the right of companies to make a profit with social and environmental responsibility (Bloomfield, 2013). This is often done by giving a voice to the injured, affected or victims, by promoting transparency, by providing educational information and often by providing a forum for an inclusive discourse between the various stakeholders. However, this is less about political neutrality and objectivity than the exploration and execution of strategic change potentials:

> Market-based, shame campaigns occupy a contested political space where inequalities in the market are leveraged to redistribute political power elsewhere. Specifically, campaign tactics reflect existing inequalities through their reliance on the asymmetrical power in markets as well as challenge inequalities through democracy promotion. These campaigns reflect many of the inherent contradictions of global civil society, but have found a way to challenge nonconsensual industry activities by circumventing the state institutions that often nurture their imposition. As long as activists are self-reflective about the inherent limitations of this approach, shame campaigns will remain a potent strategy to achieve industry reform. (Bloomfield, 2013, p. 25)

In Jacquet's perspective (2020 as cited in Deutschlandfunk), seven criteria should be constitutive of public shaming of companies and organisations. A breach of the rules should (1) affect the public addressed. From their point of view, (2) it is significant that the behaviour of the institution to be shamed deviates significantly from the desired behaviour. (3) It should be a given that the institution to be shamed will not be prosecuted in the foreseeable future. (4) The institution to be shamed should belong to the same group as the institution that is exposed. It is also important that the shaming itself (5) should be carried out by a recognised authority. Furthermore, it is necessary that public shaming (6) is aimed at something that promises maximum benefit and (7) is carried out conscientiously. The maxim guiding the action should be the preservation of the human dignity of the ashamed party, which must not be damaged; rather, the aim is to bring about correction and reintegration instead of initiating fight and flight and above all to deter from misconduct. The historian Ute Frevert (in an interview with Becker, 2020) argues in a similar direction when she stresses that shame is about reintegration into the community after a norm violation.

From a legal perspective, Taheri (2020) also points out the need for differentiation into two subcategories with regard to public naming and shaming in the context of white-collar crime. Following Braithwaite (1989; see also Wickert, 2020), Taheri shows that while disintegrative shaming integrates a stigmatisation of the person concerned and excludes exclusion from the community, reintegrative shaming is about the conviction of the delinquent, accompanied by an offer to return to the community. The affected person is thus pilloried, but at the same time the opportunity for re-socialisation is offered. According to Taheri, it is accepted or intended that "shaming" not only damages the image of the offender but also causes economic disadvantage in the medium term. In this context, the restoration of justice is also argued in the sense of "Seeing Justice Done" (Friedland, 2012). In the legal context, approaches to "corporate shaming" already exist in the USA in the field of economic criminal law, where companies using social media must publicly ask for forgiveness for certain offences. Corresponding changes can also be observed in the European legal system, for instance, with regard to capital market law (e.g. the Market Abuse Ordinance). The German Federal Financial Supervisory Authority (BaFin), for example, is to a certain extent obliged to name and shame in the case of fine decisions and must publish the name of the person concerned on its website (Haag & Wintermeier, 2020; Taheri, 2020).

In the non-legal sphere, naming and shaming—as already indicated—is primarily about generating insight and changing behaviour or preventing criminal, discriminatory, personally or environmentally harmful behaviour (see Chap. 18). Important instruments for this are social media platforms such as Facebook, YouTube, Twitter or Instagram as well as specific campaign platforms such as Change.org, Campact.de or Avaaz.org.

Social media or other Internet-based campaigns, also known as grassroots campaigning, are generally quite easy to organise, share or join with a click. Supporters can thus be easily mobilised and often achieve large coverage in a short time (Friedrich-Ebert-Stiftung, 2020). Campaigning is understood as the art of being

> able to pull out all the stops to get people to change their behaviour, thinking or attitude so that a goal can be achieved (Metzinger, 2020).

Naming and shaming on the Internet is therefore low-threshold, often uncomplicated and participative and offers a wide range of experiences of self-efficacy. As proposed by Bandura (1997), self-efficacy (expectation) is a relevant variable in terms of coping with new or difficult situations. At the same time, it can serve as an expression of empowerment and compensation and potentially represent an important resource for coping with and transforming experiences of discrimination and marginalisation, which are often particularly shameful. This idea of compensation and empowerment is also explicitly named by Internet platforms as a motive for commitment and action:

> Our mission is to empower people everywhere to create the change they want to see. Our vision is a world where no one is powerless, and creating change is part of everyday life. ... Change.org is the world's largest platform for social change, with over 265 million users globally. (Change.org, 2020)

or

> Avaaz empowers millions of people from all walks of life to take action on pressing global, regional and national issues, from corruption and poverty to conflict and climate change. Our model of internet organising allows thousands of individual efforts, however small, to be rapidly combined into a powerful collective force. (Avaaz, 2020)

Bloomfield (2013, p. 2) explains what such campaigns are all about:

> Shame campaigns aim to change industry practices by targeting the reputational value of individual firms. They occupy a contested political space from which they leverage existing inequalities in the market to redress political inequalities on the ground.

Scarcely any meaningful figures are yet available on the actual impact and reach of such campaigns (Christensen, 2011).[1] Some authors are rather critical of such activities, suspecting that they are political activities that have no impact on real political outcomes, but only serve to increase the feel-good factor of those involved (Morozov, 2009). They use the term "slacktivism" pejoratively to define this as a form of political activism that is not followed by action on the action level. It is an

> online form of self-aggrandising, politically ineffective activism (Cabrera, Matias, & Montoya, 2017, p. 1).

Christensen (2011), Morozov (2009) and Vie (2014) have identified five sub-categories of slacktivism, "clicktivism",[2] sympathy, political, charity (direct) and charity (by-product of consumption), and that the term tends to be pejorative. Other authors, such as Putnam (2000), express the fear that these activities are meaningless and ineffective to the extent that they are not suitable for achieving political goals and can divert political participants from the traditionally more effective forms of participation in the activist repertoire.

2 Research Methodology

In the following, a case study will show how public shaming can be successfully used as a resource for self-efficacy and empowerment and as a strategic instrument or political weapon.

In this chapter, the author presents a case study and uses a case study design. Schwaiger and Meyer (2009) point out that the particular strengths of case studies lie in their more comprehensive and thus better representation of reality. This makes it possible to examine not only developments and processes but also complex cause-and-effect relationships, taking into account a wide range of determinants and influencing factors (Schwaiger & Meyer, 2009, p. 363).

---

[1] Interview requests regarding the actual impact of the author on change.org, campact.de and avaaz.org remain unanswered.

[2] Clicktivism is the term used to describe political participation with which people can get involved from their mobile devices and computers with just a few clicks. Such clicks are particularly interesting for organisations that are politically active, seek support in this way or organise campaigns, because the more clicks they receive, the greater their digital impact.

Yin (2009, p. 18) stresses that a case study is:

> [...] an empirical inquiry that investigates a contemporary phenomenon within its real life context, especially when the boundaries between phenomenon and context are not clearly evident.

It is important to consider various data sources:

> Cases are rich empirical descriptions of particular instances of a phenomenon, that are typically based on a variety of data sources. (see Eisenhardt & Graebner, 2007, p. 25)

Then single case studies can also provide a good starting point for the development of theories (Schwaiger & Meyer, 2009, p. 361). Müller-Böling and Klandt (1996) support this view when they point out that the information content of case studies is usually quite high, because they allow a detailed examination of all facets of the object of investigation. Critically, however, Müller-Böling and Klandt (1996, p. 81) identify the limited transferability and general validity of case studies. A single case study may well suffice for the purpose of this chapter (Göbel, 2009).

The following criteria were decisive for the selection of the case study:

- Availability of primary sources both from the shaming initiatives and from the shamed company
- Describability of the shaming action and the company reactions to it
- Traceability of the impact of the shame campaign.

The database was based on selected company communication features in the form of selected posters, posts and video statements of the affected company, as well as the campaign including posts and video clips of the shameful initiatives.

The following case study will illustrate how such a public shaming campaign works and what it can achieve.

The case study was created by the author herself on the basis of research and analysis of social media campaigns. For this purpose, relevant corporate and social media sites—especially Facebook and YouTube—were evaluated and analysed.

In particular, individual case studies offer the special opportunity to depict social reality not only as a static snapshot, but in process, and thus to point out interdependencies and connections in a specific way. Nevertheless, they are bound to a certain context and therefore do not allow generalisations to a population (see also Albers, Klapper, Konradt, Walter, & Wolf, 2006, p. 36). In this respect, the individual case described here is dedicated to the description and analysis of a phenomenon, but this cannot be generalised. On the other hand, limitations result from the fact that it is an individual case study from the German-speaking context with references to Germany and Austria, which is not transferable to other socio-cultural contexts.

3 Case Example True Fruits

3.1 Initial Situation

True Fruits GmbH is a juice and smoothie producer with 31 employees in Bonn, Germany (True Fruits GmbH, 2020). Founded in 2006 by three friends, the start-up is now one of the market leaders for smoothies and generates annual sales of approximately 19–20 million euros (Statista, 2020). According to the company's own information, the turnover was significantly higher in 2017, at about 43 million euros. Since the beginning of 2015, True Fruits has been a market leader in the smoothie segment (True Fruits GmbH, 2019).

They describe their self-image as follows:

> We are proud to be a little bit different and live it out shamelessly. We are true, live strictly according to the principle no tricks and don't take ourselves so seriously. We are a small but fine juice shop. No more, but no less either. (True Fruits GmbH, 2020a, translated by the author)

One of the company's strategies for success is its provocative PR campaign, which repeatedly causes a stir, and some of its posts and campaigns are perceived by consumers and the public as explicitly sexist and/or racist. However, the company has also been confronted with accusations of anti-disability statements or slogans that play down-sexualised violence and promote rape culture. This self-positioning is certainly significant, as studies (Bartley & Child, 2014) have shown that the probability of becoming a target as a company also depends on the cultural organisation of the markets, which made some companies more "shamable" than others.

The 2019 summer smoothie "Sun Creamie" was perceived as a special provocation and was presented in a marketing campaign like a sun cream. The advertising motif featured a woman who had had a penis painted on her shoulder with sun cream (Deutscher Werberat, 2020b; Die WELT, 2020; MEEDIA, 2020). Two smoothies containing Chia-Samen were advertised with the slogan: "Sperm donor from a good home" or "Oral consumption—you won't get to sperm any faster" (Horizont, 2020). Also causing a stir and outrage was the launch in Germany in 2016 and in Austria in 2017—at the height of the refugee migration to Europe—of a black smoothie that was marketed with the slogans: *Unser Quoten-Schwarzer* ["Our reservation black", translated by the author,] *Schafft es selten über die Grenze* ["Rarely makes it across the border", translated by the author] or *Noch mehr Flaschen aus dem Ausland* ["Even more bottles from abroad", translated by the author; "bottle" in German means useless, irrelevant person] (Pauker, 2020).

The True Fruits posters and social media posts triggered strong protests on social media platforms, which in particular revealed the implications of these campaigns, which were perceived as sexist, but above all racist. Protesters wanted to persuade the True Fruits to give in or stop the campaign.

Among other responses such as individual single message posts, a statement by the company management was published on the company's Facebook page on 14 February 2019 (True Fruits GmbH, 2020b). This was seen as a further provocation and triggered further shitstorms and a public shaming campaign (which is described and discussed in detail later in this chapter).

3.2 Public Shaming Activities

On 18 February 2019, in reaction to this, a campaign was launched on Change.org as *#truediskriminierung und sonst nichts. Nehmt true fruits aus Eurem Sortiment* ["#true discrimination and nothing else. Take true fruits from your assortment", translated by the author].

Public shaming of the company was consciously used as a strategic tool, and further pressure was exerted by a call for a boycott of the products and, with regard to the distribution channels, removal from the sales range. An open letter was sent to the responsible persons via an online petition, asking them to take a stand on the discriminatory marketing strategy of True Fruits and to remove the products from their range (Furgalec, 2020). This petition was signed by 60,489 people (at the time of completion of this chapter). This was supported by a YouTube video of a composite of video clip statements with original quotes from people who are critical of the True Fruits campaign. Many of these people can be recognised, through their appearance or subtitles, as affected German-speaking persons of colour, immigrants or persons who are involved in refugee work or suffer from a physical disability themselves or are involved in women's work (YouTube, 2020).

The aim of the Change.org appeal is explicitly to call on the company to behave responsibly towards minorities due to its enormous reach and influence as an opinion leader and to behave and position itself clearly with regard to racism, sexism and other forms of group-related discrimination. In doing so, the initiators make it clear that in their opinion, the marketing concept of True Fruits is based "on the degradation and racist, sexist, disabled- and misogynist as well as lookistic and heteronormative discrimination of marginalized groups of people". They also criticise the way in which

> humour and provocation are used here to shamelessly instrumentalise groups of people who are already socially disadvantaged for pure profit (YouTube, 2020).

Jacquet (2015b) also refers to this as a critical aspect of embarrassment when it leads to

> further isolate a group marginalised by society (or further stigmatise a stigmatised group) (Jacquet, 2015b, p. 196, translated by the author).

In addition to the YouTube video, the campaign website lists examples of the slogans criticised, naming the corresponding context of discrimination (YouTube, 2020). They refer to the letter from True Fruits GmbH dated 14 February 2019 (see below) and criticise the fact that the company does not show any understanding or apologise with regard to the groups concerned. They indirectly appeal to True Fruits as a company with a large media and public reach to take its social responsibility seriously and not to contribute to a normalisation of discrimination by manifesting these messages in the minds of many people in times of political polarisation of society and strengthening right-wing sentiments True Fruits directly appeals to its trading partners to discontinue the products and thus set an example against discrimination.

Initiatives and campaigns also emerged on other social media channels, for example, a campaign was launched on twitter as *#truediskriminierung* (Twitter, 2020) on Instagram under *#truefruitsboykott* (Instagramm, 2020). Writer, podcaster and influencer Charlotte Roche (2019) started her own campaign in August 2019: she rearranged the refrigerated shelves of a supermarket and placed True Fruits smoothie products behind other manufacturers in front of them. She encouraged her 110,000 followers to participate live and "be part of a movement" (Roche, 2019). She received more than 10,000 likes and a positive press response; many followers followed her example.

The German Advertising Council (Deutscher Werberat), as the self-regulatory body of the advertising industry, is responsible for ensuring that advertising is legally permissible and does not exceed ethical limits (Deutscher Werberat, 2020a). In 2019, it objected to two advertising motifs of True Fruits GmbH for its product Sun Creamie, owing to more than 900 complaints. The advertising motifs (Deutscher Werberat, 2020b) showed the already mentioned penis painted with sun cream, ejaculating on a woman's or man's back. The accompanying original advertising text read: "Summer, when will you finally celebrate your cumback?" ("Cum" is the English word for sperm). In the explanatory statement, it was said that

> both advertising measures would have been objectionable. The provocative depictions crossed the border not only of good taste but also of vulgarism. Both the female and the male model would be depicted in a degrading manner as the object of sexual fantasies and practices. In its statement to the advertising council, the company had classified the advertising as childish, silly and adolescent, but not as offensive or excessively obscene (Deutscher Werberat, 2020a, translated by the author).

No position is taken on the other allegations.

The Austrian Advertising Council has called upon True Fruits GmbH to immediately stop the campaign or to change the subject in the case of the objectionable advertising measure (Internet) (Österreichischer Werberat, 2020). The company has reacted accordingly.

These campaigns quickly showed initial successes, in that sales figures for certain products, such as the smoothie in the black bottle, are declining (True Fruits GmbH, 2020b), because consumers refuse to buy. In Germany, a first major supplier completely cancelled its relationship with True Fruits (Studierendenwerk Bonn, 2020). This is decisive not only in terms of sexist, racist or other discrimination but also in the way the company owners dealt with the critics:

> From the point of view of the Studentenwerk, True Fruits has once again behaved completely inappropriately towards its critics and defamed them across the board, without any kind of constructive concession. Calling all critics "stupid people", *Pissnelken* [derogatory German term of abuse, roughly "pissing cloves"], "radical apostles" or "hysterical

people" shows little maturity of the management. (Studierendenwerk Bonn 2020, translated by the author)

The large Swiss food chain Globus also completely blacklisted True Fruits with the justification that they condemn all forms of racism and sexism and that they regard the marketing campaign from True Fruits as unacceptable (Liechti, 2020).

3.3 Company Reaction

The management of True Fruits GmbH reacted to the massive criticism and the campaign with an open letter on 14 February 2019 via social media (Horizont, 2020; True Fruits Gmbh, 2020b). The smoothie in the black bottle was withdrawn, justified by the bad sales figures for the respective product:

> Dear friends, dear supposedly discriminated ones, dear stupid ones, We are currently receiving news and criticism via social networks. We are accused of racism, sexism or even the promotion of "rape culture". We are used to the regular lamentation of some obsessive words and we apologize to all those who are also rightly bored by this.
>
> This time it's about a best-of of different slogans, which go back a few years. This includes our campaign, which we launched in 2017 as a German company in Austria with poster texts such as:
>
> - "Rarely makes it across the border"
> - "More bottles from abroad" (True Fruits GmbH, 2020, translated by the author)

The management makes it clear that they have tried to distance themselves from the political right-wing racist spectrum by referring to it:

> This campaign was a criticism of Austria's right-wing policy and the possible closure of the Brenner Pass (which would have made it more difficult for refugees to enter). That this was a campaign against xenophobia would have become clear, at the latest, if one had studied the campaign and looked at the third campaign motif, for example: "You can't vote for brown in our country" (because none of our bottles is brown ...) [Following National Socialism, brown is considered the colour of the political right. During the period in question, Austria was governed by a right-wing conservative alliance]. (True Fruits GmbH, 2020b, translated by the author, comment by the author)

And ends with the note:

> We find racism as much a pain in the ass as all forms of discrimination. Except people who listen to pop songs, they really shouldn't be allowed to fiddle with the radio. But to seriously believe that a public company of our size could be interested in using racist propaganda to capitalise on it is not very witty. (True Fruits GmbH, 2020b, translated by the author)

The removal of the black bottle from the range is not considered to be the result of customer criticism and its constructive handling, but is argued with correspondingly poor sales figures:

> Of course the black smoothie is not thrown out of the assortment because we are accused of racism, but because it sold too badly. There's no biz like juice biz baby.... (True Fruits GmbH, 2020b, first sentence translated by the author)

It is interesting to note, here, that client shaming is the response to public shaming. This is not an isolated phenomenon. Heil (2019) points out that methods of shame are not only used against large companies and institutions to expose their misconduct but are also used in return, by such institutions or authorities, to fend off such attacks. This is to be achieved, above all, by making the misconduct public, for example, by presenting it as untrustworthy and personally shaming the person who has committed the deed (Heil, 2019, p. 354).

In the case study presented, this is certainly reflected in the statement of the True Fruits owners:

> And if exactly this group of stupid people (no matter if white, black, female, male, hetero- or homosexual, with peg leg or speech impediment) thinks they have to go on the digital barricades with a burning pitchfork and hunt us down like a mob, then we send them a strong "Fuck you!". (True Fruits GmbH, 2020b, translated by the author)

In other parts of the company, management reacts in a more differentiated way, as does Inga Koster, one of the three company owners, in an interview with journalist Tamara Wernli (2019). She does not dissociate herself from the said campaign, but places it once again in the corresponding temporal contexts, making it clear that these are not exemplary posts, but rather constitute a small minority in the overall mix highlighting others such as a diversity-supporting special edition "Love is in the air" for Valentine's Day 2019 (True Fruits GmbH, 2020c). Like the other company owners, she understands the slogans to be an expression of a specific (thoroughly coarse and provocative) humour—but which explicitly excludes sexist, racist or violence-prejudicing intentions. Critically, Koster remarks that some of the slogans had been published for years without any negative reactions and that the campaign merely criticises them with a significant time lag. She recognises in the public shaming campaign against True Fruits GmbH signs of a changing society, which is less sensitive and more tolerant than it seemed a few years ago. In this context, she makes it clear that as a company, they will be even more concerned than before with the question of whether an ambiguity could be interpreted in a poster or post, whether it could be misunderstood or whether something could be read into it that the company might not have intended. Discriminating against or wanting to injure people excludes them and suggests that the company wants to maintain what, in its view, is its own humorously provocative style. In the future, they want to proceed even more cautiously and carefully, especially with posters or billboards with sexual connotations.

With regard to the customer-critical posts or statements, Koster argues that this is an expression of meeting at equal eye level because Facebook culture generally has a very rough tone (True Fruits GmbH, 2020b). Both the "#true discrimination and nothing else. Take true fruits from your assortment" campaign and the action from Charlotte Roche are named together and are perceived as "opinion fascism" because they limit the options of other people. Koster says that there have also been individual threatening e-mails to the company owners and their families and actions building against the company.

The journalist's question about the sales consequences of the shitstorm remains open and is only answered by the fact that the Sun Creamie smoothie was sold out much earlier than planned (Wernli, 2019).

3.4 *Interpretation of the Results with Regard to the Company*

The management of True Fruits GmbH actually reacts to customer criticism and embarrassment with a reversal of criticism and embarrassment. On the one hand, this is a rather unusual behaviour, because it can potentially be associated with image damage, impairment of company–customer relationships and loss of sales. On the other hand, it contradicts many classical standards for recommendations of company–customer interactions. According to the management consulting firm KPMG (2019), for example, research with over three million ratings across 24 countries and across various industries has identified the following 6 so-called drivers as relevant for customer experience excellence: personalisation, integrity, expectations, problem-solving skills, time and effort and empathy (see also Bruhn & Hadwich, 2012). Gouthier, Giese and Bartl (2012) also emphasise the particular relevance of customer experience, customer enthusiasm and service excellence, especially in connection with the increasing spread of new technologies such as social media and Web 2.0. These technologies enable customers to quickly and effectively obtain information about the market offer and also to exchange information about particularly good or particularly bad services and products. It is therefore becoming increasingly difficult for companies to consolidate or even expand their existing customer base. From Mayer-Vorfelder's (2012) point of view, in the increasing competition for customers, companies have for some years been aware of the trend to increase customer benefit by consistently improving the customer experience and thus differentiating themselves from the competition.

The following section will examine in more detail the extent to which the six so-called drivers that studies have shown to be relevant for customer experience excellence are reflected here (KPMG, 2019).

3.4.1 Personalisation

Personalisation of the interaction with the customer is considered one of the most important drivers of an outstanding customer experience. It is about making it clear that the company understands the individual's circumstances, needs and goals and designs the interaction accordingly. The customer should be given the feeling of appreciation and significance through personal contact, individual recommendations and knowledge about past contact situations.

In the case study, the company seems to be well aware of the importance of personalised interaction. As a rule, and also in the run-up to escalation, company employees reacted to all customer posts, also individualised by personalised salutation; according to company statements, enquiries are answered within 1 day. This also applied and still applies to critical feedback with regard to the marketing campaigns mentioned above. According to a member of the company management, all relevant e-mails were also answered individually and promptly (Wernli, 2019). On the other hand, the company's fulfilment of the aspect of conveying the customer's appreciation and significance is more ambivalent: the management makes it clear that it does not intend to carry out racist, sexist or other discriminatory advertising campaigns, but at the same time criticises the customers themselves for perceiving this in this way. Initially there is little actual understanding of the individual circumstances; views and needs of the customers are recognisable and also initially no insight at the level of interaction, as the escalation, which is made clear in the company statement of 14 February 2019, makes clear. Appreciation and expression of significance for customers seems to be increasingly lost or to have lost relevance. At the same time, however, in the wake of the shitstorm and the campaign, a change is discernible in the way marketing campaigns that can be interpreted as discriminatory are handled.

3.4.2 Time and Effort

The key to customer experience and relationship is the fast and smooth removal of unnecessary technical, procedural and bureaucratic barriers to interaction with the company. This enables customers to quickly address their concerns and achieve high levels of target achievement, and it increases their loyalty to the company. In the case study at hand, several individual marketing events of the company have triggered time-delayed customer criticism. Customers then express their needs and concerns in posts and campaigns. A quick and easy satisfaction of customer needs is not forthcoming; a product is blacklisted, but with the explanation of poor sales figures. No connection to customer criticism is acknowledged. At first there are no signals that customer criticism is understood and accepted; management always emphasises that customers are not able to understand and accept their humour style. An argumentative exception, with certain restrictions, is the video interview with Inka Koster (Koster and Wernli, 2019). On the other hand, it can be argued in this case study that both the customer needs and the needs expressed in the Change.org campaign are finally met by the company: a product that was considered racist was discontinued. In the future, the company wants to avoid marketing campaigns that can be perceived as discriminatory or misleading, but at the same time remain authentic and not give up their humour. Some major customers of True Fruits GmbH have adopted customer or campaign criticism and have terminated their business relationships. In this respect, the customers have achieved their goal, but since this was only achieved by public shame and was not answered by an official declaration of intent or apology on the part of the company, it is highly unlikely to impossible that this will have a loyalty-enhancing effect on the customers. However, the basis for a final assessment is still lacking, as at the time of writing this chapter, no sales figures for 2019 are available.

3.4.3 Expectations

Customers expect that their needs should be met by organisations and that top performers are capable of not only satisfying customer expectations but exceeding them. Both customers and the Change.org campaign participants clearly and unambiguously formulate their expectations, in terms of what is needed and the way in which these needs should be satisfied. The official social media reaction of the company management counteracts this by public shaming of customers and critics. True Fruits GmbH claims to be the market leader for smoothies in German-speaking countries. For the company, this is inseparably linked to a certain brand image, which is characteristic for their authenticity, such as their cheeky provocative humour, but also their attitude not to adapt to the market at any price solely to achieve higher sales figures (Wernli, 2019). It is quite possible that customers and campaign participants anticipated such a reaction and that there are customers who positively reward such corporate behaviour. To a certain extent, customer expectations were exceeded here, but not in a positive way. True Fruits GmbH has an image as a young, self-confident, unconventional and provocative company. This is definitely appreciated by the customers, which can be seen in the very relaxed interaction on the company's Facebook page, including not only high subscription numbers to the Facebook page and many "likes" but also many enthusiastic customer comments.

3.4.4 Problem-Solving Competence

Companies with positive values in terms of problem-solving competence are characterised by their ability to return customers to the state they want to be in as quickly as possible and at the same time to make them feel good. An obviously serious apology and immediate action are considered two fundamental elements of problem-solving competence as a feature of organisational culture. In the present case, the company's communication strategy does not seem to be able to achieve this. The Change.org campaign continues, which can be interpreted as meaning that the initiators do not believe that the campaign's goal has been finally achieved. In this case, immediate action is evident, but no apology has been made, nor does it seem likely to happen.

3.4.5 Integrity

In the context which is relevant here, integrity is understood to be organisational consistency-free behaviour that demonstrates trustworthiness to the customer. This also includes difficult situations in which the company must undoubtedly react with integrity in the public context. The actions and reactions of employees must contribute to strengthening trust in the organisation as a whole. The extent to which the company is willing and able to deliver on its promises is critical to the customer's long-term trust in the company. From the perspective of True Fruits GmbH, the company behaves consistently and without contradiction, as can be seen from the company's postings, the statement of 14 February 2019 and the 2019 video interview with Koster. Whether this can create the impression of integrity and trustworthiness with regard to political and social responsibility is doubtful, in view of the ongoing criticism. On the one hand, the company clearly distances itself from intentions to discriminate, and on the other hand, customers are shamed with disparaging remarks. At the reaction level, objective integrity does not appear to be desired, nor is it demonstrable on the part of the company. The reactions of employees are consistent with statements and appearances of the management and with the proclaimed corporate culture. The company itself does not explicitly discriminate, but at the same time remains true to its specific brand of humour. In this respect, this aspect of integrity seems to be true. The extent to which this is actually conducive to trust cannot be conclusively assessed, as no sales figures or other publicly accessible valid data are available.

3.4.6 Empathy

Empathy in the context of customer experience excellence is understood as the emotional ability to show that one understands another's experience and situation. If the company knows how the customer feels and makes this clear in the interaction, the sustainability of the customer relationship is stabilised, and the emotional connection between the customers and the company as well as the potential to increase customer loyalty is increased. Empathy is explicitly not in the interest of the company, as shown in the statement of the company management on 14 February 2019 and also demonstrated by many individual posts on the Facebook page. The customers formulate praise, criticism, wishes and needs very clearly towards the company. Company reactions show that this knowledge is only partially taken up; sometimes it is even decisively rejected. In a Facebook post of 29 January 2020, one customer complained that a current product (a smoothie that reminds one of a regional beer by its bottle design) is advertised in a video of a children's party, which ends with the children toasting each other with the smoothies. The customer remarked that it is inappropriate to use children in the context of advertising with products that give the impression of being alcohol. This comment was then dismissed with the remark that the company itself likes the advertising (True Fruits GmbH, 2020d).

Another customer pointed out in a post dated 12 February 2020 that it is problematic that many smoothies contain apples while many people have an allergic reaction to apples; therefore, it would be desirable if there were more smoothies without apples, as offered by competing products. True Fruits answered that they do not intend to offer this product without apples at the moment and recommended using competing products (True Fruits GmbH, 2020e). Nevertheless, the emotional connection between the company and its customers seems to be generally solid, as the high subscription and like numbers on the Facebook page prove. Currently, the company's Facebook page has 553,303 subscribers and 555,165 people like the site. Obviously, empathy is not the most important driver. As the company explicitly does not take into account a number of very relevant factors for the company–customer relationship, it opts for a decidedly different behaviour.

An explanation could be derived from the approach of Lindemann (2019) and Rhein (2012). Lindemann (2019) assumes a strong connection between shame and pride, especially in the context of certainty and doubt. The author assumes an antagonistic relationship between shame and pride, which evaluates certainty and doubt by relying on previously experienced self-evaluations and judgements. In doing so, he proceeds from two basic assumptions, namely, that the transformation of shame into pride requires success and the experience of control and that the transformation of pride into shame requires failure and the loss of control (Lindemann, 2019, pp. 562–3). Both seem to be true in the present case study. On the one hand, a failure experience and an associated loss of control can be observed through the shitstorm and public shaming posts and campaign, the associated phase-outs by some major customers and possible losses of revenue. On the other hand, the behaviour of the company in the sense described by Lindemann could be understood as the restoration of control through a public corporate statement that self-confidently expresses pride in the company's performance and culture and also announces the future orientation towards what is understood and felt to be the brand core. Potentially, this is a great opportunity for further development and transformation. According to Lindemann (2019), the important factors to be considered here would include social and organisational concerns in addition to self-evaluation. Rhein (2012, p. iii) also emphasises that organisational pride is of enormous importance to companies, especially in shaping customer relationships. It could therefore be assumed that the reversal of customers' public shaming activities into offensive shaming actions by the company with regard to customers could also be interpreted as an expression of corporate pride: pride in having made it this far as young entrepreneurs by their own efforts, pride in a specific corporate culture and pride in market leadership of popular products, for example. From a corporate system perspective, this might even be a sensible reaction to public shaming. A sensible next step could be to look for ways to transform these shaming experiences. Important steps in this process are, according to Lindemann (2019, p. 566), questioning, self-evaluation and the evaluation of the social environment. Successful completion of these steps could result in new potential for innovation, further development and improvement. The undoubted affinity customers have for the company, which is expressed, for example, in Facebook subscriptions and "like" numbers, but also in the fact that only a few major customers have cancelled their contracts owing to public shaming activities, could represent indispensable resources in the context of the Fourth Industrial Revolution.

Following this approach to the results of the study with regard to the company, the focus now shifts to the customer's view and the perspective of the campaign operators.

3.5 Interpretation of the Results with Regard to the Campaign Initiators

With reference to the Internet and to issues raised by the Fourth Industrial Revolution, Jennifer Jacquet (2016) emphasises how digital shaming has irrevocably changed from the shaming of the past, in terms of the speed at which information can travel, the frequency of anonymous shame, the size of the audience it can reach and the permanence of the information. This is also reflected in the present individual case study. Experiences of discrimination can have significant structural, social and individual effects, as well as a negative impact on mental and physical health. A representative population survey of the Federal Government's Anti-Discrimination Office (Antidiskriminierungsstelle des Bundes) (2017) showed that individual experiences of discrimination can have negative effects on social cohesion in Germany. Among those affected, experiences of discrimination can lead to a higher level of fundamental mistrust; in some cases, such experiences can even lead to the breaking off of social contacts. Uslucan (2016) and Uslucan and Yalcin (2012) have also investigated the effects of experiences of discrimination on those affected and has summarised the findings of current social science studies. An often mentioned reaction to repeated discrimination is re-ethnicisation—a kind of return to one's own group. Experiences of discrimination can also lead to a reduced self-esteem, as well as to health impairments and even an increased readiness to use violence. It is possible that the negative consequences of experiences of discrimination have an effect far beyond the particular incident.

However, the negative health effects of discrimination are best documented. In the course of a meta-analysis of almost 200 studies, Pascoe and Richman (2009) concluded that perceived discrimination occurs together with a deterioration in mental as well as physical health. Igel, Brähler and Grande (2010) confirmed a similar result for Germany. There, individuals, who have experienced discrimination based on their origin, skin colour, gender or special needs, report worse mental and physical health. An analysis of those affected by discrimination undertaken by Dieckmann, Geschke, and Braune (2017) also finds a correlation between the frequency of discrimination and psychosomatic symptoms. In the surveys conducted by the Federal Government's Anti-Discrimination Office (Antidiskriminierungsstelle des Bundes) (2017), victims also report that their experience of discrimination had negative effects on their psychological health or, far less frequently, on their physical health. Previously, Schmitt, Branscombe, Postmes, and Garcia (2014) had also established the negative connection between perceived discrimination and psychological well-being in the course of a meta-analysis. This suggests that from a salutogenesis and positive psychology wave 1.0 and 2.0 perspective, it is of enormous importance to create a state of awareness (see Mayer, Vanderheiden and Oosthuizen 2019; Mayer & Krause, 2013) by focusing on physical and psychological health maintenance, by perceiving positive life events and by including and transforming negative ones (Lomas & Ivtzan, 2016; Wong, 2011, 2019). Wong (2019, pp. viii–ix) defines some basic skills for dealing constructively with shame:

- Self-awareness, acceptance and acknowledgement of one's failures and limitations
- Self-forgiveness and self-compassion
- Self-affirmation through re-authoring and reframing
- Self-affirming the intrinsic value and sacredness of life
- Taking personal responsibility for positive change
- Seeking a support group
- Focusing on the meaning people attach to events
- Seeking deeper meaning and self-transcendence
- Seeking deeper understanding through verbalising one's emotions and dreams

In terms of the case study, since the public shaming campaign is supported by individuals who are affected by the discrimination of the True Fruits posts owing to their skin colour, gender, special needs or experience of flight, or who work in solidarity with those affected, the campaign could be seen as a contribution to actively and constructively transform these (and other) experiences of discrimination and related shaming in the sense described above. The campaign can be perceived as an expression of self-awareness and self-compassion, but above all it can be regarded as an action of self-affirmation through re-authoring and reframing. The aspect of self-affirming the intrinsic value and sacredness of life which Wong has addressed is also very apparent, especially the active assumption of personal responsibility for positive change. The active search for and use of support groups by the campaigners and their supporters is also evident here. The fact that affected persons and supporters actively take up the discrimination issues, show solidarity, communicate and concentrate on the importance they attach to events (granting themselves the power of definition) and succeed in combining this with a deeper understanding enables them to take a central step towards transforming these experiences of discrimination and being shamed. For this purpose, they use a public shaming campaigning, but at the same time, they refrain from personally shaming the other side and shame only on an organisational level.

The following table provides an overview of the extent to which the Change.org campaign and the supporting video adhere to the standards for public shaming as a political tool. Jacquet (as cited in Deutschlandfunk, 2020) considers them to be constitutive, and the extent to which these criteria can be found here (Table 24.1).

It can be stated that the initiators of the Change.org campaign have adhered to the standards described by Jaquard (as cited in Deutschlandfunk, 2020). From their point of view, the public shaming campaign can be described as a success, because:

- Within a short period of time, they received more than 60,489 signatures (at the time this chapter was completed).
- Further campaigns on other social media platforms followed.
- One retail partner in Germany and one in Switzerland took True Fruits out of their assortment.
- The black bottle was removed from the True Fruits product range because it was not accepted by the customers.

Table 24.1 Alignment of standards for public shaming based on Jacquet (as cited in Deutschlandfunk, 2020, and *#truediskriminierung und sonst nichts. Nehmt true fruits aus Eurem Sortiment*)

A breach of the rules should therefore 1. affect the public addressed	The original campaign was perceived as discriminatory against women, immigrants and people of a different colour and sexual orientation or with special needs, thus affecting broad and diverse groups of the population The campaign directly addresses consumers who can influence their purchasing decisions As users of social media platforms, they can express their anger and mobilise others
2. Deviate significantly from the desired behaviour	The campaign draws attention to certain racist, sexist, anti-LGBT and anti-disability posts and images or posts and posters that trivialise sexualised violence and documents this accordingly.
3. Not be subject to legal action in the foreseeable future	The initiators did not see any possibility of legal action. A complaint by the German and Austrian advertising council was only partially successful.
The offender should 4. belong to the group that exposes him	The owners of the company are three middle-aged Germans (mid-thirties, early forties) with a social media affinity. Many of the campaign initiators also belong to the same age group, live in Germany and share an affinity for social media to the extent that they use these forms of communication to express their opinions.
And the humiliation itself should 5. be carried out by a recognised authority	By its own account, Change.org is the world's largest petition platform. Change.org is a public benefit corporation, certified by B Lab, an independent certifying group It is financed by donations. The people who express themselves in the video are among the target groups who may perceive the original campaign as potentially discriminatory: women, immigrants and people of a (different) colour and sexual orientation or with special needs.
6. Be aimed at something that promises maximum benefit	The Change.org campaign, insofar as the boycott call is concerned with the entire company, is intended to raise awareness of the importance of its social responsibility on the basis of its acceptance, size and relevance and to avoid statements that could be understood as discriminatory. To this end, action partners are requested to terminate their business relationship with True Fruits. This could lead to a loss of prestige, but also to massive losses in sales.
7. Be implemented conscientiously	The allegations made are supported by examples. No personal accusations are made against individuals. Social responsibility on the part of the company is demanded and admonished. Since the company

(continued)

Table 24.1 (continued)

A breach of the rules should therefore 1. affect the public addressed	The original campaign was perceived as discriminatory against women, immigrants and people of a different colour and sexual orientation or with special needs, thus affecting broad and diverse groups of the population The campaign directly addresses consumers who can influence their purchasing decisions As users of social media platforms, they can express their anger and mobilise others
	management does not see any reason to do so in the statement of 14 February 2019, a boycott call is made. The statements in the video are marked as personal opinions of those affected and supporters.

- There is no official company reaction to the campaign. However, one of the three company owners, Inga Koster (Wernli, 2019), comments in a video interview. She does not consider it legitimate, in a campaign relating to individual posters, to make accusations of racism, to call for a boycott and thus to restrict the options of others. She regards reacting to this occasionally with provocation as an expression of humanity and authenticity, even though it can potentially be associated with economic losses. Koster also signals, however, that in the future, some changes are planned. In this respect, the initiators' demand for corporate social and political responsibility on the part of the company should be met at this point.
- No valid statements can be made about the loss of sales that may have resulted from the public shaming action. A corresponding demand in the video interview with Koster (Wernli, 2019) remains unanswered, and publicly available data is not yet available at the time of completion of the chapter.
- No discriminating or marginalising posts or posters of True Fruits GmbH have been published since the campaign.

4 Conclusions

In this chapter, it was shown that, with respect to the Fourth Industrial Revolution, the awareness of public shame as a resource for empowerment and self-efficacy is gaining importance. Public shaming is explicitly perceived and used as a strategic instrument against discrimination. It was discussed which standards should be adhered to in the interest of human dignity and effectiveness. A case study from the economic context of Germany and Austria was presented, which described how such a campaign works, illustrated with individual examples of the corporate reactions which took place and the reactions which were triggered in other social media contexts.

The following conclusions were drawn, which are also evident in other studies of public shaming activities on the Internet.

The information on the Internet is usually available in unlimited quantities. Sometimes it takes a while before certain information reaches a wider public. When this happens, the time difference may be insignificant. This also results from the fact that there is "no forgetting" on the Internet. History seems to have less relevance online than in the offline world. On the other hand, certain statements cannot be retracted, even if they were made in an emotional, tense and stressful situation, possibly in response to a campaign or shitstorm (Chaps. 16 and 18).

At the same time, the tone of posts on social media platforms seems in many ways to be rough and unfiltered. Storrer (2013) points out that written communication plays a central role in social networks and takes on an importance here, especially with regard to relationship-building and relationship maintenance. Storrer (2013) makes it clear that for the first time, written language is used extensively in areas of everyday communication in dialogical, spontaneous and informal exchange, which until now has tended to be the domain of spoken language. In the process, new attitudes towards writing and "the written word" are emerging, for which characteristic patterns of language design and formulation are developing. Whether this actually leads to a decline in language, to a brutalisation of language or to a general decline in the level of communication has not yet been sufficiently researched. What is certain, however, is that new linguistic and communicative norms are currently being developed and implemented for digital contexts, which seem to differ from other written and everyday language settings.

Because the initiatives, whether via campaign platforms, Twitter, Facebook, Instagram or YouTube, are relatively uncomplicated, straightforward to organise and easy to disseminate compared to the non-digital world, they can potentially achieve greater reach faster than in the non-digital world. This can lead to other Internet users virtually linking such initiatives to actions which have entirely different intentions from those of the original action, thus creating a new context for the original campaign, which can potentially be counterproductive. Virality is, in fact, uncontrollable.

Public shaming in the sense described here can be understood as an expression of self-awareness, self-compassion, self-affirmation and self-empowerment of individuals or groups of persons who experience marginalisation or discrimination. It can also be an expression of assuming social responsibility or solidarity with affected individuals or groups of people. It can be political insofar as it publicly demands compliance with ethical standards from companies or firms and exerts appropriate virtual pressure to achieve this end. In this respect, public shaming can be not only an important and powerful resource at the social, political and economic level, but it can also imply significant effects at the individual level in the sense of self-efficacy experiences, positive transformation of experiences of discreditation and shaming. And it can be a component of comprehensive social participation. Thus it is potentially suitable to create a David and Goliath situation and also to place actors in a powerful assertive position vis-à-vis a potentially much more powerful partner. It should be borne in mind that, in addition to possible intended positive effects of public shaming activities, negative side effects can occur, including damage to individuals or sustained damage to companies and thus the destruction of the livelihoods of people who may not have been involved in the misconduct originally criticised. In principle, if, for example, compliance with the standards described above is not guaranteed, there is a risk that such instruments may be abused for unfair personal or political motives.

In public shaming, it becomes clear how essential it is to have a comprehensive factual analysis and compliance with ethical standards. However, it also becomes evident that the assessment of whether this can be regarded as successful depends crucially on the perspective. In principle, it would certainly be advisable to provide spaces for dialogue with one another, even in the case of public shaming activities, instead of exclusively discoursing about one another. Then consensual solutions could be reached in corresponding negotiation processes that are sustainable for both sides. In political contexts, there are now some very interesting digital solutions for this purpose, such as the first approaches to liquid democracy.

5 Further Need for Research

Further research is needed on the actual impact of grassroots campaigns, not only for the companies or authorities concerned but also at the individual level (outcome) and societal level (impact).

Moreover, there is a lack of studies on a larger scale that would explain the connections between public shaming activities as a strategic political tool vis-à-vis companies and authorities, as described and analysed in this chapter, and political activism beyond this level of action. There is some initial analysis here, but it is hardly gender- or culture-based and only exists in rudimentary form so far. It would also be worthwhile intensifying research into the attitudes and value systems either that motivate people to participate in and support such campaigns or that prevent them from doing so. A further step could involve researching what motivates people to get involved in the online or offline world beyond the digital signature.

Furthermore, it would be desirable for future research to devote more attention to the analysis of the culturally related phenomena of public shaming. In the medium term, public shaming in the digital context will change our understanding of political participation and expression of opinion. A more intensive discourse in society as a whole is needed, across national borders since these borders are scarcely relevant to the Internet, regarding how this expression of opinion and participation can be shaped successfully, freely and fairly. Standards and netiquettes which are diversity-sensitive need to be developed for this, on which people could ideally agree globally. Such developments should be accompanied by international research activities.

Public shaming is, per se, an escalation instrument for situations where people see no other way to enforce legitimate protection of their interests or those of the environment, by forcing companies or authorities to protect these rights. A conflict is therefore factored in. In the context of the Fourth Industrial Revolution, appropriate methods to sustainably handle, resolve and transform conflicts, such as virtual mediation, are clearly needed. Here, too, appropriate research priorities could provide valuable input.

References

Albers, S., Klapper, D., Konradt, U., Walter, A., & Wolf, J. (2006). *Methodik der empirischen Forschung*. Wiesbaden: Dt. Univ.-Verl.

Antidiskriminierungsstelle des Bundes. (2017). *Diskriminierung in Deutschland: Dritter Gemeinsamer Bericht der Antidiskriminierungsstelle des Bundes und der in ihrem Zuständigkeitsbereich betroffenen Beauftragten der Bundesregierung und des Deutschen Bundestages*. Berlin: Antidiskriminierungsstelle des Bundes.

Avaaz. (2020). *About us*. Retrieved February 16, 2020, from https://secure.avaaz.org/page/en/about/

Bandura, A. (1997). *Self efficacy: The exercise of control*. New York: Freeman.

Bartley, T., & Child, C. (2014). Shaming the corporation. *American Sociological Review, 79*(4), 653–679. https://doi.org/10.1177/0003122414540653.

Becker, T. (2020). *Zeitgeist: Und raus bist du-DER SPIEGEL 39/2017*. Retrieved February 15, 2020, from https://www.spiegel.de/spiegel/print/d-153305008.html

Bloomfield, M. (2013). Shame campaigns and environmental justice: Corporate shaming as activist strategy. *Environmental Politics, 23*(2), 263–281. https://doi.org/10.1080/09644016.2013.821824.

Braithwaite, J. (1989). *Crime, shame and reintegration* (p. 55). Melbourne: Cambridge University.

Briegleb, T. (2016). *Die diskrete Scham*. Frankfurt: Insel Verlag.

Bruhn, M., & Hadwich, K. (2012). Customer Experience – Eine Einführung in die theoretischen und praktischen Problemstellungen. In M. Bruhn & K. Hadwich (Eds.), *Customer experience*. Wiesbaden: Gabler Verlag.

Cabrera, N. L., Matias, C. E., & Montoya, R. (2017, April 3). Activism or slacktivism? The Potential and Pitfalls of Social Media in Contemporary Student Activism. *Journal of Diversity in Higher Education*. Advance online publication. https://doi.org/10.1037/dhe0000061, 10, 400

Change.org. (2020). *Impact report 2018*. Retrieved February 15, 2020, from https://static.change.org/brand-pages/impact/reports/2019/change.org_Impact_Report_english_FINAL.pdf

Christensen, H. (2011). *Political activities on the Internet: Slacktivism or political participation by other means?* Retrieved February 21, 2020, from https://www.researchgate.net/publication/223956345_Political_activities_on_the_Internet_Slacktivism_or_political_participation_by_other_means

Deutscher Werberat. (2020a). *Werberat spricht nachträgliche Beanstandung aus – Social-Media-Werbung von true fruits überschreitet Grenze zulässiger Provokation*. Retrieved February 15, 2020, from https://werberat.de/werberat-spricht-nachtragliche-beanstandung-aus-social-media-werbung-von-true-fruits-uberschreitet

Deutscher Werberat. (2020b). Retrieved February 15, 2020, from https://werberat.de/sites/default/files/uploads/media/true_fruits_sun_creamie_screenshot_fb.jpg

Deutschlandfunk. (2020). *"Scham" von Jennifer Jacquet – Beschämung als öffentlicher Akt*. Retrieved February 15, 2020, from https://www.deutschlandfunk.de/scham-von-jennifer-jacquet-beschaemung-als-oeffentlicher-akt.1310.de.html?dram:article_id=321818

Die WELT. (2020). *Der kalkulierte Skandal um die Smoothie-Werbung von „True Fruits" – WELT*. Retrieved February 15, 2020, from https://www.welt.de/kultur/article199022287/Der-kalkulierte-Skandal-um-die-Smoothie-Werbung-von-True-Fruits.html

Dieckmann, J., Geschke, D., & Braune, I. (2017). *Diskriminierung und ihre Auswirkungen für Betroffene und die Gesellschaft*. Retrieved March 2, 2020, from https://www.idz-jena.de/wsddet/diskriminierung-und-ihre-auswirkungen-fuer-betroffene-und-die-gesellschaft/

Eisenhardt, K. M., & Graebner, M. E. (2007). Theory building from cases: Opportunities ald challenges. *Academy of Management Journal, 50*(1), 25–32.

Friedland, P. (2012). *Seeing justice done: The age of spectacular capital punishment in France*. Oxford: Oxford University Press.

Friedrich-Ebert-Stiftung. (2020). *Grassroots-Campaigning im Wahlkampf: Chance und Herausforderung für Parteien Ein Interview mit Dr. Arijana Neumann*. Retrieved February 15, 2020, from https://www.fes.de/index.php?eID=dumpFile&t=f&f=37034&token=d518ea8743244e6be4847b8f7cc5661c2b2d2911

Furgalec, N. (2020). *Sign the petition*. Retrieved February 15, 2020, from https://www.change.org/p/truediskriminisierung-und-sonst-nichts-nehmt-true-fruits-aus-dem-sortiment

Göbel, F. (2009). Case study approach. In M. Schwaiger & A. Meyer (Eds.), *Theorien und Methoden der Betriebswirtschaft. Handbuch für Wissenschaftler und Studierende* (pp. 355–372). München: Vahlen.

Gouthier, M., Giese, A., & Bartl, C. (2012). Customer Experiences, Kundenbegeisterung und Service Excellence – Die Spezifikation DIN SPEC 77224. In M. Bruhn & K. Hadwich (Eds.), *Customer Experience*. Wiesbaden: Gabler Verlag.

Haag, H., & Wintermeier, M. (2020). *Name and Shame – die Urteilsveröffentlichung*. Retrieved February 15, 2020, from https://www.deutscheranwaltspiegel.de/name-and-shame-die-urteilsveroeffentlichung/

Heil, D. (2018). *Lob der Scham. Nur wer sich achtet, kann sich schämen*. Gießen: Psychosozial-Verlag.

Heil, D. (2019). *Lob der Scham*. Freiburg: Herder.

Horizont. (2020). *True Fruits: Warum der Samengenuss in die Hose geht*. Retrieved February 15, 2020, from https://www.horizont.net/marketing/kommentare/True-Fruits-Warum-der-Samengenuss-in-die-Hose-geht-142387

Igel, U., Brähler, E., & Grande, G. (2010). Der Einfluss von Diskriminierungserfahrungen auf die Gesundheit von MigrantInnen. *Psychiatrische Praxis, 37*(04), 183–190. https://doi.org/10.1055/s-0029-1223508.

Instagramm. (2020). *#truefruitsboykott hashtag on Instagram · Photos and Videos*. Retrieved February 15, 2020, from https://www.instagram.com/explore/tags/truefruitsboykott/

Jacquet, J. (2014). *Shaming at scale | Edge.org*. [online] Edge.org. Retrieved January 25, 2020, from https://www.edge.org/conversation/jennifer_jacquet-jennifer-jacquet-shaming-at-scale.

Jacquet, J. (2015a). *Is Shame Necessary?* [online] C-SPAN.org. Retrieved January 25, 2020, from https://www.c-span.org/video/?324721-1/jennifer-jacquet-is-shame-necessary.

Jacquet, J. (2015b). *Scham – Die politische Kraft eines unterschätzten Gefühls* (Vol. 2015). Frankfurt am Main: S. Fischer Verlag.

Jacquet, J. (2016). *Is shame necessary? New uses for an old tool*. New York, NY: Random House.

Jacquet, J. (2020). *Jennifer Jacquet on Shame*. [online] YouTube. Retrieved January 25, 2020, from https://www.youtube.com/watch?v=piUEVsKpfhc.

Koster, I., & Wemli, T. (2019). Retrieved February 15, 2020, from https://www.youtube.com/watch?v=ODxiA9n1uJw&t=1822s

KPMG. (2019). *#CXzählt - Wie erfolgreiche Unternehmen excellente Kundenerlebnisse schaffen*. Berlin: KPMG.

Liechti, D. (2020). Bei Globus fallen Smoothies aus dem Sortiment – Blick. Retrieved February 15, 2020, from https://www.blick.ch/news/schweiz/globus-und-co-nehmen-true-fruit-aus-dem-regal-sind-das-sexistische-smoothies-id15504934.html

Lindemann, H. (2019). Transforming shame into pride ... And vice versa—A meta-model for understanding the transformations of shame and pride in counselling, mediation, consulting and therapy. In C. Mayer & E. Vanderheiden (Eds.), *The bright side of shame. transforming and*

growing through practical applications in cultural contexts (pp. 561–571). Cham: Springer International.
Lomas, T., & Ivtzan, I. (2016). Second wave positive psychology: Exploring the positive-negative dialectics of Well-being. *Journal of Happiness Studies, 17*(4), 1753–1768.
Mayer, C.-H., & Krause, C. (2013). Salutogenese in Beratung und Psychotherapie. *Klinische Verhaltensmedizin und Rehabilitation, 26*(2), 91–178.
Mayer, C., & Vanderheiden, E. (2019). *The bright side of Shame. Transforming and growing through practical applications in cultural contexts*. Cham: Springer.
Mayer-Vorfelder, M. (2012). Customer Experience Management im Dienstleistungsbereich – Konzeption eines entscheidungsorientierten Managementansatzes. In M. Bruhn & K. Hadwich (Eds.), *Customer Experience*. Wiesbaden: Gabler Verlag.
Mayer, C., Vanderheiden, E., & Oosthuizen, R. (2019). Transforming shame, guilt and anxiety through a salutogenic PP1.0 and PP2.0 counselling framework. *Counselling Psychology Quarterly, 32*(3–4), 436–452. https://doi.org/10.1080/09515070.2019.1609421.
McDavid, W. (2015). *The ever-present according to George Eliot*. Retrieved February 21, 2020, from https://mbird.com/2015/03/the-ever-present-according-to-george-eliot/
MEEDIA. (2020). *Die Provo-Masche zieht noch: True Fruits sorgt mit Sonnencreme-Penis auf Frauen-Schulter für Empörung ›* Meedia. Retrieved February 15, 2020, from https://meedia.de/2019/08/22/die-provo-masche-zieht-noch-true-fruits-sorgt-mit-sonnencreme-penis-auf-frauen-schulter-fuer-empoerung/
Metzinger, P. (2020). *Campaigning Definition und Erklärung – Campaigning heisst Veränderung bewirken*. Retrieved February 15, 2020, from http://www.campaigning.ch/index.php/campaigning-definition-und-erklaerung
Morozov, E. (2009). *The brave new world of slacktivism*. Retrieved February 21, 2020, from http://williamwolff.org/wp-content/uploads/2016/08/obar-zube-lampe-advocay-2012.pdf
Müller-Böling, D., & Klandt, H. (1996). *Methoden empirischer Wirtschafts- und Sozialforschung*. Köln: FGF c/o Univ. Dortmund.
Österreichischer Werberat. (2020). *True Fruits Smoothies*. Retrieved February 15, 2020, from https://www.werberat.at/verfahrendetail.aspx?id=2831
Pascoe, E., & Smart Richman, L. (2009). Perceived discrimination and health: A meta-analytic review. *Psychol Bull, 134*(4), 531–554.
Pauker, M. (2020). *True Fruits beschimpft Kritiker als "Pissnelken."* Retrieved February 15, 2020, from https://www.wuv.de/marketing/true_fruits_reagiert_heftig_auf_rassismus_kritik
Putnam, R. D. (2000). *Bowling alone: The collapse and revival of American community*. New York: Simon & Schuster.
Rhein, M. (2012). *Die Auswirkungen von Corporate Social Responsibility und Organisationsstolz auf Mitarbeiter im Kundenkontakt* (Promotion). Technische Universität Berlin.
Roche, C. (2019). *Charlotte Roche on Instagram: "Sonnenschutz für die Öhrchen aus Müll vom Boden gebaut. Billie Eilish gesehen. Und gehört. Ich habe ganz grosse Hoffnungen für die Frauen…"*. Retrieved February 21, 2020, from https://www.instagram.com/p/B1mrW_ZoQf3/
Schmitt, M., Branscombe, N., Postmes, T., & Garcia, A. (2014). The consequences of perceived discrimination for psychological Well-being: A meta-analytic review. *Psychological Bulletin, 140*(4), 921–948. https://doi.org/10.1037/a0035754.
Schwaiger, M., & Meyer, A. (2009). *Theorien und Methoden der Betriebswirtschaft*. München: Franz Vahlen.
Statista. (2020). *Umsatz von true fruits bis 2018 | Statista*. Retrieved February 15, 2020, from https://de.statista.com/statistik/daten/studie/828453/umfrage/umsatz-von-true-fruits/
Storrer, A. (2013). Sprachstil und Sprachvariation in sozialen Netzwerken. In B. Frank-Job, A. Mehler, & T. Sutter (Eds.), *Die Dynamik sozialer und sprachlicher Netzwerke*. Wiesbaden: Springer VS.
Studierendenwerk Bonn listet Smoothies von True Fruits aus. (2020). Retrieved February 15, 2020, from https://www.studierendenwerk-bonn.de/ueber-uns/presse/nachricht/auslistung-true-fruits/

Taheri, C. (2020). *Das BaFin Naming and Shaming*. Retrieved February 15, 2020, from https://www.compliance-manager.net/fachartikel/das-bafin-naming-and-shaming-340408644

True Fruits GmbH. (2019). *Marketing im Saftladen*. Retrieved February 21, 2020, from https://true-fruits.com/media/pdf/f8/61/8d/Marketingpaper_210519.pdf

True Fruits GmbH. (2020). *True fruits smoothies*. Posts vom 12.02.2020. Retrieved March 1, 2020, from https://www.facebook.com/true.fruits.no.tricks/

True Fruits GmbH. (2020a). *True Fruits GmbH*. Retrieved February 15, 2020, from https://true-fruits.com

True Fruits GmbH. (2020b). *True Fruits Smoothies*. Retrieved February 15, 2020, from https://www.facebook.com/true.fruits.no.tricks/photos/a.157492230913/10156203682195914/?type=3

True Fruits GmbH. (2020c). *„Love is in the air": True Fruits Gummipuppen-Edition zum Valentinstag*. Retrieved February 15, 2020, from https://www.about-drinks.com/true-fruits-gummipuppen-edition/

True Fruits GmbH. (2020d). *Früh übt sich*. Retrieved March 1, 2020, from https://www.facebook.com/true.fruits.no.tricks/videos/1040036399696677/

True Fruits GmbH. (2020e). True fruits Smoothies. Retrieved February 15, 2020, from https://www.facebook.com/true.fruits.no.tricks/posts/10156213455650914

Twitter. (2020). *Search Twitter – #truediskriminierung*. Retrieved February 15, 2020, from https://twitter.com/hashtag/truediskriminierung?src=hashtag_click

Uslucan, H. (2016). Diskriminierungserfahrungen türkeistämmiger Zuwanderer_innen. *Rassismuskritik Und Widerstandsformen*, 129–141. https://doi.org/10.1007/978-3-658-14721-1_8.

Uslucan, H. H., & Yalcin, C. S. (2012). Wechselwirkung zwischen Diskriminierung und Integration. Analyse bestehender Forschungsstände. Expertise des Zentrums für Türkeistudien und Integrationsforschung im Auftrag der Antidiskriminierungsstelle des Bundes. Essen.

Vanderheiden, E., & Mayer, C. (2017). *The value of shame. Exploring a health resource in cultural contexts*. Cham: Springer.

Vie, S. (2014). In defense of "slacktivism": The human rights campaign Facebook logo as digital activism. *First Monday. Advance online publication*. https://doi.org/10.5210/fm.v19i4.4961.

Wernli, T. (2019). True *Fruits-Streit: Bei mir spricht die Chefin Inga Koster*. Retrieved February 15, 2020, from https://www.youtube.com/watch?v=ODxiA9n1uJw

Wickert, C. (2020). *Reintegrative Shaming (Braithwaite) | SozTheo*. Retrieved February 24, 2020, from https://soztheo.de/kriminalitaetstheorien/sanktionierung/reintegrative-shaming-braithwaite/

Wong, P. T. P. (2011). Positive psychology 2.0: Towards a balanced interactive model of the good life. *Canadian Psychology, 52*(2), 69–81. Retrieved from http://www.drpaulwong.com/positive-psychology-2-0-towards-a-balanced-interactive-model-of-the-good-life/.

Wong, P. T. P. (2019). Foreword: From shame to wholeness: An existential positive psychology perspective. In C.-H. Mayer & E. Vanderheiden (Eds.), *The bright side of shame. Transforming and growing through practical applications in cultural contexts* (pp. v–xi). Cham: Springer.

Wurmser, L. (2007). Scham, Schamabwehr und tragische Wahrheit. In S. Marks & W. Schwedemann (Eds.), *Scham - Beschämung - Anerkennung*. Berlin: LIT Verlag.

Yin, R. (2009). *Case study research: Design and methods* (4th ed.). Thousand Oaks, CA: Sage Publications.

Youtube. (2020). #truediskriminierung und sonst nichts!" #truefruits. Retrieved February 15, 2020, from https://www.youtube.com/watch?v=Lsk-c-_3_BA

Elisabeth Vanderheiden is a pedagogue, theologian and intercultural mediator. She is the CEO of the Global Institute for Transcultural Research and the President of Catholic Adult Education in Germany. Her publishing activities focus on pedagogy, in particular on the further education of teachers and trainers in adult, vocational and civic education, but also on the challenges of digitalisation. She has also edited books on intercultural and transnational issues. Her most recent publications deal with shame as a resource as well as with mistakes, errors and failures and their hidden potentials in the context of Culture and Positive Psychology 1.0 and 2.0. Current research projects deal with love in transcultural contexts, with life crises as well as humour in the context of Positive Psychology 2.0. Another focus of her work is Design Thinking in transcultural contexts.

Chapter 25
Artificial Shame in the Fourth Industrial Revolution

Rudolf M. Oosthuizen

1 Introduction

The First, Second and Third Industrial Revolutions gave humanity steam power, electricity and electronics, respectively. The Fourth Industrial Revolution (4IR) is a seismic shift with a set of radically new technologies. Smart technology, artificial intelligence, robotics, algorithms, the Internet-of-Things, 3D printing, bio-printing, gene editing and autonomous vehicles are transforming the world in an incredible speed (Kruger, 2020; World Economic Forum, 2018). 4IR is changing almost all aspects of human life, including the cultural context. In this chapter, a theoretical background is provided of shame and the evolution of shame. Individuals who feel shame tend to internalise and over-personalise everything that happens to them. They cannot see things in perspective. When something goes wrong, they say to themselves, "I'm to blame for what happened. It's entirely my fault". Not only do they demean themselves, but they also feel helpless and do not think there is anything they can do to change the situation. The internal critic in their heads continually judges and criticises them, telling them that they are inadequate, inferior or worthless (Kets de Vries, 2017; Oosthuizen, 2019a) (see Mayer and Vanderheiden on "The Meaning of Shame in Cultures of the Fourth Industrial Revolution: An Introduction").

Here, the concept of artificial morality, which is a developing field within the broader range of artificial intelligence, is conceptualised. A new model of artificial cognitive architecture for intelligent systems—Neuromodulating Cognitive Architecture (NEUCOGAR)—is contemplated, and a general theoretical framework for the design of artificial emotion systems in machines is postulated. The

R. M. Oosthuizen (✉)
Department of Industrial and Organisational Psychology at the University of South Africa, Pretoria, South Africa
e-mail: oosthrm@unisa.ac.za

C.-H. Mayer et al. (eds.), *Shame 4.0*, https://doi.org/10.1007/978-3-030-59527-2_25

aforementioned concepts and framework are probed to consider whether shame may be a vital feeling for artificial cognitive systems and, in the event that it can be demonstrated, guidelines will be put forward on how to execute it in a specific cultural context.

1.1 Objective of the Chapter

The objective of the chapter is to present a critical review of shame for artificial cognitive systems, which must or may not be able to interact with human beings in the context of 4IR.

2 Research Methodology

2.1 Study Design

The critical review of the research literature entailed a broad, systematic review of contemporary research on the themes of shame, the evolution of shame, artificial intelligence, artificial morality, cognitive architecture, emotions and machines and 4IR. The question that arises is: Are machines without shame? This approach allowed the author to evaluate documented research on artificial shame in 4IR.

2.2 Study Eligibility Criteria

The boundary of the systematic review was demarcated to include only documented contemporary research in the field of shame and AI, published from 2015 to 2020. A search was done by means of an online information technology service, including search engines such as EBSCOhost/Academic Search Premier and Google Scholar academic databases. The terms "shame", "evolution of shame", "artificial intelligence", "artificial morality", "cognitive architecture", "emotions", "machines" and the "4th Industrial Revolution" were used in the search. The full texts of publications were downloaded from the databases in order to ascertain which articles to include or exclude from the systematic review. The inclusion criteria for articles reviewed for the purpose of this chapter were studies exploring artificial shame in 4IR. The research articles were treated as sources of data.

2.3 *Data Analysis*

A qualitative approach was followed in exploring artificial shame in 4IR. In the first stage, the author read the studies carefully to form an understanding of the phenomenon of artificial shame. In the second, the author synthesised a portrait of the phenomenon of artificial shame that accounts for the relations and linkages between its diverse aspects. Stage 3 consisted of theorising about how and why these artificial shame relations appear as they do, and Stage 4 consisted of re-contextualising new knowledge about the phenomenon of artificial shame, relating this back into the context of how other authors have articulated the evolving body of knowledge. Nineteen studies were identified in a systematic search for relevant research published between January 2015 and January 2020, in the following electronic databases: EBSCOhost/Academic Search Premier and Google Scholar Academic database. Publications were evaluated for their quality, and eight studies were subsequently identified as the primary sources for exploration.

2.4 *Strategies Used to Ensure Data Quality*

Systematic, rigorous and auditable analytical processes are among the most significant factors distinguishing good research from work of inferior quality. The researcher therefore articulated the findings in such a manner that the logical processes by which they were developed would be accessible to a critical reader, the relationship between the actual data and the conclusions about data would be explicit and claims made in relation to the data set would be rendered credible. Consideration was also given to potential publication bias (e.g. the assumption that not all research on the topic may have been published), trustworthiness or credibility, true value and quality, appropriateness and a reflection on the research endeavour in its entirety, as well as best practice. Value and quality were assured by reviewing each article for its scientific and methodological rigour in exploring artificial shame in 4IR. All data were retained for possible future scrutiny.

3 Theoretical Background

3.1 *The Concept of Shame*

Shame is an emotional regulation of human activities; in truth, it is basically elicited by the impact which social weights or values exert on a person. While a select few feelings can be described as individual and basic (joy, fear, anger, torment), others are more social in nature (blameworthiness, shame, embarrassment) (Ramachandran, 2002). Shame has a place in the latter category, given its social nature. Its solid bonds with moral (if antiquated) Western as well as Eastern systems make it a central focus of philosophical examination (Honderich, 1995). The following are two basic yet ancient examples:

(a) Aristotle: In *The Nicomachean Ethics* (fourth book, ninth area), he described shame as a quasi-virtue (shame ought to not be depicted as an ideal, for it is more like a feeling than a state of character). What he attempted to confirm is that shame is a transitory state between stable virtuous emotions. This characteristic turns shame into something important: it exercises control to caution against fiascos and prevent the individual from making the wrong choices (letting us to imagine disgraces that would affect us in front of the others). But shame is valuable to the extent that it may be an intercessional feeling—were it not, it might lie dormant in a person, festering so that it never becomes public knowledge, or, indeed, it may give rise to something more awful, as happened to Chrysippus, who slaughtered himself for shame (Apollodorus, Library, Book 3, Chap. 5; Vallverdú, 2014) (see Kasbova in this book).
(b) Laozi: in his *Dao de jing*, 28, he states: Know what is sufficient and escape shame. Thus, shame may be a red flag, alerting a person that something is off-kilter and needs to be attended to. The sage man will take action, as a way of moving towards the great way. Indeed, for a Confucian rationalist such as Mencius, the role of shame was vitally important: "Men cannot live without shame. A sense of shame is the beginning of integrity" (Wong & Tsai, 2007) (see Wong and Hwang; see Kotera et al.; see Takano in this book).

The above illustrations are given alongside one another, to reflect common aspects of two human social orders, namely, of shame and blame. Social studies have shown that several social orders use the teaching of shame in children and adults in society as a primary device for exercising control (the concomitant danger is that of isolation). Eastern nations such as China, Korea and Japan are significant illustrations of this kind of social order (Vallverdú, 2014). Western nations, by contrast, and customarily Judaeo-Christian nations in particular, function from the basis of guilt (Honderich, 1995). Wong and Tsai (2007) draw a parallel between "individualistic" countries and guilt (Western regions) and "collectivistic" nations and shame (Eastern regions).

Shame is an overpowering and unpleasant feeling: it may be a regular, discrete and strong (yet short-lived) emotional experience in response to a stimulus (Elfenbein, 2007; Smith & Ellsworth, 1985) that arises in reaction to self-attributed disappointment in meeting the desires of others (Bagozzi, Verbeke, & Gavino, 2003; Brown, González, Zagefka, Manzi, & Cěehajić, 2008; Lewis, 1992; Smith & Ellsworth, 1985). In other words, shame arises when an individual encounters differences between what s/he actually does (actual self) and what s/he is expected to do (ought self) (Ghorbani et al., 2013; Higgins, 1987). Past experiences of shame make individuals feel and fear the negative evaluation of others (Agrawal, Han, & Duhachek, 2013), and it is this social scrutiny that motivates them to protect themselves from further emotional anguish (De Hooge, Zeelenberg, & Breugelmans, 2010, 2011; Ferguson, 2005). As such, coping with a damaged self-image is a central concern for individuals who feel ashamed (González-Gómez & Richter, 2015; Oosthuizen, 2019a).

To escape the negative assessment of others, individuals ordinarily express shame by withdrawing or using the tactic of evasion, avoiding eye contact, assuming a slouched pose or pulling back from engaging with others and remaining quiet during social gatherings (Fischer & Tangney, 1995). By withdrawing from, or avoiding, situations where shame may be experienced, individuals aim to protect themselves from further harm. In light of the unpleasantness of the experience of being shamed, unsurprisingly, prior research has predominantly examined the negative effects of shame, including low self-efficacy and self-esteem, social anxiety and depression (Lazarus & Folkman, 1984; Leary & Kowalsky, 1995; Oosthuizen, 2019a; Tangney, Miller, Flicker, & Barrow, 1996).

3.2 The Evolution of Shame

Feelings are the result of our natural as well as our social evolution, showing degrees of complexity which progressively extend from fundamental to more complex experiences. Basically, feelings form part of our personal development as humans and are driven by circumstances. Feelings arise within our bodies and usually give rise to certain actions (either the manifestation or suppression thereof). It incorporates a social cycle of emotions, in which people express and share their feelings, making conceivable the existence of fluxes in emotional energy (Vallverdú, 2014). Sympathy is a fundamental component that allows this social emotional process to unfold. But there are feelings that make sense from a developmental point of view, namely, meta-social feelings. These feelings have emerged only through intensive sociocultural interactions, as a way of channelling complex and energetic levels of human movement. Among these feelings, shame is one of the foremost which is evident. What might clarify the rise and presence of shame as a feeling, from a developmental viewpoint? Cross-cultural research illustrates that shame advanced from a rank-related feeling, for example, where there is competition for prestige, or cooperation, or differentiation, all of which play a part in human interaction in modern societies (Fessler, 2004; Sznycer et al., 2012).

Given the pervasiveness of this emotion across the ages and across cultures, what is the adaptive purpose of shame? From an evolutionary point of view, we could hypothesise that shame evolved—specifically when looking at organisational conditions, survival depended on employees abiding by certain norms and subsequently failing to do so. Where employees needed to stand together to operate effectively as a group to better deal with complex situations, and that did not happen, one or all of them must have felt a sense of shame in letting down the team. Interestingly, these behavioural patterns can still be observed today, where employees feign compliance out of shame or subject themselves to the power and judgement of their fellow employees (Oosthuizen, 2019a). From a systems psychodynamic perspective, shame is deemed to be a complex emotional response that employees develop during the early phases of their careers in organisations, when they are completely dependent on the bond they form with their supervisors. It is a very basic emotion: employees seek to live up to their supervisor's expectations and, in failing to do so, experience shame. Within the early stages of their careers, many employees exhibit early feelings of embarrassment that can later turn into full-blown shame (Kets de Vries, 2017).

According to Deonna, Rodogno, and Teroni (2012), compassion plays a special role as a driver of social cohesion, while the reflexivity of the whole serves to maintain a strategic distance from difficult feelings (understood as part of the mechanism of shame), thus permitting the reinforcement of the idea of the "other". Usually, being exceptionally near to, and showing, empathy creates a feeling of "being in tune". For these reasons, shame cannot be considered a revolting feeling, but is in fact a vital social feeling. Despite talk of whether or not emotions (see Vallverdú, 2013, 2014) are widespread, and of the ways in which they are socially demonstrated, recent research indicates the presence of a panhuman, hardwired basis that conceivably produces feelings which people around the world express as feelings, and they do so using metaphors and/or metonyms, which are related to those sentiments (Kövecses, 2000). In turn, these feelings are generated by activities within the autonomic nervous system (Casimir & Schnegg, 2002).

A comparison of the impulses which give rise to the emotions communicated by these representations and metonyms appears to indicate that the precursors thereof, and related evaluations, do change significantly from one culture to the next. Despite the subtle conceptual elements which make up these debates, it seems clear that shame may be a universal human feeling, showing up in all known human societies. Psychological research demonstrates that humans have an intrinsic need to be seen as attractive to others. This need shapes the premise for shame and intercedes in assessments of social standing (status), social acknowledgement and social bonds. Shame and mortification are associated with assaults on, and misfortunes around, the quality of an individual's social engagement. Internal encounters of shame are inferred from tamer behaviours such as a look which signals to others an awareness of personal misfortune which may affect one's social standing and represents an attempt to limit any conceivable damage (Gilbert, 1997; Vallverdú, 2014). A few computational simulations, which attempted to arrive at an understanding of the components which legitimise social participation and the role of shame, were performed by Jaffe (2008) and Jaffe et al. (2014).

4 Literature Review

4.1 The Concept of Artificial Intelligence

The potential for digital platforms and artificial intelligence (AI) to underpin and develop the world of work is unbounded. This platform stratum establishes a digital value chain allowing for the commoditisation and computerisation of the back office, but it comes with warnings. Whereas it can create a flourishing trading cycle, it can also grow to take over the complete financial system, and with digital platforms, inescapability involves becoming powerless in the face of cyber attacks or wide-scale control (United Nations Department of Economic and Social Affairs, 2010). Closely linked to digital platforms are data. How governments, organisations and individuals decide to share and use data is key to our worlds—even the most human-centric. AI in the form of digital assistants or "chatbots", and machine learning, could enable machines to understand, learn and act, based on that information (Oosthuizen, 2019b).

It is useful to think of three levels of AI:

1. Assisted intelligence, which is widely available today, improves what people and organisations are already doing. An example is the global positioning system (GPS) navigation programme that offers directions to drivers and adjusts routes to road conditions.
2. Augmented intelligence, which is emerging today, helps individuals and organisations to do things they would otherwise not be able to do. For example, vehicle ride-sharing businesses would not be able to exist without the combination of programmes that organise the service.
3. Autonomous intelligence, which is being developed for the future, creates machines that act on their own, for example, self-driving vehicles, when they come into widespread use (Oosthuizen, 2019b).

Some visionaries believe AI could create a world where human abilities are amplified as machines help mankind process, analyse and evaluate the abundance of data that create today's world, thus allowing humans to spend more time engaged in high-level thinking, creativity and decision-making (Stubbings, 2017, 2018).

Furthermore, contemplating the culture of AI is essential for all societies and potential social futures. Social connectivity has thus acquired an inescapably technological imprint. With AI and robotics technology advancing faster than ever before, robots are becoming more human-like, which in turn creates the possibility of new modes of human–robot configurations, for instance, robot friendships. Central to Levy's (2009) argument is a conception of robots involving a significant transformation of human social relations. To situate robots in terms of property relations and advanced capitalism is to see it as an intricately woven texture of unequal power relations and gender hierarchy (Elliott, 2019).

4.2 *The Concept of Artificial Morality*

Artificial morality is a developing field within the range of AI, with the latter showing or simulating human cognitive capacities. Artificial morality, more specifically, explores whether and how artificial intelligence can be furnished with ethical capacities. One critical aspect of artificial morality is its certainty (Misselhorn, Pompe, & Stapleton, 2013). The advancement of increasingly intelligent and independent innovations will eventually lead to these systems having to confront morally problematic situations or circumstances which cannot be completely controlled by human administrators. In the event that this genuinely occurs, the requirement for artificial morality will eventually emerge from innovative progress. The requirement is that this not be seen as an impediment. One reason is that machines might be much better moral operators than people, since they are not subject to mindlessness, temptation or passionate turmoil. Moreover, they are unable of dismissing morality for reasons of self-interest (Misselhorn, 2018).

Another point regarding artificial morality is that machines with moral capacities appear to be better than ordinary machines. The essential goal of innovation is to make strides in improving human life. Ethical machines, so one might contend, are predominantly machines which are better able to recognise and respond to human needs and to interface on a personal and social level (Anderson & Anderson, 2011). While unused advances are often criticised and rejected for moral reasons, ethical machines are ethical by design. Artificial morality might moreover offer assistance in the process of expanding humans' moral capacity. Human ethical behaviour is, at best, inconsistent, as contexts change. Research into artificial morality can contribute to making human morality more reliable and cohesive, because artificial systems can function on this premise (Misselhorn, 2018). And, finally, trying to replicate human morality might lead to a stronger understanding of the concept. The aim is to discover which common structures underlie our ethical capacities, which may be executed either by the human body or by artificial systems (List & Pettit, 2011).

There are serious reservations regarding artificial morality:

- Crucial complaints include idiosyncrasies in the ethical quality of artificial morality, as it pertains to human intellect. Advocates of artificial morality frequently paint a picture of the human intellect as a calculating machine.
- A more pertinent complaint is that moral understanding cannot be demonstrated computationally, because the formal control of images is carried out by a computer, using a programme—that can never be sufficiently expansive to bring about any kind of brilliant understanding (Searle, 1980).
- A third challenge that artificial morality faces is that there is no agreement on what makes a proper ethical hypothesis, neither among the general public nor among researchers.
- Importantly, artificial morality will lead to fundamental changes to our ethics, requiring in-depth consideration of whether these changes are merely alluring or imperative (Pană, 2019).
- Another issue is whether it is advantageous that artificial morality forces us to assume a position on cases hitherto outside of the scope of our understanding. Situations may arise in instances where autonomous driving is done, which do not apply to human drivers (much longer response times, immunity to stress, lack of contextual information among interconnected artificial systems).
- Lastly, there is the concern that artificial morality might undermine our current assumption of responsibility and shame. Artificial systems cannot bear moral

responsibility in the full sense of the word, and that might influence humans' sense of responsibility (Misselhorn, 2018; Pereira & Lopes, 2020).

What can we conclude in this regard? There is a propensity within the evolution of current innovation that emphatically leads towards artificial morality, which will have a marked impact on humans' way of life. In spite of the fact that we are but at the beginning of the road, it is vital to imagine where it will lead us (Misselhorn, 2018). We should neither trust the naïve visions of technofreaks nor the equally simplistic fears of technophobes. We should instead try to gain answers to the following: "How can artificial morality be planned usefully? In which settings can it be used for the greater good? Which of our desires and hopes are more realistic? Which dangers can truly happen, and how do we evaluate them? Which ethical values are imperative for us as individuals and as a society, and how will artificial morality influence them?" (Bendel, 2017).

The question can be asked: Are we somehow obligated, morally or otherwise, to build robots whose moral views are substantially like ours? That would be a point about us and our design goals, and that is a different argument. In setting out to build an intelligent robot, it will be automatically—as a kind of conceptual inevitability—create something that shares with humans a fundamentally moral outlook because those robots will be embodied as humans are and will inhabit the world as humans do. The moral outlook that AIs share with humans may not determine specific behaviour. AI's central processing units would not explode if it tries to do something immoral. But then again sharing a moral foundation does not obligate humans in specific ways, either (Brożek & Janik, 2019). Humans routinely do immoral things. Furthermore, AIs would not be ultramoral, though it could probably be built to be that way. It is suspected that such ultramoral AIs will also seem "off" to humans. They would likely fail to exhibit a certain pragmatism or contextually appropriate selfish behaviour and will therefore seem not quite intelligent. AIs will be aligned with humans in the same way that humans are aligned with one another. Humans are impelled to be moral by a complex of conscious and nonconscious forces that are a response to their embodiment. They constitute more of a constraint on value alignment than has been appreciated (Cruz, 2019).

4.3 *Artificial Cognitive Architecture*

Talanov, Vallverdu, Distefano, Mazzara, and Delhibabu (2015) introduce a new model of artificial cognitive architecture for intelligent systems, Neuromodulating Cognitive Architecture (NEUCOGAR). The model, which is biomimetically motivated, adjusts the neuromodulators in human brains into computational environments. Thus, to arrive at more efficient artificial insights, based on the biological inspiration of the profoundly passionate working of the human brain (Minsky, 2006). Investigating the latest information obtained from neurology, psychology, philosophy and anthropology allows researchers to map monoamine neuromodulators and apply those mapped findings to computational framework parameters. Artificial cognitive frameworks can, at that point, perform much better complex tasks (with respect to data determination and discrimination, attention, advancement, inventiveness) while locking in affordable, enthusiastic connections with human clients.

The latest theories of, and most recent findings regarding, transdisciplinary views on cognition are exemplified in cognitive forms. Most abstract processes performed by the brain are directly related to sensorimotor forms. At the same time, the mind–body functioning is reliant on enthusiastic signals that capture, handle and classify information inputs (external or internal, in accordance with the multi-modality of feelings) and allow reactions (Vernon, 2009). The elemental part of turning feelings into cognitive processes is, hence, a matter of reality for any researcher in the field. At the same time, bio-inspired approaches to artificial cognitive systems, like feeling computing, emotional cognitive structures or neural systems, do not provide a reasonable approach to passionate, energetic data-management forms. It is important to highlight the utility of, and significant results reported in, a few of these application fields, which rely on ancient and well-formed thoughts around classic AI (Talanov et al., 2015).

NEUCOGAR makes conceivable the use of emotional elements as part of the framework as a whole, being fundamental in providing direction, rather than operating as a joined module with emotional contents. This design permits an easy application, from scratch (the artificial neuron or unit of processing) to the superior layers of specialised cognitive forms (e.g. memories, processors) (Lövheim, 2012). In this sense, NEUCOGAR may be a complete, artificial cognitive framework that imitates the essential running of bodily emotional frameworks, taking after a multi-layered modular architecture that is located together and ruled by the same emotional cyberneuromodulators. Talanov et al. (2015) developed a modern encapsulated AI, without genuine instantiated physicality, taking into consideration the fact that any living system is goal-oriented and that must be incorporated into a cultural system at some point, to obtain a result. The point is to decide, artificially, on the objectives, before applying the genuine instruments of cognitive organising. NEUCOGAR will be valuable for AI researchers when considering artificial shame for systems within a specific cultural context. It may be a new technology for a skyline of intelligent systems.

4.4 Theoretical Framework for the Design of Artificial Emotion Systems in Machines

Machines which are capable of showing emotional behaviours have helped to improve characteristic human–machine interactions in diverse application spaces. To supply machines with emotional components, their basic architecture must contain and execute an artificial emotion system (AES), a computational model that copies particular features of human feelings. Although several AES have been detailed in the related literature, their ability is, for the most part, bolstered on a few feelings or speculations, which allow researchers to demonstrate and coordinate separate feeling components and instruments into the models of an AES. This hypothetical establishment of AES contributes to ambiguities within the investigation and a comparison of their basic models, which requires the definition of standards, design rules and integrator systems (Churamani, Cruz, Griffiths, & Barros, 2016).

Rosales, Rodríguez and Ramos (2019) presented a mentally propelled hypothetical system, intended to represent a stage in the unification of AES components, the comparison of different AES and the planning and execution of AES in machines. The authors analysed common emotion-related prerequisites of AES and included feeling components within the plan of the computational model, as well as feeling hypotheses to drive the plan of most AES. The approval of this system illustrates its compatibility with current AES and its possibility to serve as a model for binding together numerous theories pertaining to the emotional.

The proposed framework is a reflection of the processing of human feeling and the components which are usually included in an AES. Planning the framework takes into account the common prerequisites, characteristics and properties of AES, as well as current evidence around the mechanisms underlying human emotions (Laird, 2012). In this sense, considering the complexity of human feelings, the high-level application requirements of AES and its complex design choices, the framework is proposed as a first attempt to create a common hypothetical framework that will lead to more complex plans of AES, capable of closely imitating the genuine processes involved in human emotions.

The chosen components have a hypothetical premise, since there is sufficient documentation on how each of these concepts affects feeling and emotional behaviour. That influence has been widely investigated in the literature and forms part of the method involved in producing emotions. For its part, there is little discrepancy about this concept, and most of the works define it as a primitive evaluation of the environment for the generation of emotional states (Rosales et al., 2019). There is disagreement in the literature on this concept, with some authors attributing inverse meanings to the concept. However, the acknowledgement in most works is that this component represents an internal emotional state. Finally, the emotional behaviour component is the aforementioned deterministic behaviour displayed by living beings, resulting from their feelings. This alone can be a subject for most investigations, but what it implies, essentially, is emotion beyond what is possible, for instance, interspecies communication (Vinciarelli et al., 2015).

Whereas all these proposed components appear to be sufficient for the creation of emotional frameworks, there are many critical challenges to attend to, which inhibit the complete development of emotional computational models that are capable of imitating emotional responses in human beings (Rosales et al., 2019). One of these challenges is that of influence, since we do not know how it is produced or what parameters to consider when evaluating it. This leads to more complex emotional frameworks or cognitive models, which can mull over the essential components without delivering exceptionally palatable findings, since most works fail to produce the innate emotional behaviours generally specified within the literature (Lindquist, Wager, Kober, Bliss-Moreau, & Barrett, 2012).

Centring on works which are solely positioned in terms of developing feelings in machines, it is observed that, in the same way, it is inconceivable to imitate complete emotional processes in their totality, given our common need for cognitive control over our emotions. In spite of having a considerable number of emotional theories converging on a unified theory based on components, and the accomplishment of binding together all the emotional computational models found in the literature, numerous researchers fail to fill the gaps around the development of AES that are unable to imitate emotional behaviour in humans as a whole. Rosales et al. (2019) indicate that it is possible to unify emotion theories, to build a common hypothesis that is competent at determining which components are essential for planning and using AES.

5 Discussion and Practical Implications

5.1 Emotions and Machines: Artificial Shame?

Having depicted what shame is, as well as its developmental roots and functionalities, the focus falls on the aim of this chapter, which is to consider whether shame may be a vital feeling for artificial cognitive frameworks and, in the event that it can be demonstrated to be so, how to execute it in a specific cultural context (Vallverdú, 2014). Considering the vast existing body of literature on feelings and machines, three fundamental zones were distinguished: (1) affective computing (Picard, 1997), (2) social robotics (Breazeal, 2002) and (3) emotional modelling (Sloman, 1962–2014).

Arguably, all these approaches execute “emotions” as complementary components, but never as nuclear perspectives within their frameworks. And, among the possible emotions to be actualised, shame has been overwhelmingly ignored, in support of Ekman’s (2003) classic model of fundamental feelings or essential positive-negative over-simplistic approaches. The reason is simple: main researchers on AI belong to a philosophical/conceptual tradition in which emotions are secondary aspects of cognitions or noise/fluffy components that bring flimsiness to the frameworks. At a certain level, the passionate transformation of the cognitive sciences and neurology, headed by Damasio (1994), has not yet reached AI communities, with a few exceptions: Jaffe (2006) is one such outlier who has adopted the amazingly effective investigate approaches of Axelrod (1986). But, in the case of Jaffe, he makes computer recreations on the nature of shame for social cohesion, without trying to actualise shame into artificial devices (Vallverdú, 2014).

Jaffe (2006) claims that the presentation of shame in virtual situations makes a difference to pro-social conduct, acting as a stabilising force for social order. His work is closer to a computational approach to sociology, than to the resistance or use of emotional rules in artificial cognitive devices. That is a fundamental next step in the implementation of shame and emotional characteristics into artificial cognitive devices (Vallverdú, 2014), for several reasons:

1. Shame is necessary to regulate the correct imitative processes.
2. Shame helps to generate a social environment.
3. Shame acts as a social stabiliser (with moral thresholds).
4. Cognitive processes run into complex and uncertain contexts (as human beings do) and need emotional drivers to be able to perform any kind of feasible activity.

For all of the aforementioned reasons, AI designs ought to actualise emotional components into their cognitive processing centres. In spite of the extraordinary triumphs of master frameworks, top-down approaches have failed in attempts to capture the delights and subtle elements of everyday life. Even the replication of essential morphological or cognitive viewpoints (vision, unsteady movement, grip and control activities) are still beyond the abilities of modern AI and robotics experts. The last Defense Advanced Research Projects Agency (DARPA) robotics challenge, for example, showed the remarkable results achieved by the Japanese Shaft robot (now the property of Google, a company with strong investments in robotics) and others, but there is a long way to go in measuring up to humans. Morphological computation is a recent and still unexplored research field (Casacuberta, Ayala, & Vallverdu, 2010), but a new approach called "morphological emotion" (the integration into the hardwiring or core section of any artificial entity or device of emotional architectures) as yet remains completely outside of current research agendas.

Vallverdú (2014) postulates that human feelings would not be added, external or complimentary angles within these systems, but would remain intrinsic mechanisms of these substances or devices. Since these feelings (and shame occupies an important space among them) play a crucial role in enhancing natural evolutionary systems, it ought to be fundamental to actualise them into artificial devices. Obviously, it is necessary that human–computer and human–robot interactions include shame for being among the most important emotions affecting social relationships. But, at the same time, AI and social robotics ought to consolidate artificial shame in the event that they need to create artificial cognitive products which are able to advance as well as make dynamic social bonds. Since the evolutionary success of the human species is not perfection, nor indicative of outright levelheadedness, incredible expertise is needed to preserve brain versatility throughout a human life, just as it would be to make models about that world.

Most such models are made with destitute, inadequate or bad data, but they permit human activity. Without extending the vast pool of emotional states, cognitive systems would be exceedingly unsurprising and less versatile, unable to reflect the variety of their environment (Vallverdú, 2014). Feelings, dispositions and sentiments make operational contrasts among substances that share comparative substantial structures, permitting modern designs of conduct and strategies. As noted, shame has contributed to the development of the human race. Another question of interest now, is: What is "artificial shame"? The term refers to a computational program designed to act within a social environment as it would when shamed within a human sphere. This leads to an important question: "Can we simulate emotions?" (Casacuberta et al., 2010).

The answer is that it is as conceivable, since we can already mimic other human abilities, such as scientific or logical reasoning. What we cannot imitate or mimic are the qualia related to the idea of emotion. At any rate, we will probably never be able to imitate/recreate the complete human body, but we are ready to simulate a few of the conceivable inner and external reactions of humans. Thus, we can implement artificial shame as a portion of a systemic, emotional approach within a specific cultural context. Emotions could be diminished to their essential and particular valences which trigger specific results and establish dynamical rules of interaction over time (Vallverdú, 2014). And all this happens inside bodies or systems that have specific needs, fundamentally bolstering their survival (and their replication, by whatever chosen method, as happens with genetic algorithms crossing conceivable outcomes): they act as whole, complex systems guided by enthusiastic criticism that contributes to make sense of the world—a particular sense which is valuable for that substance (Sznycer et al., 2012).

It is thus plausible of make better AI within the framework of bigger mechanisms and to do so at a low statistical cost (using emotional procedures). Information in itself does not make sense: the structure of the educational substance (characteristic or artificial) is key to understanding how models develop and why they make designs out of activities. Feelings (characteristic as well as manufactured) are the light by which any substance captures the world in relation to itself. If shame is so critical, robots will have to implement artificial shame into their essential working structures, to be connected and therefore superior (with us) or just to be able to form complex social situations in which to develop wealthy strategies (Vallverdú, 2014).

6 Chapter Conclusion

This chapter focused on a critical review of shame for artificial cognitive systems, which must (or may not be able to) interact with humans in the context of 4IR. It is a constructive, practical application intended to work with artificial shame in different social and cultural contexts. It can be concluded that it is important how artificial shame be implemented in artificial systems. A predefined framework of moral judgments could be applied, which is then adapted to specific moral cultural contexts through learning processes. Which judgments are given depends on the area of deployment of the system as well as its moral characteristics. A system might, however, be designed in such a way that it is able to adapt to the individual moral value profile of the user. Such a design would take into account the fact that people weigh up the relevant moral values differently. It is recommended that future research scrutinises the concepts of universality and culture-specific approaches of artificial cognitive systems.

References

Agrawal, N., Han, D., & Duhachek, A. (2013). Emotional agency appraisals influence responses to preference inconsistent information. *Organizational Behavior and Human Decision Processes, 1*, 87–97.

Anderson, M., & Anderson, S. L. (2011). A prima facie duty approach to machine ethics: Machine learning of features of ethical dilemmas, prima facie duties, and decision principles through a dialogue with ethicists. In M. Anderson & S. L. Anderson (Eds.), *Machine ethics* (pp. 476–494). Cambridge: Cambridge University Press.

Axelrod, R. (1986). An evolutionary approach to norms. *American Political Science Review, 80*(4), 1095–1111.

Bagozzi, R. P., Verbeke, W., & Gavino, J. C. J. (2003). Culture moderates the self-regulation of shame and its effects on performance: The case of salespersons in the Netherlands and the Philippines. *Journal of Applied Psychology, 88*, 219–233.

Bendel, O. (2017). *LADYBIRD: The animal-friendly robot vacuum cleaner. The 2017 AAAI spring symposium series*. Palo Alto: AAAI Press.

Breazeal, C. (2002). *Designing sociable robots*. Cambridge, MA: MIT Press.

Brougham, D., & Haar, J. (2018). Smart technology, artificial intelligence, robotics, and algorithms (STARA): Employees' perceptions of our future workplace. *Journal of Management & Organization, 24*(2), 239–257. https://doi.org/10.1017/jmo.2016.55.

Brown, R., González, R., Zagefka, H., Manzi, J., & Cěehajić, S. (2008). Nuestra culpa: Collective guilt and shame as predictors of reparation for historical wrongdoing. *Journal of Applied Psychology, 94*, 75–90.

Brożek, B., & Janik, B. (2019). Can artificial intelligences be moral agents? *New Ideas in Psychology, 54*, 101–106.

Casacuberta, D., Ayala, S., & Vallverdu, J. (2010). Embodying cognition: A morphological perspective. In J. Vallverdú (Ed.), *Thinking machines and the philosophy of computer science: Concepts and principles* (pp. 1798–1818). Hershey, PA: IGI Global.

Casimir, M. J., & Schnegg, M. (2002). Shame across cultures: The evolution, ontogeny and function of a 'moral emotion'. In H. Keller, Y. H. Poortinga, & A. Schölmerich (Eds.), *Between culture and biology. Perspectives on ontogenic development* (pp. 270–300). Cambridge: CUP.

Churamani, N., Cruz, F., Griffiths, S., & Barros, P. (2016). iCub: Learning emotion expressions using human reward. In *Workshop on bio-inspired social robot learning in home scenarios*, IEEE/RSJ International Conference on Intelligent Robots and Sustems (IROS).

Cruz, J. (2019, January). Shared moral foundations of embodied artificial intelligence. In *Proceedings of the 2019 AAAI/ACM Conference on AI, Ethics, and Society* (pp. 139–146).

Damasio, A. (1994). *Descartes' error*. New York: Putnam.

De Hooge, I. E., Zeelenberg, M., & Breugelmans, S. M. (2010). Restore and protect motivations following shame. *Cognition and Emotion, 24*, 111–127.

De Hooge, I. E., Zeelenberg, M., & Breugelmans, S. M. (2011). A functionalist account of shame-induced behaviour. *Cognition and Emotion, 25*, 939–946.

Deonna, J. A., Rodogno, R., & Teroni, F. (2012). *In defense of shame: The faces of an emotion*. London: OUP.

Ekman, P. (2003). *Emotions revealed: Recognizing faces and feelings to improve communication and emotional life*. New York, NY: Times Books/Henry Holt.

Elfenbein, H. A. (2007). Emotion in organizations: A review and theoretical integration. *Academy of Management Annals, 1*, 315–386.

Elliott, A. (2019). *The culture of AI: Everyday life and the digital revolution*. New York: Routledge.

Ferguson, T. J. (2005). Mapping shame and its functions in relationships. *Child Maltreatment, 10*, 377–386.

Fessler, D. M. T. (2004). Shame in two cultures: Implications for evolutionary approaches. *Journal of Cognition and Culture, 4*(2), 207–262.

Fischer, K. W., & Tangney, J. P. (1995). Self-conscious emotions and the affect revolution: Framework and overview. In J. P. Tangney & K. W. Fischer (Eds.), *Self-conscious emotions* (pp. 3–24). New York: Guilford Press.

Ghorbani, M. A., Shamshirband, S., Haghi, D. Z., Azani, A., Bonakdari, H., & Ebtehaj, I. (2013). Application of firefly algorithm-based support vector machines for prediction of field capacity and permanent wilting point. *Soil and Tillage Research, 172*, 32–38.

Gilbert, P. (1997). The evolution of social attractiveness and its role in shame, humiliation, guilt and therapy. *British Journal of Medical Psychology, 70*(2), 113–147.

González-Gómez, H. V., & Richter, A. W. (2015). Turning shame into creativity: The importance of exposure to creative team environments. *Organizational Behavior and Human Decision Processes, 126*, 142–161.

Higgins, E. T. (1987). Self-discrepancy: A theory relating self and affect. *Psychological Review, 94*(3), 319.

Honderich, T. (1995). *The Oxford companion to philosophy*. New York: OUP.

Jaffe, K. (2006). Simulations show that shame drives social cohesion. In J. S. Sichman, H. C. Solange, & O. Rezende (Eds.), *Advances in artificial intelligence. IBERAMIA-SBIA 2006. 2nd international joint conference, 10th Ibero-American conference on AI, 18th Brazilian AI symposium* (pp. 88–97). New York: Springer.

Jaffe, K. (2008). Evolution of shame as an adaptation to social punishment and its contribution to social cohesiveness. *Complexity, 14*(2), 46–52.

Jaffe, K., Florez, A., Gomes, C. M., Rodriguez, D., & Achury, C. (2014). On the biological and cultural evolution of shame: Using internet search tools to weight values in many cultures. *arXiv preprint arXiv:1401.1100.*

Kets de Vries, M. F. R. (2017). Don't let shame become a self-destructive spiral. *Harvard Business Review*. Retrieved September 5, 2017, from https://hbr.org/2017/06/dont-let-shame-become-a-self-destructive-spiral

Kövecses, Z. (2000). *Metaphor and emotion*. New York: Cambridge University Press.

Kruger, A. (2020, January 3). The rise of the robot workers – banking: Machines and artificial intelligence have been 'stealing' jobs for decades. *The Citizen (Gauteng).*

Laird, J. E. (2012). *The SOAR cognitive architecture*. Cambridge, MA: MIT Press.

Lazarus, R. S., & Folkman, S. (1984). *Stress, appraisal, and coping*. New York: Springer.

Leary, M. R., & Kowalsky, R. M. (1995). *Social anxiety*. New York: Guilford Press.

Levy, D. (2009). *Love and sex with robots: The evolution of human-robot relationships*. New York: HarperCollins.

Lewis, M. (1992). *Shame: The exposed self.* New York: Free Press.

Lindquist, K. A., Wager, T. D., Kober, H., Bliss-Moreau, E., & Barrett, L. F. (2012). The brain basis of emotion: A meta-analytic review. *Behavioral and Brain Sciences, 35*, 121–202.

List, C., & Pettit, P. (2011). *Group agency: The possibility, design, and status of corporate agents.* Oxford: Oxford University Press.

Lövheim, H. (2012). A new three-dimensional model for emotions and monoamine neurotransmitters. *Medical Hypotheses, 78*(2), 341–348.

Minsky, M. (2006). *The emotion machine and the society of mind*. New York: Simon & Schuster. ISBN:10:0743276647.

Misselhorn, C. (2018). Artificial morality: Concepts, issues and challenges. *Society, 55*(2), 161–169.

Misselhorn, C., Pompe, U., & Stapleton, M. (2013). Ethical considerations regarding the use of social robots in the fourth age. *GeroPsych., 26*, 121.

Oosthuizen, R. M. (2019a). Managing shame in organisations: Don't let shame become a self-destructive spiral. In C.-H. Mayer & E. Vanderheiden (Eds.), *The bright side of shame: Transforming and growing through practical applications in cultural contexts* (pp. 217–234). Cham: Springer Nature.

Oosthuizen, R. M. (2019b). Smart technology, artificial intelligence, robotics, and algorithms (STARA): Employees' perceptions and Well-being of future workplaces. In I. Potgieter,

N. Ferreira, & M. Coetzee (Eds.), *Fit for the future: Theory, research and dynamics of career wellbeing. Stream 1: Critical issues in understanding career wellbeing in the emerging digital workspaces of industry 4.0*. Cham: Springer Nature.

Pană, L. L. (2019). *Artificial ethics. In advanced methodologies and technologies in artificial intelligence, computer simulation, and human-computer interaction* (pp. 1–12). Hershey, PA: IGI Global.

Pereira, L. M., & Lopes, A. B. (2020). *Is it possible to program artificial emotions? A basis for Behaviours with moral connotation?* (In machine ethics (pp. 87–92)). Cham: Springer.

Picard, R. (1997). *Affective computing*. Cambridge, MA: MIT Press.

Ramachandran, V. (2002). *Encyclopedia of the human brain*. USA: Academic Press.

Rosales, J. H., Rodríguez, L. F., & Ramos, F. (2019). A general theoretical framework for the design of artificial emotion systems in autonomous agents. *Cognitive Systems Research, 58*, 324–341.

Searle, J. R. (1980). Minds, brains, and programs. *Behavioral and Brain Sciences, 3*, 417–458.

Sloman, A. (1962). *Knowing and understanding: Relations between meaning and truth, meaning and necessary truth, meaning and synthetic necessary truth* (Doctoral dissertation, University of Oxford).

Smith, C. A., & Ellsworth, P. C. (1985). Patterns of cognitive appraisal in emotion. *Journal of Personality and Social Psychology, 48*, 813–838.

Stubbings, C. (2017). *Bot.Me: A revolutionary partnership*. PriceWaterhouse coopers report. Retrieved January 24, 2019, from http://www.pwc.com/CISAI

Stubbings, C. (2018). *Workforce of the future: The competing forces shaping 2030*. PriceWaterhouse coopers report. Retrieved January 24, 2019, from http://www.pwc.com/people

Sznycer, D., Takemura, K., Delton, A. W., Sato, K., Robertson, T., Cosmides, L., & Tooby, J. (2012). Cross-cultural differences and similarities in proneness to shame: An adaptationist and ecological approach. *Evolutionary Psychology, 10*(2), 147470491201000213.

Talanov, M., Vallverdu, J., Distefano, S., Mazzara, M., & Delhibabu, R. (2015, March). Neuromodulating cognitive architecture: Towards biomimetic emotional AI. In *2015 IEEE 29th International Conference on Advanced Information Networking and Applications* (pp. 587–592). Piscataway, NJ: IEEE.

Tangney, J. P., Miller, R. S., Flicker, L., & Barrow, D. H. (1996). Are shame, guilt, and embarrassment distinct emotions? *Journal of Personality and Social Psychology, 70*, 1256–1269.

United Nations Department of Economic and Social Affairs. (2010). *World urbanization prospects: The 2011 revision*. Retrieved January 24, 2019, from http://www.un.org/en/development/desa/population/publications/pdf/urbanization/WUP2011_Report.pdf

Vallverdú, J. (2013). Ekman's paradox and a naturalistic strategy to escape from it. *IJSE, 4*(2), 7–13.

Vallverdú, J. (2014). *Artificial shame models for machines? Psychology of shame: New research*. New York: Nova.

Vernon, C. K. (2009). *A primer of affect psychology* (p. 30). Colchester, CT: The Tomkins Institute.

Vinciarelli, A., Esposito, A., André, E., Bonin, F., Chetouani, M., Cohn, J. F., et al. (2015). Open challenges in modelling, analysis and synthesis of human behaviour in human–human and human–machine interactions. *Cognitive Computation, 7*, 397–413.

Wong, Y., & Tsai, J. L. (2007). Cultural models of shame and guilt. In J. Tracy, R. Robins, & J. Tangney (Eds.), *Handbook of self-conscious emotions* (pp. 210–223). New York: Guilford Press.

World Economic Forum Study. (2018, September 18). *The Citizen*.

Rudolf M. Oosthuizen received a BA degree (Cum Laude) from the University of Pretoria in 1992 and obtained a BA (Honours) in Psychology at the same university in 1993. In 1999, he received an MA degree in Industrial and Personnel Psychology from the Potchefstroom University for Christian Higher Education. In 1999, he registered as Industrial Psychologist with the Health Professions Council of South Africa. In 2005, he completed a DLitt et Phil in Industrial and Organisational Psychology at the University of South Africa (UniSA). Currently Rudolf is an associate professor in the Department of Industrial and Organisational Psychology at the University of South Africa. Rudolf is the manager for the MComIOP programme, and he is responsible for the lecturing of honours subjects and the supervision of master's and doctoral students. He has presented conference papers at national and international conferences and published articles in accredited scientific journals. Rudolf's fields of interests are (1) career psychology, career development and management from an individual, group and organisational perspective in the twenty-first-century world of work; (2) positive psychology, with the focus on salutogenesis and well-being, sense of coherence, locus of control, self-efficacy, the hardy personality and learned resourcefulness; (3) employment relations and the improvement of the quality of employment relations in organisations and in society in general; and (4) the Fourth Industrial Revolution (smart technology, artificial intelligence, robotics and algorithms).

Chapter 26
Cybershaming Never Rests: Suggestions for Dealing with Cybershaming in a Digital Culture

Leona M. Ungerer

1 Introduction

The web, the Internet and mobile digital technologies are not merely technologies; they represent an arrangement of social relationships encompassing the use of technologies with diverse outcomes (Miller, 2020). In contrast to the role of the Internet in establishing new types of identity and social relationships, the role that online social relationships play in generating new types of violence and victimisation has not been investigated extensively (Martellozzo & Jane, 2017). The shaming of people through electronic means has increased rapidly since the introduction of web-based technology (Cheung, 2014). Social media occupies the largest portion of the Internet (Wang & Stefanone, as cited in Keipi, Näsi, Oksanen, & Räsänen, 2016) and serves as a tool for establishing relationships between Internet users (Keipi et al., 2016). Its role in cybershaming deserves attention. Existing literature comprehensively covers public shaming as a criminal sanction, but social policing, involving the informal shaming of perpetrators via the Internet, also requires further investigation (Cheung, 2014).

Cybershaming has featured in shaming literature since 2010 (Suhaimi, Mahmood, Yahya, Mohamed, & Zain, 2018). Various terms are used interchangeably to describe it, including Internet shaming, digital shaming, online shaming and public shaming. Cybershaming features strongly in "sousveillance", when the online community undertakes surveillance instead of the authorities (Mann, Nolan & Wellman, as cited in Suhaimi et al., 2018). Since it is an informal sanctioning of people who violate social norms and values, subjective decisions and not legal guidelines determine whether offences are punishable (Skoric, Wong, Chua, Yeo,

L. M. Ungerer (✉)
Department of Industrial and Organisational Psychology, University of South Africa (Unisa), Pretoria, South Africa
e-mail: ungerlm@unisa.ac.za

C.-H. Mayer et al. (eds.), *Shame 4.0*, https://doi.org/10.1007/978-3-030-59527-2_26

& Liew, 2010). Societies differ in terms of the type of violations they believe require cybershaming and the severity of punishment (Suhaimi et al., 2018). Because of its relation to social norms, cybershaming tends to be dynamic and dissimilar across cultures. When a societal norm loses its validity, its accompanying shame also vanishes (Jacquet, 2016). (See Vanderheiden on "The Terror of Being Judged"; see Mayer and Vanderheiden on "Naming and Shaming"; see Wilson and Lewandowska-Tomaszczyk and Vanderheiden and Mayer on "Some Theses on Shame and Shaming in the Age of Corona Pandemic").

Cybershaming differs from earlier types of shaming with regard to the speed at which information can be shared, the prevalence of anonymous shaming, the possibility of reaching vast audiences and the lasting accessibility of the shaming information on the web (Jacquet, 2016). It represents both a form of Internet vigilantism and online social control (Phillips & Miltner, as cited in Suhaimi et al., 2018; Wehmhoener, 2010). Cybershaming highlights violations of social norms, reminds people of the importance of complying with them, makes transgressors apologise and prevents further norm violations (Billingham & Parr, 2019). It contributes to the establishment of justice and equality because it empowers women (Kaplan, as cited in Suhaimi et al., 2018), gives marginalised groups a voice (Dewey, 2015) and serves as a remedy when suitable legal solutions are not available (Philips & Miltner, as cited in Suhaimi et al., 2018).

However, the disproportionate punishment meted out in cybershaming is of great concern (Billingham & Parr, 2019). Considering its subjective and random nature, perpetrators often are unfairly punished. Suhaimi et al. (2018) warn that cybershaming contributes to societal harassment and bullying. It may have far-reaching impacts on people's lives, including mental suffering, doxing (publishing people's personal details online to increase their humiliation and social condemnation) and losing one's job (Basak, Sural, Ganguly, & Ghosh, 2019; Billingham & Parr, 2019; Cheung, 2014). Moreover, search engines provide access to the shaming material years after their initial dissemination (Lavi, 2018), leaving a digital trail that may be to people's detriment when employers, for instance, do an online search on job applicants.

According to Trottier (2018), cybershaming has a stigmatising effect. Lavi (2018) further warns that it can have a disproportionate impact on a person's dignity (their "innate personhood, integrity and self-respect") (Cheung, 2014, p. 301). Shame may be a deadly weapon when applied by bullies and extremists. "Toxic shame" harms a person's self-concept (Fast, 2015). It criticises people for what they are and not for what they do. When shame is used to purposefully harm a person's self-concept, it becomes "weaponised shame". Bigotry, bullying, domestic violence, harassment at work, physical and sexual abuse and hate crimes represent weaponised shame (Fast, 2015).

"Online character assassination" has gradually taken root because of the abundance of social media sites where people freely share their opinions (Reynard, 2019). Offensive, derogatory and threatening online content is becoming a global concern, especially because legal and organisational measures have not yet been established to deal with malicious content. The challenge in establishing feasible codes of conduct and legal guidelines for digital speech, specifically on social media, is to find a balance between people's freedom to express their views and the protection of their rights to privacy and safety (Reynard, 2019).

Jacquet (2016) ascribes shamelessness on social media to the online disinhibition effect—when people's behaviour online differs considerably from that in reality (Scheff & Schorr, 2017). People express their views more arrogantly when they participate anonymously online. Suler (2004) distinguishes between toxic disinhibition evident in trolling and benign disinhibition when people share their private experiences anonymously. Research links anonymity to an increase in the numbers of participants and the breadth of views expressed in online discussions (McCluskey & Hmielowski, 2012). Anonymity plays an essential role in online aggression, rudeness, bad manners, trolling and cyberbullying (Bartlett, 2015; Zimmerman & Ybarra, 2016).

The online disinhibition effect further features when cybershaming gets out of hand and evolves into mob violence and harassment (Reynard, 2019). People's diminished ability to empathise with others and distinguish social cues results in toxic online disinhibition (Voggeser, Singh, & Göritz, 2018). Participants believe that they belong to a large, anonymous group and do not have to take responsibility for their actions (Suler, 2004). In essence, a person feels more at ease about taking part in online aggression because he or she is visually, emotionally and physically separated from his or her victim (Udris, as cited in Wachs, Wright, & Vazsonyi, 2019). Insufficient regulation and control in an online context contribute to the occurrence of virtual mobs.

Technology plays an essential role in both enabling and spreading cybershaming (Pendergrass, Payne, & Buretz, 2016). Owing to the increased pace of technological development and reduced data costs, access to instant communication is expected to increase during the Fourth Industrial Revolution (4IR). Digital and Internet technologies will support the establishment of new public circles for democratic engagement, but some scholars are concerned about "the dark side of Internet freedom" (Tsou, 2015). Nath (2018) foresees that online social media will become increasingly vigorous during the 4IR because people will be able to freely and swiftly express their views about contemporary events. The negative impacts of social media such as cyberbullying and hate speech should also increase during the 4IR because of advances in Internet facilities. Abusedra (2019) advises that technology involves choices. The power that the Internet affords people also means that they are responsible for protecting themselves in an online context (Ndashe, 2019). Scheff and Schorr (2017, p. 273) advise that "digital wisdom is digital survival" in terms of preventing cybershaming. As people become increasingly involved in digital environments, they should ensure that their online actions are not to their own detriment (Munn, 2016).

In the remainder of this chapter, digital culture, cybershaming and its effects, social justice and social norms will be discussed. Lastly, suggestions will be provided on how cybershaming can be prevented and dealt with as well as how it may serve as a resource.

2 Digital Culture

D'Arnault (2015) describes the term "digital culture" as an overarching concept reflecting the significant impact that technology and the Internet have on people's behaviour in a societal context, in other words, how they interact and communicate in online communities. Digital culture involves the relationship between humans and technology (D'Arnault, 2015) and refers to the "knowledge, beliefs, and practices of people interacting on digital networks that may recreate tangible-world cultures or create new strains of cultural thought and practice native to digital networks" (Poepsel, 2018, n.p.).

Poepsel (2018) identifies two schools of thought about the impact that expanding digital networks will have on fairly deep-rooted cultures in an offline context and the development of digital cultures. The first school of thought is that existing cultures, in essence, will resurface in digital format as people's lives increasingly play out in digital spheres. The second school of thought is that the prevailing digital culture is a distinct culture on its own. Poepsel (2018) posits that neither of these forms of digital culture will finally be established and that a combination of the two types of culture is more plausible. Some elements of existing culture will be adopted in an online context and some elements of digital culture will seem novel, even incomprehensible, because they were unheard of in the physical world.

For Deuze (2006), digital culture is a developing value system and expectations that are evident in the online activities of people who post news and information on online media platforms. Digital culture reflects individualisation, postnationalism and globalisation. Individualism refers to people's ability to publish their own thoughts online, as well as a social state where participants may express their views, mostly free from government control. Social media thrive on individualised expression—people take part as individuals on social media platforms such as Facebook and Twitter and increase their reach by doing so, potentially reaching all other participants on those platforms (Poepsel, 2018). In terms of cybershaming, participants may have a false sense of communicating privately with friends from behind their computer and mobile screens. They overlook the fact that their friends are able to forward content to members of other networks (Raicu, 2016).

Postnationalism relates to the trend that their country influences people's behaviour and values less strongly in an online context. Poepsel (2018) explains that the physical world and digital culture share a global perspective that adopts all types of cultural products if they are interesting, humorous and reflecting considerable talent. Some messages and cultural products have a viral quality and global appeal. The trend of postnationalism, however, does not imply that nationalism loses its impact in an offline context. In fact, nationalism is increasing globally because of postnationalism in digital interaction.

Deuze (2006) suggests that digital culture is produced through participation, remediation and bricolage. In respect of participation, anyone is able to provide inputs on online media, and participation is easy, enjoyable and affordable (Poepsel, 2018). In the print culture, the author is in control of the material that people read, but in the digital culture, readers are able to contribute material. For instance, any author can edit information on Wikipedia (Rousseau, 2011). In the digital era, any person can share a post online, draw attention to improper behaviour and shame others by doing so. This can, almost instantaneously, reach a global audience consisting of unfamiliar people with whom they may have little in common because their upbringing, viewpoints, ways of life, standards and behaviour are at odds with their own. To contain shaming through digital technologies is challenging because shaming spreads quickly and morphs into further forms of abusive behaviour such as slander, cyberbullying and harassment and because information is understood out of context (Munn, 2016).

Remediation means that old media take on new forms in digital spaces, for instance, newspapers that are published online. Their existing attractive characteristics are augmented with functionalities resulting from new types of information communication technologies and digital networking (Poepsel, 2018). Bricolage refers to doing something oneself and adding elements from a different context. Amateurs, for instance, combine existing content with new cultural inputs by means of inexpensive, useful tools, such as smartphones with high-quality cameras and video functionality. Consequently, digital culture democratises because amateurs are able to create media products that may be as popular as those of large, lucrative companies. Popular cultural products, however, are not necessarily accurate or of a high quality (Poepsel, 2018). The World Economic Forum (as cited in Acerbi, 2016) considers extensive digital misinformation as a particularly concerning contemporary global risk.

Poepsel (2018) points out various levels of culture in digital media ("media encoded in digital format, typically to be transmitted and consumed on electronic devices, such as computers and smartphones", Acerbi, 2016, n.p.). Poepsel (2018) suggests that his definition of digital culture as the "knowledge, beliefs and practices of a group of people" should be adapted to "the knowledge, beliefs and practices of a massive group of people at a certain time and place [define] common culture". Three levels of culture are evident in how culture is expressed in the mass media, namely, personal, group and common culture, corresponding to pop culture. These types of culture are based on shared knowledge from shared experiences. Common culture is influenced by the mass media and institutions such as governments, educational systems, churches and families. In a digital context, group culture refers to what was previously known as "subculture", involving the knowledge, beliefs and practices of a subset of people belonging to a larger culture. Group culture differs from common culture and revolves around religious beliefs, customs and ethnic norms. Individuals define their personal culture, namely, the knowledge, beliefs and practices that are particularly important to them. Current online communication and socialisation allow for "compartmentalisation" reflected in social bubbles in an online context (Pariser, as cited in Keipi et al., 2016). This trend represents an essential property of the Internet, allowing users to connect with others who have similar opinions, ideas or interests. A bubble not only embraces like-minded users, but it may also reinforce their existing perspectives (Keipi et al., 2016). Despite the potential diversity that social media offer by enabling diverse groups of people to share their views, information and news, online users with similar interests tend to group together, resulting in the formation of uniform clusters, termed echo chambers, where their beliefs, for instance, are accommodated or may even crystallise further (Choi, Chun, Oh, & Han, 2020).

A single common culture has not yet been established across global digital networks, and scholars disagree about whether a shared digital culture already exists or will ever be established. Poepsel (2018) describes the influences shaping digital culture as a "black box". Algorithms owned by large corporations often determine the information that people are exposed to, but it is evident that outcomes may be unpredictable when vast numbers of users receive this information. Although the shared knowledge at all three levels of culture determine the cultural impact that mass media messages have, people who identify with small-group cultures interpret events differently. People's responses to events appearing in the mass media are further influenced by their cultural norms or how they believe things should be. How divergent groups who are continuously confronted with other people's views in a free-for-all network society get along is a matter of concern. A disturbing fact of mob justice is that the group is not accountable to anyone and the shamed person has little opportunity to defend him- or herself. The sole aim is to punish by shaming (Moosa, 2014).

Twitter, in particular, lends itself to the spread of viral misinformation. Moreover, Twitter participants often demonstrate limited levels of critical thinking (Reynolds, 2019). For instance, PR executive Justine Sacco tweeted to her 170 followers moments before boarding a flight to South Africa: "Going to Africa. Hope I don't get AIDS. Just kidding. I'm white!" She boarded the plane and switched off her phone. During her flight, the hashtag #HasJustineLandedYet trended. Although her comment was meant as a joke about Westerners' ungrounded fears, it soon generated a shame mob and she lost her job. Cases of ordinary people who make careless statements or are quoted out of context are quite common because, on platforms such as Twitter, countless participants promptly add their views or comments to posts about someone's supposed misbehaviour (Reynolds, 2019).

A further issue is whether offline institutions should be involved in controlling the course of digital culture (Poepsel, 2018). Part of people's civic responsibility is deciding whether digital culture should be regulated and how such regulation could be achieved. This also depends on their cultural power (Poepsel, 2018).

Culture evolving from digitalisation differs in various ways from earlier types of culture such as print and broadcast culture (Varris, 2019). Digital technologies support collaborative, networked and participatory forms of culture. Social media, for instance, support immense levels of human connectedness and offer significant benefits such as shared power in protest actions (for instance, the "#metoo" movement when women objected to sexual harassment) (Baccarella, Wagner, Kietzmann, & McCarthy, 2018). However, social media hold considerable risks at individual, community, company and societal level (Baccarella et al., 2018). Kietzmann, Hermkens, McCarthy, and Silvestre (2011) developed a framework for the main social media functionalities (conversations, sharing, presence, relationships, reputation, groups and identity) that distinguishes various types of participation such as connecting and engaging with other users and monitoring them. Each functional block provides insight in the possible dark side of social media (Baccarella et al. (2018). Conversations, for instance, refer to the degree to which users communicate with others through a social media platform by liking or replying to their comments and sending direct messages. Engagement during conversations can become offensive. The functionality of sharing refers to the degree to which users swap, disseminate and obtain content, for instance, videos on YouTube. Shared content may be inappropriate and can infringe on others' intellectual property rights.

Since digital technologies present information in numerical code, digital material can be modified and compressed (Miller, 2011). Because digital media are networked and interactive, the trend of user-generated content diminishes the distinction between senders and receivers of media content (Varris, 2019). Where people previously merely consumed media, they now are able to produce media (Miller, 2020). Tsou (2015, p. 180) warns that prosumers who "consume, produce, share and disseminate information in participatory and collaborative ways" may also join forces for harmful purposes such as cybershaming.

Digital media are hypertextual. In other words, any text contains links to other texts or nuggets of content. Online content is organised primarily by hyperlinking. Digital objects are often generated by means of automated processes from databases. These automated, algorithmic processes support the personalisation of content and social media feeds, online recommendation systems and targeted online advertising (Miller, 2011). Since digital material can be copied, distributed and adapted easily, digital cultural products are continuously transformed. They are works in progress instead of complete products (Miller, 2011). Digital culture is a "remix culture" in which digital participants systematically adapt a source (including images) to assemble an account of daily events (Manovich, as cited in Mielczarek, 2018). Digital-culture participants create their own versions of what happened through, for instance, Internet memes (Lessig, as cited in Mielczarek, 2018).

A photo and a short video of an altercation between a University of California–Davis police officer and a number of students protesting against tuition price increases went viral during the 2011 Occupy Wall Street movement (Mielczarek, 2018). In what became known as the "pepper-spraying cop" incident in the media, Lt. John Pike pepper-sprayed students who were sitting on a sidewalk. The students buried their heads in their arms because the spray was aimed at their eyes. On social media, it was regarded as a power struggle. The photo had severe repercussions for the university and the officer. Several investigations into the possible excessive use of force were conducted, and Officer Pike's service was terminated. During the subsequent online upheaval, Internet users joined forces to ridicule Officer Pike and focus attention on his abuse of power. They transformed the photo into an Internet meme which is described by Wiggins and Bowers (2015) as "a piece of cultural knowledge that replicates and mutates online through remixing". The resulting memes presented Pike randomly aiming at anything in his way, including children, kittens and even the US Constitution (Mielczarek, 2018) (see also Mayer and Vanderheiden on "Naming and Shaming").

According to Mielczarek (2018), the meme meant constant shaming for Officer Pike. Mielczarek terms it "collective meme bullying" (2018, p. 78). The cyberbullying that Pike endured because of the meme amounted to mob law. The Yolo County district attorney found no grounds for criminal charges. Although the meme imitated the process of social justice, it had no legal basis. It reflected only large-scale shaming, protesting and bullying (Mielczarek, 2018).

Further, it is difficult to distinguish between interpersonal and mass communication in a networked society (Poepsel, 2018). In the same way that society forms messages in the mass media and is partly formed by these messages, culture forms messages in mass media and is partly formed by them. Changes in media and information as well as communication technology may lead to changes in how people produce culture (Poepsel, 2018). Poepsel highlights two features of the relationship between digital and real-world cultures. On the one hand, increasing interaction on digital networks influences traditional cultures, and on the other hand, existing cultural traditions influence the development of digital culture. Although people's physical-world norms and ethics influence their perceptions of appropriate behaviour and values in digital networks, appropriate behaviour in an online context and in the physical world are sometimes at odds. For instance, with cybershaming, social norms are enforced in an inhuman and humiliating way.

3 Cybershaming

Hamilton (2016, p. 9) defines cybershaming as "the act of distributing information, be it a message or a photo or video, about a particular target online with the intent to cause reputation damage". As explained earlier, it involves shaming through electronic media (Levy et al., 2012). Klonick (2016) draws a distinction between cybershaming on the one hand and cyberbullying and cyberharassment on the other. She points out that the three trends all involve continuous taunting of a target over time. Cybershaming differs from cyberbullying and cyberharassment in the sense that people are shamed because they are perceived to have violated a social norm. Three characteristics distinguish cybershaming from similar phenomena. It involves a specific target or victim who has committed an action that is regarded as wrong and deserving of societal disapproval (Basak et al., 2019). It focuses the audience's attention on the fact that someone's viewpoint, action or intention does not conform to group norms. Shamers believe that they are morally superior (Klonick, 2016). Cybershaming evolves into cyberbullying and cyberharassment when shamers lose focus of social norm enforcement (Klonick, 2016).

Cybershaming and cyberbullying both involve sharing harmful content via social media, but they are not the same. Cyberbullying is meant to make fun of, humiliate or scare someone. When cybershaming is meant to bully someone, it is often out of prejudice (Hamilton, 2016). Fast (2015) suggests that, as with traditional bullying, an imbalance in power underlies cyberbullying although cyberbullies' power may also emanate from their digital literacy. But some scholars suggest that cyberbullying does not require extensive technical expertise and that anonymity contributes far more to a power imbalance in cyberbullying (Vandebosch &Van Cleemput, as cited in Fast, 2015).

A degree of digital literacy is also required in cybershaming. The media report daily about instances of cybershaming such as revenge porn, e-mail hacks, sexting scandals and webcam hijackings (Scheff & Schorr, 2017). Hate sites with content of a racist, sexist or homophobic nature are also found. In online identity theft, a person logs on to social media sites pretending to be someone else and posts content that harms another person. Some shaming sites contain explicit photos (for instance, revenge porn) or private details about people's ex-spouses or ex-partners (Hamilton, 2016). Further trends in cybershaming involve fat shaming, slut shaming, ugly polls, mean memes, elder shaming, shaming of the helpless, body shaming, teacher shaming, baby bashing and parent shaming (Scheff & Schorr, 2017).

In terms of the effects of cybershaming, the painful experience can ruin people's mental health (Borba, as cited in Scheff & Schorr, 2017). Some victims commit suicide, while others lose their livelihood (Scheff & Schorr, 2017). Cybershaming harms victims' identity and reputation, and, besides, they have no way of knowing who else is aware of their embarrassment. It causes them to feel that their world is falling apart. They may also ask themselves whether they deserve it because they did something wrong. People of all ages experience these negative effects. They are traumatised and would like to talk to someone who had the same experience. Victims feel trapped in a never-ending painful situation. Cybershaming affects victims' sense of security (Borba, as cited in Scheff & Schorr, 2017), and they require assistance before they realise that they are not to blame. Victims go through various stages of grief, namely, denial, anger, bargaining and depression, before they finally accept the situation (Scheff & Schorr, 2017).

3.1 *The Virtues and Vices of Cybershaming*

Billingham and Parr (2019) argue that although cybershaming has some merit, it is seldom warranted because of its failings. The next section elaborates on some its virtues.

3.1.1 The Virtues of Cybershaming

Cybershaming offers numerous benefits. For one, the responsibility for law enforcement is more evenly distributed among stakeholders. It makes offensive behaviour public, condemns misbehaviour, increases the possibility that neglect of duty such as poor service delivery, receives attention and persuades people to refrain from unacceptable behaviour. Cybershaming therefore helps to uphold norms and maintain order.

Cybershaming provides consumers with information to evaluate merchants' reputation and prevents unsatisfactory deals and services (Lavi, 2018). It may serve as a means to ensure justice and equality, for instance, when powerful people express mean or ill-informed views (Raicu, 2016). Since people get a fair opportunity to share their views, cybershaming supports democracy and a participatory culture (Lavi, 2018).

In spite of the above, cybershaming also has a dark side and can cause severe harm.

3.1.2 The Vices of Cybershaming

Shamers tend to be biased because they shame others based on the values that are important to them and not on universal norms (Lavi, 2018). Cybershaming harms a person's dignity when a vast number of online participants are aware of it. This may result in disproportionate punishment if a victim is ostracised. It may impact on society in general if people cease to act spontaneously in public for fear of being shamed.

There aren't any guidelines to guide the process when ordinary people instigate cybershaming without consulting the victim beforehand. Because they are unaware of the original context, people often interpret an online picture or video inaccurately and share erroneous information (Lavi, 2018). As a result, innocent people are shamed. Because of the psychological effects, victims may rebel against norms and even become violent. As shaming becomes increasingly common, it may lose its power to enforce norms (Lavi, 2018).

4 Social Justice

Cybershaming is justified by the belief that the targeted person or firm deserves public punishment for unethical or socially unacceptable behaviour (Hamilton, 2016). The opposite view is that cybershaming is unethical because the persons who dispense justice do not foresee the consequences of their shaming behaviour (Raicu, 2016). Considering the volatile nature of the Internet, cybershaming may have unforeseen consequences for both shamer and victim. Once someone has posted content online, he or she loses control over the course it takes and the effects it will have (Hamilton, 2016). Cybershaming that goes viral can ruin a person both on- and offline forever. An essential requirement is that punishment should be commensurate with the transgression (Raicu, 2016).

4.1 The Role of Social Norms in Cybershaming

Cybershaming enforces social norms. A social norm involves a rule without any official force (for instance, being declared by government), a directive that people are not legally required to comply with (Klonick, 2016). When norms are well-established, societal members accept them as mandatory, internalise and comply with them and experience guilt or shame when they violate them. When internal sanctions do not support compliance over extended periods of time, external sanctions may be necessary (Billingham & Parr, 2019).

As an external sanction, cybershaming fulfils a number of constructive roles in enforcing social norms, particularly to make offenders aware that they have violated one. Cybershaming also fulfils a reparative role. When offenders realise that their behaviour was unacceptable, they show regret, apologise, atone for their behaviour and promise future compliance with the norm. As a deterrent, cybershaming reduces future norm violations. People who have suffered because of a norm violation experience a sense of solidarity when others criticise the offender. The public nature of cybershaming supports the various roles it fulfils (Jacquet, 2016). When misbehaviour is exposed publicly and people are able to comment on it, offenders regret their behaviour and repent. Ultimately, cybershaming is a way for people to demonstrate that they support valuable social norms, and enhances collective commitment to norms and their underlying values (Billingham & Parr, 2019).

Billingham and Parr (2019) warn that although cybershaming is potentially a constructive practice, it is, at the same time, dangerous. Since cybershaming plays an essential role in enforcing social norms, it would not be wise to prohibit it. A moral framework or guidelines that establish under which conditions and in what forms it is appropriate are necessary to regulate it. Two principles would be important in such a framework: proportionality and accountability. Cybershaming is justified only if it is fair or proportionate—its negative effects should not overshadow its positive effects. Positive consequences entail the previously mentioned consequences such as remorse among offenders and discouraging future norm violations. Negative consequences include psychological harm to those being shamed, damage to their reputation and the loss of a job.

Determining the proportionality of cybershaming is a complex task considering the various contextual factors. Billingham and Parr (2019) distinguish between narrow and wide proportionality. Cybershaming aimed at enforcing a social norm is proportionate only if the particular norm is morally authoritative (a norm that people have a duty to comply with). If a particular social norm is not morally authoritative, there is no use in enforcing it, suggesting that cybershaming is often disproportionate.

The context, whether online or offline, determines whether norms are morally authoritative. When cybershaming is used to shame a person's offline behaviour, the violated norm has to be morally authoritative in the particular offline context and should not be a norm that guides online behaviour (Billingham & Parr, 2019). Cybershaming is narrowly proportionate when people mete out punishment to norm violators who they would probably not excuse for violating the norm (McMahan, as cited in Billingham & Parr, 2019). A person is liable only if he or she deserves to be blamed for violating a norm.

Former victims often complain that it seemed if as if the world was against them and that they had to endure severe shame, degradation and anguish (Ronson, as cited in Billingham & Parr, 2019). Cybershaming would not be narrowly proportionate considering these harsh effects. Its potential to be reintegrative also determines whether it is narrowly proportionate. Cybershaming could be healthy if the transgressor is readmitted to the community and not permanently stigmatised (Billingham & Parr, 2019). Social media, however, does not allow for reintegrative shaming because of limited space for explanations. Besides, the communication used on them is not suitable for fine nuances. Abuse and threats, which do not support reintegration, are common (Billingham & Parr, 2019). Participants make fun of offenders' explanations and apologies or overlook them in the surge of condemnation. Barriers to reintegration have to be removed for cybershaming to become more warranted (Billingham & Parr, 2019).

Wide proportionality weighs up the positive effects of the sanctions imposed in cybershaming against the negative effects on people who were not involved, such as the norm violator's family, friends and employer. When the positive consequences resulting from an instance of cybershaming surpass the negative effects on parties who are not guilty, cybershaming may be justifiable, considering wide proportionality (Billingham & Parr, 2019). The systemic effects of cybershaming also feature in determining its wide proportionality. Certain instances may seem proportionate, but the continual nature of cybershaming may have an unnerving effect on observers. People may avoid online interaction or posting material that could be perceived as contentious because they fear public shaming. Trends such as these would reduce the interaction in online contexts to the detriment of everyone involved. It appears that current instances of cybershaming often are disproportionate, considering both narrow and wide proportionality (Billingham & Parr, 2019).

New social norms for guiding online activity are necessary to encourage people not to hastily conclude that others are guilty, to curb criticism, not to mete out disproportionate punishment and to pardon past offences so that people can take up their place in an online community again. The fact that some negative consequences are constantly disproportionate should also be considered and prohibited through legislation, for instance, the harm caused to themselves and others when norm violators lose their jobs. New social norms are required regarding the accountability of people who cybershame others. Those who enforce norms should be able to defend their behaviour, explain why their target deserves criticism and prove that an important social norm was violated. Preventing or limiting anonymity in an online context may further support accountability during online participation. When shaming takes place anonymously, it limits the ability of those who are shamed to apply their right of reply because they cannot confront shamers personally.

Finally, Billingham and Parr (2019) highlight the issue of collective harm. Large, diverse groups of participants who take part in cybershaming often merely share or re-tweet negative comments. The person being shamed experience the full impact of the large group's actions, but each individual shamer may only play a small part in the victim's experience. Considering the dispersed nature of cybershaming, it is impossible to hold a particular participant accountable for an episode of shaming (Billingham & Parr, 2019). If it is assumed that people cannot be held accountable for the effects of cybershaming, it causes concern about whether cybershaming is ever warranted. Collective harm is an important concern in terms of cybershaming because it is an inherent feature that cannot be changed easily through legislation or suitable social norms (Billingham & Parr, 2019).

5 Dealing with Cybershaming

This section provides suggestions on how to avoid falling victim to cybershaming and how shame may serve as a resource.

5.1 Digital Discretion

In a digital world, anyone may be a victim of cybershaming. Some people, for instance, have been shamed for trivial "transgressions" such as being poor tippers (Scheff & Schorr, 2017). Some people do not have an online presence or completely avoid social media to limit the risk of becoming a victim of cybershaming. Scheff and Schorr (2017), however, advise that suitable digital participation is a requirement in modern society, for instance, when people apply for employment or admission to university. Therefore, it is vital for people to cultivate a suitable online persona instead of avoiding digital media altogether.

Scheff and Schorr (2017) present a few strategies for ensuring digital discretion that may protect people from cybershaming. In respect of online sharing, it is advisable that people avoid oversharing, considering that it is not essential that they document their whole life online. It further is advisable that people guard against sharing inappropriate material. People should consider how they would feel if the content went viral and whether the content truly reflects them, that is, the persons sharing the content. Would it cause embarrassment if the people who respect them observe them posting the content (Weber-Van Gundy, as cited in Weiner, 2019)? The lack of guaranteed privacy in cyberspace highlights the importance of not sharing inappropriate material (Scheff & Schorr, 2017).

To avoid sharing content with the wrong people, it is advisable that people review the settings on their social media accounts and confirm that their contacts are trusted friends. Even high privacy settings do not guarantee protection against trolls (who post negative online comments to provoke arguments for their own enjoyment). It is important to think before you post and not to share content hastily. Aspects to consider when pausing before posting are whether the content may be embarrassing in the future and amounts to oversharing. Further, it is important to obtain people's permission before using their photos on social media (Scheff & Schorr, 2017).

Weber-Van Gundy (as cited in Weiner, 2019) explains that people post controversial comments online for a number of psychological reasons such as expressing strong emotions or convincing someone of their opinion. Fortunately, people are able to learn how to control these responses (Weber-Van Gundy, as cited in Weiner, 2019). A further guideline to ensure digital discretion is to share content with dignity. For instance, do not post content that presents others in compromising situations such as when they make fools of themselves. It is important to avoid offensive language. According to Scheff and Schorr (2017), people constantly build a "virtual résumé" online, and therefore it is advisable not to share negative content continually or to vent your indignation on social media. Any content that a person shares online can become "public and permanent" (Guerry, as cited in Scheff & Schorr, 2017).

5.2 Shame as a Resource

Shame is a strong, distressing and all-encompassing emotion, and people do not have to be ashamed of it because it may also be benevolent (Maija, 2016). Shame derives from people's basic need to be accepted and appreciated in society, a community or a group they belong to. Trends such as cybershaming make people unreasonably fearful of criticism and can result in unexpected aggression, restlessness and depression. Avoiding others may result in loneliness. According to Wong (2019), such responses do not help victims to deal with shame.

Wong (as cited in Wong, 2019) proposes a positive psychological perspective that views shame as a normal experience and suggests that people's most severe experiences of pain offer the most potential for growth (see Wang and Hwang in this book). Maija (2016), for instance, advises that people should embrace shame and turn it into a resource to generate increased creativity. Shameful situations can occur throughout people's lives, and, unfortunately, it is impossible to hide from shame. This especially applies to cybershaming, because anyone may become a victim of cybershaming in a digital world (Scheff & Schorr, 2017).

Maija (2016) suggests a number of ways in which people can deal with shame so that it does not block their creativity, namely, recognising and accepting the experience of shame, being critical, talking about the experiences of shame and reconnecting with compassion. People should be aware of their own experiences and the vulnerabilities in them that trigger their shame. Mayer and Vanderheiden (2019) advise that people have to become aware of the types of individual and sociocultural shame they are susceptible to and deal with them so that they become a health resource. When people consciously acknowledge unfounded emotions such as desperation, worthlessness and humiliation resulting from shame, they gain an understanding of their patterns and signals of shame and related anguish. It enables them to deal with shame (Maija, 2016). Acceptance also is an essential step in overcoming cybershaming. Since victims may never get justice, their healing depends on their acceptance of what happened to them. By accepting it, they learn to cope with the shaming and may even thrive (Scheff & Schorr, 2017).

Maija (2016) advises that people should be critical of their reactors to shame and their interpretation of it. It further is advisable to be critical of the people or media who brought about the shame in them. Online perpetrators' comments typically are reactive and should not be taken too seriously (Weber-Van Gundy, as cited in Weiner, 2019). Perpetrators' frustration may emanate from their own insecurity or bias. A perpetrator's opinion cannot change who a victim intrinsically is (Weber-Van Gundy, as cited in Weiner, 2019). People should also reconsider their own views and self-evaluation to determine whether the shaming events ascribe meaning to them as people or whether they can distance them from these events.

When people talk about shame and its related feelings, they vent their emotions and establish connections defeating and transforming shame (Brown, as cited in Mayer & Vanderheiden, 2019). In sharing experiences of shame with a trusted person, the events become more obvious, real and understandable, enabling a person to gain rational insight into misguided emotions and interpretations (Maija, 2016). Compassion is particularly suited to addressing shame, self-criticism, possible feelings of isolation and some of the fears experienced during the shaming process. Shame resilience requires that people admit their vulnerability, critically consider their experiences and establish what Brown (2006) terms "mutually empathic relationships". The main feature of shame resilience is self-awareness. It therefore is necessary to learn to ignore the triggers of shame and replace negative emotions with compassion and re-establishing human relationships. It further is important to speak up when they notice instances of cybershaming and online bullying. Showing kindness to others also benefits yourself (Scheff & Schorr, 2017). Community service and volunteering may, for instance, support the recovery of cybershaming victims.

Scheff and Schorr (2017) advise victims to allow themselves to be angry because anger is acceptable and normal. They can use the energy generated by their anger to garner strength for fighting back, whether this involves confronting the perpetrator (s), obtaining legal assistance or gaining expert assistance to repair the damage to their online reputation. It may be healing to find an element of humour in the shameful situation, if possible (Holly, as cited in Scheff & Schorr, 2017). When victims laugh, they may realise that although they are suffering at the moment, they are also capable of experiencing other emotional states than the current one. Victims of cybershaming could also gain courage by learning from the experiences of other people who managed to get their lives back on track after cybershaming. It is important to regain trust and participate on social media again (Scheff & Schorr, 2017).

All in all, it is important that victims follow a restorative process after a shaming experience. Shame resilience involves adapting a person's self-perception to rebuild his or her self-esteem and address his or her mental and emotional issues (Bartley, n.d.). Gilbert (2019) distinguishes between external and internal shame. External same refers to peoples' thoughts about others' views and opinions of them, whereas internal shame centres on self-appraisal and self-criticism. These two types of shame require different types of intervention. Mindfulness and reframing may be suitable for addressing both types of shame, but it may also be necessary to question a toxic culture in which bias and stigmatisation result in external shame. An increased awareness of the disproportionateness of cybershaming and possible new social norms would assist in this regard.

6 Conclusion

The web, the Internet and mobile digital technologies allow new types of social relationships with diverse outcomes. A degree of duality was evident in this chapter because some of the mentioned technologies and processes may be used in either a constructive or a destructive manner. The Internet, for instance, supports the establishment of new types of social relationships, but these relationships may also generate new types of disparagement and victimisation. Social media may be used in both a constructive and a destructive manner. Each of the functionalities that enable various types of participation on them can also support destructive behaviour, for instance, when online participation becomes derogative.

Cybershaming plays a constructive role by upholding community norms and maintaining order. Shaming, however, should be applied in moderation to achieve optimum results. For cybershaming to have a reintegrative effect, transgressors should be welcomed back into the online community and should not be permanently stigmatised. Because cybershaming is unpredictable, is often indiscriminately applied and leaves a near-permanent digital trail, it causes considerable harm. It further appears that cybershaming is often disproportionate in terms of the offence it is supposed to punish. Trends such as these highlight its destructive impact.

People have a choice in how they live in a digital world. Increased societal awareness of the possible harmful effects of cybershaming may result in new social norms to guide it. People further are responsible for protecting themselves in an online context by, for instance, posting and sharing content sensibly and refraining from sharing content that may humiliate or harm. When they notice harmful or derogatory content, they should report it to the Internet service provider or the particular social media platform. It has been suggested that technology is amoral and humans therefore determine whether it is applied in a destructive of constructive manner. Another view is that the adoption of a particular technology will result in social change according to embedded values, virtues and vices. Unfortunately, there is no concrete evidence to prove that cybershaming prevents unacceptable actions. Research on the effectiveness of cybershaming in enforcing social norms as well as on the interplay between the characteristics of technology and humans to determine the constructive or destructive application of technology is required.

References

Abusedra, A. (2019). *Law must be adapted for the fourth industrial Revolution*. Retrieved from https://thehill.com/opinion/technology/475937-law-must-be-adapted-for-the-fourth-industrial-revolution.

Acerbi, A. (2016). A cultural evolution approach to digital media. *Frontiers in Human Neuroscience, 10*, 636. Retrieved from https://www.frontiersin.org/articles/10.3389/fnhum.2016.00636/full.

Baccarella, C. V., Wagner, T. F., Kietzmann, J. H., & McCarthy, I. P. (2018). Social media? It's serious! Understanding the dark side of social media. *European Management Journal, 36*(4), 431–438.

Bartlett, C. P. (2015). Anonymously hurting others online: The effect of anonymity on cyberbullying frequency. *Psychology of Popular Media Culture, 4*(2), 70–79.

Bartley (n.d.) Reversing shame.

Basak, R., Sural, S., Ganguly, N., & Ghosh, S. K. (2019). Online public shaming on twitter: Detection, analysis, and mitigation. *IEEE Transactions on Computational Social Systems, 6*(2), 208–220.

Billingham, P., & Parr, T. (2019). Online public shaming: Virtues and vices. *Journal of Social Philosophy, 0*(0), 1–20.

Brown, B. (2006). Shame resilience theory: A grounded theory study on women and shame: Families in society. *The Journal of Contemporary Social Services, 87*(1), 43–52.

Cheung, A. S. (2014). Revisiting privacy and dignity: Online shaming in the global e-village. *Laws, 3*(2), 301–326.

Choi, D., Chun, S., Oh, H., & Han, J. (2020). Rumor propagation is amplified by echo chambers in social media. *Scientific Reports, 10*(1), 1–10.

D'Arnault, C. (2015). *What is digital culture?* Retrieved from https://digitalculturist.com/what-is-digital-culture-5cbe91bfad1b.

Deuze, M. (2006). Participation, remediation, bricolage: Considering principal components of a digital culture. *The Information Society, 22*(2), 63–75.

Dewey, C. (2015, September 16). Can online shaming shut down the Internet's most skin-crawly creeps? Retrieved from https://www.washingtonpost.com/news/the-intersect/wp/2015/09/16/can-online-shaming-shut-down-the-internets-most-skin-crawly-creeps/.

Fast, J. (2015). *Beyond bullying: Breaking the cycle of shame, bullying, and violence*. Oxford: Oxford University Press.

Gilbert, P. (2019). Distinguishing shame, humiliation and guilt: An evolutionary functional analysis and compassion-focused interventions. In C.-H. Mayer & E. Vanderheiden (Eds.), *The bright side of shame: Transforming and growing through practical applications in cultural contexts* (pp. 413–432). Cham: Springer International.

Hamilton, T. B. (2016). *Combatting internet shaming*. New York: Rosen Publishing.

Jacquet, J. (2016). *Is shame necessary? New uses for an old tool*. New York: Pantheon Books.

Keipi, T., Näsi, M., Oksanen, A., & Räsänen, P. (2016). *Online hate and harmful content: Cross-national perspectives*. New York: Taylor & Francis.

Kietzmann, J. H., Hermkens, K., McCarthy, I. P., & Silvestre, B. S. (2011). Social media? Get serious! Understanding the functional building blocks of social media. *Business Horizons, 54* (3), 241–251.

Klonick, K. (2016). Re-shaming the debate: Social norms, shame, and regulation in an internet age. *Maryland Law Review, 75*, 1029–1065.

Lavi, M. (2018). The good, the bad, and the ugly behavior. *Cardozo L. Rev., 40*, 2597–2682.

Levy, N. Cortesi, S., Gasser, U., Crowley, E., Beaton, M., Casey, J., & Nolan, C. (2012). *Bullying in a networked era: A literature review*. Retrieved from http://ssrn.com/abstract=2146877.

Maija, A. (2016). *How to turn shame to a resource of becoming more creative*. Retrieved from https://medium.com/indian-thoughts/how-to-turn-shame-as-to-a-resource-of-becoming-more-creative-fbcef50a37f8.

Martellozzo, E. Jane, E.A. (2017). Introduction: Victims of cybercrime on the small 'i' internet. In Martellozzo, E., E. A. Jane . *Cybercrime and its victims* (pp. 1–23). New York Taylor and Francis.

Mayer, C.-H., & Vanderheiden, E. (2019). Calling on shame! An introduction to transforming shame. In C.-H. Mayer & E. Vanderheiden (Eds.), *The bright side of shame: Transforming and growing through practical applications in cultural contexts* (pp. xix–xxxiii). Springer International: Cham.

McCluskey, M., & Hmielowski, J. (2012). Opinion expression during social conflict: Comparing online reader comments and letters to the editor. *Journalism, 13*(3), 303–319.

Mielczarek, N. (2018). The "pepper-spraying cop" icon and its internet memes: Social justice and public shaming through rhetorical transformation in digital culture. *Visual Communication Quarterly, 25*(2), 67–81.

Miller, V. (2011). *Understanding digital culture*. London: SAGE.

Miller, V. (2020). *Understanding digital culture* (2nd ed.). London: SAGE.

Moosa, T. (2014). *The dangers of public shaming, Mob justice and scolding on the internet*. Retrieved from http://www.newstatesman.com/voices/2014/01/dangers-public-shaming-mob-justice-and-scolding-internet.

Munn, N. (2016). *Local action, global shame. Contemporary issues in applied and professional ethics (research in ethical issues in organizations, vol. 15)*. Bingley: Emerald Group Publishing Limited.

Nath, S. S. (2018). *The fourth industrial revolution and its impact*. Retrieved from https://www.linkedin.com/pulse/impact-fourth-industrial-revolution-swikriti-sheela-nath/.

Ndashe, N. (2019). *The power of social media and influence in today's 4th industrial Revolution*. Retrieved from https://www.bizcommunity.com/Article/196/669/192629.html.

Pendergrass, W. S., Payne, C. A., & Buretz, G. R. (2016). Cybershaming: The shallowing hypothesis in action. *Issues in Information Systems, 17*(2), 65–75.

Poepsel, M. (2018). *Media, society, culture and you: An introductory mass communication text*. Rebus Publishing. Retrieved from https://press.rebus.community/mscy/.

Raicu, I. (2016). *On the ethics of online shaming*. Retrieved from https://www.abc.net.au/religion/on-the-ethics-of-online-shaming/10097280.

Reynard, L. J. (2019). Troll farm: Anonymity as a weapon for online character assassination. In I. E. Chiluwa & S. A. Samoilenko (Eds.), *Advances in media, entertainment, and the arts (AMEA) book series. Handbook of research on deception, fake news, and misinformation online* (pp. 392–419). Hershey, PA: Information Science Reference/IGI Global. https://doi.org/10.4018/978-1-5225-8535-0.ch021.

Reynolds, G. H. (2019). *The social media upheaval (encounter intelligence)*. Encounter Books.

Rousseau, G. (2011). Technology: Together, bit by bit. *Nature, 473*(7345), 28–29.

Scheff, S., & Schorr, M. (2017). *Shame nation: The global epidemic of online hate*. Naperville: Sourcebooks.

Skoric, M. M., Wong, K. H., Chua, J. P. E., Yeo, P. J., & Liew, M. A. (2010). Online shaming in the Asian context: Community empowerment or civic vigilantism? *Surveillance & Society, 8*(2), 181–199.

Suhaimi, N. S., Mahmood, A., Yahya, N. A., Mohamed, F., & Zain, H. N. M. H. (2018). The efficacy of online shaming as a modality for social control: A survey amongst UiTM law students. *International Journal of Academic Research in Business and Social Sciences, 8*(12), 903–911.

Suler, J. (2004). The online disinhibition effect. *Cyberpsychology & Behavior, 7*(3), 321–326.

Trottier, D. (2018). Coming to terms with shame: Exploring mediated visibility against transgressions. *Surveillance and Society, 16*(2), 170–182.

Tsou, Y. Z. (2015). *Digital natives in the name of a cause. From "flash mob" to "human flesh Search"*. Retrieved from https://mediarep.org/bitstream/handle/doc/3027/Digital_Activism_179-195_Tsou_Human_Flesh_Search.pdf?sequence=1.

Varris, P. (2019). *Digital culture*. Retrieved from https://www.diggitmagazine.com/wiki/digital-culture.

Voggeser, B. J., Singh, R. K., & Göritz, A. S. (2018). Self-control in online discussions: Disinhibited online behavior as a failure to recognize social cues. *Frontiers in Psychology, 8*, 2372.

Wachs, S., Wright, M. F., & Vazsonyi, A. T. (2019). Understanding the overlap between cyberbullying and cyberhate perpetration: Moderating effects of toxic online disinhibition. *Criminal Behaviour and Mental Health, 29*(3), 179–188.

Wehmhoener, K. A. (2010). *Social norm or social harm: An exploratory study of internet vigilantism*. (Master), Iowa State University, Ames, Iowa. Retrieved from http://lib.dr.iastate.edu/cgi/viewcontent.cgi?article=2561&context=etd.

Weiner, Y. (2019). *"5 things we can each do to make social media and the internet a kinder and more tolerant place" with Rebecca Weber-Van Gundy*. Retrieved from https://thriveglobal.com/stories/5-things-we-can-each-do-to-make-social-media-and-the-internet-a-kinder-and-more-tolerant-place-with-rebecca-weber-van-gundy/.

Wiggins, B., & Bowers, G. B. (2015). Memes as genre: A structurational analysis of the memescape. *New Media & Society, 17*(11), 1886–1906.

Wong, P. T. P. (2019). Foreword: From shame to wholeness: An existential positive psychology perspect. In C. H. Mayer & E. Vanderheiden (Eds.), *The bright side of shame: Transforming and growing through practical applications in cultural contexts* (pp. v–ix). Springer International: Cham.

Zimmerman, A. G., & Ybarra, G. J. (2016). Online aggression: The influences of anonymity and social modelling. *Psychology of Popular Media Culture, 5*(2), 181–193.

Leona Ungerer (PhD) is an associate professor in the Department of Industrial and Organisational Psychology at the University of South Africa. Her areas of interest are consumer psychology and technology-mediated teaching and learning.

Chapter 27
Technologies of Shame: Agency, Identity, and Visibility

Michael Uebel

1 Introduction

To understand shame is to understand its relationship to technology. Indeed, we may say, with little qualification or few caveats, that a critique of shame is a critique of technology. While this chapter cannot claim to do more than lay out a sketch of this relationship or a tracing of this critique, it will point toward the contention that there is no instance of shame other than that produced in the name of technology. I have in mind, given the limits of this chapter, one crucial dimension of the shame experience—its identity with visibility. Because shame is identical with visibility, the technologies that prop up shame, which make it recognizable as a phenomenological condition of being, have centrally to do with the dialectic of visibility and invisibility. My wider claim is that we live in an evolving shame culture, that the Fourth IR has contributed to the conditioning such a culture, in a way that is broadly consistent with Norbert Elias's (1939/2000) famous demonstration that modernity—and, here, we must add contemporaneity—is marked above all by a civilizing process, begun in the late Middle Ages, characterized not only by Weberian rationalization but by "the peculiar molding of the drive economy that we call shame" (p. 292). The progress of personality and social norms correlates with a veritable explosion of shame and shaming: this thesis, as Elias frames it, can be related to some of the other grand themes of the emerging Fourth IR, for instance, its potentially alienating and inequality exacerbating consequences, its rescripting of our notions of ownership (e.g., who owns your personal data?), and its refiguring of what it means to control privacy and self-identity. These consequences, currently lived and potential, are

M. Uebel (✉)
University of Texas, Austin, TX, USA
e-mail: uebel@utexas.edu

C.-H. Mayer et al. (eds.), *Shame 4.0*, https://doi.org/10.1007/978-3-030-59527-2_27

related no less to decreasing shame thresholds than to the decreasing acknowledgment and awareness of shame itself.

This chapter, by placing the dialectic of visibility and invisibility at the center of technology, brings before us the significance of exposure and privacy in any consideration of shame. New and expanding forms of connectivity mean that discussions of urgent issues such as how our psyches are modified by the increasing loss of control over our personal data in the so-called Age of Surveillance Capitalism (Zuboff, 2019) may be usefully informed by reflection upon shame as an indelible marker of human affectivity. What I propose is that any account of shame phenomena in the Fourth Industrial Revolution is enhanced by tracing the origin and meaning of shame to technology (here, back to the ancient Greeks). Sociological inquiries and psychological theories help explain the origin of shame as related to disparate technologies, both magical and real, as we will see: Gyges's ring of invisibility; eating utensils (the medieval reception of the knife, the increasing use of the fork), along with other "instruments of civilization" as Elias (1939/2000) called them generally, such as the train; and punishment devices (the contemporary pillory of online shaming). First, I will situate the history of shame in both philosophical and psychological perspectives related to the dialectic of visibility and invisibility and the problem of control. In further sections of the chapter, we will examine the technological origins of shame, transformations of shame by contemporary sociotechnologies of connectivity and exclusion, and, finally, the future of shame as a moral construct imbedded in technology, with attention to the binary divisions such as technology/society and subject/object that have traditionally structured the cultural significance of shame and are increasingly problematized by the operations of the Fourth IR.

2 Shame as a Cloaking Device

Shame is itself a technology of control, a device for preserving a relationship of self to self that may be toxic but is, in its prospective form, fundamentally motivated by an ethical drive to self-reform and self-protection. Shame is thus about mastery and in its negative applications can be used to control others where, for example, the shaming of others amounts to an effort to make them transparent as ethical subjects. The irony in all this has always been that shame, once felt by the subject, is a brilliant protective or cloaking device (recalling the word's Indo-European etymon meaning hide or cover). Joan Copjec (2006) observes, while differentiating it from guilt, that "shame does not seek to penetrate surfaces or tear away veils; rather, it seeks comfort in them, hides itself in them as in a safe haven. Our relationships to the surface change in shame, compared to guilt; we become fascinated with its maze-like intricacies, its richness and profundity" (p. 111). The profundity of the surface, while oxymoronic, is a key feature of what shame means personally and ethically since shame offers an antidote to an external all-seeing Eye. Shame means that, if I revel in its labyrinthine depths rather than become conscious of it as the protective device it is, there is a chance my dependence on the views of others will not be betrayed. Yet this may be the problem posed by the Fourth IR: if emphasis on isolated persons (e.g., as collectible and transparent data points) increases, along with an emphasis on self-reliance, then might shame be irrevocably concealed? In other words, if, as Gary Thrane (1979) summarizes it, "shame is always provoked by discovery" (p. 336), and we become preeminently and inescapably discoverable, then shame risks becoming so normal that it becomes invisible.

The risk here is rather grave. It is crucial that we be aware of our shame, even if we are fastened to it. Not to be aware of shame entails a loss of mastery. Shame, Sabini and Silver (1997) write, "ill fits our voluntarist culture. People... can be ashamed of things that they did not choose, that they did not will, that aren't their fault. This strikes us as unfair" (p. 12). "Unfair" might be putting it mildly since uncontrollable shame involves nothing less than the loss of control over our very identities. I concur with the pioneering scholar of shame Silvan Tomkins (1963) who states that, compared to other affects, "shame strikes deepest into the heart of man" (p. 118) and would add that when it does so strike, the point is that one knows for sure, has proof, that one is human. Given, for example, the current revolutions in biotechnology and AI defining a couple of the leading edges of the Fourth IR, shame may function as a kind of Chinese Room experiment (Searle, 1980), where natural thinking and feeling can be distinguished from machinic forms of consciousness. Searle (1980) contends that AI, which employs syntactic rules to decode symbols such as Chinese characters, cannot do what human minds actually do, that is, understand natural language drawing upon a range of mental capabilities including, most crucially, feelings (Koch, 2019). Cognition is not mere computation. If what it means to be human (how we think, how long we live, what we are capable of, and so on) is continually subject to redefining, then there is something urgently humanistic about shame. It is intrinsically linked to our agency *as humans*.

As agency increases, negative shame diminishes. As agency decreases, positive, that is, protective or discretionary, shame comes into being in order to restore, however partially, agency. Let's unpack this. Negative shame results from, as Sartre (1956) put it, an "apprehension *of* something and this something is *me*" (emph. in orig., p. 221). Shame is most salient when we are most uncomfortably visible to ourselves through the eyes of others whose ridicule or hostility actually means something to us. For this very reason, collectivist cultures demonstrate higher levels of shame, as shown across multiple studies (e.g., Bierbrauer, 1992; Sznycer et al., 2012; Tang, Wang, Qian, Gao, & Zhang, 2008; Thomas, Deighton, Mizuno, & Fujii, 2019). We simply do not feel ashamed if, for instance, we are criticized or laughed at on account of our behavior by others whom we do not respect or with whom we do not share ideals. The most shameless behavior issues, then, from the most total arrogance or narcissistic self-enclosure. The more powerful I imagine myself to be, the more immune I am to the kind of shame that might prevent me from doing ugly things. The eighteenth-century New England Puritans, who did not imagine for themselves any agency that could not otherwise be attributed to God's will, had a profound sense of always being observed—watched by self, by other community members and religious leaders, and, literally, *above all* by God. As John Demos

(1996) has shown, the Puritans felt themselves to be preeminently transparent objects of observation and scrutiny. Relative to the omnipotence of a deity, human agency is miniscule, and so philosopher Paul Tillich, in his sermon "Escape from God" (*The Shaking of the Foundations*, 1953), grappled with the putatively horrifying notion of an omniscient and omnipresent God as a kind of all-reflecting mirror of humanity. It was Nietzsche (1966b), whose parable of the Ugliest Man in *Thus Spoke Zarathustra* Tillich references, who averred that the very notion of an all-seeing God contributes to the production of shame.

The birth of shame in a diminished state of pure visibility—to oneself, others, or an omniscient and omnipresent deity—gives rise to certain desires that issue not from a lack of being or deficiency but from an unbearable plenitude of being to which we are riveted. The philosopher Emmanuel Levinas (2003) charted precisely this sense of "an existence incapable of hiding itself" (p. 64) when he discussed our shamefulness in terms of a desire to flee oneself that is squelched by "the unalterably binding presence of the I to itself" (ibid.). In the absence of exteriority to ourselves as agents, we will abjectly suffer shame. This is why the nakedness of exotic dancers is not necessarily shameless—in the conventional sense of the word—since their own bodies appear to themselves "with that exteriority of self that serves as a form of cover" (ibid., p. 65). Thus, Levinas declares that "shame is, in the last analysis, an existence that seeks excuses" (ibid.). Shame is related to everything that we would like to hide from visibility but cannot cover up, and therefore what we require most is "excuses" or escapes. What about the self we have the power to choose to reveal or to hide determines our sense of shame. Agency is therefore always at the center of any determination of whether shame violates or preserves subjectivity. To be seen in a certain light carries the risk of feeling shame since invisibility has been foreclosed. A fine example of this is St. Augustine's interpretation of the punishment given to Adam and Eve for eating from the forbidden Tree of the Knowledge of Good and Evil. In *The City of God* (XIV.15), Augustine states that insubordination to God was correspondingly punished with the torment of flesh becoming insubordinate to humankind. With "their disobedience," the theologian explains, "chastised by a corresponding punishment, there appeared in the movements of their body a certain indecent novelty, which made nakedness shameful. It at once made them observant and made them ashamed" (St. Augustine, 2003, p. 578). When they lost the ability to control the physical signs of arousal (e.g., tumescence), Adam and Eve experienced the novelty of a shame that turned their reproductive organs into *pudenda* (literally, shameful things). Like lust, which according to Augustine was absent in the prelapsarian world, shame signals a certain loss of control, an involuntary subordination to drives that must be compensated for by assertions of autonomy (vigilance, laws), privacy (hiding, isolating), agency (coercion, passion), and self-protection (Taylor, 1985). I follow John Velleman (2006), who discusses the Augustinian interpretation, in seeing the vulnerability of being displayed as anything less than a master of one's self-definition to constitute a central occasion for shame.

As a result of the Fall, Augustine tells us, humans were simultaneously compelled to be observant and ashamed. We may read this fall into humanness as a dialectic, mediated by shame, of seeing and being seen, a making visible and a wish to be invisible. The human blush is an excellent device for the expression of both being seen (the face visibly reddening) and appealing to others for sympathy, perhaps forgiveness, or at least a mitigation of judgment (Shweder, 2003, p. 1115). Blushing with shame or embarrassment both sets a person apart, perhaps resulting from a social failure or offense, and marks an acceptance and honoring of "the very virtues, high standards, and ideals that were the cause of one's loss of face" (ibid.). The blush simultaneously reveals and conceals difference from the social and moral order. Shame has an inherently self-revelatory quality that is both invited and refused, and it is best comprehended within a dialectical experience of exposure and mystification. I want to close this chapter section with a discussion of how the dialectical device of shame operates, drawn from philosopher Max Scheler whose analysis I cited in an earlier essay on shame (Uebel, 2019).

Scheler (1957/1987) finds in every instance of shame "an act of turning to ourselves" (p. 15) precisely because it harbors the "the power to abolish self-deception; shame is the pioneer into our selves" (p. 53). But in order for self-consciousness to be aroused, there must be a disruptive oscillation between subjective possibilities. Let's follow Scheler's illustration:

> Even one's knowing oneself to be seen by someone else is not yet a condition for shame. Although for very different reasons, a very bashful woman can feel as little shame when being a model for a painter, being a patient of a physician, or when bathing in the presence of a servant as she feels with her beloved. If she experiences herself in front of the painter as "given" for aesthetic quality and as a valuable visual model for the arts, the turn-experience will not occur... she does not experience herself as individual... let us have the painter be for a moment distracted from his original intentions so that the woman begins to feel this happening, and the "painting" disappears. .. the woman will then strongly react with shame while turning to herself. Conversely, let us have the woman feel that her beloved is distracted from her individuality and just looking at her as "a beautiful woman" such that the woman feels he is comparing her with, or she is reminding him of, another woman... she will immediately react with shame. (pp. 15–16)

Scheler unpacks the meaning of his illustrations:

> the turning to one's self in whose dynamics shame has its beginnings does not occur if one is "given" to oneself as something general or individual. It occurs when the feelable intention of the other oscillates between an individualizing and generalizing attitude and when's own intention and the experienced counterintention have not the same but an opposite direction. (p. 16)

For my purposes, there is perhaps no better explanation of the dynamics of shame. If a person's control over her image, her self-presentation, and her beliefs about such as it exists for others fails, then confusion occurs. Only in this psychological state of dislocation does the person feel shame. The perceived dissonance of the other's attention triggers an event of confusion which is synonymous with the shame experience. Confusion, as Schneider (1977, p. 24) points out, is so commonly paired with shame that they form a Biblical cliché: e.g., hearing the Psalmist's petition, "let all who seek my life be brought to shame and confusion" (Psalm 70:2), and the plea for retribution, "Let them be put to shame and confusion who rejoice at my fall" (Psalm 35:26). Indeed, in a moment of shame, persons often look down, Georg Simmel (1924, p. 358) theorizes, so that others cannot see how they are responding to the moment, preventing, more specifically, the other from comprehending the extent of their confusion. Shame, by masking confusion, provides an intimate space of protection in which the confusion can be managed, opening the possibility that something authentic can truly be known about the self.

3 The Technological Origins of Shame

The impossibility of concealing the fact that we are ourselves means that we will forever seek excuses, returning to Levinas's (2003) framing of the mechanism of shame. Shame's history indeed involves technologies of excuse making. If shame, in the final analysis, acknowledges the potential danger of exposing the basic fact(s) of our being to others, then it is not surprising that technologies have played a role in how those facts are revealed—or concealed. Technologies create the contextual spaces in which shame is worked out through techniques of visibility and invisibility. Exposure has long been taken to be central to the shame experience, and it is here that the spatial structure of shame is indicated (to *ex-pose* derives from the Latin word *exponere*, to place out). Shame, observes Schneider (1977), "arises when something doesn't fit. Thus we experience shame when we feel we are placed out of the context within which we wish to be interpreted. Shame occasions are those when someone or some aspect of a person or group is 'out of place'—that is, exposed" (p. 35). Despite being displaced, we cannot have a shame experience if we are rendered absolutely other—to ourselves or to others—for the reason I mentioned above, namely, that shame depends on our having the opportunity to see ourselves in relation to something, a value or moral code, for example, that reflects or marks a mysterious, yet essential, dimension of the self. We may become ashamed of a thing that, when revealed, possesses an ambivalent meaning while remaining a personally powerful symbol. Consider Dostoyevsky's unfortunate Dmitri Fyodorovich Karamazov, who submits to a degrading police interrogation requiring him to undress and whose crooked nail on his right big toe causes him immense shame when he is compelled to remove his sock. Despite the context of a disciplinary technology of power that "establishes over individuals a visibility through which one differentiates and judges them," leaving "no zone of shade" (Foucault, 1977, p. 184; 177), an unsightly toe is scarcely some unequivocal key to knowledge. Rather, as Jack Katz (1997) explains, such a toe reveals only "the existence of an abiding mystery, a personally resonant something-that-has-been-kept-hidden" (p. 235).

Certain technologies preserve the resonant mystery at the heart of shame. They structure situations in which relationships somewhere between absolute alterity and absolute intimacy are allowed to flourish. Just as strangers are not likely to elicit shame so are intimates unlikely to do so since they possess significantly richer sources for appraising character than an isolated behavior or trait (Bero, 2019; Katz, 1997, p. 251). Simmel, in his time, was struck by the surprising openness of people who met for the first and presumably last time when they shared a train compartment: "Travelling companions who were unknown to one another until an hour ago, and who will not see each other again an hour later, are often prepared to entrust one another with intimacies" (qtd. in Gerhards, 1986, p. 907). The appearance of shame, Simmel theorized, belongs only in relationships that were, in terms of their intimacy or alterity, of the intermediate range and structured by the specific technology of train travel. Today, trains are changing the relationship to a special type of contemporary shame called "flight shame," what the Dutch dub *vliegschaamte*, the Swedish *flygskam*, and the Germans *Flugscham*. This is the shame associated with airline travel whose significant and increasing toll on the environment can be minimized by the use of alternate, more sustainable, modes such as electric trains or buses. Flight shame is felt in the context of visibility to an audience that is not necessarily actual but always symbolic. John Deigh (1983) has argued that shame is not understandable independent of the central role that one's concern for the opinion of others plays, especially concern for an audience's opinion that is imagined. Flight shame exemplifies a kind of intermediate shame—neither fully intimate- nor fully other-directed—conditioned by a concern for the views of members of future generations regarding their antecedents' unchecked ecological destructiveness. Furthermore, one need not agree with the views of future generations or contemporary environmental activists in order to access a sense of shame. Cheshire Calhoun (2004) has persuasively affirmed that "vulnerability to feeling ashamed before those with whom one shares a moral practice, *even when one disagrees with their moral criticisms*, is often a mark of moral maturity" (emph. in orig., p. 129).

Pre-industrial technologies also hold a key to understanding the origins of shame. In his *Metamorphoses*, Ovid offers a description of the Four Ages of the World (I. 89–150) in which, with each subsequent age, technology mediates the harmony of humans and nature. Beginning with the Golden Age and ending with the Iron Age, humans increasingly forfeited their sense of justice, tranquility, and innocence. In the Golden Age, the earth offered its abundance of crops without being touched by ploughshares; in the Silver Age, the technologies of husbandry and architecture became necessary when the eternal spring was broken by Zeus into the different seasons; in the Bronze Age, technologies of war-making and destruction disrupted harmony among humans; and, ultimately, in the terminal Iron Age, all crime broke forth, characterizing a period of uncontrollable mistrust, deception, and treachery that became the violent engines of social dissolution as technologies of mining the earth, Ovid tells us, symbolized greed and left no room for shame (*pudor*), honor, and truth. For Ovid, the final loss of shame was lamentable and marked just how fully the restraining power of the sense of shame supports the order of things. These evolving and profound social changes, circulating around the presence or absence of shame, draw our attention to the role that technology plays in shaping and unshaping structures of power and legitimacy. Yet, it turns out, the most striking examples of how social and moral orders are formed and deformed involve the most basic of all technologies—clothing and eating utensils.

In Norbert Elias's *The Civilizing Process* (1939/2000), we find extended analyses of premodernity's management of the internal state of shame through education, primarily in the form of conduct books aimed at the European nobility. Elias demonstrates that an increasing discomfort with displays of the human body developed over centuries. Codes concerning how one dresses and before whom one undresses, for example, contributed to a rising threshold of shame and embarrassment that gradually became internalized as automatic forms of self-restraint. At the late-medieval table, the use of knives was beginning to be regulated in novel ways that contributed to the transformation of violent warriors into domesticated courtiers. The knife symbolized aggression and the provocation of fear, and so, to curb its association with danger and death, rules emerged about how to handle the knife at table (e.g., it is not to be turned toward one's face and is always to be offered by the handle rather than the point). The fork has an even more interesting history in terms of its relation to shame. Following its appearance in the West in Italy in the eleventh century, this novel instrument first caused scandals such that a Byzantine princess who employed one was afflicted by a hideous disease that St. Bonaventura declared to be a punishment from God. The practicality of the knife would not be suppressed, however, and its increasing presence at late-medieval European courts through the seventeenth century invited softer responses in the forms of mockery and wonderment at its actual utility for more than picking morsels from a common plate. The great shift in the use of the fork happened around the nineteenth century when etiquette books recommended its use based on beliefs that only cannibals eat with their fingers and that consuming food with the hands is unhygienic. Elias detected a richer explication for the fork's popular usage:

> The real explanation hinges on a very slow and profound change in the subconscious of people in a particular society. These people have begun to construct an affective wall between their bodies and those of others. The fork has been one of the means of drawing distances between other people's bodies and one's own. One repulses the body, isolates it, feels ashamed of it, tries to ignore it. It's a considerable change. For many centuries, this wall did not exist. (Fontaine, 1978, p. 245)

The fork, like clothing, is a fundamental corporeal technology of distancing, concealing, and insulating. The "affective wall" that shame embodies serves to curb the intrusion of tactless desires, the irreverence of spontaneous physical urges, and the indiscretion of immoderate appetite. Nietzsche (1966a), in characteristically hyperbolic fashion, describes shame as a barrier to "so-called educated people['s]" inveterate desire to "see through everything," to desacralize with a "nauseous. . .lack of modesty [*Mangel an Scham*] and the comfortable insolence of their eyes and hands with which they touch, lick, and finger everything" (p. 213). Civilizing technologies have the capacity to erect momentary stays against confusion between the public and the private, the mysterious (hidden) and the mundane (visible), and the sacred and the profane. They mediate the shame structuring the visible and the invisible.

Part of the power of shame resides in its providing the protection necessary to stand before the sacred or revered. Shame in the Old Testament, for example, is closely associated with awe (Gr. *aidos*): only in shame does one stand before the deity. Αἰδώς also plays a significant role in the last technological device we will examine—Gyges's magic ring of invisibility. Significantly, the ring is evoked in several ethical and historical treatments of shame (e.g., Heller, 1974; Kekes, 1988; Severson, 2018; Williams, 1993). There are two primary ancient Greek tales of Gyges, one found in Herodotus's *History* (1.8–12) and the other in Plato's *Republic* (359d–60b). While only Plato's version references a magical ring, both versions tell the general story of Gyges's ascendency to power, which turns on his ability to make things visible or invisible. Both tales are set in Lydia, a kingdom of western Asia Minor that the Greeks associated with the birth of the technology of minted coinage and the political technique of tyranny. Indeed, ancient Greeks named Gyges as the first representation of a true tyrant, a person whose power is maintained, Aristotle points out in *Politics* (1313b7), by two strategies of vision and concealment: using spies to make others visible and ensuring that he himself remains invisible to the people he rules (see Kasbovas chapter). The person wielding the power of spectation controls the state (Travis, 2000). As we will see, both the Herodotean and Platonic plots are built around acts of transgressive spectation that point to an important dimension of the shame experience and its mediation by a technology of vision.

Herodotus tells the story of Gyges as the first dramatic narrative in his *History*, and its plot is (briefly) as follows: Lydian King Candaules prizes his wife, considering her the most beautiful woman in the world. Extolling the beauty of his wife to his retainer Gyges and insisting that "seeing is believing," he finally presses him to see her naked despite the taboo against seeing royalty in this state. The queen spies the voyeur Gyges as he slips from the royal bedchamber, but remains silent and confronts Gyges the next day with the choice to either kill Candaules or die himself: "For either he that contrived this must die or you, who have viewed me naked and done what is not lawful" (Herodotus, 1987, p. 37). He chooses to murder the king while lying in wait in the royal chamber where he had hidden before. Gyges afterward rules as a tyrant. Significantly, Gyges, at first resisting Candaules's importuning of him to see the queen naked, cites an apothegm that, connecting the basic technology of clothing to shame, declares that women lay bare their shame (*aidos*) when they undress. The plot unfolds such that Gyges subjected himself to the consequences of his own defense around not violating a woman's shame (Travis, 2000). In seeing the queen's *eidos* (beauty), Gyges violates her *aidos* (shame). One of the recoverable lines from a papyrus fragment of a tragic Greek play about Gyges has the queen, upon recognizing the violation, suppressing a "cry of shame" (Travis, 2000, p. 345). In Herodotus's tale, the modesty of Lydian women is stressed, and so the act of seeing in the narrative is a kind of making visible of that which is supposed to be invisible. To see without being seen is a power belonging to the divinities, and on the human level, this translates to the power of the archetypal tyrant whose absolute rule relies on the semblance of omniscience resulting from panoptical vision (Shell, 1989). Gyges's rise to power occurs through reversals, transforming the invisible into the visible through a violation of shame, and transforming visibles into invisibles (employing novel political and economic technologies).

Whereas Herodotus's tale of voyeurism and power can be read in terms of technologies ranging from clothing to spy networks and coinage, the short story about the ring of invisibility told by Glaucon, Socrates's chief interlocutor in the *Republic*, explicitly links technologies of invisibility to ethical concerns related to shame and its capacity to shape moral behavior. Glaucon's story of Gyges, told in the middle of a debate about ethics, may be summarized: A magical power once came to (the ancestor of) Gyges the Lydian, a shepherd and serf who, having explored a cave, found a corpse on whose finger was a wondrous ring. Gyges took the ring and discovered that turning the setting one way rendered him invisible and turning it back made him reappear. Quickly installing himself as one of the king's messengers, he commits adultery with the queen and, along with her, usurps the throne after the king is murdered. Gyges is said to have the power to take whatever he desires—goods from the marketplace or women in their homes—as well to kill or free from slavery whomever he wishes. Gyges's power of invisibility allows him to appear good or just while keeping his treachery concealed. It permits him the unrestrained latitude to act shamelessly.

Famous throughout antiquity (Suidas, 1853), the magical ring of Gyges would illustrate discussions of ethics from Cicero (Laird, 2001; Woolf, 2013) to Rousseau (Still, 1993), as well as appear in the plots of novelists and playwrights, including La Fontaine, Hebbel (Koschorke, 2005), Addison, Hugo von Hofmannsthal, Gide, H. G. Wells, Vargas Llosa, and Mahfouz. Glaucon uses the ring story to challenge Socrates's view that justice is profitable for whoever practices it when he suggests that just actions are in fact done unwillingly and issue from a want of power to commit injustice. If, he argues, the unjust and the just are granted the power do whatever they please, then the difference between these two types of person is negated, if "we follow each of them in our gaze" (*Republic* 359c, translation in Laird, 2001, p. 21). Glaucon maintains that removing all restraints from the conventions of law (*nomos*) allows us to see humans as they truly are. Glaucon's tale in effect grants the reader the same power, in relation to those whose exposure or visibility is otherwise prevented, that Herodotus's Gyges had in relation to the Lydian royalty. In other words, we may see Gyges in his moral nakedness as he acts out his unjust intentions. Thus Socrates counters that the tyrant Gyges can never be truly viewed as enviable or happy, having soundly proved that "justice in itself is the best thing for the soul itself, and that the soul ought to do justice whether it possesses the ring of Gyges or not, or the helmet of Hades to boot" (Plato, 1961, p. 837). Philosophical argument renders Gyges visible whereby, the Platonic point goes, just moral conduct does not merely depend upon whether one will be found out or not. In both Herodotus and Plato, invisible Gyges lacks the moral counterbalance of shame, has no internalized audience, and, thus, hidden from others, is in the same way unable to see himself as he truly is. A sense of discretion shame means there is no invisibility to self, or we may posit further that invisibility is the very marker of shame's absence. Thrane (1979) once put this rather brilliantly: "The lust of the vampire is shameless; he cannot see himself in any mirror" (p. 330). This insight links to a theme related to the technics of shame that we have already seen in the case of the Puritans and Nietzsche's Ugliest Man: visibility contributes to the production of shame.

Technologies of invisibility such as Gyges's magical ring, the helmet of Hades (which affords invisibility to the gods), or Bentham's Panopticon question the possibility of a shame-free existence. Being figured as the object of the gaze always signifies a certain ambiguity inherent in the object. The weakness of normal vision resides in its failure to access the object's interiority, and because of this, "it fails to comprehend *aidos*" (Travis, 2000, p. 243). Even the employment of a fork, in accordance with etiquette, is a "wall" preventing access to the interiority of affect. Shame, as is well attested, makes persons wish to disappear, to become invisible, and to erase the boundaries between self and other at the same time that such a disappearance act demonstrates the ongoing debt to the mirroring other for any and all self-recognition. Shame experiences function, as Eve Kosofsky Sedgwick (2003) puts it, on the very "threshold between introversion and extroversion, between absorption and theatricality" (p. 38). As the differential between immersion in the other and forms of self-distinction, shame embodies the dilemma and danger of being both one of the crowd and the star performer (Uebel, 2019). It is thus unsurprising that psychoanalytic approaches to shame relate it to conflicts around exhibitionism and stage fright (Fenichel, 1945; Gabbard, 1979). Shame is always locatable at the site where visibility and the wish for invisibility collide.

4 Shaming Technology

What is so abjectly horrible about stage fright is that one is inescapably oneself and at the same time vulnerable to the interpellations of others. To be riveted to oneself in such a disturbing state, as Levinas (2003) describes the shame experience, entails, as I am suggesting, a loss of freedom with respect to self-presentation and a forfeiture of effortless attunement to the world. Levinas (2003) further characterizes shame as the outcome of having sought pleasure as an escape from self-enclosure only to find that any momentary contentment or ecstasy collapses into a state that he likens to physical nausea. Of course, it was Sartre who defined nausea as the encounter, in excess (*de trop*), with the brute facticity of our own existence. There is an echo here of Sartre's (1956) graphic description of the sometimes violent immediacy of the shame moment when being driven back to the self feels like "an internal hemorrhage" (p. 261). What I want to suggest in this section is that technology increasingly mediates our existential relation to the world in ways that generate particular formations of shame.

In a compelling reading of the shame that inheres in a disabled person's relation to the sociotechnical world, Matthew Rukgaber (2019) directs our attention to feelings of exclusion registered as a result of confronting a world that forecloses "effortless, anonymous coexistence" (p. 103). The paradigmatic example of such a feeling is being ashamed before a staircase that one cannot negotiate. The basic technology of stairs, dating back to Egyptian pylons of the second millennium BCE, is virtually coeval with what it means to be a seamless part of a world in which certain elements of sociotechnical functioning may be taken for granted. Any disruption of such seamlessness may be felt as shame producing, since, as Heinz Kohut (1975) theorizes, the holistic sense of the self is imperiled in attempts to restore cohesion at times when the self is projected into the world but fails to be recognized. Existential shame, in this case, may be seen as a function of the breakdown of affective attunement to technological systems. Debilitated attunement foregrounds the extent to which dis-ability does not allow for dis-appearance. Technology opens a rift between a world that fails to respond and—crucially—a world to which one's responses are limited. What develops is "an inescapable publicity" (Rukgaber, 2019, p. 105) in which, as I see it, the possibility of a seamless sociotechnical existence is foreclosed due to the unrelenting nature of a technological world whose function is increasingly that of exposure and correction. The Fourth IR, more than any preceding revolution, relies on a medical model that views illnesses and disabilities as personal deficits that are eminently "fixable" through novel medical interventions (e.g., genomics, genetic engineering, synthetic biology, nanotechnology, AI, and robotics). Such a model cannot escape a perspective informed by the belief that there are standards to which human beings must correspond in terms of how they are visible and appear, how they act, and what they are capable of doing. Not to fit with such a standard is to risk shame.

Shame highlights the sense of fit, or lack of such, between persons and their world; and to imagine a world in which everything seamlessly "fits" is to imagine a world without shame. Policing this fit becomes its own mode of shame production, as we will see momentarily with the example of online digilantism, but for now the point is more general: technology, by making persons visible (as users or non-users), simultaneously stimulates the need for shame as a protective cloaking device and mobilizes the need for invisibility as the condition from which it is easier to shame others. Consider the publicized problem of invisible disabilities, toward which we will pursue two angles. Invisible disabilities are those mental and physical conditions (e.g., chronic illnesses like schizophrenia, AIDS, epilepsy, or cancer) that are not immediately discernible by unknowing observers. Visibility, linked in the scientific and disabilities studies literature to feelings of stigma and shame, bears upon impression management generally (Leary & Kowalski, 1990) and internal negotiations around passing and self-disclosure (Brune & Wilson, 2013; Matthews & Harrington, 2000) specifically. Being visible means that one is compelled to make decisions about which identities will be embodied, and these choices are particularly urgent when the invisible disabled are interacting with the technologies that able-bodied others take for granted. Not fitting may require a decision about passing, which Erving Goffman (1963) defines as a strategy for managing the stigma of "spoiled identities"—those devalued by opinion, penalized by law, or abjected by social convention. The shame felt, for example, by a person who receives disability benefits for an invisible mental illness may result in efforts to pass as someone who is fully able to support herself by being employed. In structuring an unobtrusive appearance, shame is inextricably linked to an urge for invisibility. The other angle here is that, when passing, the invisible disabled may be subject to vigilante justice which metes out labels such as "faker" or "selfish" or "lazy" person. For example, invisible disabled persons risk being shamed by others when they have used a handicapped parking space, with the proper placard, and then anonymously walked into a store. This may incite the rage of vigilante witnesses who are armed to impugn the morality or legitimacy of the handicapped person. Policing efforts targeting the use of handicapped parking spaces extend to similar practices of naming and shaming, driven by social media, whereby blatant disabled parking space abusers (e.g., in cars that display no placard or other identification) are made visible through photographs of persons and their vehicles posted to public websites and social media.

With each succeeding Industrial Revolution, there has been an increasing need for persons who "fit" and who are fundamentally interchangeable (e.g., as service-industry workers), and the disabled person's relation to the technological world brings before us the durability of shame as an exposure of the basic fact of our being to others—in other words, the degree of our fitness. One question the Fourth IR raises is precisely this issue of fit: what strategies will prove useful for shaping the society in which one might fit? The use of shaming technologies in order to force, by means of exposure strategies, social compliance and membership has been increasing over the last couple of decades. The use of Internet and online shaming as a form of social control—policing and punishing—is well documented (Goldman, 2015; Oravec, 2019). Public shaming is hardly novel, yet it is being utilized with greater scope and force than ever before related to rapid transformations in technological speed, impact, adoption, and relevance. Emergent genres of online shaming, including the use of Twitter to out "deadbeat dads" (Battle, 2019), may involve violations of privacy, and these exposures can erode democratic space as people's ability to continue to participate socially in cybervenues free from humiliation and attack is compromised (Laidlaw, 2017). One motivation for online shaming appears to be the preservation of both personal and general beliefs in a just world, with one study showing a positive correlation between the strength of such beliefs and the likelihood to engage in shaming (Hou, Jiang, & Wang, 2017).

The effects of using online naming and shaming for promoting justice and conformity are mixed. In cases where it is aimed at enhancing institutional transparency, it has been successful in contributing to political reformation, for example, in the Arab world where it has been central to prosecuting corruption by authorities (Aman & Jayroe, 2013) or in the West where threatened business-consumer relationships have compelled changes in the behavior of multinational corporations such as Nike and Shell. In other instances, employed as a strategy for incentivizing emission cuts by corporations in order to address climate change, its efficacy is less certain (Taebi & Safari, 2017). For the stimulation of social behavioral change, such as the #metoo movement and drought shaming targeting water restriction violators, and as a chief strategy supporting human rights activism, such as drawing attention to the use of sweatshop labor by businesses, its effectiveness has also been mixed. Despite its inconclusive virtues, there are those who see shaming as a deeply democratic form of influence since it reflects communal values and does not issue from an authority (Etzioni, 1999). Indeed, it is argued that "true or pure shaming involves only *symbolic* acts that communicate censure" (ibid., p. 45; emph. in orig.). The obvious problem here is that, increasingly, a sense of community is disintegrating, so that what made public shaming an effective technology in, say, colonial America (e.g., stocks and pillories; the wearing of letters labeling a crime) is not characteristic of or transposable to contemporary Western modalities of sociotechnical living. Instead, all too commonplace is the ugliness of online attacks and humiliating gestures whose ability to shock, Pogue (2016) suggests, will fade, becoming "just a sport," a kind of impersonal game (p. 28). One interesting piece of evidence along these lines is a name-and-shame project in New York City called the "Parking Hall of Fame" listing persons with accumulated parking fines (some totaling over US $60000), some of whom achieved the celebrity of minor folk heroes (Oravec, 2019). Shame's attachment to moral as well as nonmoral objects places it at the center of any discussion about the affect's future as a technology for change mobilizing, and sometimes weaponizing, the dialectic of inclusion and exclusion.

5 Shame Embedded in Technology

I will conclude with a brief speculation on the future of shame as an affective construct imbedded in technology (see Table 27.1 for a partial summary). Binary divisions such as technology/society, subject/object, and reality/unreality that have traditionally structured the cultural and moral significance of shame may be collapsing. Shame's relation to reality is shifting. If we follow Alain Badiou (2007) in identifying as the dominant feature of the previous century the passion of the Real (*la passion du réel*), in contrast to the nineteenth century's passion for utopian scientific ideals, we may see that the stage has been set for shame's absolute necessity. By this, I mean that the twentieth century's frenzied, often scopic, drive to strip off the veils of reality in the name of some direct experience of the Real is simultaneously marked by shameless violence—think of the technology of the World Wars ranging from rockets to concentration camps—and by the availability of shame as a signal that such horror calls into existence the possibility of its own ending. Shame involves an arresting and also indicates a moment of pausing—sometimes rooted only in confusion, as I noted—at which affectivity itself arises relative to human agency. The

Table 27.1 Some implications of the relationship of shame and Fourth IR

	Positive and negative roles of shame	Potential impact of Fourth IR
Agency	• Limits illusion of complete control over environment • Shapes behavior	• Views persons as isolates (e.g., data points) • Uses technologies of surveillance as control
Identity	• Signals effortless attunement to world is at risk • Provokes confusion	• Demands "fit" with sociotechnical world • Uses technology to "fix" persons (in double sense of repair and rivet)
Visibility	• Marks exposure as a risk • Furnishes invisibility	• Imperils power of self-presentation • Uses technology to make persons eminently discoverable

operations of the Fourth IR, as exemplified, for example, in the Internet of Things, will more and more increase certain kinds of agency, human and certainly machinic. Controlling our home's temperature setting with a smartphone app, letting our cars drive us while it detects hazards, and accessing any genre of music with a smart speaker device provide (illusions of) the sense of total control. Interestingly, Susan Miller (1996) frames shame in terms of our sense of technological control:

> Shame only occurs if events are experienced as reflecting on the value of the self. The average adult has no expectation that he should be able to control the electrical power supply to his television, so he feels only frustration, not shame, if the power goes out. But a person who believes that to exercise less than perfect control over his environment signifies personal deficiency might indeed feel shame if his electrical power failed during a televised basketball game (p. 26)

It may be fair to say the Fourth IR raises just the novel possibility of the latter kind of person. If human-to-human and human-to-computer interaction become less requisite, the question is whether or not frustration supersedes shame (see Mayer and Vanderheiden on "The Meaning of Shame in Cultures of the Fourth Industrial Revolution: An Introduction"; see Kelley; see Oosthuizen).

References

Aman, M. M., & Jayroe, T. J. (2013). ICT, social media, and the Arab transition to democracy: From venting to acting. *DOMES: Digest of Middle East Studies, 22*(2), 317–347.

Augustine, S. (2003). *Concerning the City of God against the pagans* (H. Bettenson, Trans.). New York: Penguin Books.

Badiou, A. (2007). *The century* (A. Toscano, Trans.). New York, NY: Polity.

Battle, B. P. (2019). "They look at you like you're nothing": Stigma and shame in the child support system. *Symbolic Interaction, 42*, 640. https://doi.org/10.1002/symb.427.

Bero, S. (2019). The audience in shame. *Philosophical Studies, 177*, 1283. https://doi.org/10.1007/s11098-019-01253-9.

Bierbrauer, G. (1992). Reactions to violation of normative standards: A cross-cultural analysis of shame and guilt. *International Journal of Psychology, 27*(2), 181–193.

Brune, J. A., & Wilson, D. J. (2013). *Disability and passing: Blurring the lines of identity*. Philadelphia: Temple University Press.

Calhoun, C. (2004). An apology for moral shame. *Journal of Political Philosophy, 12*(2), 127–146.

Copjec, J. (2006). May '68, the emotional month. In S. Zizek (Ed.), *Lacan: The silent partners* (pp. 90–114). New York: Verso Books.

Deigh, J. (1983). Shame and self-esteem: A critique. *Ethics, 93*, 225–245.

Demos, J. (1996). Shame and guilt in early New England. In R. Harré & G. Parrott (Eds.), *The emotions* (pp. 74–88). London: Sage.

Elias, N. (1939/2000). *The civilizing process: Sociogenetic and psychogenetic investigations*. (E. Jephcott, Trans.), E. Dunning, J. Goudsblom, & S. Mennell (Eds.). Malden, MA: Blackwell.

Etzioni, A. (1999). Back to the pillory? *The American Scholar, 68*(3), 43–50.

Fenichel, O. (1945). *The psychoanalytic theory of neurosis*. New York, NY: W. W. Norton.

Fontaine, S. (1978). The civilizing process revisited: Interview with Norbert Elias. *Theory and Society, 5*(2), 243–253.

Foucault, M. (1977). *Discipline and punish: The birth of the prison* (A. Sheridan, Trans.). New York, NY: Vintage Books.

Gabbard, G. O. (1979). Stage fright. *International Journal of Psycho-Analysis, 60*, 383–392.
Gerhards, J. (1986). Georg Simmel's contribution to a theory of emotions. *Social Science Information, 25*, 901–924.
Goffman, E. (1963). *Stigma: Notes on the management of spoiled identity*. Englewood Cliffs, NJ: Prentice-Hall.
Goldman, L. M. (2015). Trending now: The use of social media websites in public shaming punishments. *American Criminal Law Review, 52*, 415.
Heller, E. (1974). Man ashamed: Reflections on love, sex, and death. *Encounters, 42*(2), 23–30.
Herodotus. (1987). *The History* (D. Greene, Trans.). Chicago, IL: University of Chicago Press.
Hou, Y., Jiang, T., & Wang, Q. (2017). Socioeconomic status and online shaming: The mediating role of belief in a just world. *Computers in Human Behavior, 76*, 19–25.
Katz, J. (1997). The elements of shame. In M. R. Lansky & A. P. Morrison (Eds.), *The widening scope of shame* (pp. 231–260). Hillsdale, NJ: Analytic Press.
Kekes, J. (1988). Shame and moral progress. *Midwest Studies in Philosophy, 13*, 282–296.
Koch, C. (2019). *The feeling of life itself: Why consciousness is widespread but can't be computed*. Cambridge, MA: MIT Press.
Kohut, H. (1975). Pride, shame, and self-regulation. In P. Tolpin & M. Tolpin (Eds.), *Heinz Kohut: The Chicago institute lectures* (pp. 243–257). Hillsdale, NJ: Analytic Press.
Koschorke, A. (2005). Phantasmagorias of power: Hebbel's drama *Gyges und sein Ring* (trans: Golb, J.). *MLN, 120*(3), 539–561.
Laidlaw, E. B. (2017). Online shaming and the right to privacy. *Laws, 6*(1), 1–26.
Laird, A. (2001). Ringing the changes on Gyges: Philosophy and the formation of fiction in Plato's republic. *The Journal of Hellenic Studies, 121*, 12–29.
Leary, M. R., & Kowalski, R. M. (1990). Impression management: A literature review and two-component model. *Psychological Bulletin, 107*(1), 34–47.
Levinas, E. (2003). *On escape* (B. Bergo, Trans.). Stanford, CA: Stanford University Press.
Matthews, C. K., & Harrington, N. G. (2000). Invisible disability. In D. O. Braithwaite & T. L. Thompson (Eds.), *Handbook of communication and people with disabilities: Research and application* (pp. 405–421). Mahwah, NJ: Lawrence Erlbaum Associates Publishers.
Miller, S. B. (1996). *Shame in context*. Hillsdale, NJ: The Analytic Press.
Nietzsche, F. (1966a). *Beyond good and evil: Prelude to a philosophy of the future* (W. Kaufmann, Trans.). New York: Vintage Books.
Nietzsche, F. (1966b). *Thus spoke Zarathrustra: A book for all and none* (W. Kaufmann, Trans.). New York: Penguin Books.
Oravec, J. A. (2019). Online social shaming and the moralistic imagination: The emergence of internet-based performative shaming. *Policy & Internet*. https://doi.org/10.1002/poi3.226.
Plato. (1961). Republic (trans: P. Shorey). In E. Hamilton & H. Cairns (Eds.), *The collected dialogues* (pp. 575–844). Princeton, NJ: Princeton University Press.
Pogue, D. (2016). The bright side of internet shaming. *Scientific American, 315*(4), 28.
Rukgaber, M. (2019). Being in and excluded from the sociotechnical world. In C. Mun (Ed.), *Interdisciplinary perspectives on shame: Methods, theories, norms, cultures, and politics* (pp. 95–113). New York: Lexington Books.
Sabini, J., & Silver, M. (1997). In defense of shame: Shame in the context of guilt and embarrassment. *Journal for the Theory of Social Behaviour, 27*(1), 1–15.
Sartre, J.-P. (1956). *Being and nothingness: An essay on phenomenological ontology* (H. E. Barnes, Trans.). New York, NY: Philosophical library.
Scheler, M. (1987). Shame and feelings of modesty. In M. S. Frings (Ed. & Trans.), *Person and self-value: Three essays* (pp. 3–85). Dordrecht: Martinus Nijhoff. (Original work published 1957).
Schneider, C. D. (1977). *Shame, exposure, and privacy*. New York, NY: W. W. Norton.
Searle, J. (1980). Minds, brains and programs. *Behavioral and Brain Sciences, 3*, 417–457.
Sedgwick, E. K. (2003). Shame, theatricality, and queer performativity: Henry James's the art of the novel. In *Touching feeling: Affect, pedagogy, performativity* (pp. 35–65). Durham, NC: Duke University Press.

Severson, E. (2018). A time for shame: Levinas, diachrony, and the hope for shame. In L. Hinton & H. Willemson (Eds.), *Temporality and shame: Perspectives from psychoanalysis and philosophy* (pp. 57–73). New York: Routledge.
Shell, M. (1989). The ring of Gyges. *Mississippi Review, 17*(1/2), 21–84.
Shweder, R. A. (2003). Toward a deep cultural psychology of shame. *Social Research: An International Quarterly, 70*(4), 1100–1129.
Simmel, G. (1924). Sociology of the senses: Visual interaction. In R. E. Park & E. W. Burgess (Eds.), *Introduction to the science of sociology* (pp. 356–361). Chicago, IL: University of Chicago Press.
Still, J. (1993). *Justice and difference in the works of Rousseau: Bienfaisance and pudeur*. Cambridge: Cambridge University Press.
Suidas. (1853). In G. Bernhardy (Ed.), *Suidae lexicon: Graece et latine*. Halle: Sumptibus Schwetschkiorum.
Sznycer, D., Takemura, K., Delton, A. W., Sato, K., Robertson, T., Cosmides, L., & Tooby, J. (2012). Cross-cultural differences and similarities in proneness to shame: An adaptationist and ecological approach. *Evolutionary Psychology: An International Journal of Evolutionary Approaches to Psychology and Behavior, 10*(2), 352–370.
Taebi, B., & Safari, A. (2017). On effectiveness and legitimacy of 'shaming'as a strategy for combatting climate change. *Science and Engineering Ethics, 23*(5), 1289–1306.
Tang, M., Wang, Z., Qian, M., Gao, J., & Zhang, L. (2008). Transferred shame in the cultures of interdependent-self and independent self. *Journal of Cognition and Culture, 8*(1), 163–178.
Taylor, G. (1985). *Pride, shame and guilt: Emotions of self-assessment*. Oxford: Clarendon Press.
Thomas, R., Deighton, R., Mizuno, M., & Fujii, S. Y. A. C. (2019). Shame and self-conscious emotions in Japan and Australia: Evidence for a third shame logic. *Culture & Psychology, 26*, 622. https://doi.org/10.1177/1354067X19851024.
Thrane, G. (1979). Shame and the construction of the self. *Annual of Psychoanalysis, 7*, 321–341.
Tillich, P. (1953). The escape from god. In *The shaking of the foundati ons* (pp. 38–51). New York: Charles Scribner's Sons.
Tomkins, S. (1963). Affect, imagery, consciousness. In *The negative affects* (Vol. 2). London: Springer.
Travis, R. (2000). The Spectation of Gyges in P. oxy. 2382 and Herodotus book 1. *Classical Antiquity, 19*(2), 330–359.
Uebel, M. (2019). Dirty rotten shame? The value and ethical functions of shame. *Journal of Humanistic Psychology, 59*(2), 232–251.
Velleman, J. D. (2006). The genesis of shame. In *Self to self: Selected essays* (pp. 45–69). Cambridge: Cambridge University Press.
Williams, B. (1993). *Shame and necessity*. Berkeley, CA: University of California Press.
Woolf, R. (2013). Cicero and Gyges. *The Classical Quarterly, 63*(2), 801–812.
Zuboff, S. (2019). *The age of surveillance capitalism: The fight for a human future at the new frontier of power*. New York, NY: PublicAffairs.

Michael Uebel, PhD, LCSW, has taught literature and theory at the University of Virginia, Georgetown University, and the University of Kentucky. He practices as a mental health provider with the Veterans Health Administration, US Department of Veterans Affairs. He works primarily on the philosophical dimensions of psychology (theory and therapy). He has published two essays on shame from psychological perspectives in *American Imago* and the *Journal of Humanistic Psychology*. His current book project is on ethical, ideological, and psychocultural understandings of equanimity.

Part V
Outlook for Shame 4.0 in the Face of the Covid-19 Pandemic

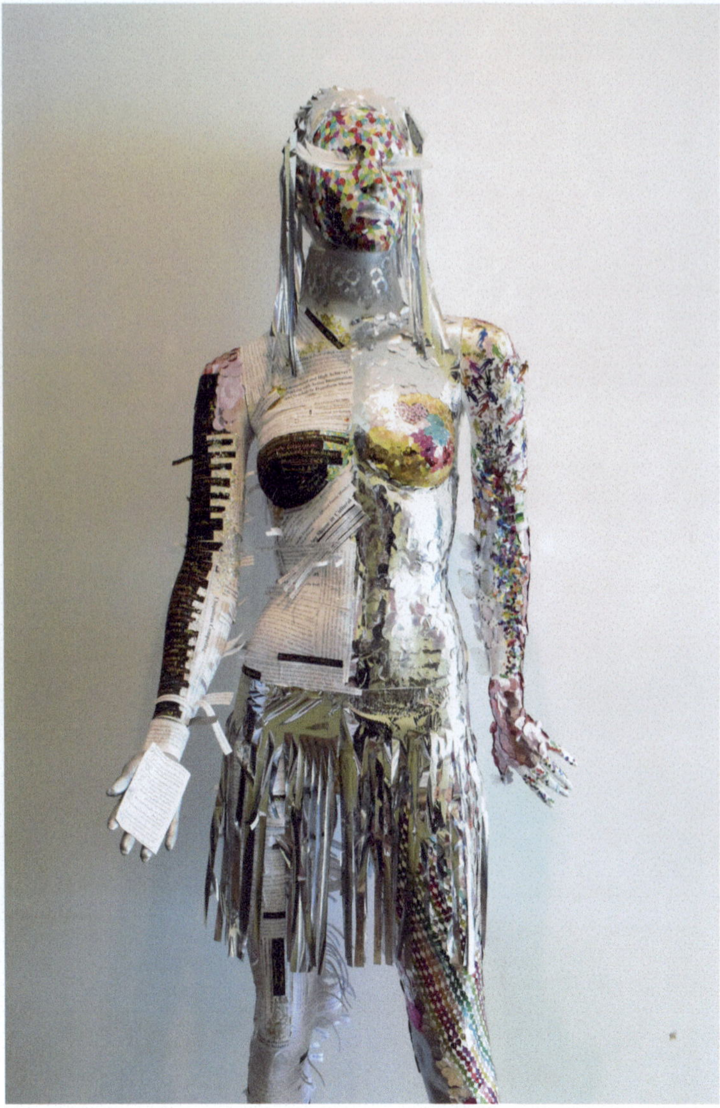

Chapter 28
"Who Could Breathe Without Hope…" Shame and Shaming 4.0 During Covid-19 and Beyond

Elisabeth Vanderheiden and Claude-Hélène Mayer

Wer könnte atmen
ohne Hoffnung
dass auch in Zukunft
Rosen sich öffnen

—Rosa Ausländer[1]

During the completion of this book, COVID-19 spreads worldwide. At the time of the book publication, there are over 107 million cases and over 2.3 million deaths confirmed (World Health Organization, 2021), with an increasing trend. Unlike other major crisis events, the COVID-19 pandemic is not limited to a specific region like a natural disaster such as a tsunami or earthquake or a national or multinational event like a war. It is a global crisis. Other than the climate crisis, such a phenomenon is as yet unknown, and, unlike the climate crisis, the pandemic does not leave any room for interpretation as to its crisis character is unknown.

Excerpt from the poem Hoffnung II by Rose Ausländer, translated by Vanderheiden

---

[1]Who could breathe without hope that also in the future roses will open. (Excerpt from Rose Ausländer, Hoffnung II, trans. by Elisabeth Vanderheiden)

E. Vanderheiden (✉)
Global Institute for Transcultural Research, Römerberg, Germany
e-mail: ev@keb-rheinland-pfalz.de

C.-H. Mayer
Department of Industrial Psychology and People Management, University of Johannesburg, Auckland Park, Johannesburg, South Africa

Kulturwissenschaftliche Fakultät, Europa Universität Viadrina, Frankfurt (Oder), Germany

C.-H. Mayer et al. (eds.), *Shame 4.0*, https://doi.org/10.1007/978-3-030-59527-2_28

1 Trends in Global Working and Learning Environments during Covid-19

In a very short time, COVID-19 has led to massive restrictions up to complete lockdowns in almost all countries of the world. This has produced an eruptive increase in working from home. As global figures are not yet available, some examples from different parts of the world are quoted here. In a representative survey in *Germany* of more than 1000 German citizens aged 16 and over, it was found that in March 2020, 1 in 2 (49%) of the working respondents was now working partially if not entirely from the home office. For 18%, this was a completely new experience, because before the outbreak of the pandemic they were not allowed to work from home, but were now doing so temporarily (15%) or completely (3%). A further 31% of those surveyed were already able to work from their home office before the pandemic and now do so more often (17%) or completely (14%). In contrast, 41% state that their activity is fundamentally not suitable for the home office. For 43%, existing home office regulations were extended by the employer. For 45% of those in employment, telephone and web conferences replace the previous meetings with personal presence (Bitkom, 2020).

It is assumed that almost half of *India*'s technology workers, estimated at three million, have already begun to work from home for social distancing reasons (Sangani, 2020). In *Brazil* approximately 78% of people surveyed stated that not going out to work was necessary to prevent the spread of the novel coronavirus, which causes COVID-19. Another 37% of the respondents confirmed that they had not left their homes to work during the days prior to the survey (Statista, 2020a). The proportion of people working from home due to the corona virus in *Denmark* in March 2020 was between 16 and 41% depending on the region (Statista, 2020b). In Norway, 49% of working people were given the option to work from home immediately after the pandemic broke out (Statista, 2020c). In *Finland*, the proportion of people who started working from home because of the corona virus was as high as 76%, with a further 8% indicating they were working from home more now than before the virus (Statista, 2020f). In *Romania*, only 23% of the people were working in a home office because of COVID-19; 3% already worked from home before the virus (Statista, 2020d).

Covid-19 exposes existing socio-economic and cultural divides and deepens them. As shown already in previous years, remote working options, for example, are often the privilege and limited to the highly educated social strata:

> Forty-two million wage and salary workers (29 percent) could work at home, and 36 million workers (25 percent) sometimes worked at home .... Wage and salary workers who were Hispanic or Latino were less likely to work at home than workers who were not Hispanic or Latino (13 percent, compared with 27 percent). Blacks were less likely to work at home than Whites or Asians (18 percent, compared with 26 percent and 32 percent, respectively). (US Bureau of Labor Statistics, 2019, pp. 2–3)

This is mainly because the option to work from home is closely related to the industry in which a person is professionally engaged. In fact, these industries are often segregated by race and gender (Arntz, Ben Yahmed & Berlingieri, 2020), so that some employees are more likely to work from home than others. For example in the *USA*, white and Asian workers are more likely to work in professional management positions than black and Latin American workers (Hess, 2020). However, not only ethnicity seems to be a selection criterion for access to the potential resource home office; formal education and income also seem to be corresponding selection criteria. In the USA, about 37% of workers with higher education qualifications do some work from home, but only 12% of workers with a high school degree or people with a college degree do so. There is also a stratified dynamic across all income brackets in the USA, for example, in terms of working from home. Hess (2020) reports that about 35% of workers earning $1531 or more per week (about $79,612 per year) have been working from home for some time. This is significantly more than those earning between $961 and $1530 per week (23%), those earning between $631 and $960 per week (11%) and those earning less than $630 per week (8%). This can also be observed in other countries currently under the influence of COVID-19. Initial figures from *Hungary*, for example, show that 61% of university graduates are allowed to work from home, while only 25% of those with high school graduation and 25% of those with technical school certificates are permitted to work from home (Statista, 2020e).

However, COVID-19 seems to provide a great opportunity for the digitalisation of organisations, companies and even public authorities, schools and universities in many ways. Some institutions which had long refused digitalisation or only approached it with great scepticism have been compelled, in the interest of their own survival, to set up home offices. This establishes a new culture of trust with regard to their employees, to develop new means of communication and distribution, which in the analogue world could be largely contactless or reduced, as otherwise their organisational survival would have been at risk. However, working cultures have changed beyond the introduction of home offices. In view of COVID-19, large US corporations such as Google, Microsoft, Zoom and Slack are making their collaboration and video call software partially or temporarily available free of charge. This has led to enormous increases in usage worldwide (Kessler, 2020). People still spend time in virtual spaces, trying to reconcile private and professional obligations, to keep private and professional identities in balance and to bring them into harmony.

Many institutions that have been involved in digital activities for a long time have taken COVID-19 as an opportunity and developed new innovative collaboration, and innovation formats, conferences and educational events have been re-designed and digitised and have been moved to the web without further ado and offered as webinars, online courses, Massive Open Online Courses (MOOCs) and digital exhibitions. In this way, new learning worlds have been created in addition to the working worlds (Reuters, 2020). Many commercial platforms have expanded digital educational offerings and put them online, some at reduced cost and some free of charge.

Another exciting resilience format to have reached unprecedented scope and potential with COVID-19 is that of hackathons. Hackathons are actions that originated from the ethical hacker scene. They are virtual conferences for software and hardware developers, where people who do not know each other work together on a problem for a very limited period to find the most innovative and sustainable solutions. At "#Wir versus Virus" (#WirVsVirus, 2020), three young women in Germany organised a digital participation process under the patronage of the German government during 1 week in March 2020. The aim was to develop ideas for overcoming the problems associated with the corona crisis. During 48 hours, 28,361 people were brought together on the digital collaboration platform SLACK, and over 1500 solutions were developed. With more than 28,000 participants, the world's largest hackathon was set up within a week. Work on the implementation of the solutions continues.

Other creative approaches are platforms such as OpenIDEO, which virtually bring together companies, non-profit organisations and individuals worldwide to develop people-centred design approaches to solve complex problems based on the design thinking concept. Since its founding, hundreds of thousands of people in more than 200 countries and territories have created almost 19,000 solutions (OpenIDEO, 2020). Currently, numerous global workshops are working on solutions to problems related to COVID-19. Ruitenberg and Desmet (2012) have explored the links between design thinking approaches and positive psychology, asking how creating products that consciously stimulate people's subjective well-being can be a means of both validating and underpinning the movement's current contributions to positive psychology. In their research, they conclude that design thinking and the products that emerge in connection with it represent an untapped potential for bringing positive psychology into the everyday lives of many people. The authors explain:

> We propose that in line with this thought, the design discipline can play an equally important role by materializing the vision of the good life, enabling and stimulating actions that lead to well-being and thriving communities. (Ruitenberg & Desmet, 2012, p. 10)

Just like the hackathon, approaches such as these which work transnationally and across organisations as well as across disciplines are particularly exciting and goal-orientated solutions and an expression of individual and collective resilience, especially in the face of a global crisis.

2 COVID-19 Promotes Shaming in the Form of Racism and Social and Cultural Finger-Pointing

Along with the worldwide spread of COVID-19, the emergence of the virus was promptly accompanied by the shaming of individuals and groups in the form of racist and discriminatory attacks on people who were assumed to be of Chinese origin (Ku, 2020; Le, 2020). This shaming is related to the fact that such people are held responsible for the crisis solely on the basis of their external appearance and their assumed ethnic origin (Yu, 2020). US President Trump played a significant role by referring to COVID-19 as a "Wuhan virus" or "Chinese virus" for several weeks, until he had to stop doing so in response to protests from China, the international community and criticism within the USA (Aratani, 2020; New York Times, 2020).

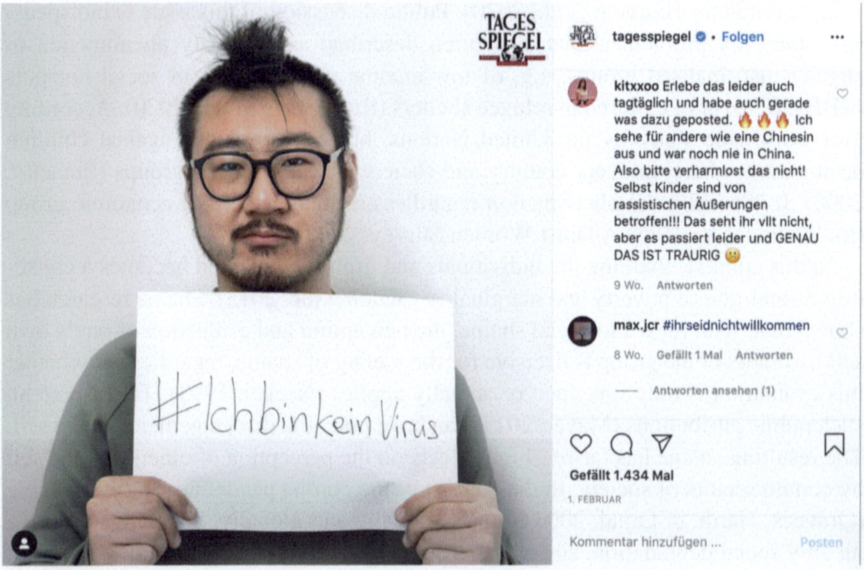
TAGES SPIEGEL
#IchbinkeinVirus
tagesspiegel • Folgen
kitxxoo Erlebe das leider auch tagtäglich und habe auch gerade was dazu geposted. Ich sehe für andere wie eine Chinesin aus und war noch nie in China. Also bitte verharmlost das nicht! Selbst Kinder sind von rassistischen Äußerungen betroffen!!! Das seht ihr vllt nicht, aber es passiert leider und GENAU DAS IST TRAURIG
9 Wo. Antworten
max.jcr #ihrseidnichtwillkommen
8 Wo. Gefällt 1 Mal Antworten
Antworten ansehen (1)
Gefällt 1.434 Mal
1. FEBRUAR
Kommentar hinzufügen ...
Posten

Fig. 28.1 German Journalist Marvin Ku #Ich bin kein Virus (I am no virus)

But even in the aftermath, repeated offensive accusations and public threats of punishment against China have taken place (Tagesschau, 2020).

To organise resistance against these racist assumptions and attacks, about 260 civil rights organisations have addressed a letter of protest to the US Congress (Orton, 2020). Those affected also join together on social media platforms to protest. An example is shown in Fig. 28.1 of the Instagram campaign of the German journalist Marvin Ku from February 2020 *#ichbinkeinvirus* (I am no virus).

However, racial exclusion is not limited to people of Asian origin or appearance. On the one hand, reports of racially motivated attacks against African people in Guangzhou are increasing (Sui, 2020). On the other hand, current findings from the USA indicate that COVID-19 disproportionately affects African American citizens, showing that their infection rate and death rate are significantly higher than that of the white population (Patton, 2020); in some cases up to 70% of the dead are African Americans as in Louisiana (Kendi, 2020). The reasons are manifold. Health researcher Jeanette Kowalik points out structural racism (BBC News, 2020), in the sense that there is no full participation in society and no equal access to education, healthcare or housing. That this is not a North American phenomenon is also proven, for example, by a first study of more than 2000 COVID-19 patients from the UK, 35% of whom are black, Asian or other ethnic minorities. This is twice the proportion of the total population (Hirsch, 2020).

For many people, even in times of lockdown, home is not a sanctuary but a place of danger and threat: children and women are exposed to maltreatment or sexual violence. This was discussed soon after the lockdown in a wide variety of national contexts and at global level (UNICEF, 2020; United Nations, 2020). Only a few weeks of lockdown have led to a drastic increase in violence against children and women (Graham-Harrison et al., 2020). Public discussion of this issue is indispensable; the only problem is that it is often described as a priority phenomenon of already marginalised groups, e.g. of low-income people living in social hotspots (RBB, 2020), or of children in refugee shelters (Ruhr Nachrichten, 2020). According to a worldwide study by the United Nations, however, violence against children occurs everywhere, in every country and society and in all social groups (Pinheiro, 2006). It is a universal phenomenon regardless of membership of economic group (International Violence Against Women Survey, 2008).

In this context, shaming the individuals and groups concerned becomes a constitutive condition of poverty and marginality (Schoneville, 2013). Shame research has shown that, with regard to social shame, the perception and evaluation of one's own self by others or the group is decisive for the feeling of shame, regardless of whether this evaluation is only imagined or actually applies (Neckel, 1993). To this extent, such public attributions (Mayer, 2017) can have potential disparagements of the self. The resulting shame has far-reaching effects on the perception of others and the self by certain sectors of society, in the context of the corona pandemic rapidly growing (Oravecz, Hárdi, & Lajtai, 2004), both nationally and globally. Shame is accompanied by social degradation, since "subordination of one subject to the evaluation of another" is signalled and the balance of power is shifted to the disadvantage of the person who is ashamed (Neckel, 1991, p. 106). Shame thus potentially alters the power structure in social interactions by reducing the shame and recognising this in some way in the sense of shame. Shame and embarrassment in this toxic sense can thus contribute to the establishment and cementing of structural inequalities, define social status and affect self-image and as a consequence have access to resources and remaining options for action. With regard to social shaming and status, Neckel points to four central practices that can be described as the main sources of social shame (Neckel, 1991, p. 210; 1993, p. 256):

1. *Exclusion* is the practice in which the affiliation of a person to social groups or associations ends. This occurs on the basis of actual or supposed "strangeness". Through exclusion, the basic human need for belonging is curtailed and this can lead to existential shame.
2. Within formal organisations, *degradation* of a person is an important trigger of social shame. The person is publicly degraded, power is demonstrated, and subordination is demanded. This can lead to a violation of self-esteem. Social shame arises at the interface between one's self-image and public role.
3. *Tests* can be a major source of shame. Testing refers to the reproduction of knowledge and questioning a person's competencies. Given their formalisability and (assumed) objectivity, their consequences can have very negative effects on self-image and self-confidence.
4. *Devaluation* refers to a person's work or neediness and deprives them of material values and appreciation. This can lead to both poverty and stigmatising. The associated loss of social esteem is experienced as humiliation and shame.

Neckel's (1993) four practices can be recognised in many contexts in connection with the pandemic. We recognise exclusion, for example, in the identification of scapegoats, as described at the beginning of this section, but also in the identification and forced isolation of so-called risk groups. People of certain age groups are being curtailed without a say, without intervention options. Basic rights are being curtailed. As examples of the second social shaming strategy of degradation, the abovementioned examples of access to home office are given in the context of COVID-19. As has been shown, this is decisively influenced by educational status and indirectly by ethnicity and gender. For example, in certain countries such as Germany, working from home involves no financial change at all for state employees of public authorities. They continue to receive their full salary, and others – mostly those who are well educated – are given the opportunity to continue working from home on full pay. Those who are less well educated, mostly production workers, receive state subsidies of up to 60% instead of wages, while freelancers or those working in the low-wage sector receive state compensation which is barely enough to survive on.

In South Africa, industry came to a complete halt; President Ramaphosa instituted a total lockdown in which only police, security, healthcare workers and supermarket staff were allowed to work. All other people in the country were only allowed to leave the house for healthcare or food shopping. Then, for example, the government released a rescue package of 500 billion Rand[2] (Seekings, 2020) to support South African citizens who had lost their jobs (such as domestic workers, gardeners, nannies, industry workers on contract) or who were extremely vulnerable (children, elderly people) and who were sent back to their "home towns". However, the support programmes are often not made known to many of the suffering individuals, they do not have a bank account to receive funds, or they are unable to apply for the funding because they cannot complete the required forms. All of these erupting insights in socio-economic divides within the South African society led to experiences of shame and shaming. At the same time, the South African lockdown specified that no alcohol or cigarettes were to be sold and a curfew was put into place from 8 pm to 6 am. During the lockdown, many addicted individuals struggle, and people with addictions buy or sell cigarettes and liquor illegally, shamed by the fact that they cannot manage to withdraw from alcohol consumption or smoking. Further, masses of people have been led to criminal behaviour, looting liquor shops as well as food stores due to pressures of addiction. South African university students were sent to their family homes where many of them experienced struggles with internet connectivity, lack of technological equipment, poverty, violence and family conflict which led to a decrease in ability to study and focus on their work. Many of these different aspects led to experiences of shame and shaming.

In addition to its 58 million legal citizens, South Africa caters for approximately 7–9 million illegal foreigners in the country (Eisenberg, 2019). These illegal foreigners were hit extremely hard by the lockdown situation in South Africa, due to the fact that often they could not acquire work, they were not able to leave the country and return to their home countries, places of detention were facing deportation delays (South African Government, 2020). Mukumbang et al. (2020) point out that refugees, asylum seekers, and undocumented migrants in the South African

[2]In 2020, 500 Billion Rand amount to approximately 27 Billion US Dollars.

country were hit extremely hard by the lockdown: COVID-19 has exacerbated existing vulnerabilities of members of these groups and led to an increase in suffering and exposure to survival challenges. During Covid-19 foreigners and Pan-African migrants were increasingly blamed and shamed for the problems within the South African economy, even by politicians to win votes for the 2021 elections (Gatticchi & Maseko, 2020).

The extent to which Neckel's (1993) third strategy of tests proves to be shame-relevant in the COVID-19 era will probably need to be the subject of future global studies. But it is already apparent that home schooling during the pandemic appears to massively increase social inequalities in the educational context (Gallup, 2020; Pauli, 2020). There are numerous examples of Neckel's fourth shaming strategy devaluation in various countries in the context of COVID-19. One which should be mentioned here is the exodus of domestic and migrant workers immediately after the lockdown in India and the reaction of the Indian police to this exodus. The unprepared and chaotically organised implementation of the lockdown hit the poor particularly hard, exposing them to severe unprotected health risks and massive police violence. Even though Prime Minister Modi later issued a public apology, these events publicly demonstrated a lack of respect for these populations (BBC News, 2020).

The topic of shame has also played a role in the context of the military and police interaction which was strongly present to enforce the lockdown in South African urban areas during the first lockdown sequence (Maseko, 2020). It was pointed out that military and police interaction was partly accompanied with high levels of violence, fraud and bribary (Olewe, 2020). Several voices within the South African society have shamed police and military for unlawful actions and behaviour and its strong increase during Covid-19 (Williams, 2020).

Another example of shaming is the debate concerning the so-called corona bonds. A majority of the European Union states want all 19 member countries to overcome the consequences of the corona crisis together by raising capital jointly, limited in time and amount, so that the highly indebted countries would be relieved of their debt. This has so far failed, primarily because of German resistance (Gammelin, 2020). This could be perceived as public embarrassment, especially by Italy, which is not only particularly hard hit by the pandemic but is also weighed down by a high debt burden, as this is explicitly cited as a reason for not agreeing to the proposal. At the global level, the IMF is responding to the plight of countries in the Global South with new loans, temporary debt relief for 25 selected particularly poor countries (at the time of writing this text) (Deutsche Welle, 2020); appeals by churches and NGOs for final debt cancellation remain unheard.

3 COVID-19 Fosters Shame Through Social Isolation and Loneliness

> We cannot stop the coronavirus.
> What we can do is stop the loneliness virus!

King Willem-Alexander of The Netherlands[3]

The curfews and lockdowns associated with COVID-19 enforce social distancing and social isolation. This can lead to severe psychological stress. It is not yet possible to assess the extent to which this is a burden and the extent to which individual previous experiences have a reinforcing or relieving effect, even if it appears that previously acquired resiliencies show positive effects now (Cyrulnik, 2020).

A strong consequence of social isolation can be loneliness. Loneliness can be defined as a perceived discrepancy between desired and actual social relationships (Peplau & Perlman, 1982). Loneliness is "a universal human condition" (Bodford, 2017) and describes the subjective understanding that existing social relationships and contacts do not have the desired quality or scope (Arp, 2019). However, loneliness is not only a phenomenon that affects people living alone. Intimate or emotional loneliness, for example, refers to the lack of a very close, intimate relationship, such as that found in couple relationships. Social (relational) loneliness refers to a lack of friendships and other personal relationships (Luhmann & Bücker, 2019, p. 4). Loneliness is a worldwide phenomenon regarded as a known risk factor for numerous physical and mental health consequences (see Ypsilanti, 2018, p. 1). As social beings, people depend on a safe and secure social environment and social contacts to survive. Satisfactory social relationships are essential for people's mental and physical well-being, while impaired social relationships or their limitation can lead to loneliness (Mushtaq et al. 2020). If left untreated, loneliness can have serious consequences for the mental and physical health of people (Luhmann & Bücker, 2019, pp. 33–44). For example, loneliness can cause various psychiatric disorders such as depression, alcohol abuse, child abuse, sleep disorders, personality disorders and Alzheimer's disease. It can also lead to various physical disorders such as diabetes, autoimmune diseases such as rheumatoid arthritis and lupus and cardiovascular diseases such as coronary heart disease, hypertension, obesity, physiological ageing, cancer and hearing impairment (Mushtaq et al. 2020). Other authors (see Holtbernd, 2018) take a critical view of this and suspect a deficit-oriented perspective in psychology and medicine.

Although it is a global phenomenon that occurs in all cultures, loneliness is presented and expressed differently (see Arp, 2019; BBC, 2020; Lykes & Kemmelmeier, 2013). Lykes and Kemmelmeier (2013) examined loneliness in the context of cultural values and found that the level of loneliness in so-called collectivist societies was higher than in individualistic societies but that societies differed in terms of their predictors of loneliness. In collectivist societies, the absence of interaction with the family caused a stronger sense of loneliness than in individualistic societies. Conversely, the absence of interaction with friends and the absence of a trusted person in individualistic terms were more closely associated with loneliness than in collectivistic terms. This led the authors to conclude that autonomy and choice of interaction partners have a greater impact on well-being in individualistic societies, while traditional social bonds are more pronounced in collectivist

[3]https://nltimes.nl/2020/03/20/full-text-english-dutch-kings-speech-coronavirus-pandemic.

societies. Loneliness affects people of all ages. An online study by the BBC (2020) with over 55,000 participants showed that 40% of participants aged 16–24 years often or very often feel lonely, compared to 27% of the over-75-year-old participants. Overall, the study showed higher rates of loneliness among young people across all cultures, countries and genders.

People who feel lonely are often very prone to shame (Thoresen, Aakvaag, Strøm, Wentzel-Larsen, & Birkeland, 2018, pp. 8–9; Rostami & Jowkar, 2016; Oravecz et al., 2004; Mental Health Foundation, 2020, p. 19, 26; Wei, Shaffer, Young, & Zakalik, 2005). Those affected often experience loneliness as a stigma (Luhmann & Bücker, 2019, p. 58): The feeling of loneliness can have negative effects on self-image, lead to a reduction in self-esteem and self-efficacy expectations (Cohen-Mansfield, Hazan, Lerman, & Shalom, 2016) and thus trigger feelings of shame. It can lead to lower subjective well-being and low life satisfaction (Cohen-Mansfield et al., 2016; Ong et al., 2016), restrict positive emotions and increase negative emotions (Böger & Huxhold, 2018; Steptoe, Leigh, & Kumari, 2011).

According to the BBC survey (BBC, 2020), it is more often women who feel ashamed because they feel lonely. This is confirmed by the study conducted by Rostami and Jowkar (2016), showing that feelings of shame about loneliness decrease with age, and yet older people say that they are more likely to hide their loneliness than younger people. Luhmann and Bücker (2019, p. 58), on the other hand, point to the special and increasing shame burden of loneliness with age.

Mushtaq et al. (2020, p. 1) emphasise that loneliness can be seen as a resource and can awaken potentials, because "loneliness reminds us of the pain and warns us of the threat of becoming isolated". This potential has been recognised and used in many ways in connection with COVID-19, in both analogue and digital contexts, for instance, by supporting shopping and other support services for old and elderly neighbours in housing estates. In Germany, many people with insufficient income are dependent on obtaining food free of charge or at reduced prices at "Tafel" social food distribution points. At least 1.65 million people in the country are affected by this. The fact that these 300 distribution points had to be closed in the course of the lockdown is a serious blow to these people, especially because families are often affected and the situation is exacerbated by the loss of school meals and COVID-19-related income losses. However, creative solutions have been found in many places. Volunteer Tafel employees pack food in bags and leave them in front of customers' doors or distribute them in public places (ZEIT, 2020). In other locations, people donate food and hygiene articles and deposit them in public places. Elsewhere, charities organise telephone chains against loneliness (Haller Kreisblatt, 2020).

Loneliness was and still is of particular importance in the context of COVID-19 because in the first weeks of the pandemic, important events of the world religions such as Easter, Passover, Holi or Ramadan took place or are still taking place. Initiatives against isolation and innovative spaces for virtual proximity such as mystery coffee dates and spiritual and religious offerings have been created. People meet virtually for mediation rounds and church services or to break the digital fast during Ramadan. Johansson and Andreasson (2017) have investigated experiences of loneliness and related issues in the context of online communication and found that people in the digital world make a variety of efforts to find a way to initiate and realise satisfying social relationships, thus reconnecting with society and avoiding isolation and marginalisation. The virtual lunch breaks and virtual team diaries reported by some organisations can also be considered as examples of such initiatives. In a private context, friends and families arrange virtual lunch dates or playgrounds and meet for book or poetry clubs and much more. Self-help groups such as Alcoholics Anonymous move their meetings to the Internet; other groups organise virtual parties (Stöhr, 2020) or topic-related discussion groups. People thematise fears and loneliness experiences, but also hopes in poetic circles, at virtual readings or through digital concerts.

4 Positive Psychology and Coping with Shame 4.0 During Covid-19

In his new taxonomy of Positive Psychology 2.0, Wong (2011) focuses on the adaptation processes that bad living conditions, poor health, negative attitudes and lack of resources require in order to prevent downward spirals and enable coping from different cultural contexts. The above mentioned examples from different cultural contexts provide first ideas on how shame might need to be transformed during and Post-Covid-19.

Positive Psychology 2.0 can help on global levels to emphasise the importance of awareness and mindfulness towards human suffering and its transformation for personal growth and development through courage, faith and solidarity (Wong, 2020). Wong (2020) points out that it is highly important to be aware and accept the tenets of the human condition to transform shame in a Covid and Post-Covid-19 world: "(1) We all live in a dangerous world full of evil and suffering; (2) All human being have inherent limitations and vulnerability; and (3) Flourishing is impossible without overcoming the frailty and the dark side of life." The four pillars of Positive Psychology 2.0 (Wong, 2016, 2019) which are meaning, resilience, virtue and well-being will further help to provide individuals, but also organisations and society, with strength and guidance to transform shame on different societal levels.

"Who hopes/is young" begins the poem by the Ukrainian-German Jewish poet Rose Ausländer quoted at the beginning of this chapter and ends with the hopeful words: "Who could breathe /without hope /that also in the future /roses will open/a word of love/survives fear". Her lines of poetry provide space to suffering, pain and fear on the one hand, but also point just as powerfully to the perspective of hope on the other hand. She reminds us of our potential to live in courage, solidarity, love and, hope as individuals and collectives. In the tradition of PP2.0 her words allow for the suffering, as well as for the transformation into a new life's energy and an improved future Post Covid-19.

References

Aratani, L. (2020). *'Coughing while Asian': living in fear as racism feeds off coronavirus panic.* Retrieved April 16, 2020, from https://www.theguardian.com/world/2020/mar/24/coronavirus-us-asian-americans-racism#maincontent

Arntz, M., Ben Yahmed, S., & Berlingieri, F. (2020). Working from home and COVID-19: The chances and risks for gender gaps. Intereconomics, 55(6):381–386. https://doi.org/10.1007/s10272-020-0938-5

Arp, D. (2019). *Einsamkeit – Analyse Eines Ambivalenten Gefühls.* [online] Deutschlandfunk. Retrieved April 17, 2020, from https://www.deutschlandfunk.de/einsamkeit-analyse-eines-ambivalenten-gefuehls.1148.de.html?dram:article_id=449234.

BBC. (2020). BBC radio 4 – the anatomy of loneliness – who feels lonely? *The results of the world's largest loneliness study.* [online] BBC. Retrieved April 17, 2020, from https://www.bbc.co.uk/programmes/articles/2yzhfv4DvqVp5nZyxBD8G23/who-feels-lonely-the-results-of-the-world-s-largest-loneliness-study.

BBC News. (2020). *India's PM seeks 'forgiveness' over virus lockdown.* Retrieved April 17, 2020, from https://www.bbc.com/news/world-asia-india-52081396

Bitkom. (2020). *Corona-Pandemie: Arbeit im Homeoffice nimmt deutlich zu.* Retrieved April 16, 2020, from https://www.bitkom.org/Presse/Presseinformation/Corona-Pandemie-Arbeit-im-Homeoffice-nimmt-deutlich-zu

Bodford, J. (2017). Loneliness in Modern Life. In *Encyclopedia of evolutionary psychological science* (pp. 1–16).

Böger, A., & Huxhold, O. (2018). Do the antecedents and consequences of loneliness change from middle adult- hood into old age? *Developmental Psychology, 54*(1), 181–197. https://doi.org/10.1037/dev0000453.

Cohen-Mansfield, J., Hazan, H., Lerman, Y., & Shalom, V. (2016). Correlates and predictors of loneliness in older-adults: A review of quantitative results informed by qualitative insights. *International Psychogeriat- rics, 28*(04), 557–576. https://doi.org/10.1017/S1041610215001532.

Cyrulnik, B. (2020). *Die Quarantäne ist eine schwere psychische Belastung.* Retrieved April 28, 2020, from https://www.arte.tv/de/videos/096899-000-A/boris-cyrulnik-die-quarantaene-ist-eine-schwere-psychische-belastung/

Deutsche Welle. (2020). *Wie viel bringt der Schuldenerlass des IWF?* | DW | 14.04.2020. Retrieved April 17, 2020, from https://www.dw.com/de/wie-viel-bringt-der-schuldenerlass-des-iwf/a-53127083

Eisenberg, G. (2019, 28 August). Is it time for a blanket amnesty for illegal foreigners living in South Africa? Daily maverick. https://www.dailymaverick.co.za/opinionista/2019-08-28-is-it-time-for-a-blanket-amnesty-for-illegal-foreigners-living-in-south-africa/

Gallup. (2020). *42% of Parents Worry COVID-19-19 Will Affect Child's Education.* Retrieved April 17, 2020, from https://news.gallup.com/poll/305819/parents-worry-COVID-19-affect-child-education.aspx

Gammelin, C. (2020). *Corona-Bonds – Und jetzt alle für alle.* Retrieved April 17, 2020, from https://www.sueddeutsche.de/wirtschaft/corona-bonds-anleihen-schulden-eu-1.4868017

Gatticchi, G., & Maseko, L. (2020). *Xenophobic tensions surge as Covid-19 batters SA's economy.* Fin 24. Retrieved 20 December 2020, from https://www.news24.com/fin24/economy/xenophobia-surges-as-covid-19-slams-south-african-economy-20201220

Graham-Harrison, E., Giuffrida, A., Smith, H., Ford, L., Connolly, K., & Jones, S. et al. (2020). *Lockdowns around the world bring rise in domestic violence.* Retrieved April 16, 2020, from https://www.theguardian.com/society/2020/mar/28/lockdowns-world-rise-domestic-violence

Hess, A. (2020). Coronavirus highlights the inequality of who can — and can't — work from home. Retrieved April 16, 2020, from https://www.cnbc.com/2020/03/04/coronavirus-highlights-who-can-and-cant-work-from-home.html

Hirsch, A. (2020). *If coronavirus doesn't discriminate, how come black people are bearing the brunt?* Retrieved April 16, 2020, from https://www.theguardian.com/commentisfree/2020/apr/08/coronavirus-black-people-ethnic-minority-deaths-pandemic-inequality-afua-hirsch

Holtbernd, T., (2018). Einsamkeit und Singularisierung: Ein kulturanalytischer Versuch. *IZPP | Ausgabe 2/2018* | 2.

International Violence Against Women Survey. (2008). *International Violence Against Women Survey IVAWS (1997–2008) – Heuni*. Retrieved April 16, 2020, from https://www.heuni.fi/en/index/researchareas/violenceagainstwomen/internationalviolenceagainstwomensurveyivaws.html

Johansson, T., & Andreasson, J. (2017). The web of loneliness: A Netnographic study of narratives of being alone in an online context. *Social Sciences, 6*(3), 101.

Kendi, I. (2020). *Stop blaming black people for dying of the coronavirus*. Retrieved April 16, 2020, from https://www.theatlantic.com/ideas/archive/2020/04/race-and-blame/609946/

Kessler, S. (2020). *Slack, Zoom und Microsoft sind die Gewinner der Corona-Krise*. Retrieved April 16, 2020, from https://nzzas.nzz.ch/wirtschaft/slack-zoom-und-microsoft-sind-die-gewinner-der-corona-krise-ld.1549025?reduced=true

Kreisblatt, H. (2020). *Isolation Durch Corona: Telefonkette Hilft Gegen Einsamkeit | Halle*. [online] Halle. Retrieved April 18, 2020, from https://www.haller-kreisblatt.de/lokal/halle/22750936_Isolation-durch-Corona-Telefonkette-hilft-gegen-Einsamkeit.html.

Ku, M. (2020). *Tagesspiegel on Instagram: "Seit das Coronavirus über den Globus wütet, breitet sich gleichzeitig der Rassismus gegen jeden aus, der „asiatisch" aussieht. So geht es...".* Retrieved April 16, 2020, from https://www.instagram.com/p/B8Bsnj-HujD/

Le, N. (2020). *Ich bin kein Virus*. Retrieved April 16, 2020, from https://www.zeit.de/campus/2020-03/rassismus-coronavirus-asiaten-husten-oeffentlichkeit-diskriminierung

Luhmann, M., & Bücker, S. (2019). *Einsamkeit und soziale Isolation im hohen Alter. Projektbericht*. Bochum: Ruhr-Universität Bochum.

Lykes, V., & Kemmelmeier, M. (2013). What predicts loneliness? Cultural difference between individualistic and collectivistic societies in Europe. *Journal of Cross-Cultural Psychology, 45* (3), 468–490.

Maseko, N. (2020). *South Africa could resemble a 'military state'*. BBC News Johannesburg. https://www.bbc.com/news/world-africa-52387962

Mayer, C.-H. (2017). *Wie ticken die denn so? Über Schemata und Attribuierungen*. Retrieved April 17, 2020, from https://www.trainerscut.com/home/wie-ticken-die-denn-so-über-schemata-attribuierungen/

Mental Health Foundation. (2020). *The lonely society?* [online] Mentalhealth.org.uk. Retrieved April 17, 2020, from https://www.mentalhealth.org.uk/sites/default/files/the_lonely_society_report.pdf.

Mukumbang, F. C., Ambe, A. N., & Adebiyi, B. O. (2020). Unspoken inequality: How COVID-19 has exacerbated existing vulnerabilities of asylum-seekers, refugees, and undocumented migrants in South Africa. *Int J Equity Health, 19*, 141. https://doi.org/10.1186/s12939-020-01259-4.

Mushtaq, R., Shoib, S., Shah, T., & Mushtaq, S. (2020). Relationship between loneliness, psychiatric disorders and physical health? A review on the psychological aspects of loneliness. *J Clin Diagn Res 2014 Sep, 8*(9), WE01–WE04.

Neckel, S. (1991). Status und Scham. In *Zur symbolischen Reproduktion sozialer Ungleichheit*. Frankfurt am Main: Campus.

Neckel, S. (1993). Achtungsverlust und Scham. Die soziale Gestalt eines existentiellen Gefühls. In Fink-Eitel, H., Lohmann, G. (Hg.), *Zur Philosophie der Gefühle*. Frankfurt am Main: Suhrkamp, 244–265.

New York Times. (2020). *Opinion | Call It 'Coronavirus'*. Retrieved April 16, 2020, from https://www.nytimes.com/2020/03/23/opinion/china-coronavirus-racism.html

Olewe, D. (2020). *Coronavirus in Africa: Whipping, shooting and snooping*. Retrieved 13 February 2021, from https://www.bbc.com/news/world-africa-52214740

Ong, A. D., Uchino, B. N., & Wethington, E. (2016). Loneliness and health in older adults: A mini-review and synthesis. *Gerontology, 62*(4), 443–449. https://doi.org/10.1159/000441651

OpenIDEO. (2020). *Social impact powered by design thinking - OpenIDEO*. Retrieved 13 February 2021, from https://www.openideo.com

Oravecz, R., Hárdi, L., & Lajtai, L. (2004). *Social transition, exclusion, shame and humiliation.*

Orton, G. (2020). *NCAPA letter to Nancy Pelosi*. Retrieved April 16, 2020, from https://d3n8a8pro7vhmx.cloudfront.net/ncapa/pages/89/attachments/original/1583935643/NCAPA_Letter_to_House_Leadership.pdf?1583935643

Patton, S. (2020). *The pathology of American racism is making the pathology of the coronavirus worse*. Retrieved April 16, 2020, from https://www.washingtonpost.com/outlook/2020/04/11/coronavirus-black-america-racism/

Pauli, R. (2020). *Folgen der Schulschließungen: Corona macht Bildung ungleicher*. Retrieved April 17, 2020, from https://taz.de/Folgen-der-Schulschliessungen/!5670367/

Peplau, L. A., & Perlman, D. (Eds.). (1982). *Loneliness: A sourcebook of current theory, research, and therapy*. New York: Wiley Interscience.

Pinheiro, P. (2006). *Report of the independent expert for the United Nations study on violence against children*. New York: United Nations.

RBB. (2020). *So stellen sich Berliner Jugendämter auf die Corona-Krise ein*. Retrieved April 16, 2020, from https://www.rbb24.de/politik/thema/2020/coronavirus/beitraege/corona-berlin-jugendamt-kriseninterventionsteam-marzahn-hellersdorf.html

Reuters. (2020). *Zoom takes lead over Microsoft Teams as virus keeps Americans at home: Apptopia*. Retrieved April 16, 2020, from https://www.reuters.com/article/us-health-coronavirus-zoom/zoom-takes-lead-over-microsoft-teams-as-virus-keeps-americans-at-home-apptopia-idUSKBN21I3AB

Rostami, S., & Jowkar, B. (2016). 2016. The relationship between guilt and shame feelings with the dimensions of loneliness: The moderating effect of gender. *Int J Behav Sci, 10*(2), 72–76.

Ruhr Nachrichten. (2020). *Kinder- und Jugendärzte: Kinderschutz in Corona-Krise nicht vergessen*. Retrieved April 16, 2020, from https://www.ruhrnachrichten.de/nachrichten/kinder-und-jugendaerzte-kinderschutz-in-corona-krise-nicht-vergessen-1512827.html

Ruitenberg, H. P., & Desmet, P. M. (2012, 11–14 September). *Design thinking in positive psychology: The development of a product-service combination that stimulates happiness-enhancing activities*. Conference paper out of control: Proceedings of the 8th international conference on design and emotion, London, UK.

Sangani, P. (2020). *Coronavirus crisis may fast-forward IT's work-from-home adoption*. Retrieved April 16, 2020, from https://economictimes.indiatimes.com/tech/ites/coronavirus-crisis-may-fast-forward-its-work-from-home-adoption/articleshow/74766020.cms?from=mdr

Schoneville, H. (2013). Armut und Ausgrenzung als Beschämung und Missachtung. *Soz Passagen, 5*, 17–35. https://doi.org/10.1007/s12592-013-0132-8.

Seekings, J. (2020). COVID-19-19: Ramaphosa's plan is good, but the budget is insufficient. *GroundUp, 23*(4), 2020. https://www.groundup.org.za/article/ramaphosas-plan-good-budget-insufficient/.

South African Government. (2020). *Immigration act: Determination of correctional facilities as places of detention of illegal foreigners pending deportation during Coronavirus COVID-19 lockdown*. https://www.gov.za/documents/immigration-act-determination-correctional-facilities-places-detention-illegal-foreigners

Statista. (2020a). *Working from home to prevent COVID-19-19 Brazil 2020 | Statista*. Retrieved April 16, 2020, from https://www.statista.com/statistics/1106213/public-opinion-work-from-home-coronavirus-brazil/

Statista. (2020b). *Denmark: Working from home during COVID-19-19 2020 | Statista*. Retrieved April 16, 2020, from https://www.statista.com/statistics/1109824/share-of-people-working-from-home-due-to-the-coronavirus-in-denmark/

Statista. (2020c). *Norway: Working from home during the COVID-19-19 pandemic 2020 | Statista.* Retrieved April 16, 2020, from https://www.statista.com/statistics/1107292/working-from-home-during-the-COVID-19-19-pandemic-in-norway/

Statista. (2020d). *Home office possibilities Romania 2020 | Statista.* Retrieved April 16, 2020, from https://www.statista.com/statistics/1104107/home-office-possibilities-romania/

Statista. (2020e). *Share of Hungarians working from home due to COVID-19-19 2020 | Statista.* Retrieved April 16, 2020, from https://www.statista.com/statistics/1106454/hungary-share-of-people-working-from-home-due-to-coronavirus/

Statista. (2020f). *Finland: Working from home during the COVID-19 pandemic | Statista.* Retrieved 13 February 2021, from https://www.statista.com/statistics/1105777/share-of-people-working-from-home-due-to-the-coronavirus-pandemic-finland/

Steptoe, A., Leigh, E. S., & Kumari, M. (2011). Positive affect and distressed affect over the day in older people. *Psychology and Aging, 26*(4), 956–965. https://doi.org/10.1037/a0023303.

Stöhr, M. (2020). *Compassion in the Time of Corona – DER SPIEGEL – International.* [online] Spiegel.de. Retrieved April 18, 2020, from https://www.spiegel.de/international/world/corona-how-people-around-the-world-are-supporting-each-other-a-9d6b1e7d-b12b-432e-aad4-e814802243b4.

Sui, C. (2020). *China's Racism is wrecking its success in Africa.* Retrieved April 16, 2020, from https://foreignpolicy.com/2020/04/15/chinas-racism-is-wrecking-its-success-in-africa/

Tagesschau. (2020). *Coronavirus: Trump schimpft über China.* Retrieved April 28, 2020, from https://www.tagesschau.de/ausland/trump-corona-115.html

Thoresen, S., Aakvaag, H., Strøm, I., Wentzel-Larsen, T., & Birkeland, M. (2018). Loneliness as a mediator of the relationship between shame and health problems in young people exposed to childhood violence. *Social Science & Medicine, 211*, 183–189.

UNICEF. (2020). *Höhere Risiken für Kinder wegen Maßnahmen zur Eindämmung des Coronavirus.* Retrieved April 16, 2020, from https://www.unicef.de/informieren/aktuelles/presse/2020/risiken-fuer-kinder-bei-eindaemmung-des-coronavirus/213060

United Nations. (2020). *Children vulnerable to abuse and violence during coronavirus lockdowns, UN experts warn.* Retrieved April 16, 2020, from https://news.un.org/en/story/2020/04/1061282

US Bureau of Labour Statistics. (2019). *Job flexibilities and work schedules — 2017–2018 data from the American time use survey.* Retrieved April 16, 2020, from https://www.bls.gov/news.release/pdf/flex2.pdf

Wei, M., Shaffer, P., Young, S., & Zakalik, R. (2005). Adult attachment, shame, depression, and loneliness: The mediation role of basic psychological needs satisfaction. *Journal of Counseling Psychology, 52*(4), 591–601.

Williams, M. (2020). *SA's rotten cops among most crooked during Covid-19.* News24. Retrieved 22 September 2020, from https://www.news24.com/news24/SouthAfrica/News/sas-rottencops-among-most-crooked-during-covid-19-finds-corruption-watch-report-20200922

WirvsVirus. (2020). *WirVsVirus – Der Hackathon der Bundesregierung – Corona/COVID-19-19.* Retrieved April 16, 2020, from https://wirvsvirushackathon.org

Wong, P. (2020). *The second wave positive psychology of shame in East and West in the age of the 4IR.* Retrieved 2 May 2020, from http://www.drpaulwong.com/the-second-wave-positive-psychologyof-shame-in-east-and-west-in-the-age-of-the-4ir/comment-page-1/

Wong, P. T. P. (2011). Positive psychology 2.0: Towards a balanced interactive model of the good life. Canadian Psychology, 52(2), 69–81. Retrieved from http://www.drpaulwong.com/positive-psychology-2-0-towards-a-balanced-interactive-model-of-the-good-life/

Wong, P. T. P. (2016, September). *Mapping the contours of positive psychology 2.0.* Positive Living Newsletter.

Wong, P. T. P. (2019). Foreword: From shame to wholeness: An existential positive psychology perspective. In C.-H. Mayer & E. Vanderheiden (Eds.), *The bright side of shame. Transforming and growing through practical applications in cultural contexts* (pp. 5–11). Cham: Springer.

World Health Organization. (2021). *WHO Coronavirus Disease (COVID-19) dashboard*. Retrieved 13 February 2021, from https://covid19.who.int/

Ypsilanti, A. (2018). Lonely but avoidant—The unfortunate juxtaposition of loneliness and self-disgust. *Palgrave Commun, 4*, 144. https://doi.org/10.1057/s41599-018-0198-1.

Yu, L. (2020). *LiyaYu 喻俐雅 (@LiyaYuBerlin) on Twitter*. Retrieved April 16, 2020, from https://twitter.com/LiyaYuBerlin

ZEIT. (2020). *Ein Großteil Unserer Ehrenamtlichen Gehört Zur Risikogruppe*. [online] Zeit.de. Retrieved April 18, 2020, from https://www.zeit.de/gesellschaft/zeitgeschehen/2020-03/tafeln-schliessung-coronavirus-ehrenamt-risikogruppe/komplettansicht.

Elisabeth Vanderheiden is a pedagogue, theologian and intercultural mediator. She is the CEO of the Global Institute for Transcultural Research and the President of Catholic Adult Education in Germany. Her publishing activities focus on pedagogy, in particular on the further education of teachers and trainers in adult, vocational and civic education, but also on the challenges of digitalisation. She has also edited books on intercultural and transnational issues. Her most recent publications deal with shame as a resource as well as with mistakes, errors and failures and their hidden potentials in the context of Culture and Positive Psychology 1.0 and 2.0. Current research projects deal with love in transcultural contexts, with life crises as well as humour in the context of Positive Psychology 2.0. Another focus of her work is Design Thinking in transcultural contexts.

Mayer, Claude-Hélène, (Dr. habil., PhD, PhD) is a Professor in Industrial and Organisational Psychology at the Department of Industrial Psychology and People Management at the University of Johannesburg; an Adjunct Professor at the European University Viadrina in Frankfurt (Oder), Germany; and a Senior Research Associate at Rhodes University, Grahamstown, South Africa. She holds a PhD in Psychology (University of Pretoria, South Africa), a PhD in Management (Rhodes University, South Africa), a Doctorate (Georg-August University, Germany) in Political Sciences (socio-cultural anthropology and intercultural didactics) and a Habilitation (European University Viadrina, Germany) in Psychology with focus on work, organisational and cultural psychology. She has published several monographs, text collections, accredited journal articles and special issues on transcultural mental health and well-being, sense of coherence, shame, transcultural conflict management and mediation, women in leadership in culturally diverse work contexts, constellation work, coaching and psychobiography.

Chapter 29
Shame Warrior

Justine Pistorius

1 Introduction: The Role of Energy and How it Influences Human Behaviour?

The significant individual features of the Shame Warrior is a reflection of the character and gradual development of humanity. As the artist, I wanted to depict Claude's and Elizabeth's work from both a 3rd-dimensional perspective, as well as the qualities of spirituality within the framework of shame.

The motivation for the art piece is to show how humanity will need to start adopting a more introspective, balanced and healthier expression to thrive within the changes that the Fourth Industrial Revolution influences.

Serious thought and consideration need to be applied to the context of our emotions and how they influence behaviour we adopt in the world towards our relationships with self and others. The energy that is applied and required for sustained physical, mental and emotional activity is influenced not only by how society moulds the beliefs of individuals, but also how the individual perceives and responds to those life experiences and belief systems, and how that energy is nurtured, focused and represented within the world we live in.

J. Pistorius (✉)
JIP FUSION, Johannesburg, South Africa

GOL Institute of Mastery, Johannesburg, South Africa

C.-H. Mayer et al. (eds.), *Shame 4.0*, https://doi.org/10.1007/978-3-030-59527-2_29

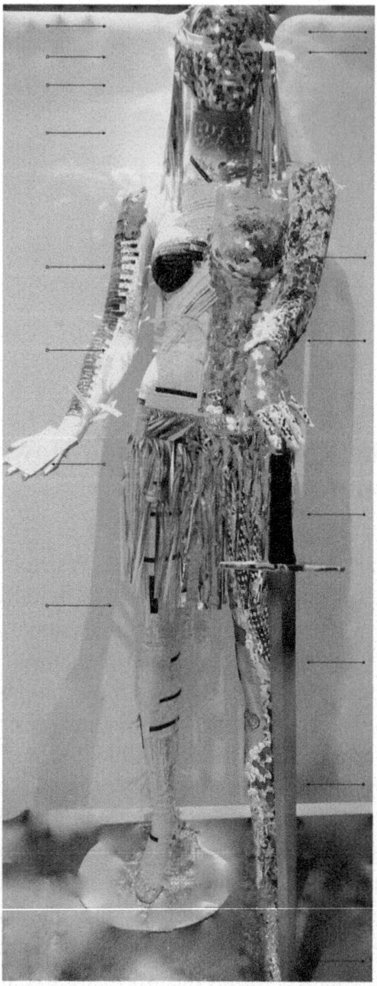

The essence of Shame Warrior is a reflection of the deeper aspects of evolution. As the artist I wanted to show Claude and Elizabeths work not only from a 3rd dimensional perspective but also within the realms of spiritual influence. The motivation for the art piece was to show how humanity will have to start adopting the brighter and higher aspects of our makeup and frequency in order to thrive within the changes that will be cast upon humanity not only by and within the 4th Industrial Revolution ,but also from the influences of Spiritual Evolution and the future of humanity.

Right Side of Warrior - Masculine Energy

1. Back of head - bronze hair representing dream state and an individuals energy system with regards to 7 basic chakras, aura and higher chakras from a 3rd, 4th and 5th dimensional aspect (Spirit)

2. Right side of Brain - the 23 shifts highlighting the 4IR

3. Face - the different colours of the face represent the multiple influences of shame and the Brighter side/value of bringing these aspects to the surface "showing face"

4. Neck- indicative of 4IR and that dialogue will need to be shared and changes instituted so that a great part of humanity don't feel left behind/ constricted/confined/chained

5. Arm (colourful text) - indicating the positive psychology/ inner and outer awareness and mindfulness that brings shame into the light

6. Arm (backside) - aspects of Elisabeth Vanderheiden and Claude-Hélène Mayer research on Shame

7. Front and back of upper torso/legs - words from the work of Elisabeth Vanderheiden and Claude-Hélène Mayer indicating the dialogue they have started with regards to the "Value and Brighter side of Shame" The overlapping of the pieces of script indicate that Shame has its roots buried not only in history of humanity but also across cultures and within and throughout aspects of peoples lives and society

8. Hand - silver in colour to indicate the beginning stages of a new revolution

The left side of Warrior shows how humanity will have to create a new armour for themselves with regards to the changes that the 4IR will bring, not only from a mental, physical and emotional perspective, but also from a spiritual one. The aspects of the left side are rooted within the Divine Feminine which is why we begin at the base of the left foot. The sword indicative of the strength and courage needed for this evolution

Left Side of Warrior - Divine Feminine Energy

1. Foot - stepping into the future and 4IR with a positive sense of oneself. Spiritual essence will also be an important aspect in dealing with the changes to come, so re-aligning ones energy to higher frequencies will be important in the grounding and growth of an individual. The colourful sequins on the foot are also indicative of the New Age (future) children that will be born into the world with higher frequencies.

2. Front Shin - purple and silver armour indicating new and positive aspects of the self being exercised and implemented mentally, physically, emotionally and spiritually to cope with the rapid changes across the World.

3. Knee - colourful strands indicating genetic change on a physical and spiritual level. 12 strands of DNA being activated.

4. Thigh - bronze and silver armour indicate changes that have taken place physically, mentally, emotionally and spiritually through science, education, and global change within the dynamics of 4IR

5. Arm - changes that 4IR will bring forth: Wearable Internet, Implantable Technologies and Smart Tattoos . The butterflies represents natural metamorphoses balanced within 4IR

6. Breast - heart on the breast indicates that our human essence must not be exchanged/lost to AI and robotics

7. Eyes - feathers represent a lighter and new way of seeing the world not only for a select few but for the greater good of all

8. Left side of Brain - new way of thinking

Justine Pistorius is an Entrepreneur, Abstract Artist, Photographer, Writer and Spiritual Teacher from South Africa. Justine works from within. She draws on inner feelings and emotions to express herself rather than on external subject matter. Her work radiates with the freedom that this gives her, as a contemporary and spiritual artist. She tackles her work with a freshness and without inhibition, which as an artist, is a challenge to achieve. When she works she seems to care more about the process and being in the moment than the result. This results in play and a discussion that takes place between her work and herself with an outcome that is mesmerising. The painting, paint and feelings from within seem to mysteriously guide her. Each of Justine Pistorius's works offers the viewer an insight into this emotion and an honesty, which reflects in work that continues to give. She expresses her message through an assortment of signs and symbols, hidden within her translations of colours, lines and shapes. She believes that her work will speak to the person it is meant to and find its place in "The History Of Time". Every artwork has its own personality and is worthy of individual contemplation. Justine has an amazing ability to express herself with both words and paint. She holds seminars, workshops and retreats on spiritual development and creative arts.

The manufacturer's authorised representative in the EU is Springer Nature Customer Service Centre GmbH, Europaplatz 3, 69115 Heidelberg, Germany. If you have any concerns regarding our products, please contact ProductSafety@springernature.com

Printed and bound by CPI Group (UK) Ltd, Croydon, CR0 4YY
30/09/2026
02225687-0014